PROTECTING INFANTS THROUGH HUMAN MILK

Advancing the Scientific Evidence

ADVANCES IN EXPERIMENTAL MEDICINE AND BIOLOGY

Recent Volumes in this Series

Volume 546
COMPLEMENTARY AND ALTERNATIVE APPROACHES TO BIOMEDICINE
Edited by Edwin L. Cooper and Nobuo Yamaguchi

Volume 547
ADVANCES IN SYSTEMS BIOLOGY
Edited by Lee K. Opresko, Julie M. Gephart, and Michaela B. Mann

Volume 548
RECENT ADVANCES IN EPILEPSY RESEARCH
Edited by Devin K. Binder and Helen E. Scharfman

Volume 549
HOT TOPICS IN INFECTION AND IMMUNITY IN CHILDREN
Edited by Andrew J. Pollard, George H. McCracken, Jr., and Adam Finn

Volume 550
BRAIN DEATH AND DISORDERS OF CONSCIOUSNESS
Edited by Calixto Machado and D. Alan Shewmon

Volume 551
POST GENOMIC PERSPECTIVES IN MODELING AND CONTROL OF BREATHING
Edited by Jean Champagnat, Monique Denavit-Saubie, Gilles Fortin, Arthur S. Foutz, and Muriel Thoby-Brisson

Volume 552
TYPE I DIABETES: Biomedical Science and Technology
Edited by George Eisenbarth

Volume 553
BIOMEDICAL SCIENCE AND TECHNOLOGY
Edited by Nesrin Hasirci and Vasif Hasirci

Volume 554
PROTECTING INFANTS THROUGH HUMAN MILK: Advancing the Scientific Evidence
Edited by Larry K. Pickering, Ardythe L. Morrow, Guillermo M. Ruiz-Palacios, and Richard J. Schanler

---

A Continuation Order Plan is available for this series. A continuation order will bring delivery of each new volume immediately upon publication. Volumes are billed only upon actual shipment. For further information please contact the publisher.

PROTECTING INFANTS THROUGH HUMAN MILK

Advancing the Scientific Evidence

Edited by

Larry K. Pickering
Centers for Disease Control and Prevention
Atlanta, Georgia

Ardythe L. Morrow
Cincinnati Children's Hospital Medical Center
Cincinnati, Ohio

Guillermo M. Ruiz-Palacios
Instituto Nacional de Ciencias Médicas y Nutrición
Mexico City, Mexico

and

Richard J. Schanler
Schneider Children's Hospital at North Shore
Manhasset, New York

Springer Science+Business Media, LLC

Proceedings of the 11th International Conference of the International Society for Research in Human Milk and Lactation (ISRHML) held October 4–8, 2002, in Mexico City, Mexico

ISBN 978-1-4419-3461-1 ISBN 978-1-4757-4242-8 (eBook)
DOI 10.1007/978-1-4757-4242-8

Originally published by Kluwer Academic / Plenum Publishers, New York in 2004.
Softcover reprint of the hardcover 1st edition 2004

http://www.wkap.nl/

10 9 8 7 6 5 4 3 2 1

A C.I.P. record for this book is available from the Library of Congress

DEDICATION

This book reflects the science of the International Society for Research in Human Milk and Lactation (ISRHML) meeting held in 2002 in Mexico City. We dedicate this book to our friend and colleague of many years, Dr. Margit Hamosh, whose scientific leadership in research on human milk has paved the way for many others to follow. Margit was the organizer of the international conference on research in human milk and lactation held in Oaxaca, Mexico in 1986. The Oaxaca conference served as the foundation for collaborations of the editors of this book. The science of that conference was captured in another book, *Human Lactation: Maternal and Environmental Factors*, Hamosh M, Goldman AS, editors, New York: Plenum Press, 1986. Both conferences were plagued by natural disasters. In 1986, the Oaxaca conference was delayed by a few months because of an earthquake, and in 2002, a hurricane hit Merida, Mexico, days before our conference, which resulted in quickly re-siting the conference to Mexico City. Margit was unable to attend the 2002 meeting, but she sympathized with our challenges by email, and somehow, that helped. In the end, with hard work and good will, both conferences turned out to be successful and memorable, marked by a healthy mix of science, lively discussion, and camaraderie. Margit's enjoyment of the company of her ISRHML friends is evident in the photograph below. She says the picture was taken in 1985 by Mary Frances Picciano at the international meeting in Kiel on "Recent Research on Human Milk," to illustrate that she engaged in drinking beverages other than milk.

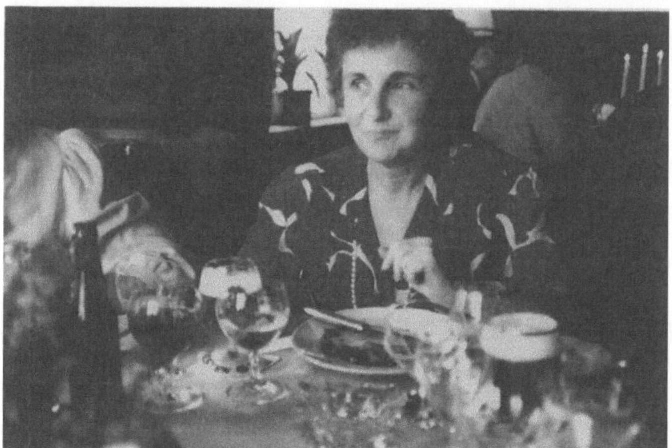

An active participant in the formation of ISRHML, Margit was elected the first president of the society in 1988, and was honored in 1999 with the Macy-György Award. Over the years, Margit helped bring human milk research to a high level of scientific quality and acceptance. Her own research interests have focused on the role of lipids in human milk, including understanding lipoprotein lipase, the lipid composition of preterm and full-term milk, enzymes in human milk, the anti-infective functions of milk fat globule components, long-chain polyunsaturated fatty acids, and the effects of storage on human milk. She contributed to many ISRHML conference books, published 115 original scientific articles, 104 chapters or reviews, wrote or edited 5 books, co-authored 5 special reports for the Institute of Medicine or USAID, and has helped ensure that human milk/lactation issues have remained on the radar screen at the National Institutes of Health. Dr. Hamosh is Professor emeritus of Georgetown University School of Medicine and continues to contribute to the literature on human milk and lactation.

PREFACE

Approximately every two years the International Society for Research in Human Milk and Lactation (ISRHML) organizes a conference during which various aspects of research into human milk and lactation are presented and discussed. ISRHML is a non profit organization dedicated to the promotion of excellence in research and the dissemination of research findings in the field of human milk and lactation. The Society has accomplished dissemination of research findings by publication of the proceedings of the ISRHML scientific meetings that are discussed below. Additional information about the Society can be found at www.isrhml.org.

In 1982, well before the official formation of the Society, a conference was held in Elk Ridge, Maryland, dealing with methodologies in human milk banking. The next conferences dealing with human milk research were held in 1984 in Winter Park, Colorado, under the auspices of the National Institute of Child Health, and 1986 in Oaxaca, Mexico. Presentations from these meetings were organized into books that were published in 1985 and 1986, respectively, and subsequently, were followed by publication of eight such books on human milk, including this volume. In 1988 ISRHML was formed officially. Since 1988, meetings have been held in Costa Rica (1988); Asilomar, California (1990); Stockholm, Sweden (1992); Tlaxcala, Mexico (1995); Plymouth, Massachusetts (1997); Irsee, Germany (1999); Tucson, Arizona (2000); and Mexico City, Mexico (2002). Most meetings have resulted in publication of books of meeting proceedings that advance multidisciplinary research on human milk bioactive factors, lactation, and breastfeeding.

The editors of this book are indebted to the ISRHML Board of Directors, members, and supporters, and the authors of manuscripts who made this edition possible. We also thank individuals who assisted us with funding, editing, and/or conference planning and management, including Dr. Margaret Neville; Ms. Roxana Remus Galván and staff; Dr. Frank Greer; Dr. David Newburg; Dr. Mary Frances Picciano; Dr. M. Lourdes Guerrero; Mr. Kim Jerger; Ms. Jareen Meinzen-Derr; and Dr. Kathleen Rasmussen, whose judicious decision-making regarding the change of conference venue will always be appreciated. We gratefully acknowledge support of the 2002 ISRHML conference in Mexico by the National Institutes of Health, Office of Dietary Supplements for trainee travel awards and the National Institute of Child Health and Human Development (HD 13021), which supported travel for some of the scientific presenters. We also gratefully acknowledge the generous sponsorship of Telmex, Inc.; Cincinnati Children's Research Foundation; Wyeth Nutritionals International; Baby Care Division, The Procter and Gamble Co.; Mead Johnson Nutritionals; Yakult, Inc.; and Medela International, which provided support for the conference and preparation of this book. This book could not have been prepared without the dedication and expert support of Kathryn Newburg, Jareen Meinzen-Derr, Stephanie Renna, and Kristi Martin. The editors particularly appreciate the constant encouragement of Mimi Pickering, Beatriz Ruiz-Palacios, Mary Schanler, and our children: Maggie and Andy; Winona, Justin, and Michael; Rodrigo, Betty, and Alonso; and Daniel, Susan, and Sariel, who serve as a constant source of support, pride, and happiness.

Larry K. Pickering, MD
Ardythe L. Morrow, PhD
Guillermo M. Ruiz-Palacios, MD
Richard J. Schanler, MD

Published Monographs of the Society's International Meetings:

1. Jensen RG, Neville MC, editors. Human Lactation: Milk Components and Methodologies. New York: Plenum Press, 1985.
2. Hamosh M, Goldman AS, editors. Human Lactation: Maternal and Environmental Factors. New York: Plenum Press, 1986.
3. Goldman AS, Atkinson SA, Hanson LA, editors. Human Lactation: The Effects of Human Milk on the Recipient Infant. New York: Plenum Press, 1987.
4. Atkinson SA, Hanson LA, Chandra RK, editors. Breastfeeding, Nutrition, Infection and Infant Growth in Developed and Emerging Countries. St. John's, Newfoundland: ARTS Biomedical Publishers and Distributors, 1990
5. Picciano MF, Lönnerdal B, editors. Mechanisms Regulating Lactation and Infant Nutrient Utilization. Contemporary Issues in Clinical Nutrition, Vol. 15. New York: Wiley-Liss, 1992.
6. Allen L, King J, Lönnerdal B, editors. Nutrient Regulation during Pregnancy, Lactation, and Infant Growth. New York: Plenum Press, 1994.
7. Koletzko B, Michaelsen KF, Hernell O, editors. Short and Long Term Effects of Breast Feeding on Child Health. Advances in Experimental Medicine and Biology, Vol. 478. New York: Kluwer Academic/Plenum Publishers, 2000.
8. Newburg DS, editor. Bioactive Components of Human Milk. Advances in Experimental Medicine and Biology, Vol. 501. New York: Kluwer Academic/Plenum Publishers, 2001.
9. Davis MK, Isaacs C, Hanson LA, Wright AL, editors. Integrating Population Outcomes, Biological Mechanisms and Research Methods in the Study of Human Milk and Lactation. Advances in Experimental Medicine and Biology, Vol. 503. New York: Kluwer Academic/Plenum Publishers, 2002.
10. Pickering LK, Morrow AL, Ruiz-Palacios GM, Schanler RJ, editors. Protecting Infants through Human Milk: Advancing the Scientific Evidence. New York: Kluwer Academic/Plenum Publishers, 2004.

CONTRIBUTORS

Anderson, Alex K.
University of Connecticut
Nutritional Science Department, U4017
Storrs, CT 06269 USA
Tel 860 486 0113
Fax 860 486 3674
Email fianko@hotmail.com

Azeredo, Vilma Blondet de
Laboratório de Bioquimica
Nutricional e de Alimentos
Instituto de Quimica
Universidade Federal do
Rio de Janeiro, Brazil
Email vilmab@provide.psi.br

Bernabe-Garcia, Mariela
Instituto Mexicano del Seguro Social
Unidad de Investigación Médica
en Nutrición
Av. Cuauhtémoc N° 330 Col. Doctores
México DF, Mexico 06720
Tel 56 27 6900 ext 3417 or 3416
Fax 56 27 69 44
Email mariela_bernabe@yahoo.com

Caire, Graciela
Centro de Investigación en
Alimentación y Desarrollo, A. C.
Departamento de Nutrition
Carretera a la Victoria
Hermosillo, Sonora 8300 Mexico
Tel 662 289 2400
Fax 662 280 0094
Email gcaire@cascabel.ciad.mx

Casanueva, Esther
Instituto Nacional de Perinatología
Instituto Nacional de Ciencias Médicas
y Nutrición Salvador Zubirán, and
Universidad Iberoamericana
México DF, México
Email casanuev@servidor.unam.mx

Chapman, Donna
University of Connecticut
Nutritional Science Department, U4017
Storrs, CT 06269 USA
Tel 860 486 5073
Email donna.chapman@uconn.edu

Cleary, Thomas
University of Texas Medical School
Department of Pediatrics
Div. of Infectious Diseases
6431 Fannin
Houston, TX 77030 USA
Tel 713 500 5714
Fax 713 500 5688
Email Thomas.g.cleary@uth.tmc.edu

Cregan, Mark
The University of Western Australia
Dept. Biochem. & Molec. Biology
School of Biomedical & Chem. Sci.
35 Stirling Highway
Nedlands, Perth Western Australia
Australia 06009
Tel 61 41 2455 206
Fax 61 8 6488 1148
Email Mark.Cregan@uwa.edu.au

Davidson, Barbara
Cincinnati Children's Hospital
Medical Center
Center for Epidemiology & Biostatistics
3333 Burnet Avenue
Cincinnati, OH 45229 USA
Tel 513 636 1833
Fax 513 636 7509
Email Barbara.Davidson@cchmc.org

Dewey, Kathryn G.
University of California, Davis
Department of Nutrition
One Shields Avenue
Davis, CA 95616-8669 USA
Tel 530 752 0851
Fax 530 752 3406
Email kgdewey@ucdavis.edu

Domellöf, Magnus
Umeå University
Clinical Sciences, Pediatrics
SE 901 85
Umeå, Sweden SE 90185
Tel 46 90 785 2128
Fax 46 90 123 728
Email magnus.domellof@pediatri.umu.se

Dvorak, Bohuslav
University of Arizona
Department of Pediatrics
1501 N. Campbell Avenue
PO Box 245073
Tucson, AZ 85724 USA
Tel 520 626 6553
Fax 520 626 5009
Email dvorakb@peds.arizona.edu

Eidelman, Arthur I.
Shaare Zedek Medical Center
Hebrew University School of Medicine
Department of Pediatrics
PO Box 3235
Jerusalem, Israel 91031
Tel 972 2 655 5197
Fax 972 2 563 6789
Email eidel@cc.huji.ac.il

Guerrero, M. Lourdes
Instituto Nacional de Ciencias Médicas
y Nutrición Salvador Zubirán
Department of Infectious Diseases
Vasco de Quiroga No. 15, Col. Tlalpan
Mexico DF, Mexico14000
Tel 52 55 5655 9675
Fax 52 55 5513 0010
Email mlga@quetzal.innsz.mx

Habicht, Jean-Pierre
Cornell University
Department of Nutritional Science
Savage Hall
Ithaca, NY 14853 USA
Tel 607 255 4419
Fax 607 255 2608
Email JH48@cornell.edu

Hadsell, Darryl
Baylor College of Medicine
Department of Pediatrics
1100 Bates, Room 10072
Houston, TX 77030 USA
Tel 713 798 7043
Fax 713 798 7057
Email dhadsell@bcm.tmc.edu

Hale, Thomas W.
Texas Tech University
School of Medicine
Department of Pediatrics
1400 Coulter
Amarillo, TX 79106 USA
Tel 806 354 5776
Fax 806 354 5536
Email tom@ama.ttuhsc.edu

Haney, Peter M.
Baylor College of Medicine
Department of Pediatrics
1100 Bates, Room 10018
Houston, TX 77030 USA
Tel 713 798 7067
Fax 713 798 7057
Email phaney@neo.bcm.tmc.edu

Hawkes, Joanna
Flinders Medical Centre
Department of Child Nutrition
Research Centre, Bedford Park
Adelaide, South Australia
Australia 5042
Tel 61 8 8204 5755
Fax 618 8204 3945
Email jo.hawkes@flinders.edu.au

Hovey, Russell C.
University of Vermont
Department of Animal Science
Terrill Hall #121
570 Main Street
Burlington, VT 05405 USA
Tel 802 656 1122
Fax 802 656 8196
Email rhovey@zoo.uvm.edu

Innis, Sheila M.
Department of Paediatrics
Research Institute for Children's and
Women's Health
University of British Columbia
950 West 28th Avenue
Vancouver, Canada V5Z 4H4
Tel 604 875 2431
Fax 604 875 2226
Email sinnis@interchange.ubc.ca

Isaacs, Charles E.
Institute of Basic Research
Dept. of Developmental Biochem.
10050 Forest Hill Road
Staten Island, NY 10314 USA
Tel 718 494 5227
Fax 718 698 7916
Email chisi@cunyvm.cuny.edu

Jarjou, Landing M.A.
MRC Keneba
PO Box 273, The Gambia and
MRC Human Nutrition Research
Elsie Widdowson Laboratory
Fulbourn Road, Cambridge CB1 9NL
United Kingdom
Email c/o Ann Prentice:
ann.prentice@mrc dunn.cam.ac.uk

Jiang, Xi
Cincinnati Children's Hospital
Medical Center
Division of Infectious Diseases
3333 Burnet Avenue
Cincinnati, OH 45229 USA
Tel 513 636 0119
Fax 513 636 7655
Email jason.jiang@cchmc.org

Kalkwarf, Heidi J.
Cincinnati Children's Hospital
Medical Center
Department of General and
Community Pediatrics
3333 Burnet Avenue
Cincinnati, OH 45229 USA
Tel 513 636 3803
Fax 513 636 4402
Email heidi.kalkwarf@cchmc.org

Kirsten, Gert F.
Tygerberg Hospital and
The University of Stellenbosch
Department of Paediatrics
Private Bag 3
Tygerberg Cape, South Africa 7505
Tel 27 21 938 6480
Fax 27 21 938 7138
Email gfk@sun.ac.za

Kramer, Michael S.
1020 Pine Avenue West
Montreal, Quebec
Canada H3A 1A2
Tel 514 398 6261
Fax 514 398 4503
Email michael.kramer@mcgill.ca

Lau, Chantal
Baylor College of Medicine
Department of Pediatrics
One Baylor Plaza
Houston, TX 77030 USA
Tel 713 798 6710
Fax 713 798 7187
Email clau@bcm.edu

Le Pendu, Jacques
INSERM U419, Institut de Biologie
9 Quai Moncousu
44035, Nantes Cedex, France
Tel 33 02 40 08 40 99
Fax 33 02 40 08 40 82
Email jlependu@nantes.inserm.fr

Li, Ruowei
Centers for Disease Control
and Prevention
Division of Nutrition and
Physical Activity
Mail Stop K 25
4770 Buford Hwy, NE
Atlanta, GA 30341 USA
Tel 770 488 6033
Fax 770 488 5369
Email ril6@cdc.gov

Lien, Eric
Wyeth Nutrition
Department Research & Development
500 Arcola Road (2 North)
Collegeville, PA 19426 USA
Tel 484 865 2362
Fax 484 865 9391
Email liene@wyeth.com

Lonnerdal, Bo
University of California, Davis
Department of Nutrition
One Shields Avenue
Davis, CA 95616 USA
Tel 530 752 8347
Fax 530 752 3564
Email bllonnerdal@ucdavis.edu

López-Alarcón, Mardya
Instituto Mexicano del Seguro Social
Nutrition Research Unit
PO Box C-029, CSPI,
Coahuila #5 Col. Roma
Mexico DF, Mexico 06703
Tel 52 55 5627 6944
Fax 52 55 5627 6944
Email marsau@prodigy.net.mx

Lovelady, Cheryl A.
University of North Carolina
Department of Nutrition
PO Box 26170
Greensboro, NC 27402-6170 USA
Tel 336 256 0310
Fax 336 334 4129
Email cheryl_lovelady@uncg.edu

Marquis, Grace S.
Iowa State University
Food Science and Human Nutrition
1127 Human Nutritional Sciences Bldg
Ames, IA 50011 USA
Tel 515 294 9231
Fax 515 294 6193
Email gmarquis@iastate.edu

Mast, Eric E.
National Center for Infectious Diseases
Centers for Disease Control and
Prevention, Division of Viral
Hepatitis, Mailstop G37
1600 Clifton Road
Atlanta, GA 30333 USA
Tel 404 371 5910
Fax 404 371 5488
Email emast@cdc.gov

McManaman, James L.
University of Colorado Health
Science Center
Dept. of Physiology and Biophysics
4200 E. Ninth Avenue
Denver, CO 80262 USA
Tel 303 315 7093
Fax 303 315 8110
Email jim.mcmanaman@uchsc.edu

Meier, Paula
Rush-Presbyterian St. Luke's Medical
Center, Special Care Nursery
Director, Clinical Research & Lactation
1653 W. Congress Parkway
Suite 625 Jones
Chicago, IL 60612 USA
Tel 708 383 3318
Fax 708 383 3374
Email pmeier@rush.edu

Meinzen-Derr, Jareen K.
Cincinnati Children's Hospital
Medical Center
Center for Epidemiology & Biostatistics
3333 Burnet Avenue
Cincinnati, OH 45229 USA
Tel 513 636 7789
Fax 513 636 7509
Email Jareen.meinzen-derr@cchmc.org

Meneses, Flavia
Instituto de Quimica
Universidade Federal do Rio de Janeiro
CT bloco A, lab 528, Ilha do Fundao
Rio de Janeiro 21949-900
Tel 55 21 2562 7352
Fax 5521 2295 6876
Email flakes@acd.ufrj.br

Miracle, Donna J.
Rush University
818 Longford Way
Noblesville, IN 46060 USA
Tel 315 877 2407
Email miracle@anderson.edu

Mitoulas, Leon
The University of Western Australia
Dept. of Biochem. & Molec. Biology
School of Biomedical and
Chemical Science
35 Stirling Highway
Nedlands Perth WA Australia 06009
Tel 61 8 9380 3327
Fax 61 8 9380 1148
Email Leon.Mitoulas@edu.au

Morrow, Ardythe L.
Cincinnati Children's Hospital
Medical Center
Center for Epidemiology & Biostatistics
3333 Burnet Avenue
Cincinnati, OH 45229 USA
Tel 513 636 7626
Fax 513 636 7509
Email ardythe.morrow@cchmc.org

Newburg, David S.
Univ. of Massachusetts Medical School
Shriver Center, 200 Trapelo Road
Waltham, MA 02452 USA
Tel 781 642 0025
Fax 781 642 0126
Email david.newburg@umassmed.edu

Ochoa, Theresa J.
University of Texas Medical School
Department of Pediatrics
6431 Fannin
Houston, TX 77030 USA
Email Theresa.j.ochoa@uth.tmc.edu

Oddy, Wendy H.
Telethon Institute for Child Research
Curtin University of Technology
Department of Nutrition,
PO Box 855, West Perth
Perth, Western Australia Australia 6872
Tel 61 8 9266 3716
Fax 61 8 9266 2258
Email wendyo@ichr.uwa.edu.au

Pérez-Escamilla, Rafael
The University of Connecticut
Nutritional Science Department, U4017
Storrs, CT 06269 USA
Tel 860 486 5073
Fax 860 486 3674
Email rperez@canr.uconn.edu

Piwoz, Ellen G.
Academy for Educational Development
1825 Connecticut Avenue, NW
Washington, DC 20009 USA
Tel 202 884 8816
Fax 202 884 8447
Email epiwoz@aed.org

Rea, Marina Ferreira
Instituto de Saude, São Paulo
Department of Mother and Child Health
R. Santo Antonio 590
São Paulo 01314-000 Brazil
Tel 11 30 64 5235
Fax 11 31 06 7328
Email marifrea@usp.br

Santos-Torres, Maria Irene
Hospital General de Occidente
Secretaría de Salud
Zapopan, Jalisco, México
Email isantos@cucs.udg.mx

Savino, F.
Department of Pediatrics
University of Turin
Piazza Polonia, 94
Torino, Italy 10126
Tel 0039 11 3135257
Fax 0039 11 677082
Email savino@pediatria.unito.it

Schack-Nielsen, Lene
The Royal Veterinary and Agricultural University
Research Dept. of Human Nutrition
Rolighedavej 30, Frederiksberg C
DK 1958 Denmark
Tel 45 35 28 2537
Fax 45 35 28 2483
Email lsn@kvl.dk

Sellen, Daniel W.
Emory University
Department of Anthropology
1557 Pierce Drive, NE
Atlanta, GA 30322 USA
Tel 404 727 4777
Fax 404 727 2860
Email dsellen@emory.edu

Sievers, Erika
University of Kiel
Department of Pediatrics
Schwanenweg 20
D-24105 Kiel, Germany
Tel 49 431 336837
Fax 49 431 5971831
Email Erika.Sievers@t-online.de

Sisk, Paula M.
Univ. of North Carolina, Greensboro
Department of Nutrition and Foodservice Systems
1102 Rockridge Road
Asheboro, NC 27205 USA
Tel 336 626 4954
Fax 336 718 9765
Email pmsisk@novanthealth.org

Springer, Skadi
University of Leipzig
Children's Hospital
Osistraze 21-25
D-04317 Leipzig, Germany
Tel 0049 341 9726 075
Fax 0049 341 9726 089
Email skspr@medizin.uni-leipzig.de

Torres, Alexandre G.
Instituto de Quimica, Universidade Federal do Rio de Janeiro
CT bloco A, UFRJ, Ilha do Fundao
Rio de Janeiro, RJ 21949-900 Brazil
Tel 55 21 25627351
Fax 55 21 25627266
Email agtorres@attglobal.net

Trott, Josephine F.
University of Vermont
Department of Animal Science
Terrill Hall #121
570 Main Street
Burlington, VT 05405 USA
Tel 802 656 1122
Fax 802 656 8196
Email trottj@mac.com

Urdaneta, Sandra L.
Pennsylvania State University
College of Medicine
M.S. Hershey Medical Center
Dept. of Microbiology & Immunology
500 University Drive, H107
Hershey, PA 17033 USA
Tel 717 531 4056
Fax 717 531 0665
Email surdaneta@psu.edu

Viveros-Rogel, Monica
Instituto Nacional de Ciencias Médicas
y Nutrición Salvador Zubirán
Departament of Infectious Diseases
Vasco de Quiroga No. 15, Col. Tlalpan
México DF 14000 Mexico
Tel 52 55 56 55 9675
Fax 52 55 55 13 0010
Email moviveros@yahoo.com.mx

Wagner, Carol L.
Medical University of South Carolina
Department of Pediatrics
Division of Neonatology
171 Ashley Avenue
PO Box 250917
Charleston, SC 29425 USA
Tel 843 792 2401
Fax 843 792 8801
Email wagnercl@musc.edu

Walker, W. Allan
Depts of Nutrition and Pediatrics
Harvard Medical School
260 Longwood Ave, TMEC 367
Boston, MA 02115 USA
Tel 617 432 3081
Fax 617 432 2988
Email allan_walker@hms.harvard.edu

Willeitner, Andrea
University of Wisconsin
Dept. of Neonatal/Perinatal Medicine
Meriter Hospital, 6 Center
202 S. Park Street
Madison, WI 53715 USA
Tel 608 262 6561
Fax 608 267 6377
Email aswilleitner@wisc.eedu

Wills-Karp, Marsha
Cincinnati Children's Hospital
Medical Center
Department of Immunology
3333 Burnet Avenue
Cincinnati, OH 45229 USA
Tel 513 636 7641
Fax 513 636 5355
Email wilde7@chmcc.org

CONTENTS

SECTION I
INTRODUCTION AND SPECIAL SESSIONS

SECTION II
SCIENCE AND POLICY: OPTIMAL DURATION OF EXCLUSIVE BREASTFEEDING

SECTION III

BREASTFEEDING FROM THE MOTHER'S PERSPECTIVE

SECTION IV

INNATE AND ACQUIRED IMMUNE SYSTEMS OF HUMAN MILK

SECTION V

RISK OF VIRAL TRANSMISSION BY BREASTFEEDING

SECTION VI

CELLULAR AND MOLECULAR BIOLOGY OF MAMMARY GLAND DEVELOPMENT AND LACTATION

SECTION VII

EXTENDED ABSTRACTS

FACTORS ASSOCIATED WITH BREASTFEEDING INITIATION AND DURATION

BREASTFEEDING IN RELATION TO CHILD DEVELOPMENT, NUTRITION, AND CHRONIC DISEASE OUTCOMES

BIOACTIVE FACTORS IN HUMAN MILK

ANTI-INFECTIVE PROPERTIES OF HUMAN MILK AND VIRAL TRANSMISSION VIA HUMAN MILK

OTHER TOPICS

SECTION I

INTRODUCTION AND SPECIAL SESSIONS

INTRODUCTION

Improving breastfeeding practices has been identified as the most effective child survival intervention worldwide, with the potential to save over a million infant lives each year, mostly in low-income developing countries (Jones et al. 2003). In these regions of the world, questions about breastfeeding and infant health tend to focus on survival, prevention of infectious diseases, adequate nutrition, and growth. In other regions of the world, the questions about breastfeeding tend to focus more on its relation to reducing the plagues of "over-development": obesity, cardiovascular disease, asthma, and related disorders. The title of this book, "Protecting Infants through Human Milk: Advancing the Scientific Evidence," reflects our perception that scientific investi-gation of human milk relevant to infant health has significantly advanced in recent years in relation to infectious, chronic, developmental, and nutritional outcome measures. Progress in the field has been due in part to the proliferation of technology but also to the growing understanding of the importance of breastfeeding to child survival and healthy development, as well as the increasingly strong multidisciplinary collaborations found among researchers in this field that provide the depth of expertise and cross-talk necessary for innovative research. This book represents a balanced integration of basic science with the study of health outcomes relevant to diverse populations.

Many aspects of human milk and lactation were presented and vigorously discussed at the 11th International Conference of the International Society for Research on Human Milk and Lactation (ISRHML) held in Mexico City, Mexico, on October 4-8, 2002. This book includes seven major sections and consists of 19 chapters. The first section of the book, described as **special sessions,** begins with the Macy-György Lecture given by Bo Lönnerdal, the 2002 honoree. His paper discusses the species specificity of human milk proteins; these unique milk proteins and peptide components include many that are biologically active. The next article, by Sheila Innis, presents polyunsaturated fatty acids in human milk and represents the keynote address of the conference. This article provides current information about variations in polyunsaturated fatty acids in human milk due to maternal diet and implications for infant development. The third article in this section, by Pérez-Escamilla and Guerrero, deals with advances and multidisciplinary applications of epidemiology to research on breastfeeding. Presented as a workshop prior to the conference, the article is recommended as a methodologic reference, because it covers appropriate research designs, analytical methods that are useful for epidemiologic studies of human milk, strengths of multidisciplinary teams that link aspects of breastfeeding behavior and biomedical outcomes, and the availability of innovative analytical approaches applicable to human milk research.

The next section, on **science and policy**, contains two articles that provide a point and counterpoint. The first article, by Kramer and Kakuma, describes a systematic review of the optimal duration of exclusive breastfeeding. The systematic review that they describe was the foundation for an expert consultation on the optimal duration of exclusive breastfeeding, which is the subject of the article by Habicht. Taken together, these articles review the rationale for and the process behind the World Health Organization (WHO) recommendation of exclusive breastfeeding for six months. This WHO policy has had global impact. The papers provide important insight into the formation of policy recommendations regarding breastfeeding based on the research undertaken by the scientific community, notably including research by members of ISRHML.

To balance the attention given to infant health in this book, the third section of the book deals with **breastfeeding from the mother's perspective**. Addressing the needs of lactating mothers also helps support successful breastfeeding. The first article in this section, by Dewey, addresses the impact of lactation on weight loss postpartum and on maternal micronutrient status. The second article, by Kalkwarf, addresses concern about long-term effects of lactation on maternal bone health and potential future risk of osteoporotic bone fracture. The effect of exercise and energy restriction on maternal bone health, immune status, and the composition of human milk is addressed by Lovelady in the third article in this section. The last article in this section, by Rea and Morrow, discusses the special needs of women who work outside the home with regard to protection, promotion, and support of breastfeeding.

The fourth section of this book provides an overview of different dimensions of the **innate and acquired immune systems of human milk**. The first of four articles in this section, by Le Pendu, describes the relationship between genetic polymorphisms in relation to host risk of infectious diseases and control of the expression of protective oligosaccharides in human milk. In the second article in this section, Cleary presents three principles involved in human milk protection of the nonimmune infant exposed to a new pathogen. The third article, by Walker, provides insight into the effects of breastfeeding on intestinal development and host defense. The final article in this section, by Wills-Karp et al., addresses a different dimension of human milk immunobiology. This article provides an overview of the current understanding of asthma pathogenesis and the potentially controversial role of breastfeeding in relation to asthma pathogenesis.

The fifth section deals with an issue of concern in certain populations and environments: the **risk of viral transmission by breastfeeding**. In this section, the first article, by Piwoz et al., addresses issues pertaining to the transmission of human immunodeficiency virus (HIV) via human milk. The second article, by Mast, addresses concern about transmission of hepatitis C virus (HCV) via human milk. In the HIV chapter, data are reviewed regarding current knowledge about HIV transmission during breastfeeding, as well as experience of programs that have counseled HIV-infected women about various feeding options and public health considerations. The HCV chapter deals with data on HCV transmission from mother to infant, focusing on studies of breastfeeding, and reviews recommendations for counseling pregnant and lactating women and management of infants born to HCV-infected mothers.

The sixth section contains four articles pertaining to the **cellular and molecular biology of mammary gland development and lactation**. The first article, by Hovey and Trott, discusses the dynamic process of morphogenesis of mammary gland development, while the second, by Hadsell, reviews genetic control of mammary gland development and lactation. The last two chapters in this section deal with the complex issues of glucose transport in lactation (Haney) and the molecular and cellular framework for understanding milk lipid formation and secretion (McManaman et al.).

In the seventh section of the book, we have included 53 **extended abstracts** describing research presented at the meeting on a variety of current topics. These abstracts are organized in relation to seven themes: Factors associated with breastfeeding initiation and duration; nutrition in lactating women; breastfeeding in relation to child development, nutrition, and chronic disease outcomes; bioactive factors in human milk; anti-infective properties of human milk; viral transmission via human milk; and other topics.

The common theme of this book is advancing our understanding of how human milk contributes to infant health outcomes, whether infectious, chronic, developmental, and/or nutritional. The combination of scientific articles and extended abstracts in this book provides a review of the current thinking in the field of human milk and lactation research, and represents a breadth of basic and clinical sciences. Following this introduction, we share an inspired photograph of a mother-infant pair taken in the San Pedro Martir area of Mexico City, where some of the editors and contributors to this book (GMR-P et al.) have for years conducted studies of human milk protection against infectious disease. In our eyes, the photograph provides inspiration for the theme of this book, as it vividly conveys the love of the breastfed infant for his mother. As scientists, we seek to improve our understanding of the gifts that mother's milk conveys to her beloved infant through breastfeeding. And through advances in our understanding about human milk and lactation, we hope to contribute substantial information and support to mothers, health care professionals, and policymakers worldwide to guide their decisions about breastfeeding.

Jones G, Steketee RW, Black RE, Bhutta ZA, Morris SS. How many child deaths can we prevent this year? Lancet 2003;362:65-71.

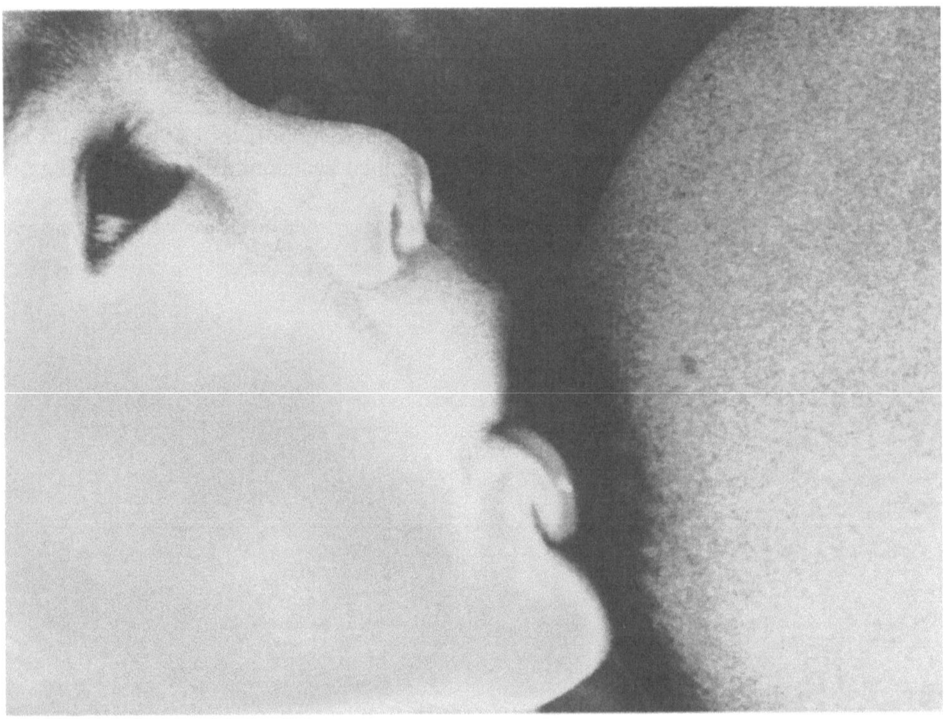

Photograph by Patricia Lagarde (January 2004, San Pedro Martir, Mexico City)

EHRLICH-KOLDOVSKY YOUNG INVESTIGATOR AWARD

The Society recognizes investigators at the junior faculty level who have begun to make outstanding, original scientific contributions to the study of human milk and lactation with the EHRLICH-KOLDOVSKY YOUNG INVESTIGATOR AWARD FOR RESEARCH IN HUMAN MILK AND LACTATION. Paul Ehrlich was known for his work on the principles of immunology and theories of antibody responses as magic bullets which would go straight to the organisms at which they were aimed. Otakar Koldovsky studied intestinal maturation during the suckling period and the importance of mammalian milk for its growth-promoting properties, exclusive of the known nutrients present. This led him to develop the concept of "Biologically Active Substances" in milk and to explore what these substances might be and how they might act using artificially reared animals, the 'pup in the cup' model. Ehrlich-Koldovsky Young Investigator awardees are listed below. Additional information about Dr. Koldovsky can be found on the Society website at www.ISRHML.org.

EHRLICH-KOLDOVSKY YOUNG INVESTIGATOR AWARDEES

2002	Joanna Hawkes, PhD; Michelle McGuire, PhD
2000	Bohuslav Dvorak, PhD; Cheryl Lovelady, PhD
1999	Rafael Perez-Escamilla, PhD
1997	Ardythe L. Morrow, PhD; Henry F. Gomez, MD
1995	Sharon Donovan, PhD

MACY-GYÖRGY AWARD

At each bi-annual international meeting since 1995, the Executive Committee of the International Society for Research in Human Milk and Lactation has honored outstanding investigators in the field of human milk and lactation. Senior scientists whose work has been recognized internationally and whose many papers have appeared in prominent peer-review journals are candidates for the MACY-GYÖRGY AWARD FOR RESEARCH IN HUMAN MILK AND LACTATION. This award honors individuals who have made outstanding, original scientific contributions to the study of human milk and lactation. This award is appropriately named for two outstanding scholars in the field of human milk and lactation, Drs. Icie G. Macy and Paul György.

Icie G. Macy was a physiological chemist who conducted fundamental research into the metabolism of women during the reproduction cycle, evaluation of food purchasing and preparation, nutrition and infant growth and development, and secretion and composition of human milk. She demonstrated a love of the search for scientific truth, independence of thought, and respect for the guidance to be found in the history of science.

Paul György studied the unique biological properties of human milk, a unique food that contians what we now designate as bioactive compounds. In that respect, he was one of the first scientists to point out the superiority of human milk for human infants and ecological factors of disease and their relationships to breastfeeding.

The awards and the biographies of Drs. Macy and György can be found on the Society website at www.ISRHML.org/. Macy-György awardees are listed below.

MACY-GYÖRGY AWARDEES

2002	Bo Lönnerdal, PhD
2000	Armond S. Goldman, MD
1999	Margit Hamosh, PhD
1997	Stuart Patton, PhD
1995	Robert G. Jensen, PhD

HUMAN MILK PROTEINS
Key Components for the Biological Activity of Human Milk

Bo Lönnerdal

1. ABSTRACT

Human milk contains a wide array of proteins that provide biologic activities ranging from antimicrobial effects to immunostimulatory functions. Proteins like lactoferrin, secretory IgA, κ-casein, lactoperoxidase, haptocorrin, lactadherin and peptides formed from human milk proteins during digestion can inhibit the growth of pathogenic bacteria and viruses and therefore protect against infection. At the same time, proteins like lactoferrin, bile-salt stimulated lipase, haptocorrin, κ-casein, and folate-binding protein can facilitate the absorption of nutrients in the neonatal gut. However, the proteins in human milk themselves also provide adequate amounts of essential amino acids to the growing infant. This suggests a highly adapted digestive system, which allows the survival of some proteins and peptides in the upper gastrointestinal tract, while still allowing amino acid utilization from these proteins further down in the gut. It is now possible to produce recombinant human milk proteins in transgenic plants and animals, which makes it possible to further study the bioactivity of these proteins. Provided these proteins can be produced in large scale at low cost, that they show biologic activity and pose no safety concerns, it may be possible to add some human milk proteins to infant diets, such as formula and complementary foods. Human milk proteins produced in rice or potatoes, for example, could be added without much purification, because these staples commonly are used in weaning foods. Thus, some qualities provided by human milk may be included into other diets, although it is highly unlikely that all unique components of human milk can be copied this way.

2. INTRODUCTION

The advantages of breastfeeding are plentiful and the benefits provided include long-lasting effects on development and prevention against chronic diseases. There are numerous components in human milk that are absent or only present in low concentrations in

Department of Nutrition & Program of International Nutrition, University of California, One Shields Avenue, Davis, CA 95616

Protecting Infants through Human Milk, edited by Pickering *et al.*
Kluwer Academic/Plenum Publishers, 2004

infant formula, which may help to explain differences in growth, nutritional status, health, and long-term outcome between breastfed and formula-fed infants. A majority of these components, and also most of those likely to have physiologic activity in breastfed infants, are proteins. By using different fat blends and adding arachidonic and docosahexenoic acid (DHA), formula manufacturers have been able to make the fatty acid profile of infant formula very similar to that of human milk. Quantitatively minor components of the fat fraction, though, such as sphingomyelin and very long-chain polyunsaturated fatty acids, are still lacking in formula. The major carbohydrate in human milk is lactose, which is usually the same in formulas, but the very complex oligosaccharide fraction in human milk, which is likely to be involved in the defense against infection, is absent in infant formula. Minerals, trace elements, and vitamins are added to infant formula at concentrations similar to or higher than in human milk, although the chemical form may vary somewhat.

The proteins of human milk are species specific with bovine proteins being different from their human counterparts. It has not been possible to add bovine proteins, a blend of cow milk proteins, or protein fractions to obtain a protein pattern similar to that of human milk. Thus, there is a wide variety of unique proteins in human milk, and many of the biologic activities ascribed to human milk are believed to be provided by protein or peptide components.

3. PHYSIOLOGIC SIGNIFICANCE OF HUMAN MILK PROTEINS

Human milk provides a wide array of proteins that contribute to defense against infections in the newborn infant. Several proteins (e.g., lactoferrin, lysozyme, κ-casein, and haptocorrin) have been shown to have both bacteriostatic and bactericidal activity against many common bacterial pathogens, and other proteins (lactadherin, lactoferrin) are protective against viruses and yeast infection. Some of these proteins are likely to act independently, while others may act synergistically. There appears to be considerable redundancy with several components acting upon the same pathogen, suggesting a multilayered defense system, which may explain the lower prevalence of infection in breastfed infants when compared with formula-fed infants (Dewey et al. 1995).

Besides these active components, other proteins have a more passive, "prebiotic" role in establishing a "host-friendly" gut microflora, which in itself prevents proliferation of pathogenic bacteria. Immunoglobulins (primarily secretory IgA), cytokines and growth factors (EGF and IGF) participate in the mucosal defense system against infection, and also on the proliferation, development and maturation of the mucosal barrier. There are several proteins that facilitate digestion and absorption of nutrients from human milk, such as bile salt-stimulated lipase (lipids), lactoferrin (iron), haptocorrin (vitamin B_{12}), folate-binding protein (folate) and casein phosphopeptides (calcium).

4. CHANGES IN PROTEIN COMPOSITION DURING LACTATION

The protein concentration of colostrum is high and largely consists of whey proteins, because casein synthesis is absent or low during the first few days of lactation (Kunz & Lönnerdal 1987a) and the lipid content (also membrane proteins) is low. The protein concentration then decreases rapidly during the first month of lactation, and more slowly after that (Lönnerdal et al. 1976a; Dewey & Lönnerdal 1983; Dewey et al. 1984). Virtually all proteins in human milk are synthesized within the mammary gland, but a few proteins, such as serum albumin, may be transferred from maternal blood. Milk proteins usually are classified into three groups: mucins (fat globule membrane proteins), casein, and whey proteins. Mucins, enveloping the lipid globules in milk, contribute only a small fraction of the total human milk protein content (Patton & Houston 1986). The fat content of human milk does not vary much once lactation has been established, and milk mucin levels are therefore most likely relatively constant, although this has not been studied systematically. Concentrations of casein and whey proteins, however, change dramatically during lactation; the concentration of whey proteins is high, whereas casein is virtually nondetectable during the first days of lactation (Kunz & Lönnerdal 1987a, 1987b). When milk production increases, mammary gland casein synthesis and milk casein levels increase, whereas concentrations of whey proteins decrease, partially due to the increased volume of milk being secreted. Therefore, there is no "fixed" whey-to-casein ratio of human milk; the ratio varies throughout lactation. The often cited whey-to-casein ratio of 60:40 may be considered an estimate of the ratio during full lactation, but it does vary from about 80:20 in early lactation to 50:50 in late lactation. Since the amino acid composition of casein(s) and whey proteins differs, the amino acid composition of human milk also varies during lactation, which rarely is considered when estimating amino acid requirements of infants.

The true protein concentration of human milk is often overestimated, which is due to the comparatively high proportion of nonprotein nitrogen (NPN) in human milk (Donovan & Lönnerdal 1987). The fraction of NPN is low (<5%) in milk from most species, which allows a good estimate of true milk protein content by analyzing nitrogen (by the Kjeldahl method) and multiplying by a dairy protein factor of 6.38, which takes into account such a fraction of NPN. In human milk, the NPN fraction contributes about 20% to 25% of total nitrogen. The Kjeldahl nitrogen analysis using the conversion factor for dairy protein (6.38) will overestimate human milk protein content considerably. A more accurate approach is to analyze total nitrogen and NPN, subtract the NPN from total nitrogen and then multiply by the conventional Kjeldahl factor of 6.25 (Lönnerdal et al. 1976a). This slightly underestimates the total protein content (when considering protein as a source of amino acids), because small peptides and free amino acids are included in the NPN fraction, but this amount is only a few percent of the total. It is possible to determine the precise amino acid content and true protein content (alpha amino nitrogen) by amino acid analysis, but this is expensive as well as time-consuming. Determinations of true protein content by the "corrected Kjeldahl" method and amino acid analysis have been shown to be in close agreement (Lönnerdal et al. 1976a).

The true protein content of human milk, determined as described above, is 14 to 16 g/L during early lactation, 8 to 10 g/L at 3 to 4 months of lactation, and 7 to 8 g/L at 6 months and later (Lönnerdal et al. 1976b; Kunz & Lönnerdal 1987b). These protein concentrations and, consequently, the corresponding intakes may not accurately reflect the utilizable amounts of amino acids provided to the breastfed infant. This argument is based on the observation that intact human milk proteins can be found in stools of breastfed infants (Davidson & Lönnerdal 1987); thus, these proteins are incompletely digested and do not represent utilizable amino acids. It has therefore been suggested that such proteins (lactoferrin, sIgA) should be subtracted from the protein concentration of human milk to derive a true "digestible" protein content. However, it is not correct to assume that these proteins are completely undigestible; even if they have properties that make them more resistant towards proteolytic enzymes than most other proteins. Only a minor fraction escapes digestion. For example, 6% to10% of lactoferrin is estimated not to be digested by breastfed infants (Davidson & Lönnerdal 1987). The quantitatively most significant of the relatively "indigestible" human milk proteins are lactoferrin and secretory IgA. The total concentration of these two proteins in mature milk (>30 days of lactation) is approximately 2 g/L; assuming that 6% to 10 % is undigested, this corresponds to a potential loss of ~0.12 to 0.2 g/L, or about 1.2% to 2 % of total protein intake, which may be within the margin of error for the analysis used (Lönnerdal 2003). Thus, while undigested, biologically active proteins may have physiologic significance for the breastfed infant, the impact of the loss of these amino acids on meeting the infant's requirements may be insignificant.

Biologically active peptides that are formed during digestion of several human milk proteins, such as casein phosphopeptides, also represent "undigestible" protein and it could therefore be argued that they should not be included in the total protein content of human milk. However, no such peptides have been detected in the stools of breastfed infants and it is possible that they are formed transiently during digestion in the upper part of the gastrointestinal tract. Thus, they may be formed in the duodenum/upper jejunum to exert their physiologic activity locally, to subsequently be completely digested and absorbed in the lower jejunum and ileum. Further studies are needed to support this potential sequence of events.

5. CASEINS

5.1. β-Casein

The major constituent of the human casein micelle is β-casein, a highly phosphorylated protein (Greenberg & Groves 1984). Clusters of phosphorylated serine and threonine residues are located close to the N-terminal end and are capable of complexing Ca^{2+} ions (Sato et al. 1991). When β-casein is digested, small peptides with several phosphorylated amino acids are formed and such phosphopeptides have been shown to keep Ca^{2+} soluble, thus enhancing its absorption (Sato et al. 1986). It is therefore likely that phosphopeptides released from β-casein contribute to the high bioavailability of calcium from human milk. Casein phosphopeptides also may facilitate the absorption of other divalent cations, such as zinc (Hansen et al. 1996).

5.2. K-Casein

K-casein, a minor casein subunit in human milk, is a heavily glycosylated protein containing several charged sialic acid residues (Brignon et al. 1985). In vitro, κ-casein has been shown to inhibit the adhesion of *Helicobacter pylori* to human gastric mucosa (Strömquist et al. 1995). *H. pylori* infection has been shown to occur in increasingly younger age groups, but breastfeeding seems to provide some protection. The glycan component of κ-casein may be responsible for this activity, since sIgA (which is also glycosylated) has similar activity, and both proteins lost their activity when deglycosylated (Strömquist et al. 1995). K-casein has been shown to prevent the attachment of pathogenic bacteria to the mucosa by acting as a receptor analog (Newburg 1997). Oligosaccharide structures on the glycans of these glycoproteins thus act as "decoys" for similar surface-exposed carbohydrate structures on the gastric mucosa, thereby inhibiting adhesion, and, subsequently, infection.

5.3. α_{s1}-Casein

It was believed for quite some time that α_{s1}-casein is totally absent in human milk. However, an "α_{s1}-casein-like" protein in human milk was isolated and characterized in 1994 (Cavaletto et al.), but its concentration is low (~0.06% of total protein). *Escherichia coli* has been used to express recombinant human α_{s1}-casein (Kim et al. 1999). Three peptides resulting from trypsin digestion of this recombinant human α_{s1}-casein were found to exhibit angiotensin-I-converting enzyme inhibitory activity in a dose-dependent manner. Whether the concentrations of such peptides, formed from a minor component of human milk, are sufficient to exert physiologic activity in the infant is not yet known.

5.4. Casein-Derived Peptides

A multitude of small peptides have been generated from human casein, particularly β-casein, that have been shown to have biologic activity. Most of these have been generated in vitro, but some also have been isolated from intestinal contents, suggesting that they may be formed in vivo. Among the biologic effects that have been demonstrated in experimental systems are antithrombotic, antihypertensive, and opioid activities (Brantl 1984; Fiat et al. 1993; Kim et al. 1999; Schlimme & Meisel 1995). Whether such activities also are present in infants is not yet known, but opioid peptides have been implicated to have both local effects by affecting fluid transport in the small intestine and systemically by affecting sleep habits of infants (Brantl 1984).

6. WHEY PROTEINS

6.1. α-Lactalbumin

Human α-lactalbumin has been shown to bind Ca^{2+} (Lönnerdal & Glazier 1985) and under some circumstances bind Zn^{2+} (Ren 1993). Although the proportion of total calcium bound to α-lactalbumin in human milk is less than 1% (Lönnerdal & Glazier 1985), α-lactalbumin may exert a positive effect on mineral absorption, possibly by the generation of peptides that facilitate absorption of divalent cations. We have observed that infant formula supplemented with bovine α-lactalbumin increased the absorption of zinc and iron in infant rhesus monkeys as compared to monkeys fed regular formula (Kelleher et al. 2003). Whether human α-lactalbumin affects mineral absorption in breastfed infants has not yet been studied.

The potential antimicrobial activity of α-lactalbumin has received limited attention. However, three polypeptide fragments from α-lactalbumin have been found to have antimicrobial activity against *E. coli, Klebsiella pneumoniae, Staphylococcus aureus, S. epidermis, Streptococci* and *Candida albicans* (Pellegrini et al. 1999). These peptides were generated by treating α-lactalbumin with proteolytic enzymes known to be present in the gastrointestinal tract. This observation may explain our finding of an inhibitory effect of α-lactalbumin-supplemented infant formula on enteropathogenic *E. coli* (EPEC)-induced diarrhea in infant rhesus monkeys (Kelleher et al. 2003). The primary structure of bovine and human α-lactalbumin is similar, but whether identical antimicrobial peptides are being formed during digestion has not yet been studied.

6.2. Immunoglobulins

The major immunoglobulin class in human milk is secretory IgA (>90% of total immunoglobulins), a dimer of IgA linked together with a secretory component and a joining chain (Goldman 1993). This structure makes the secretory IgA molecule comparatively resistant towards digestion by proteolytic enzymes (Lindh 1985) and, as mentioned above, small quantities of secretory IgA have been found intact in stools of breastfed infants (Davidson & Lönnerdal 1987). Concentrations of secretory IgA in human milk are remarkably high, about 1 to 2 g/L during early lactation, and remain at 0.5 to 1 g/L up to 2 years of lactation (Goldman 1993). Maternal immunity against several pathogens can be transferred to her breastfed infant in the form of secretory IgA, mediated via the so-called "enteromammary pathway" (Telemo et al. 1996). This allows the immature immune system of the newborn to be "boosted" by acquired immunity in the mother. Secretory IgA antibodies against bacterial pathogens such as *E. coli, V. cholerae, H. influenzae, S. pneumoniae, C. difficile,* and *Salmonella,* viruses like rotavirus, CMV, HIV, influenza virus and RSV, as well as yeasts, like *C. albicans,* have been found in human milk (Goldman 1993), illustrating the versatility of this defense.

6.3. Lactoferrin

A major protein in human milk is lactoferrin, an iron-binding protein capable of binding two ferric ions (Lönnerdal & Iyer 1995). Lactoferrin binds a significant proportion of iron in human milk (Fransson & Lönnerdal 1980) and facilitates the uptake of this bound iron by human intestinal cells in culture, which is most likely mediated by enterocyte receptors specific for human lactoferrin (Kawakami & Lönnerdal 1991; Suzuki et al. 2001). This is supported by the observation that transfection of Caco-2 cells with cDNA for the lactoferrin receptor significantly enhanced cellular iron uptake as well as of lactoferrin, suggesting endocytosis of the protein with iron bound to it (Suzuki et al. 2001). Supplementation of infant formula with bovine lactoferrin, however, has not resulted in any enhancing effect on iron absorption or iron status (Fairweather-Tait et al. 1987; Chierici et al. 1992), which may be due to the fact that bovine lactoferrin does not bind to the human lactoferrin receptor (Davidson & Lönnerdal 1988). However, there is usually little information provided in these studies with regard to the bioactivity of the lactoferrin prior to being added to the formula, how the lactoferrin was added to the formula, and how the formula was heat-treated, all steps possibly affecting the resulting activity of lactoferrin when fed as part of the diet to an infant. It also is possible that a positive effect of lactoferrin is found only when it is present in human milk; when added to infant formula, other constituents of the formula may interfere with the ability of lactoferrin to interact with its receptor.

Lactoferrin has been shown to exhibit several antimicrobial activities (Lönnerdal & Iyer 1995). It was first assumed that lactoferrin, which in human milk is largely in the iron-unsaturated form, could withhold iron from iron-requiring pathogens due to its high affinity for iron, thereby having a bacteriostatic effect (Bullen et al. 1972). This is a possible scenario, but other studies have demonstrated strong bactericidal activity of lactoferrin against a variety of pathogens, which is not dependent upon the degree of iron-saturation of lactoferrin (Arnold et al. 1980). Some, if not all, of this activity may be the result of generation of lactoferricin, a potent bactericidal peptide, formed during proteolytic digestion of lactoferrin (Tomita et al. 1991). Studies also have shown that lactoferricin can inhibit attachment of enteropathogenic *E. coli* (EPEC) to intestinal cells

(Edde et al. 2001), which may be mediated by serine protease activity of lactoferrin (Plaut et al. 2000). By degrading protein structures of EPEC needed for attachment and invasion of the bacteria, infection may be blocked. Thus, several activities of lactoferrin may contribute to the defense against bacterial infection. In vitro studies also show that lactoferrin can exert inhibitory activity against viruses, such as HIV and cytomegalovirus (Harmsen et al. 1995), and fungi, such as *C. albicans* (Andersson et al. 2000); however, the mechanisms behind these activities are not known.

Binding of lactoferrin to its receptor in the small intestine may explain its effect on cytokine expression. Lactoferrin has been shown to increase the production and release of cytokines such as TNF-α, IL-1β, IL-8, and nitric oxide (Kelleher & Lönnerdal 2001), which in turn may affect immune function. It is possible that this is caused by signaling events triggered by the interaction with the receptor, but it also is possible that internalized lactoferrin can bind to the nucleus, affecting NF-Kβ, and subsequently cytokine expression (He & Furmanski 1995). Human lactoferrin has been shown to activate the transcription of IL-1β (Son et al. 2002), suggesting that lactoferrin may directly interact with the nucleus. The released cytokines may then have immunomodulatory effects, similar to what was described above for cytokines in milk.

Lactoferrin has been shown to increase proliferation of intestinal cells in experimental animals and to affect crypt cell development (Nichols et al. 1987). This mitogenic effect of lactoferrin has been hypothesized to be in part responsible for the rapid development of the intestinal mucosa of the suckling newborn (Berseth et al. 1983; Heird et al. 1984). Weight gain of infants fed formula supplemented with bovine lactoferrin has been shown to be higher than in infants fed regular formula (Hernell & Lönnerdal 2002), which would be in agreement with this proposed function of lactoferrin. Further studies on the potential growth-stimulatory effect of lactoferrin are needed.

6.4. Lysozyme

Human milk contains unusually high concentrations of lysozyme, an enzyme capable of breaking down the outer cell wall of Gram-positive bacteria by hydrolyzing β1,4 linkages of *N*-acetylmuramic acid and 2-acetylamino-2-deoxy-D-glucose residues (Chipman & Sharon 1969). Studies show that addition of recombinant human lysozyme produced in rice (see also below) to chicken feed could serve as a natural "antibiotic" (Humphrey et al. 2002), suggesting that it may be possible to replace currently used antimicrobial agents with this human milk protein.

Lysozyme also has been shown to kill Gram-negative bacteria in vitro, in a synergetic action with lactoferrin (Ellison & Giehl 1991). Lactoferrin is capable of binding lipopolysaccharide (LPS) tightly and can thus remove LPS from the outer cell membrane of bacteria, thereby allowing lysozyme to access and degrade the inner proteoglycan matrix of the membrane, hence killing the bacteria.

Lysozyme also has been shown to inhibit the growth of HIV in vitro (Lee-Huang et al. 1999), but in human milk it may only act upon the free virus and not on cell-associated virus. The mechanism of this antiviral activity still needs to be studied.

6.5. Bile Salt-Stimulated Lipase

Enzymatic activity provided by bile-salt stimulated lipase in human milk may facilitate lipid digestion in newborn infants, particularly in preterm infants who have low lipase activity and poor lipid utilization (Hernell & Bläckberg 1983; Hernell et al. 1989).

Pasteurization of human milk, which destroys the activity of bile salt-stimulated lipase, has been shown to result in decreased lipid absorption in premature infants (Fredrikzon et al. 1978). Bile salt-stimulated lipase may aid in lipid digestion in term infants, due to its uniquely wide substrate specificity; it hydrolyzes mono-, di-, and triacylglycerols, cholesterol esters and diacylphosphatidylglycerols, and micellar as well as water-soluble substrates, thus complementing endogenous digestive enzymes (Hernell & Bläckberg 1983).

6.6. Lactoperoxidase

In the presence of hydrogen peroxide (formed in small quantities by cells), lactoperoxidase catalyzes the oxidation of thiocyanate (part of saliva) forming hypothiocyanate, which can kill both Gram-positive (Steele & Morrisons 1969) and Gram-negative (Björck et al. 1975) pathogenic bacteria. Thus, lactoperoxidase in human milk may contribute to the defense against infection already in the mouth and upper gastrointestinal tract. Human milk contains bioactive lactoperoxidase (Shin et al. 2001), but its physiological significance is not yet known. For cow milk, however, the lactoperoxidase system has been used by the dairy industry in developing countries for decades to preserve microbial quality.

6.7. Haptocorrin

Vitamin B_{12} in human milk is almost exclusively bound to haptocorrin, previously called vitamin B_{12}-binding protein (Sandberg et al. 1981). There is considerably more haptocorrin than vitamin B_{12} on a molar basis in human milk, resulting in the protein being largely in its unsaturated form (Gullberg 1973), which may be important for its antimicrobial activity. Holo-haptocorrin has been shown to bind in a saturable manner to human intestinal brush-border membranes. In addition, vitamin B_{12} bound to haptocorrin is taken up by human intestinal (Caco-2) cells in culture (Adkins & Lönnerdal 2002), suggesting that haptocorrin may be involved in vitamin B_{12} absorption during early life. Intrinsic factor (IF) is present in stools of breastfed infants at a young age, but the concentration of haptocorrin is low and it may not be adequate to facilitate uptake of vitamin B_{12} via the IF receptor (Adkins & Lönnerdal 2002).

Vitamin B_{12}-binding protein (haptocorrin) has been suggested to inhibit bacterial growth by tightly binding and withholding the vitamin from the bacteria (Gullberg 1973). The structure and activity of haptocorrin were maintained after in vitro digestion with pepsin and pancreatic enzymes, demonstrating that haptocorrin may resist digestion in the gastrointestinal tract. Whether the tight binding of vitamin B_{12} is the inhibitory mechanism, how broad its antimicrobial activity is, and whether haptocorrin quantitatively contributes to the defense against infection in breastfed infants remain to be explored. Recent studies in vitro show that both apo- and holo-haptocorrin can inhibit growth of EPEC, but the mechanism behind this vitamin B_{12}–independent activity is not yet known (Adkins & Lönnerdal 2003).

6.8. Folate-Binding Protein

A folate-binding protein (FBP) has been found in both particulate and soluble form in human milk (Antony et al. 1982). The soluble FBP is glycosylated to about 22%, which may help it to survive proteolytic digestion. Folate-binding proteins have been shown to tolerate low gastric pH and resist proteolysis in newborn goats (Salter &

Mowlem 1983). The human milk FBP may be equally stable in human infants. Experiments using rat intestinal cells have shown that folate uptake was higher when it was complexed to FBP than in the free form (Colman et al. 1981), suggesting that FBP may facilitate folate uptake. It has also been proposed that FBP may actually slow the release and uptake of folate in the small intestine to allow a gradual release and absorption of folate that may increase tissue utilization (Said et al. 1986).

6.9. Growth Factors

Several growth factors, such as insulin-like growth factors (IGFs) and epidermal growth factor (EGF) have been found in human milk (Donovan & Ogle 1994). IGF-I and IGF-II were shown to stimulate DNA synthesis and to promote the growth of various cells in culture (Klagsburn 1978; Corps et al. 1987a, 1987b), suggesting that they may promote the development of the neonatal gastrointestinal tract. Effects on intestinal mucosal growth has been demonstrated and development of biologic functions may be affected, as shown by stimulation of intestinal enzyme expression and maturation (Ma & Xu 1997; Young et al. 1990).

EGF also has been shown to affect maturation of intestinal function in newborns (Read et al. 1984), possibly by interacting with EGF receptors in the small intestine (Menard & Pothier 1991).

6.10. IGF-Binding Proteins

IGF-I and IGF-II are present in human milk and primarily are found associated with IGF-binding proteins (Donovan et al. 1991). These binding proteins may protect IGF-I and IGF-II from being digested, prolong their half-life and modulate their interaction with intestinal receptors (Morgan et al. 1996). Following binding of IGF-I and IGF-II to the enterocyte, they may exert activity locally and, possibly, be transported and act systemically.

6.11. α_1-Antitrypsin

The protease inhibitors α_1-antitrypsin and antichymotrypsin are present in human milk at concentrations that may be of physiologic significance (Lindberg et al. 1982). Together they may limit the activity of pancreatic enzymes in the breastfed infant (Lindberg 1979; Hamosh 1995), therefore acting as modulators of digestion. Some milk proteins, including α_1-antitrypsin, have been shown in part to escape digestion and are found in stools of breastfed infants (Davidson & Lönnerdal 1987, 1990). In vitro experiments show that addition of α_1-antitrypsin to human milk resulted in a larger proportion of lactoferrin resisting proteolytic degradation (Chowanadisai & Lönnerdal 2002). Although the inhibitory activity of α_1-antitrypsin and antichymotrypsin against proteolytic enzymes may have relevance for the slower rates of digestibility of specific proteins, this may only delay their eventual breakdown. Data on total nitrogen balance of breastfed infants suggest that net protein utilization is high.

6.12. Amylase

Human milk contains a significant concentration of α-amylase (Lindberg & Skude 1982). This enzyme is active also at low pH and is relatively stable against pepsin degradation (Hamosh 1995). While there is no natural substrate for amylase in human milk, the amylase in human milk may compensate for low salivary and pancreatic amylase activity in the newborn and aid in digestion of complex carbohydrates when complementary foods are being fed in proximity to nursing (Heitlinger et al. 1979). Whether this contributes significantly to carbohydrate utilization in mixed-fed infants is not yet known.

6.13. Cytokines

Human milk has been shown to contain several cytokines, such as IL-1β, IL-6, IL-8, IL-10, TNF-α and TGF-β (Grosvenor et al. 1993). Although all of these have immunomodulatory activities, it appears that most of them are anti-inflammatory, thereby possibly lessening the impact of infections. These cytokines can be released from cells in human milk but also are found in their free form. The combined action of these potent signal molecules on the immature immune system, and its variation among infants, needs to be studied further, as well as their suggested effect on Th2 and Th1 switching and development of allergy.

6.14. "Prebiotic" Components

The microbial flora in the gut of breastfed infants is different from that in formula-fed infants by having fewer potentially pathogenic bacteria such as *E. coli, Bacteroides, Campylobacter,* and *Streptococci*, but more *Lactobacilli* and *Bifidobacteria* (Kleesen et al. 1995). While antimicrobial components in human milk are likely to inhibit the growth of pathogens, some components are likely to stimulate the growth of host-friendly bacteria, i.e., have prebiotic activity. This factor(s), originally called "*bifidus* factor," may promote the growth of *Lactobacilli* and *Bifidobacteria*, which can limit the growth of several pathogens by decreasing intestinal pH. One possible substance identified was *N*-acetylglucosamine (György 1971). Subsequently, several oligosaccharides have been shown to have this activity (Newburg 1997), but it is possible that milk proteins also can have such prebiotic activity.

Recently, bifidogenic peptides were purified by chromatography following in vitro digestion of human milk with pepsin (Liepke et al. 2002). Two of these peptides were found to originate from lactoferrin and one from the secretory component of sIgA, and were found to be stable upon further digestion with pepsin, trypsin, and chymotrypsin. They showed activity at low concentrations; the bifidogenic effect was about 100 times stronger than that of *N*-acetylglucosamine, a known "bifidus factor." A synthetic lactoferrin-derived peptide was shown to have as strong bifidogenic activity as the native peptide, verifying the results from the generation of peptides in vitro.

7. RECOMBINANT HUMAN MILK PROTEINS

Since many of the physiologic activities provided by human milk are linked to specific protein constituents, the possibility exists to produce recombinant versions of these proteins in various production systems (Lönnerdal 1994). These systems include transgenic animals (cows, goats, sheep, pigs), transgenic plants (tobacco, potatoes, rice) and microorganisms (*Aspergillus*, yeast). In principle, the amino acid sequences of the recombinant proteins will be identical to those of their native counterpart; however, if the protein is glycosylated or phosphorylated, there will likely be differences in the extent and composition of their post-translational modification (Lönnerdal 2002). For many proteins such variances may have no effect on their physiologic activities because they are not dependent on such modifications, but this needs to be evaluated (Adkins & Lönnerdal 2003).

Recombinant human milk proteins produced in transgenic animals have not reached commercialization for infant food products, possibly due to excessive cost. Similarly, microorganism-produced recombinant human milk proteins (e.g., lactoferrin), have not been included into infant formula, most likely due to the extensive purification required to avoid any contaminant proteins, also making the protein expensive. Plant-produced recombinant human milk proteins are more likely to be an economically and safe approach, due to the enormous production capacity (Lönnerdal 2002). In addition, with the exception of proteins produced in tobacco plants, which contain many toxic compounds and therefore also will require extensive purification, the plants used (rice, potatoes) are commonly among the first foods introduced in the weaning diet of infants, and thus unlikely to cause any adverse effects. Therefore, the proteins do not need to be purified; allergies towards rice and potato proteins are not common.

We have produced recombinant human lactoferrin (Nandi et al. 2002; Suzuki et al. 2003) and lysozyme (Huang et al. 2002a, 2002b) in rice at high expression levels, ~5% of total protein. These proteins were chosen because lactoferrin has been proposed to have several functions in the newborn and lysozyme has antimicrobial activity. Further, Ellison & Giehl (1991) have shown that these two proteins have synergistic activity; lactoferrin binds lipopolysaccharide (LPS) from the outer cell membrane of Gram-negative bacteria, literally "poking holes" in this membrane and allowing lysozyme to access the inner bacterial membrane and degrading it, thus causing lysis. We have shown in vitro that the recombinant lactoferrin binds and releases iron in a manner similar to that of human milk lactoferrin, that it binds to lactoferrin receptors on human intestinal cells in culture, and that it inhibits the growth of enteropathogenic *E. coli* (EPEC) to an extent similar to human milk lactoferrin (Suzuki et al. 2003). Further, the recombinant and native lactoferrin resisted low pH treatment and proteolytic enzymes (in vitro digestion), suggesting that they may be active in the infant gut. In addition, there were limited and similar effects on the two forms following moderate heat treatment at a temperature and duration used for infant formula processing. Results from the same tests on recombinant lysozyme were similar (Huang et al. 2002b). Thus, recombinant lactoferrin and lysozyme produced in rice appear to have stability and biologic activities similar to those of the human milk proteins. Further extensive safety and efficacy studies in animal models and clinical trials are needed before these proteins may be used in infant foods. Finally, even if some of the properties of human milk may be transferred to infant formula, it will most likely never be possible to copy all the numerous beneficial qualities of human milk.

8. ACKNOWLEDGMENTS

I would like to express my gratitude to Professor Leif Hambraeus who directed me into research on human milk composition. I also would like to sincerely thank all my graduate students, post-docs, and colleagues who have greatly contributed to the work presented in this review and made the research both enjoyable and fascinating – "Breast is Best"!!

9. REFERENCES

Adkins Y, Lönnerdal B. Mechanisms of vitamin B12 absorption in breast-fed infants. J Pediatr Gastroenterol Nutr 2002;35:192-198.

Adkins Y, Lönnerdal B. Potential host-defense role of a human milk vitamin B_{12}-binding protein, haptocorrin, in the gastrointestinal tract of breast-fed infants assessed with porcine haptocorrin in vitro. Am J Clin Nutr 2003;77:1234-1240.

Adkins Y, Lönnerdal B. Biotechnology Strategies to Produce Specific Food Ingredients: Proteins and Peptides. In: Eds. German B (in press)

Andersson Y, Lindquist S, Lagerqvist C, Hernell O. Lactoferrin is responsible for the fungistatic effect of human milk. Early Hum Dev 2000;59:95-105.

Antony AC, Utley CS, Marcell PD, Kolhouse JF. Isolation, characterization, and comparison of the solubilized particulate and soluble folate binding proteins from human milk. J Biol Chem 1982;257:10081-10089.

Arnold RR, Brewer M, Gauthier JJ. Bactericidal activity of human lactoferrin: sensitivity of a variety of microorganisms. Infect Immun 1980;28:893-898.

Berseth CL, Lichtenberger LM, Morriss FH. Comparison of the gastrointestinal growth-promoting effects of rat colostrum and mature milk in newborn rats in vivo. Am J Clin Nutr 1983;37:52-60.

Björck L, Rosen CG, Marshall V, Reiter B. Antibacterial activity of lactoperoxidase system in milk against pseudomonas and other gram-negative bacteria. Appl Microbiol 1975;30:199-204.

Brantl V. Novel opioid peptides derived from human β-casein. Eur J Pharmacol 1984;106:213-214.

Brignon G, Chtourou A, Ribadeau-Dumas B. Preparation and amino acid sequence of human k-casein. FEBS Lett 1985;188:48-54.

Bullen JJ, Rogers HJ, Leigh L. Iron-binding proteins in milk and resistance to Escherichia coli infection in infants. Br Med J 1972;1:69-72.

Cavaletto M, Cantisani A, Giuffrida G, Napolitano L, Conti A. Human α_{S1}-casein like protein: purification and N-terminal sequence determination. Biol Chem Hoppe-Seyler 1994;375:149-151.

Chierici R, Sawatzki G, Tamisari L, Volpato S, Vigi V. Supplementation of an adapted formula with bovine lactoferrin. 2. Effects on serum iron, ferritin and zinc levels. Acta Paediatr 1992;81:475-479.

Chipman DM, Sharon N. Mechanism of lysozyme action. Science 1969;165:454-465.

Chowanadisai W, Lönnerdal B. Alpha-1-antitrypsin and antichymotrypsin in human milk: origin, concentrations, and stability. Am J Clin Nutr 2002;76:828-833.

Colman N, Hettiarachchy N, Herbert V. Detection of a milk factor that facilitates folate uptake by intestinal cells. Science 1981;211:1427-1428.

Corps AN, Brown KD. Stimulation of intestinal cell proliferation in culture by growth factors in human and ruminant mammary secretions. J Endocrinol 1987;113:285-290.

Corps AN, Blakeley DM, Carr J, Rees LH, Brown KD. Synergistic stimulation of Swiss mouse 3T3 fibroblasts by epidermal growth factor and other factors in human milk. J Endocrinol 1987;112:151-159.

Davidson LA, Lönnerdal B. Persistence of human milk proteins in the breast-fed infant. Acta Paediatr Scand 1987;76:733-740.

Davidson LA, Lönnerdal B. Specific binding of lactoferrin to brush border membrane: ontogeny and effect of glycan chain. Am J Physiol 1988;254:G580-G585.

Davidson LA, Lönnerdal B. Fecal alpha1-antitrypsin in breast-fed infants is derived from human milk and is not indicative of enteric protein loss. Acta Paediatr Scand 1990;79:137-141.

Dewey KG, Lönnerdal B. Milk and nutrient intake of breastfed infants from 1 to 6 months: relation to growth and fatness. J Pediatr Gastroenterol Nutr 1983;2:497-506.

Dewey KG, Finley DA, Lönnerdal B. Breast milk volume and composition during late lactation (7-20 months). J Pediatr Gastroenterol Nutr 1984;3:713-720.

Dewey KG, Heinig MJ, Nommsen-Rivers LA. Differences in morbidity between breast-fed and formula-fed infants. J Pediatr 1995;126:696-702.

Donovan SM, Lönnerdal B. Isolation of the non-protein nitrogen fraction from human milk by gel-filtration chromatography and its separation by fast protein liquid chromatography. Am J Clin Nutr 1987;50:53-57.

Donovan SM, Ogle J. Growth factors in milk as mediators of infant development. Annu Rev Nutr 1994;14:147-167.

Donovan SM, Hintz RL, Rosenfeld RG. Insulin-like growth factors I and II and their binding proteins in human milk: effect of heat-treatment on IGF and IGF binding protein stability. J Pediatr Gastroenterol Nutr 1991;13:242-253.

Edde L, Hipolito RB, Hwang FF, Headon DR, Shalwitz RA, Sherman MP. Lactoferrin protects neonatal rats from gut-related systemic infection. Am J Physiol Gastrointest Liver Physiol 2001;281: G1140-G1150.

Ellison RTJ, Giehl TJ. Killing of Gram-negative bacteria by lactoferrin and lysozyme. J Clin Invest 1991;88:1080-1091.

Fairweather-Tait SJ, Balmer SE, Scott PH, Ninski MJ. Lactoferrin and iron absorption in newborn infants. Pediatr Res 1987;22:651-654.

Fiat AM, Migliore-Samour D, Jollès P, Drouet L, Sollier CB, Caen J. Biologically active peptides from milk proteins with emphasis on two examples concerning antithrombotic and immunomodulating activities. J Dairy Sci 1993;76:301-310.

Fransson G-B, Lönnerdal B. Iron in human milk. J Pediatr 1980;96:380-384.

Fredrikzon B, Hernell O, Bläckberg L, Olivecrona T. Bile salt-stimulated lipase in human milk: evidence of activity in vivo and of a role in the digestion of milk retinol esters. Pediatr Res 1978;12:1048-1052.

Goldman AS. The immune system of human milk: antimicrobial, anti-inflammatory, and immunomodulating properties. Pediatr Infect Dis J 1993;12:664-672.

Greenberg R, Groves ML. Human β-casein. Amino acid sequence and identification of phosphorylation sites. J Biol Chem 1984;259:5128-5132.

Grosvenor CE, Picciano MF, Baumrucker CR. Hormones and growth factors in milk. Endocrinol Rev 1993;14:710-728.

Gullberg R. Possible influence of vitamin B_{12}-binding protein in milk on the intestinal flora in breast-fed infants. Scand J Gastroenterol 1973;8:497-503.

György P. The uniqueness of human milk. Biochemical aspects. Am J Clin Nutr 1971;24:970-975.

Hamosh M. Enzymes in human milk. In: Jensen RG, editor. Handbook of Milk Composition. San Diego: Academic Press, 1995; pp 388-427.

Hansen M, Sandström B, Lönnerdal B. The effect of casein phosphopeptides on zinc and calcium absorption from high phytate diets assessed in rat pups and Caco-2 cells. Pediatr Res 1996;40:547-552.

Harmsen MC, Swart PJ, Debethune MP, Pauwels R, Declercq E, The TH, Meijer DKF. Antiviral effects of plasma and milk proteins: Lactoferrin shows potent activity against both human immunodeficiency virus and human cytomegalovirus replication in vitro. J Infect Dis 1995;172:380-388.

He J, Furmanski P. Sequence specificity and transcriptional activation in the binding of lactoferrin to DNA. Nature 1995;373:721-724.

Heird WC, Schwarz SM, Hansen IH. Colostrum-induced enteric mucosal growth in beagle puppies. Pediatr Res 1984;18:512-515.

Heitlinger LA, Lee PC, Dillon WP, Lebenthal E. Mammary amylase: a possible alternate pathway of carbohydrate digestion in infancy. Pediatr Res 1979;13:969-972.

Hernell O, Bläckberg L. Digestion of human milk lipids: physiologic significance of sn-2-monoacylglycerol hydrolysis by bile salt-stimulated lipase. Pediatr Res 1983;16:882-885.

Hernell O, Lönnerdal B. Iron status of infants fed low iron formula: no effect of added bovine lactoferrin or nucleotides. Am J Clin Nutr 2002;76:858-864.

Hernell O, Bläckberg L, Lindberg T. Human milk enzymes with emphasis on the lipases. In: Lebenthal E, editor. Textbook of Gastroenterology and Nutrition in Infancy. New York: Raven Press, 1989; pp 209-217.

Huang J, Wu L, Yalda D, Adkins Y, Kelleher SL, Crane M, Lönnerdal B, Rodriguez RL, Huang N. Expression of functional recombinant human lysozyme in transgenic rice culture. Transgenic Res 2002a;11:229-230.

Huang J, Nandi S, Wu L, Yalda D, Bartley G, Rodriguez RL, Lönnerdal B, Huang N. Expression of natural antimicrobial human lysozyme in rice grains. Mol Breeding 2002b;10:83-94.

Humphrey BD, Huang N, Klasing KC. Rice expressing lactoferrin and lysozyme has antibiotic-like properties when fed to chicks. J Nutr 2002;132:1214-1218.

Kawakami H, Lönnerdal B. Isolation and function of a receptor for human lactoferrin in human fetal intestinal brush-border membranes. Am J Physiol 1991;261:G841-G846.

Kelleher SL, Lönnerdal B. Immunological activities associated with milk. In: Woodward B, Draper HH, editors. Immunological Properties of Milk. New York: Plenum Publishers. Adv Nutr Res 2001;10:39-65.

Kelleher SL, Chatterton D, Nielsen K, Lönnerdal B. Effects of glycomacropeptide and α-lactalbumin supplementation of infant formula on growth and nutritional status in infant rhesus monkeys. Am J Clin Nutr 2003;77:1261-1268.

Kim Y-K, Yu D-Y, Lönnerdal B, Chung B-H. Novel angiotensin-I-converting enzyme inhibitory peptides derived from recombinant human α_{s1}-casein expressed in Escherichia coli. J Dairy Res 1999;66:431-439.

Klagsburn M. Human milk stimulates DNA synthesis and cellular proliferation in cultured fibroblasts. Proc Natl Acad Sci USA 1978;75:5057-5061.

Kleesen B, Bunke H, Tovar K, Noack J, Sawatzki G. Influence of two infant formulas and human milk on the development of the fecal flora in newborn infants. Acta Paediatr 1995;84:1347-1356.

Kunz C, Lönnerdal B. Human-milk proteins: analysis of casein and casein subunits by anion-exchange chromatography, gel electrophoresis, and specific staining methods. Am J Clin Nutr 1987a;51:37-46.

Kunz C, Lönnerdal B. Re-evaluation of the whey protein/casein ratio of human milk. Acta Paediatr 1987b;81:107-112.

Lee-Huang S, Huang PL, Sun Y, Kung HF, Blithe DL, Chen HC. Lysozyme and RNAses as anti-HIV components in beta-core preparations of human chorionic gonadotropin. Proc Natl Acad Sci USA 1999;96:2678-2681.

Liepke C, Adermann K, Raida M, Mägert H-J, Forssmann W-G, Zucht H-D. Human milk provides peptides highly stimulating the growth of bifidobacteria. Eur J Biochem 2002;269:712-718.

Lindberg T. Protease inhibitors in human milk. Pediatr Res 1979;13:969-972.

Lindberg T, Skude G. Amylase in human milk. Pediatrics 1982;70:235-238.

Lindberg T, Ohlsson K, Weström B. Protease inhibitors and their relation to proteases in human milk. Pediatr Res 1982;16:479-483.

Lindh E. Increased resistance of immunoglobulin dimers to proteolytic degradation after binding of secretory component. J Immunol 1985;113:284-288.

Lönnerdal, B. Recombinant human milk proteins—an opportunity and a challenge. Am J Clin Nutr 1996;63:622S-626S.

Lönnerdal B. Expression of human milk proteins in plants. J Am Coll Nutr 2002;21(Suppl 3):218S-221S.

Lönnerdal B. Nutritional and physiologic significance of human milk proteins. Am J Clin Nutr 2003;77:1537S-1543S.

Lönnerdal B, Glazier C. Calcium binding by α-lactalbumin in human milk. J Nutr 1985;115:1209-1216.

Lönnerdal B, Iyer S. Lactoferrin: molecular structure and biological function. Annu Rev Nutr 1995;15:93-110.

Lönnerdal B, Forsum E, Hambraeus L. A longitudinal study of the protein, nitrogen and lactose contents of human milk from Swedish well-nourished mothers. Am J Clin Nutr 1976a;29:1127-1133.

Lönnerdal B, Forsum E, Hambraeus L. The protein content of human milk. I. A transversal study of Swedish normal material. Nutr Rep Int 1976b;13:125-134.

Ma L, Xu RJ. Oral insulin-like growth factor-I stimulates intestinal enzyme maturation in newborn rats. Life Sci 1997;61:51-58.

Menard D, Pothier P. Radioautographic localization of epidermal growth factor receptors in human fetal gut. Gastroenterology 1991;101:640-649.

Morgan CH, Coutts AGP, McFadyen MC, King TP, Kelly D. Characterization of IGF-I receptors in porcine small intestine during postnatal development. J Nutr Biochem 1996;7:339-347.

Nandi S, Suzuki YA, Huang J, Yalda D, Pham P, Wu L, Bartley G, Huang N, Lönnerdal B. Expression of human lactoferrin in transgenic rice grains for the application in infant formula. Plant Sci 163:713-722.

Newburg DS. Do the binding properties of oligosaccharides in milk protect human infants from gastrointestinal bacteria? J Nutr 1997;127: 980S-984S.

Nichols BL, McKee KS, Henry JF, Putman M. Human lactoferrin stimulates thymidine incorporation into DNA of rat crypt cells. Pediatr Res 1987;21:563-567.

Patton S, Houston GE. A method for isolation of milk fat globules. Lipids 1986;21:170-174.

Pellegrini A, Thomas U, Bramaz N, Hunziker P, Von Fellenberg R. Isolation and identification of three bactericidal domains in the bovine α-lactalbumin molecule. Biochim Biophys Acta 1999;1426:439-448.

Plaut AG, Qiu J, St Geme JW 3rd. Human lactoferrin proteolytic activity: analysis of the cleaved region in the IgA protease of Hemophilus influenzae. Vaccine 2000;19(Suppl 1):S148-S152.

Read LC, Upton FM, Francis GL, Wallace JC, Dahlenburg GW, Ballard FJ. Changes in the growth-promoting activity of human milk during lactation. Pediatr Res 1984;18:133-139.

Ren J. Alpha-lactalbumin possesses a distinct zinc binding site. J Biol Chem 1993;268:19292-19298.

Said HM, Horne DW, Wagner C. Effect of human milk folate binding protein on folate intestinal transport. Arch Biochem Biophys 1986;251:114-120.

Salter DN, Mowlem A. Neonatal role of folate-binding protein: studies on the course of digestion of goat's milk folate binder in the 6-d old kid. Br J Nutr 1983;50:589-596.

Sandberg, DP, Begley JA, Hall CA. The content, binding, and forms of vitamin B_{12} in milk. Am J Clin Nutr 1981;34:1717-1724.

Sato R, Noguchi T, Naito H. Casein phosphopeptide (CPP) enhances calcium absorption from the ligated segment of rat small intestine. J Nutr Sci Vit 1986;32:67-76.

Sato R, Shindo M, Gunshin H, Noguchi T, Naito H. Characterization of phosphopeptide derived from bovine beta-casein: an inhibitor to intra-intestinal precipitation of calcium phosphate. Biochim Biophys Acta 1991;1077:413-415.

Schlimme E, Meisel H. Bioactive peptides derived from milk proteins. Structural, physiological and analytical aspects. Nahrung 1995;39:1-20.

Shin K, Hayasawa H, Lönnerdal B. Purification and quantification of lactoperoxidase in human milk with use of immunoadsorbents with antibodies against recombinant human lactoperoxidase. Am J Clin Nutr 2001;73:984-989.

Son K-N, Park J, Chung C-K, Chung DK, Yu D-Y, Lee K-K, Kim J. Human lactoferrin activates transcription of IL-1β gene in mammalian cells. Biochem Biophys Res Commun 2002;290:236-241.

Steele WF, Morrisons M. Antistreptococcal activity of lactoperoxidase. J Bacteriol 1969;97:635-639.

Strömquist M, Falk P, Bergström S, Hansson L, Lönnerdal B, Normark S, Hernell O. Human milk κ-casein and inhibition of Helicobacter pylori adhesion to human gastric mucosa. J Pediatr Gastroenterol Nutr 1995;21:288-296.
Suzuki YA, Shin K, Lönnerdal B. Molecular cloning and functional expression of a human intestinal lactoferrin receptor. Biochemistry 2001;40:15771-15779.
Suzuki YA, Kelleher SL, Yalda D, Wu L, Huang J, Huang N, Lönnerdal B. Expression, characterization, and biologic activity of recombinant human lactoferrin in rice. J Pediatr Gastroenterol Nutr 2003;36:190-199.
Telemo E, Hanson LÅ. Antibodies in milk. J Mammary Gland Biol Neoplasia 1996;1:243-249.
Tomita M, Bellamy W, Takase M, Yamauchi K, Wakabayashi H, Kawase K. Potent antibacterial peptides generated by pepsin digestion of bovine lactoferrin. J Dairy Sci 1991;74:4137-4142.
Young GP, Taranto TM, Jonas HA Cox AJ, Hogg A, Werther GA. Insulin-like growth factors and the developing and mature rat small intestine: receptors and biological actions. Digestion 1990;46:240-252.

POLYUNSATURATED FATTY ACIDS IN HUMAN MILK

An Essential Role in Infant Development

Sheila M. Innis

1. ABSTRACT

The n-6 and n-3 fatty acids are essential dietary nutrients required for optimal growth and development, particularly of the brain and retina. Large amounts of the n-3 fatty acid docosahexaenoic acid (DHA) is accumulated in the brain grey matter and the visual elements of the retina during development, and reduced DHA in these tissues can result in decreased visual and psychomotor development. Although the possible importance of differences in n-6 and n-3 fatty acids, particularly DHA, between human milk and infant formulas has been the subject of intense clinical research, the variability in the essential fatty acid content of milk within and among different populations of women and implications of this to infant growth and development have received much less attention. Considerable research has shown that the DHA content of the maternal diet is the most important determinant of the amount of DHA secreted in milk, and thus the dietary intake of the breastfed infant. The DHA content of human milk varies over 10-fold, being lowest in women with no intake of DHA and highest in women with high intakes of DHA, which is found predominantly in fatty fish. The requirement for n-3 fatty acids, and the balance of n-6 and n-3 fatty acids for optimal growth and development of the brain and retina, and long-term minimization of risk of chronic disease remains as one of the most important questions in infant nutrition. Dietary recommendations to modifying dietary fat with the aim of reducing risk of chronic disease, including obesity and cardiovascular disease in adults, need to consider that when followed by pregnant women, these recommendations can have a marked effect on the amount and balance of n-6 and n-3 fatty acids secreted in milk.

Department of Paediatrics, B.C. Research Institute for Children's and Women's Health, University of British Columbia, 950 West 28th Avenue, Vancouver, B.C., Canada V5Z, 4H4

Protecting Infants through Human Milk, edited by Pickering *et al.*
Kluwer Academic/Plenum Publishers, 2004

2. INTRODUCTION

Human milk contains the dietary essential n-6 and n-3 polyunsaturated fatty acids linoleic acid (18:2n-6) and alpha linolenic acid (18:3n-3), as well as longer chain, more highly polyunsaturated fatty acids (Innis 1992; Jensen 1999). Of these longer chain fatty acids, the n-6 arachidonic acid (ARA, 20:4n-6) and n-3 docosahexaenoic acid (DHA, 22:6n-3) are of particular interest because of their important roles in infant growth and development (Innis 1991, 2003a). The importance of ARA relates to its role as a precursor for synthesis of highly active oxygenated metabolites (often collectively termed eicosanoids), in receptor-mediated cell signaling pathways and in cell division. DHA is selectively enriched in the rods and cones of the retina, brain grey matter, and heart muscle phospholipids. The n-6 and n-3 polyunsaturated fatty acids and their eicosanoid metabolites also regulate the expression of key genes of carbohydrate and lipid metabolism (Clarke 2001). Recent evidence has shown n-3 fatty acids regulate the expression of a large number of genes in the brain (Kitajka et al. 2002; Mata de Urquiza et al. 2000). Although always present, the concentrations n-6 and n-3 polyunsaturated fatty acids in human milk varies widely, both within and between different populations of women, reflecting the composition of fat in a mother's diet (Innis 1992; Jensen 1999). This variability in the polyunsaturated fatty acid composition of human milk results in considerable differences in polyunsaturated fatty acid intake among breastfed infants. This chapter provides a review of recent understanding of polyunsaturated fatty acids in human milk, the variations due to maternal diet, and the implications for infant development.

3. FUNCTIONAL ROLES OF POLYUNSATURATED FATTY ACIDS

Much of the interest in polyunsaturated fatty acids in infant nutrition over the last two decades has focused on the importance of DHA in the developing central nervous system and, more recently, on the role of ARA in growth. ARA and DHA are predominantly esterified in cell membrane phospholipids. Cell membranes are composed of a bilayer of phospholipids in which the fatty acids are oriented inwards to form the hydrophobic core of the membrane interior, and the polar head groups (such as choline, ethanolamine, inositol, or serine) are oriented outwards towards the aqueous intercellular, cytosolic, or plasma compartment. Cell membrane fatty acids, due to their chain length and degree of unsaturation, play an important role in determining the properties (such as packing density) of the membrane microenvironment, and this in turn can affect the activity of membrane-associated proteins, receptors, transport systems, and ion channels (Innis 1991, 2003a). When released by phospholipases, the n-6 and n-3 fatty acids become available as unesterified fatty acids and can function as important signaling molecules, in addition to serving as substrates for eicosanoid synthesis. Their functions include regulation of the activity of protein kinases, G-proteins, adenylate and guanylate cyclases, phospholipases, ion channels, and multiple other proteins and receptors (Innis 2003a). DHA, unlike the n-6 fatty acids, has a highly specific distribution in tissues and phospholipids. Concentrations of DHA are particularly high in the amino phospholipids, (phosphatidylserine and phosphatidylethanolamine) of neural grey matter, and in the outer segments of rod and cone photoreceptors in the retina (Giusto et al. 2000; Sastry 1985), as well as in specific phospholipids in the heart and sarcoplasmic reticulum of skeletal muscle sarcolemma (Innis 2003a). Rods and cones are highly specialized differentiated neurons that contain a stack of photosensitive membranes, known as the outer segments, at their distal end (Giusto et al. 2000). As much as 80% of the polyunsaturated fatty acids in the outer segment discs are 22:6n-3, and phospholipids in which both fatty acids are 22:6n-3 are present in these outer segment disks. The visual pigment rhodopsin (opsin + the carotenoid 11-cis retinal) functions as a photon receptor coupled to regulatory G-proteins (Giusto et al. 2000). Recent studies have provided evidence that DHA may influence photoreceptor signal transduction by influencing the ability of photons to transform rhodopsin from meta-rhodopsin l to the activated meta-rhodopsin ll state (Litman et al. 2001). The role of DHA in brain function is not well understood. Studies, have shown that n-3 fatty acids regulate the expression of genes involved in synaptic plasticity, endocytosis, signal transduction, synaptic vesicle recycling and formation, lipid metabolism, ion channel formation, energy metabolism, nuclear ligand activated transcription factor receptors, and retinoid X receptor (Kitajka et al. 2002; Mata de Urquiza et al. 2000). Decreased brain DHA also has been shown to decrease cytochrome C oxidase activity and glucose uptake (Ximenes de Silva et al. 2002), which could have important functional consequences because of the high metabolic activity of the developing brain. Other studies have explored the neurochemical link between altered behavior and learning and n-3 fatty acid deficiency. These studies have shown that decreased DHA in the developing brain alters the metabolism of dopamine at multiple levels, including dopamine concentration, expression of the vesicular monoamine transporter 2 mRNA, dopamine D_2 receptor mRNA, and immunoreactivity of tyrosine hydroxylase (the rate-limiting enzyme in dopamine synthesis) (Delion et al. 1994; de la Presa Owens & Innis 1999, 2000; Zimmer et al. 2002). Changes in serotonin metabolism also have been found (Delion et al. 1994; de la Presa Owens & Innis 1999). These findings are of particular relevance to infant development because of the major role of dopamine in many of the cognitive advances of early childhood, as a modulator of attention and motivation, and in the visual pathways (Antal et al. 1997; Basmak et al. 1999), and the possible relation of DHA with some psychological problems (Hibbeln et al. 1997).

4. POLYUNSATURATED FATTY ACID METABOLISM

The polyunsaturated fatty acids linoleic acid and alpha linolenic acid are both recognized as essential dietary nutrients (IOM/NAS 2002). This is explained by the inability of humans, as well as other animals, to insert a double bond at the n (or omega, ω) 6 or 3 position of a fatty acid carbon chain, together with the presence of clinical and biochemical signs of deficiency following feeding of a diet deficient in n-6 or n-3 fatty acids. Deficiency of alpha linolenic acid in developing animals results in decreased DHA (an n-3 fatty acid), with a reciprocal increase in n-6 fatty acids, particularly docosapentaenoic acid (22:5n-6), in the retina and brain (Innis 1991). The decrease in brain and retina DHA is accompanied by decreased amplitude in electroretinograph recordings, decreased looking and visual acuity, and changes in performance on a variety of behavioral tasks of learning (Innis 1991, 2003a). Studies in preterm infants also have shown that supplementation of formulas containing alpha linolenic acid with DHA results in an early enhancement in development of visual acuity and higher scores on some tests of neurodevelopment (O'Connor et al. 2001; SanGiovanni et al. 2000). Clinical signs of n-6 fatty acid deficiency include growth failure, increased transepidermal water loss, alopecia, and histological abnormalities in many organs. These clinical signs are prevented by a diet in which 3% to 4% of energy intake is from linoleic acid, or about 0.2% of energy intake is from ARA (Innis 1991, 2003b).

Linoleic acid and alpha linolenic acid are present in the diet in greatest concentrations in unsaturated plant, seed, and nut oils, although different oils vary considerably in content of these fatty acids (Chow 2000). Once obtained from the diet, linoleic acid and alpha linolenic acid can be further metabolized by Δ 6 desaturation, elongation, and Δ 5 desaturation to form arachidonic acid (20:4n-6) and eicosapentaenoic acid (EPA, 20:5n-3), respectively (Fig. 1). The final steps in the pathway involve two successive elongations of 20:5n-3 and 20:4n-6 to form 24:5n-3 and 24:4n-6, respectively, then desaturation at position 6 to yield 24:6n-3 and 24:5n-6. The latter two fatty acids are then translocated to the peroxisomes where partial oxidation generates DHA (22:6n-3) and docosapentaenoic acid (22:5n-6), respectively (Ferdinandusse et al. 2001; Sprecher et al. 1999; Innis 1996).

One of the most important functions of polyunsaturated fatty acids is their role as precursors for synthesis of eicosanoids and leukotrienes. The fatty acids 20:3n-6, ARA, and EPA are converted to prostaglandins by cyclo-oxygenase and to leukotrienes by lipoxygenase (Innis 1996; Jump 2002). However, ARA and EPA compete for cyclo-oxygenase and lipoxygenase, and thus tissue concentrations of these fatty acids influence the balance of eicosanoids formed from the different fatty acid families. In general, the series 2 eicosanoids and series 4 leukotrienes, which are formed from ARA, have proinflammatory and proaggregatory effects, while the series 3 eicosanoids and series 5 leukotrienes formed from EPA have weaker or opposing effects (Innis 1996; Jump 2002; Calder 2001).

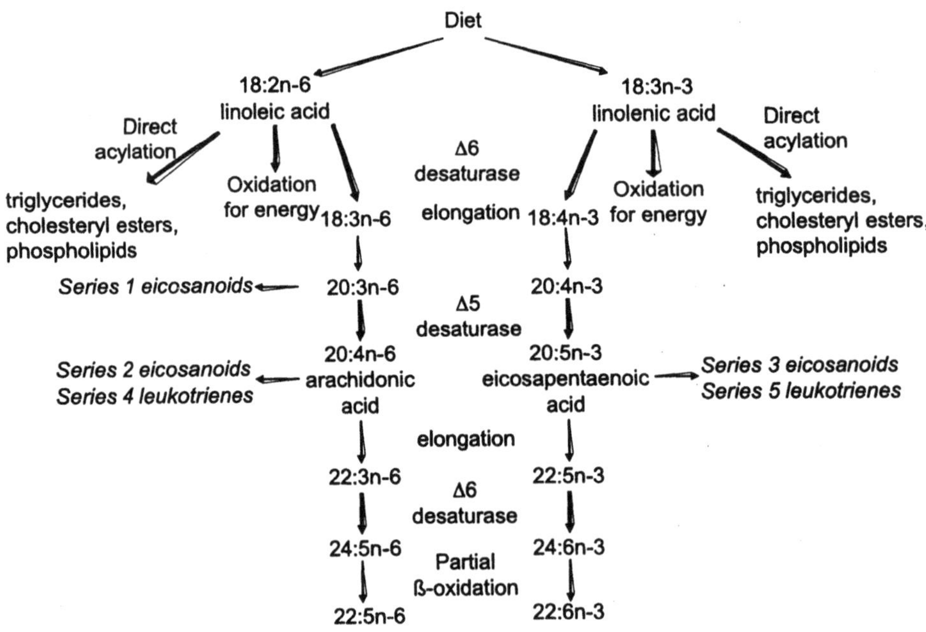

Figure 1. Schematic of n-6 and n-3 fatty acid metabolism

The synthesis of DHA and ARA from their 18-carbon precursors involves the same Δ 6 and Δ 5 desaturase enzymes (Innis 1991, 2003a). Because of this, synthesis of a given fatty acid is subject to substrate and product inhibition by the opposing n-6 or n-3 series of fatty acids, as well as product inhibition by fatty acids of the same or opposing fatty acids series. For example, high intakes of n-3 fatty acids EPA and DHA from fish oils results in decreased tissue ARA, an n-6 fatty acid. Decreased plasma ARA also has been found in preterm infants fed formula in which the fat was supplemented with EPA and DHA from fish oil (Carlson et al. 1993a). In this case, the lower ARA in the infants' blood lipids was associated with lower growth measured in terms of weight, length, and head circumference (Carlson et al. 1992, 1993b). In vitro, the first and rate-limiting step in fatty acid desaturation (Δ 6 desaturase) shows clear preference in order 18:3n-3>18:2n-6>18:1n-9 (oleic acid) (Innis 1991). However, in vivo, dietary alpha linolenic acid is preferentially oxidized rather than desaturated to DHA (Cunnane 2000; DeLany et al. 2000), and both dietary intakes and human milk levels of linoleic acid greatly exceed those of alpha linolenic acid (Innis 1992; Jensen 1999; IOM/NAS 2002; Chow 2000; Simopoulos 1999).

Tracer studies using stable isotopes have shown that preterm and term human infants are able to synthesize ARA from linoleic acid, and DHA from alpha linolenic acid (Carnielli et al. 1996; Demmelmair et al. 1995; Salem et al. 1996; Sauerwalk et al. 1996; Uauy et al. 2000). Area-under-the-curve estimates for the products of linoleic acid and alpha linolenic acid metabolism suggest preterm infants are as capable as term infants, and perhaps more so, in converting linoleic acid and alpha linolenic acid to their longer chain metabolites (Uauy 2000). Rates of conversion are lower in infants fed human milk than in infants fed formula containing linoleic acid and alpha linolenic acid from vegetable oils and no ARA or DHA. This is consistent with inhibition of fatty acid desaturation by ARA and DHA present in human milk.

The later steps in the pathway from Δ 5 desaturase leading to ARA, EPA, and DHA are found in animal, but not plant cells (Innis 2003a). As a result, these fatty acids are present in the diet in meat, fish, and eggs, with the highest concentrations of EPA and DHA present in fatty fish such as herring, mackerel, and salmon (Chow 2000). Dairy products are exceedingly low in DHA and ARA, and in their precursors linoleic acid and alpha linolenic acid. The absence of ARA, EPA, and DHA in foods of plant origin, and considerable variability in linoleic acid and alpha linolenic acid among different vegetable oils (Table 1) results in wide differences in individual intakes of n-6 and n-3 fatty acids. Modern diets in many western countries often contain relatively high amounts of linoleic acid, particularly in regions where safflower, sunflower, and corn oils are used (Simopoulos 1999). Currently available estimates suggest that linoleic acid represents about 7% of energy intake and alpha linolenic acid represents about 0.5% intake in the United States (IOM/NAS 2002); the average intake of EPA plus DHA is about 100 mg/person/day (Kris-Etherton et al. 2000). Recent analysis of dietary intake data together with analyses of n-6 and n-3 fatty acids in the food supply found intakes of 160 mg/day for DHA and 120 mg/day for ARA among women in western Canada (Innis & Elias 2003). Over 80% of the dietary supply of DHA is from fish and shellfish, with about 10% from eggs, and the remainder from meats and poultry (Innis & Elias 2003).

Table 1. Fatty acid composition of common vegetable oils (g/100 g fatty acids)

Common Oil	Palmitic 16:0	Stearic 18:0	Oleic 18:1n-9	Linoleic 18:2n-6	Linolenic 18:3n-3
Soy	11	0.5	22	54	8
Canola	4	2	58	23	10
Corn	12	2	32	52	0.8
Safflower	7	2	12	77	0.1
HOsaff[a]	4	5	81	9	<0.1
Olive	14	2	71	10	0.5
Sesame	10	5	41	43	0.2
Linseed (flax)	7	3	24	17	48
Almond	12	0.1	44	40	0.6
Walnut	2	2	16	56	16

[a]High oleic safflower oil

5. POLYUNSATURATED FATTY ACIDS IN HUMAN MILK

Prior to birth, all of the n-6 and n-3 fatty acids accumulated by the fetus must originate from the maternal circulation via placental transfer, and after birth all must be provided to the breastfed infant in human milk. DHA is accumulated actively in membrane lipids of brain grey matter during the last trimester of gestation and the first one to two years after birth (Martinez 1992). Because of this, and impairments in visual and neural development that result from reduced brain DHA (Innis 1991, 2003a), it is important that the milk diet provides the infant with the necessary amounts of n-3 fatty acids to support optimal accretion in the growing brain.

Fat, of which 98% is triglycerides, is the most variable macronutrient in human milk. Furthermore, the composition of the component fatty acids is variable, both among different populations and among individual women (Innis 1992; Jensen 1999). Over 200 different fatty acids have been identified in human milk. Most of these are present as a result of transfer from the maternal diet and are not known to have any essential role in the nutrition of the infant, other than as a source of energy. Studies on human milk fat composition conducted in the United States, Canada, and Europe generally report as a mean percentage of the total fat, 12% to 16% for linoleic acid, 1% to 1.5% for alpha linolenic acid, 0.4% to 0.7% for ARA, and 0.15% to 0.4% for DHA (Innis 1992; Jensen 1999; Innis & King 1999). However, the range of concentrations of the different fatty acids in milk fat among individual women, particularly for linoleic acid and DHA, is wide (Table 2). Concentrations of linoleic acid vary from 6% in women following omnivorous diets to over 30% among women following vegan diets (Innis & King 1999; Sanders & Reddy 1992). Current information shows that the maternal intake of DHA is the single most important determinant of the DHA content of human milk. Milk from women following vegan diets contains about 0.1% DHA, reflecting their lack of a dietary intake of DHA (Sanders & Reddy 1992), whereas much higher amounts are found among women with high habitual intakes of fish and other marine animals. For example, the average amount of DHA as a percentage of fat in human milk was 2.8% in Zhangzi, China, 1.0% in Japan, 0.8% to 0.9% on the Malay Peninsula, 0.5% in Norway and 1.4% among Inuit living on Baffin Island (Chulei et al. 1995; Hellend et al. 2001; Innis &

Table 2. Human n-6 and n-3 fatty acids (g/100 g fatty acids) following supplementation with 18:3n-3 or 22:6n-3[a]

Fatty acid[b]	Structure	18:3n-3 Supplementation			22:6n-3 Supplementation		
		Pre	14 days	Post 14 days	Pre	14 days	Post 14 days
Linolenic	18:3n-3	1.6±0.19	2.6±0.26[c]	1.4±0.16	1.4±0.12	1.7±0.13	1.4±0.02
EPA	20:5n-3	0.1±0.01	0.1±0.01	0.1±0.02	0.1±0.01	0.4±0.07[c]	0.1±0.01
DHA	22:6n-3	0.2±0.03	0.02±0.03	0.2±0.05	0.2±0.04	0.7±0.06[c]	0.2±0.02
Linoleic	18:2n-6	12.7±0.95	13.8±0.90	11.9±1.04	12.6±1.06	11.9±0.84	12.1±1.23
ARA	20:4n-6	0.4±0.02	0.4±0.02	0.4±0.02	0.4±0.02	0.4±0.03	0.4±0.02
	22:4n-6	0.1±0.01	0.1±0.01	0.1±0.00	0.1±0.00	0.1±0.00	0.1±0.01
	22:5n-6	<0.01	<0.01	<0.01	<0.01	<0.01	<0.01

[a]Milk samples were analyzed before, after 14 days supplement with 3g 18:3n-3 from flax seed oil (60% 18:3n-3) or 300 mg DHA from salmon oil (12.6% DHA), and again 14 days after the supplementation had ended, n=10 per group. All women were 2 months postpartum and exclusively breastfeeding a single, term infant. The data were analyzed by ANOVA for time and supplement.
[b]EPA, eicosapentaenoic acid; DHA, docosahexaenoic acid; ARA, arachidonic acid.
[c]Significantly different from pre-supplementation within the same group.

Kuhnlein 1988; Kneebone et al. 1985; Nakajima 2000), reflecting the high intake of DHA from fish and other marine foods among these populations. Milk fat from women following mixed diets in North America and most European countries typically has 0.2% to 0.4% DHA (Innis 1992; Jensen 1999; Innis & King 1999). Many studies have now shown that supplementation of lactating women with fish or fish oil increases the amount of DHA and EPA, while supplementation with single cell oils containing only DHA increases the DHA content of human milk (Hellend et al. 2001; Fidler et al. 2000; Gibson et al. 1997; Harris et al. 1984; Henderson et al. 1992; Jensen et al. 2000; Makrides et al. 1996; Smit et al. 2000).

In Table 2 we present results of our studies in which lactating women supplemented their diets with flax seed oil to provide 3 g of alpha linolenic acid, or salmon oil to provide about 300 mg of DHA, for 14 days (n=10 women per group). Milk samples were collected at three times: prior to supplementation, after 14 days of supplementation, and 14 days after ending supplementation. Whereas maternal dietary DHA supplementation increased the secretion of DHA in human milk, supplementation with alpha linolenic acid does not have the same effect. Furthermore, the effects of the dietary DHA on the secretion of DHA in milk is dynamic and largely dependent on current intake, rather than adipose tissue stores. This is further supported by studies showing that supplementation of lactating women with about 230, 170, or 260 mg/day of DHA from algal triglyceride (44.9% DHA), DHA-enriched eggs (3.3% DHA), or a fish oil low in EPA (4.8% EPA, 26.0% DHA) for six weeks increased both the maternal plasma phospholipid and the milk DHA (Fig. 2) (Jensen et al. 2000). Human milk concentrations of ARA, in contrast, appear to be much more tightly regulated and are not reduced by high intakes of EPA and DHA, or in vegetarian or vegan women (Sanders & Reddy 1992; Chulei et al. 1995; Hellend et al. 2001; Innis & Kuhnlein 1988; Nakajima 2000; Jensen et al. 2000; Makrides et al. 1996). We also found that the milk concentrations of ARA were not affected by supplementation of lactating women with high amounts of either alpha linolenic acid or DHA. In these studies, the milk fat consisted of about 0.4% ARA before and after 14 days supplementation with either alpha linolenic acid or DHA (Table 2).

Studies by Insull and colleagues in the late 1950s reported 7.7% linoleic acid in milk from women following their typical ad libitum diet, 10.4% linoleic acid when 40% dietary energy was from lard, and a 4-fold increase to 41.4% linoleic acid in milk when the diet had 40% energy from corn oil (which contains about 52% linoleic acid) (Insull et al. 1959). Studies in the 1960s reported mean concentrations of 9.5% linoleic acid in human milk (Tomarelli et al. 1968), and current data from many countries following western diets now report mean levels of 12% to 16% linoleic acid in human milk (Table 3) (Innis 1992; Jensen 1999). The mean levels of linoleic acid in the milk of Canadian and European women is about 2% lower than in their U.S. counterparts (Table 3) (Innis 1992; Jensen 1999; Innis & King 1999; Chen et al. 1995). The apparent increase in linoleic acid in human milk in western nations could be explained by the numerous dietary recommendations from the 1970s encouraging consumption of lower amounts of saturated animal fats in favor of higher intakes of polyunsaturated fats high in linoleic acid. In addition, whereas soybean oil (54% linoleic acid) is the major oil in the United States, canola oil (23% linoleic acid) is the most prominent vegetable oil in the Canadian food supply (Kris-Etherton et al. 2000). However, analysis of human milk from other regions of the world suggests that the relation between linoleic acid intake and the secretion of linoleic acid in milk may not be simple. A summary of analyses of human milk fat from different regions of the world shows that the concentration of linoleic acid is also high in some countries following non-western diets (Jensen 1999). Studies in

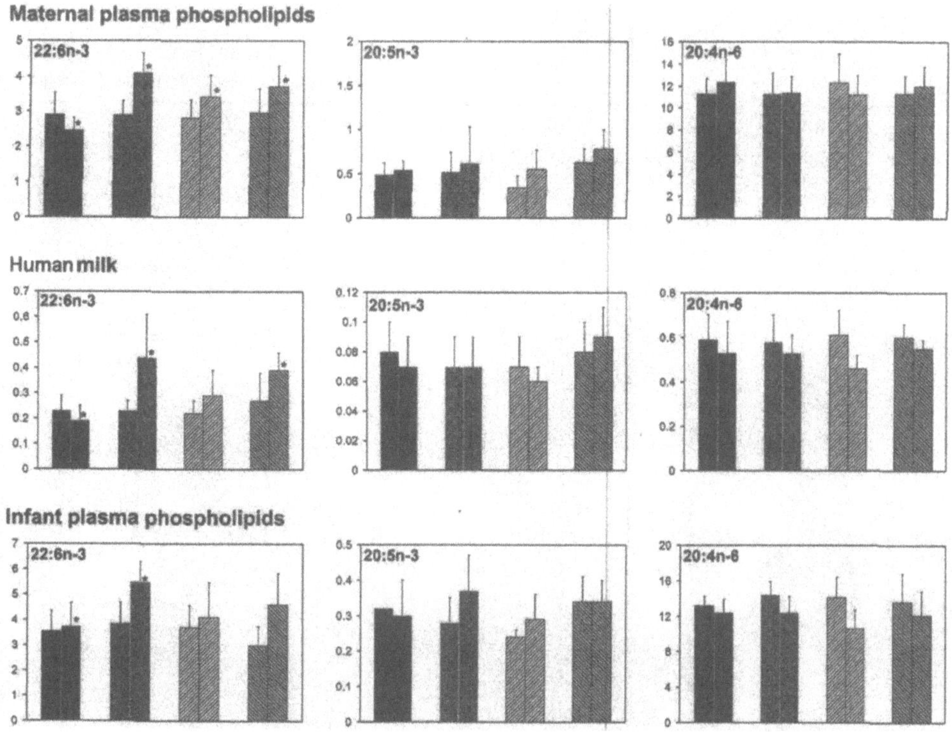

Figure 2. Concentrations of docosahexaenoic acid (22:6n-3), eicosapentaenoic acid (20:5n-3) and arachidonic acid (20:4n-6) as g/100 g fatty acids on the y axis in maternal plasma phospholipids, human milk and infant plasma phospholipids before and following (second column) 6 weeks of no supplementation [black bars], or supplementation with 230 mg [gray bars], 170 mg [ascending diagonal bars], or 260 mg [descending diagonal bars] per day 22:6n-3. Adapted from Jensen et al. 2000. *Significantly different from group before supplementation, $P<0.05$. Note the different y axis scale.

different regions of China found similar (18.4–20.5%) linoleic acid composition of the milk fat of women consuming a wide range of dietary energy as soybean oil (2–12%) in diets containing 27% to 35% total energy from fat (Chulei et al. 1995). Studies on the composition of milk from a large group of Sudanese women similarly found a mean of 18.3% (range, 9.3–32.7%) linoleic acid in human milk (Jensen 1999). However, data from ten different studies on the composition of milk fatty acids in Africa (Table 3) show a median of 12.0% linoleic acid, with a range of 5.7% to 17.2% linoleic acid (Koletzko et al. 1992). More recent studies on the composition of human milk fat from regions of Africa where fat total intakes are low and the diet is largely based on grains have also found mean concentrations of 11% to 12% linoleic acid (Okolo et al. 2000; Schmeits et al. 1999).

In addition to the increase in intake of unsaturated vegetable oils, the consumption of meat and eggs, which provide a dietary source of DHA, has decreased in North America (Gray-Donald 2000). Analysis of the changes in DHA and ARA in mature human milk collected from predominantly Caucasian women participating in our studies in Vancouver over the last decade shows a decrease of 50% in DHA from 0.4% to 0.2%,

Table 3. Major n-6 and n-3 polyunsaturated fatty acids in human milk (g/100g fatty acids) from women living in different countries

Fatty acid	Canada[a,b]	USA[c]	Europe	Africa	Japan	China, rural	China, marine
	mean (range)	mean (range)	median (range)	median (range)	mean		
18:3n-3	1.4 (0.1–3.6)	1.3 (0.5–2.1)	0.9 (0.7–1.3)	0.8 (0.1–14)	1.1	2.7	3.0
20:5n-3	0.1 (0.0[d]–0.3)	0.1 (0.0–0.2)	0.2 (0.0–0.6)	0.1 (0.1–0.5)	0.1	0.4	1.0
22:5n-3	0.2 (0.1–0.7)	0.1 (0.0–0.3)	0.2 (0.1–0.5)	0.2 (0.1–0.4)	0.6	—	—
22:6n-3	0.2 (0.1–1.0)	0.1 (0.0–0.4)	0.3 (0.3–1.8)	0.3 (0.1–0.9)	1.1	0.7	2.8
18:2n-6	12.0 (6.0–21.5)	16.6 (9.3–22.3)	11.0 (6.9–16.4)	12.0 (5.7–17.2)	13.3	18.4	18.5
20:2n-6	0.3 (0.2–0.5)	0.4 (0.3–0.6)	0.3 (0.2–0.5)	0.3 (0.3–0.8)	—	—	—
20:3n-6	0.3 (0.0–0.7)	0.3 (0.2–0.6)	0.3 (0.2–0.7)	0.4 (0.2–0.5)	0.6	—	—
20:4n-6	0.4 (0.2–0.8)	0.5 (0.3–0.9)	0.5 (0.2–1.5)	0.6 (0.3–1.0)	1.0	0.8	1.2
22:4n-6	0.1 (0.0–0.2)	0.1 (0.0–0.2)	0.1 (0.1–0.2)	0.1 (0.0–0.1)	—	—	—
22:5n-6	0.0 (0.0–0.1)	0.0 (0.0–0.1)	0.1 (0.0–0.2)	0.1 (0.1–0.3)	—	—	—

[a]Adapted from: Innis & King 1979 (Canada); Auestad et al. 2001 (USA); Koletzko et al. 1992 (Europe & Africa); Nakajima 2000 (Japan); Chulei et al. 1995 (China).
[b]Data from Innis & King 1979 excludes women taking n-3 fatty acid supplements.
[c]Composition of milk from breastfeeding mothers in Auestad et al. 2001.
[d]Values <0.05 are rounded to 0.0.

P<0.001, and a decrease in ARA from 0.7% to 0.4%, P<0.001 (Innis 2003). This decrease was not related to a concurrent increase in linoleic acid in the milk. A similar decrease in DHA in human milk in Australia has been reported (Makrides et al. 1995a). Whether this is explained by a decrease in meat, egg, and/or fish intake is not clear. However, we recently questioned if the decrease in DHA in milk from women participating in our clinical studies is representative of breastfeeding women in the general population. These studies found a wide variability in DHA in human milk from breastfeeding women in the community, which differed by ethnic background. The mean concentration of DHA in human milk of Caucasian women was 0.27±0.06% (range, 0.1–0.49%) and among women of Chinese ancestry was 0.50±0.09% (range, 0.2–1.1%). The milk from Caucasian and Chinese women both had ARA concentrations of 0.45±0.03%, but linoleic acid was lower in the milk of the Caucasian than Chinese women, 13.1±0.9% and 16.8±1.6%, respectively. The difference in n-6 and n-3 fatty acids in milk from different groups of women here raise the possibility that the decline in DHA in milk of women participating in clinical trials may reflect dietary trends among some, but not necessarily all segments of the population.

6. POLYUNSATURATED FATTY ACIDS IN MILK AND THE BREASTFED INFANT

It is known that plasma and red blood cell DHA and ARA are lower in infants fed formulas containing only vegetable sources of fat than in infants who are breastfed (Makrides et al. 1994; Ponder et al. 1992; Putnam et al. 1982). Numerous clinical studies also have shown that inclusion of ARA and DHA in formula increases the levels of these fatty acids in blood lipids of formula-fed infants (Auestad et al. 1997; Innis 1996). However, it is less well appreciated that the circulating levels of DHA and ARA in breastfed infants depend on the concentrations of DHA and ARA in the mothers' milk (Innis & King 1999). Results from our studies with 62 mother-infant pairs that show highly significant correlations between the milk concentrations of linoleic acid, alpha linolenic acid, ARA, and DHA and the concentration of the same fatty acid in infant plasma triglycerides and phospholipids are summarized in Figure 3 (Innis & King 1999). Studies on the effects of a vegan diet during lactation have reported 1.9±0.32% DHA in the red blood cell lipids of breastfed infants whose mothers followed a vegan diet (and thus devoid of DHA) compared with 6.2±0.41% DHA in the red blood cell lipids of breastfed infants whose mothers followed omnivorous diets (Sanders & Reddy 1992). For comparison, red blood cell lipids of infants in the same study who were fed formula with no DHA had 3.7±0.21% DHA. Consistent with the importance of the maternal intake of DHA in determining DHA status of the breastfed infant, several studies have shown that supplementation of lactating women with DHA results in increased secretion of DHA in milk, and higher DHA in the blood lipids of the recipient breastfed infant (Harris et al 1984; Henderson et al. 1992). This was elegantly demonstrated in the dose-response studies of Jensen and colleagues, in whose studies there was no evidence that increased intakes of DHA from human milk reduced ARA in infant blood lipids (Jensen et al. 2000).

We addressed whether the variability in DHA in human milk is of physiological significance to visual and neural development among breastfed infants (Innis et al. 2001). Infants were divided into tertiles of red blood cell phosphatidylethanolamine (PE) DHA at 2 months of age. This approach was chosen because visual acuity when measured with acuity cards is a discontinuous, rather than a continuous, data set. The red blood cell PE DHA at 2 months of age, when all infants were breastfed exclusively, varied over 2-fold from 6.3% to 13.0% fatty acids. Infants in the lowest tertile of red blood cell PE DHA had significantly lower visual acuity at both 2 and 12 months of age than infants in the highest tertile of red blood cell PE DHA (Fig. 4).

Milk from mothers with infants in the lowest, middle, and highest tertile had 0.17%, 0.2%, and 0.31% DHA, respectively. We found no evidence of any association between the infant's plasma or red blood cell DHA and scores on the Bayley II mental or motor developmental indices, novelty preference assessed using the Fagan test, or on a standardized object search task (Piaget's A not B), using multiple regression analyses,

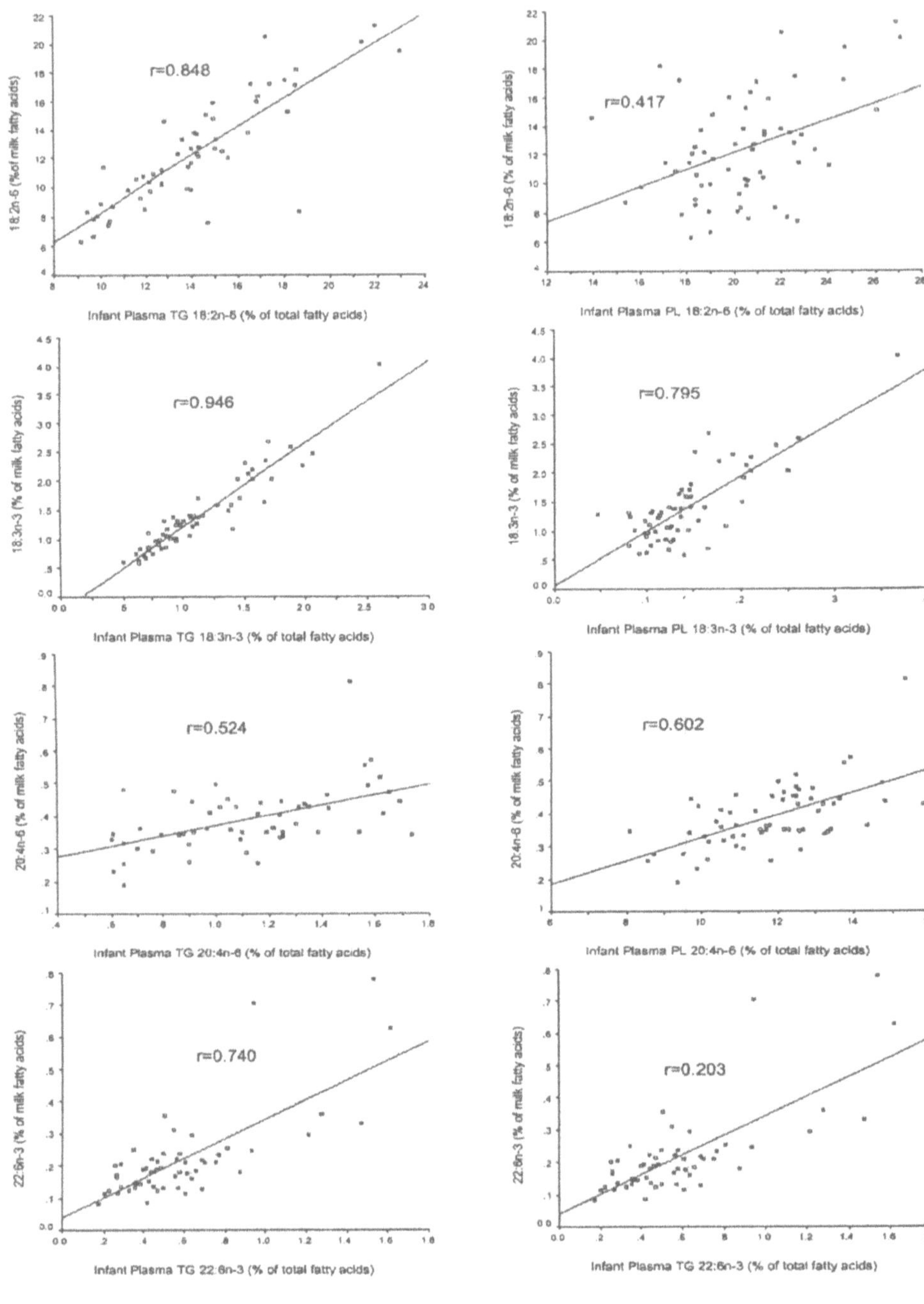

Figure 3. Correlation between milk and infant plasma levels of polyunsaturated fatty acids

which controlled for important socioeconomic and infant variables. However, the infant's plasma phospholipids and red blood cell DHA at 2 months of age was significantly related to the ability to discriminate a non-native retroflex and dental phonetic contrast at

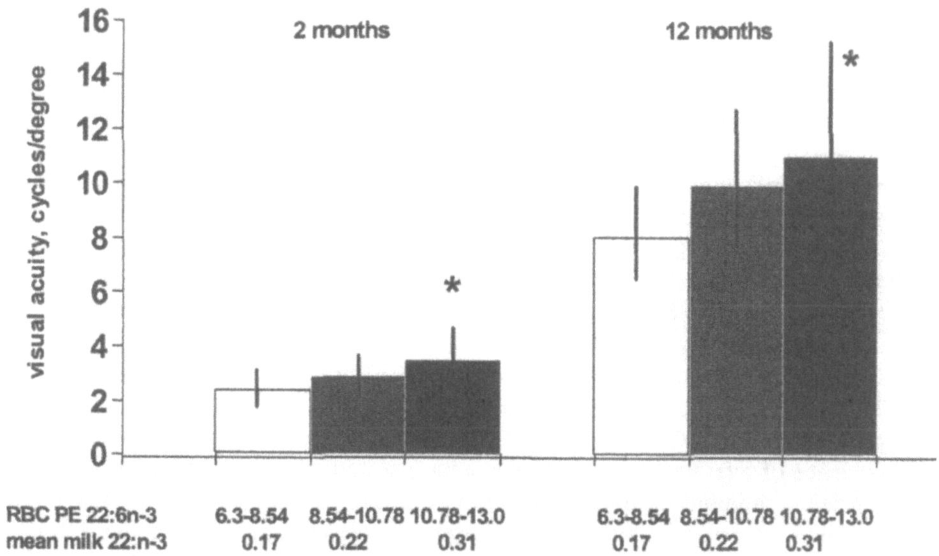

Figure 4. Relationship between milk and infant RBC PE 22:6n-3 at 2 months of age to visual acuity at 2 and 12 months of age in term infants. The infants were divided into tertiles of RBC PE 22:6n-3 at 2 months of age: 6.3-8.54, 8.54-10.78, and 10.78-13.0 g/100 g fatty acids. The mean 22:6n-3 in the mothers' milk for infants in the tertiles was 0.17, 0.22, and 0.31 g/100 g milk fatty acids. *Visual acutity at 2 and 12 months of age was significantly higher ($P<0.05$) among infants in the highest compared with the lowest tertile of RBC PE 22:6n-3 at 2 months of age. All the infants were exclusively breastfed for 4 months or longer. Adapted from Makrides et al. 1995b.

9 months of age (Innis et al. 2001). In addition, language development assessed with the MacArthur Communicative Developmental Inventories (CDI) at 18 months of age was related significantly to the plasma phospholipid, and red blood cell PE and phosphatidylcholine DHA at 2 months of age for vocabulary comprehension, $r=0.326$, $P=0.01$; $r= 0.359$, $P=0.005$; $r=0.342$, $P=0.007$, respectively, and vocabulary production, $r=0.367$, $P=0.004$; $r=0.410$, $P=0.001$; $r=0.23$, $P=0.05$, respectively, after adjusting for confounding variables (Innis 2003a, 2003b). A significant association between sweep visual evoked potential acuity and human milk DHA also was recently reported in a cross-sectional study of breastfed infants in Denmark (Jorgensen et al. 2001). These associations between DHA and visual and neural development in breastfed infants, however, should not be confused with a demonstration of causality; this requires dietary intervention that modifies the intake of DHA, but not other nutrients. However, the evidence to show dependence of infant DHA status on the supply of DHA in human milk raises important questions on the n-3 fatty acid requirements of lactating women with respect to supporting optimal visual and neural development in the infant.

Several clinical studies have reported an association between infant measures of ARA status and growth (Carlson et al. 1993; Cunnane 2001; Innis et al. 2002; Koletzko & Braun 1991). This association raises the possibility that ARA, or the balance of ARA to n-3 fatty acids in human milk, is an important modulator of growth. In our studies with breastfed infants, we found no relationships between any of the measures of ARA and growth, but infant weight at 6 months of age was related inversely to the red blood cell phosphatidylcholine DHA (P=0.01) and PE DHA (P=0.04), after adjusting for confounding variables (Innis et al. 2001). Experimental studies have shown that polyunsaturated fatty acids up-regulate the expression of genes encoding for proteins involved in fatty acid oxidation, while at the same time down-regulating genes for proteins involved in lipid synthesis in liver, heart, and skeletal muscle (Clarke 2001). The n-3 fatty acids appear to be more potent in this respect than the n-6 fatty acids, although their eicosanoid metabolites are several-fold more potent in altering gene expression than the polyunsaturated fatty acids themselves. The n-6 fatty acids and ARA eicosanoid products also are involved in adipogenesis during development by pathways involving peroxisome proliferator activated-receptor gamma (PPARγ2) (Forman et al. 1995; Gregoire et al. 1998; Ntambi et al. 1988; Reginato et al. 1998). Both mature adipocytes and preadipocytes produce significant amounts of PGE_2, PGD_2, $PGF_{2\alpha}$, PGI_2, $PGF_{2\alpha}$, and $PGI_{2\alpha}$ have been shown to modulate preadipocyte differentiation. Eicosanoids derived from EPA, however, inhibit fat cell differentiation and down-regulate genes involved in adipocyte differentiation (Okuno et al. 1997). Several studies have provided evidence of a lower incidence of overweight conditions among children who were breastfed as infants rather than fed with infant formula (Toschke et al. 2002; Von Kries et al. 1999). Whether the n-6 and n-3 fatty acids in human milk, through a role in regulating metabolic energy flux or effects on adipose tissue growth, are related to long-term effects on growth is unknown.

In summary, while the possible importance of the differences in n-6 and n-3 fatty acids, particularly DHA, between human milk and infant formula has been the subject of intense clinical research for over two decades, their variability in human milk, and the marked effects of maternal diet in determining the intake of the breastfed infant has received much less attention. The requirement for n-3 fatty acids, and the balance of n-6 and n-3 fatty acids for optimal growth and long-term minimization of risk of chronic disease remains as one of the most important questions in infant nutrition. Dietary guidelines aimed at reducing risk of chronic disease, including obesity and cardiovascular disease, need to be cognizant that when followed by pregnant women, they also can have a marked effect on the amount and balance of n-6 and n-3 fatty acids transferred to the breastfed infant.

7. REFERENCES

Antal A, Keri S, Bodis-Wollner J. Dopamine D2 receptor blockade alters the primary and cognitive components of visual evoked potentials in the monkey, Macaca fasciliaris. Neurosci Lett 1997;232:179-181.

Auestad N, Montalto MB, Hall RT, Fitzgerald KM, Wheeler RE, Connor WE, Neuringer M, Connor SE, Hartmann EE. Visual acuity, erythrocyte fatty acid composition, and growth in term infants fed formulas with long chain polyunsaturated fatty acids for one year. Pediatr Res 1997;41:1-10.

Auestad N, Halter R, Hall RT, Blatter M, Bogle ML, Burks W, Erickson JR, Fitzgerald KM, Dobson V, Innis SM, Singer LT, Montalto MB, Jacobs JR, Qui W, Bornstein MH. Growth and development in term infants fed long-chain polyunsaturated fatty acids: a double-blind, randomized, parallel, prospective, multivariate study. Pedaitrics 2001;108:372-381.

Basmak H, Yildirim N, Erdinc O, Ywdakul S, Ozdemir G. Effect of leuodopa therapy on visual evoked potentials and visual acuity in amblyopia. Ophthalmologica 1999;213:110-113.

Calder PC. Polyunsaturated fatty acids, inflammation, and immunity. Lipids 2001;36: 1007-1024.

Carlson SE, Cooke RJ, Werkman SH, Tolley EA. First year growth of preterm infants fed standard compared to marine-oil n-3 supplemented formula. Lipids 1992;27:901-907.

Carlson SE, Werkman SH, Rhodes PG, Tolley EA. Visual-acuity development in healthy preterm infants, effect of marine-oil supplementation. Am J Clin Nutr 1993a;58:35-42.

Carlson SE, Werkman SH, Peeples JM, Cooke RJ, Tolley EA. Arachidonic acid status correlates with first year growth in preterm infants. Proc Natl Acad Sci USA 1993b;90:1073-1077.

Carnielli VP, Wattimena DJ, Luijendijk IH, Boerlage A, Degenhost HJ, Sauer PJ. The very low birthweight premature infant is capable of synthesizing arachidonic and docosahexaenoic acids from linolenic and linolenic acids. Pediatr Res 1996;40:169-174.

Chen Z-Y, Pelletier G, Hollywood R, Ratnayake WMN. Trans fatty acid isomers in Canadian human milk . Lipids 1995;30:15-21.

Chow C, editor. Fatty Acids in Foods and Their Health Implications. 2nd Edition. New York: Marcel Dekker, 2000.

Chulei R, Xiafang I, Hongseng M Xiulan M, Guizheng I, Gianhong D, DeFrancesco CA, Connor WE. Milk composition in women from five different regions of the China, the great diversity of milk fatty acids. J Nutr 1995;125:2993-2998.

Clarke SD. Polyunsaturated fatty acid regulation of gene transcription, a molecular mechanism to improve metabolic syndrome. J Nutr 2001;141:1129-1132.

Cunnane SC. New developments in alpha-linolenate metabolism with emphasis on the importance of beta-oxidation and carbon recycling. World Rev Nutr Diet 2001;88:178-183.

de la Presa Owens S, Innis SM. Docosahexaenoic and arachidonic acid reverse changes in dopaminergic and sertoninergic neurotransmitters in piglets frontal cortex caused by a linoleic and alpha linolenic acid deficient diet. J Nutr 1999;129:2088-2093.

de la Presa Owens S, Innis SM. Diverse, region specific effects of addition of arachidonic and docosahexaenoic acid to formula with low or adequate linoleic and alpha linolenic acid on piglet brain monoaminergic neurotransmitters. Pediatr Res 2000; 48:125-130.

DeLany JP, Windhauser MM, Champagne CM, Bray GA. Differential oxidation of individual dietary fatty acids in humans. Am J Clin Nutr 2000;72:905-911.

Delion S, Chalon S, Herault J, Guilloteau D, Besnard JC, Durand G. Chronic dietary α-linoleic acid deficiency alters dopaminergic and serotinergic neurotransmitters in rats. J Nutr 1994;124:2466-2476.

Demmelmair H, Schenck UV, Behrendt E, Sauerwalk T, Koletzko B. Estimation of arachidonic acid synthesis in full term neonates using natural variation of 13 C content. J Pediatr Gastroenterol Nutr 1995;21:31-36.

Ferdinandusse S, Denis S, Mooijer PAW, Zhang Z, Reddy JK, Spector AA, Wanders RJA. Identification of the peroxisomal β-oxidation enzymes involved in the biosynthesis of docosahexaenoic acid. J Lipid Res 2001;42:1987-1995.

Fidler N, Sauerwald T, Pohl A, Demmelmair H, Koletzko B. Docosahexaenoic acid transfer into human milk after dietary supplementation: a randomized clinical trial. J Lipid Res 2000;41:1376-1383.

Forman BM, Tontonoz P, Chen J, Brun RP, Spiegelman BM, Evans RM. 15-Deoxy-delta 12, 14-prostaglandin J2 is a ligand for the adipocyte determination factor PPAR gamma. Cell 1995; 83:803-812.

Gava VK, McKean CM. Role of 5-hydroxytryptamine in the modulation of acoustic brainstem (far-field) potentials. Neuropharmacol 1997;16:447-449.

Gibson RA, Neuman MA, Makrides M. Effect of increasing breast milk docosahexaenoic acid on plasma and erythrocyte phospholipid fatty acids and neural indices of exclusively breast fed infants. Eur J Clin Nutr 1997;51:578-584.

Giusto NM, Pasquare SJ, Salvador GA, Castagnet PI, Roque ME, Ilincheta de Boschero MG. Lipid metabolism in vertebrate retinal rod outer segments. Prog Lipid Res 2000;39:315-391.

Gray-Donald K, Jacobs-Starkey L, Johnson-Down L. Food habits of Canadians: reduction in fat intake over a generation. Can J Public Health 2000;91:381-385.

Gregoire FM, Smas CM, Sul HS. Understanding adipocyte differentiation. Physiol Rev 1998;78:783-809.

Harris WS, Connor WE, Lindsay S. Will dietary omega -3 fatty acids change the composition of human milk? Am J Clin Nutr 1984;40:780-785.

Helland IB, Saugstad OD, Smith L, Saarem K, Solvoll K, Ganes T, Drevon CA. Similar effects on infants of n-3 and n-6 fatty acids supplementation to pregnant and lactating women. Pediatrics 2001;108:E82-E91.

Henderson RA, Jenson RG, Lammi-Keefe CJ, Ferris AM, Dardick KR. Effect of fish oil on the fatty acid composition of human milk and maternal and infant erythrocytes. Lipids 1992;27:863-869.

Hibbeln JR, Umhau JC, Gorge DT, Salem N Jr. Do plasma polyunsaturates predict hotility and depression? World Rev Nutr Diet 1997;82:175-186.

Innis SM. Essential fatty acids in growth and development. Prog Lipid Res 1991;30:39-103.

Innis SM. Human milk and formula fatty acids. J Pediatr 1992;120:S56-S61.

Innis S.M. Present Knowledge in Nutrition: Essential Dietary Lipids. Pub Int Life Sci Inst, 1996. Chapter 7, pp 58-66.

Innis SM. Perinatal biochemistry and physiology of long chain polyunsaturated fatty acids. J Pediatr 2003a;143(4 Suppl):S1-S8.

Innis SM. Essential fatty acid metabolism during early development. In: Biology of Metabolism in Growing Animals. Burrin DG, editor. Amsterdam: Elsevier Science B.V., 2003b.

Innis SM, Kuhnlein HV. Long chain n-3 fatty acids in breast milk of Inuit consuming traditional foods. Early Hum Dev 1988;18:185-189.

Innis SM, King DJ. Trans fatty acids in human milk are inversely associated with levels of essential all-cis n-6 and n-3 fatty acids, and determine trans, but not n-6 and n-3 fatty acids in plasma of breast-fed infants. Am J Clin Nutr 1999;70:383-390.

Innis SM, Auestad N, Siegman JS. Blood lipid docosahexaenoic and arachidonic acid in term gestation infants fed formulas with high docosahexaenoic acid, low eicosapentaenoic acid fish oil. Lipids 1996;31:617-25.

Innis SM, Gilley J, Werker J. Are human-milk long-chain polyunsaturated fatty acids related to visual and neural development in breast-fed infants? J Pediatr 2001;139:532-538.

Innis SM, Adamkim DH, Hall RT, Kalhan SC, Lair C, Lim M, Stevens DC, Twist PF, Diersen-Schade DA, Harris CL, Merkel KL, Hansen JW. Docosahexaenoic acid and arachidonic acid from single cell triglycerides enhance growth with no adverse effects in preterm infants fed formula. J Pediatr 2002;140:547-554.

Innis SM, Elias SL. Essential n-6 and n-3 polyunsaturated fat intakes among Canadian pregnant women. Am J Clin Nutr 2003;77:473-478.

Insull W, Hirsch J, James J, Ahrens EH. The fatty acids of human milk. II. Alterations produced by manipluation of calorie balance and exchange of dietary fats. J Clin Invest 1959;38:443-450.

[IOM/NAS] Institute of Medicine of the National Academies. Dietary reference intakes for energy, carbohydrate, fiber, fat, fatty acids, cholesterol, protein and amino acids. Washington, DC: The National Academies Press, 2002.

Jensen RG. Lipids in human milk. Lipids 1999;34:1243-1271.

Jensen CL, Maude M, Anderson RE, Heird WC. Effect of docosahexaenoic acid supplementation of lactating women on the fatty acid composition of breast milk lipids and maternal and infant plasma phospholipids. Am J Clin Nutr 2000;71:292S-299S.

Jorgensen MH, Hernell O, Hughes EL, Michaelsen KF. Is there a relation between docosahexaenoic acid concentration in mothers' milk and visual development in term infants? J Pediatr Gastroenterol Nutr 2001;32:293-296.

Jump DB. The biochemistry of n-3 polyunsaturated fatty acids. J Biol Chem 2002;11:8755-9858.

Kitajka K, Puskas LG, Zvara A, Hackler L Jr, Barcelo-Coblijn G, Yeo YK, Farkas T. The role of n-3 polyunsaturated fatty acids in brain: modulation of rat brain gene expression by dietary n-3 fatty acids. Proc Nat Acad Sci USA 2002;99:2619-2624.

Kneebone GM, Kneebone R, Gibson RA. Fatty acid composition of breast milk from three racial groups from Penang, Malaysia. Am J Clin Nutr 1985;41;765-769.

Koletzko B, Braun M. Arachidonic acid and early human growth, is there a relation? Ann Nutr Metab 1991;35:128-131.

Koletzko B, Thiel I, Abiodun PO. The fatty acid composition of human milk in Eurpoe and Africa. J Pediatr 1992;120:S62-S70.

Kris-Etherton PM, Taylor DS, Yu-Poh S, Huth P, Moriarty K, Fishell V, Hargrove RL, Zhao G, Etherton TD. Polyunsaturated fatty acids in the food chain in the United States. Am J Clin Nutr 2000;71:179S-188S.

Le Moal M, Simon H. Mesocorticolimbic dopaminergic networks. Physiol Rev 1991;71:155-234.

Litman BJ, Niu SL, Polozova A, Mitchell DC. The role of docosahexaenoic acid containing phospholipids in modulating G protein-coupled signaling pathways: visual transduction. J Mol Neurosci 2001;16:237-242.

Makrides M, Neumann MA, Byard RW, Simmer K, Gibson RA. Fatty acid composition of brain, retina, and erythrocytes in breast- and formula-fed infants. Am J Clin Nutr 1994;60:189-194.

Makrides M, Neumann MA, Simmer K, Gibson RA. Erythrocyte fatty acids of term infants fed either breast milk, standard formula, or formula supplemented with long-chain polyunsaturates. Lipids 1995b;30:941-948.

Makrides M, Simmer K, Neuman M, Gibson R. Changes in the polyunsaturated fatty acids of breast milk from mothers of full-term infants over 30 wk of lactation. Am J Clin Nutr 1995a;51:1231-1233.

Makrides M, Neumann MA, Gibson RA. Effect of maternal docosahexaenoic acid (DHA) supplementation on breast milk composition. Eur J Clin Nutr 1996;50:352-357.

Martinez, M. Tissue levels of polyunsaturated fatty acids in early human development. J Pediatr 1992;120:129-138.

Mata de Urquiza A, Liu S, Sjoberg M, Zetterstrom RH, Griffiths W, Sjovall J, Perlman T. Docosahexaenoic acid, a ligand for the retinoid X receptor in mouse brain. Science 2000;290:2140-2144.

Nakajima H. Comparison of the fatty acid compositon of total lipids and phospholipids in breast milk from Japanese women. Pediatr Int 2000;42:14-20.

Ntambi JM, Buhrow SA, Kaestner KH, Christy RJ, Sibley E, Kelley TJ, Lane MD. Differentiation and induced gene expression in 3T3-L1 preadipocytes: characterization of a differentially expressed gene encoding stearoyl-CoA desaturase. J Biol Chem 1988;263:17291-17300.

O'Connor DL, Auestad N, Jacobs J. Growth and development in preterm infants fed long-chain polyunsaturated fatty acids, a prospective randomized controlled trial. Pediatrics 2001;108:359-372.
Okolo SN, VanderJagt TJ, Vu T, VanderJagt TA, VanderJagt DJ, Okonji M, Chuang L-T, Onwuanaku C, Glew RH. The fatty acid composition of human milk in Northern Nigeria. J Hum Lact 2000;16:28-35.
Okuno M, Kajiwara K, Imai S, Kobayashi T, Honma N, Maki T, Suruga K, Goda T, Takase S, Muto Y, Moriwaki H. Perilla oil prevents the excessive growth of visceral adipose tissue in rats by down-regulating adipocyte differentiation. J Nutr 1997;127:1752-1757.
Ponder DL, Innis SM, Benson JD, Siegman JS. Docosahexaenoic acid status of term infants fed breast milk or infant formula containing soy oil or corn oil. Pediatr Res 1992;32:683-688.
Putnam JC, Carlson SE, DeVoe PW, Barness LA. The effect of variations in dietary fatty acids on the fatty acid composition of erythrocyte phosphatidylcholine and phosphatidylethanolamine in human infants. Am J Clin Nutr 1982;36:106-114.
Reginato MJ, Krakow SL, Bailey ST, Lazar MA. Prostaglandins promote and block adipogenesis through opposing effects on peroxisome proliferator-activated receptor gamma. J Biol Chem 1998;273:1855-1858.
Salem N Jr, Wegher B, Mena P, Uauy R. Arachidonic and docosahexaenoic acids are biosynthesized from their 18-carbon precursors in human infants. Proc Natl Acad Sci USA 1996;93:49-54.
Sanders TAB, Reddy S. The influence of vegetarian diet on the fatty acid composition of human milk and essential fatty acid status of the infant. J Pediatr 1992;120:71S-77S.
SanGiovanni JP, Parra-Cabrera S, Colditz GA, Berkey CS, Dwyer JT. Meta-analysis of dietary essential fatty acids and long-chain polyunsaturated fatty acids as they relate to visual resolution acuity in healthy preterm infants. Pediatrics 2000;105:1292-1298.
Sastry PS. Lipids of nervous tissue: composition and metabolism. Prog Lipid Res 1985;24:169-176.
Sauerwald TU, Hachey DL, Luijendijik IHT, Boerlage A, Degerhart HJ, Sauer PJJ. New insights into the metabolism of long chain polyunsaturated fatty acids during infancy. Eur J Med Res 1996;2:88-92.
Schmeits BL, Okolo SN, VanderJagt DJ, Huang Y-S, Chuang L-T, Mata JR, Tsin AATC, Glew RH. Content of lipid nutrients in the milk of Fulani women. J Human Lact 1999;15:113-120.
Simopoulos AP. Evolutionary aspects of omega-3 fatty acids in the food supply. Prostaglandins Leukot Essent Fatty Acids 1999;60:421-429.
Smit EN, Koopmann M, Boersma ER, Muskiet FAJ. Effect of supplementation of arachidonic acid (AA) or a combination of AA plus docosaehxaenoic acid on breastmilk fatty acid composition. Prostaglandins Leukot Essent Fatty Acids 2000;62:335-340.
Sprecher H, Luthria DL, Mohammed BS, Baykousheva SP. Reevaluation of the pathways for the biosynthesis of polyunsaturated fatty acids. J Lipid Res 1995;36:2471-2477.
Sprecher H, Chen Q, Yin FQ. Regulation of the biosynthesis of 22:5n-6 and 22:6n-3: a complex intracellular process. Lipids 1999;34:S153-S156.
Tomarelli RM, Myer BJ, Weaber JR, Bernhart FW. Effect of positional distribution on the absorption of the fatty acids of human milk and infant formulas. J Nutr 1968;95:583-590.
Toschke AM, Vignerova J, Lhotska L, Oscancova K, Koletzko B, von Kries R. Overweight and obesity in 6- to 14- year old Czech children in 1991: protective effect of breastfeeding. J Pediatr 2002;141:764-769.
Uauy R, Mena P, Wegher B, Nieto S, Salem N Jr. Long chain polyunsaturated fatty acid formation in neonates: effect of gestational age and intrauterine growth. Pediatr Res 2000;47:127-135.
Von Kries R, Koletzko B, Sauerwald T, Von Mutius E, Barnert D, Grunet V, von Voss H. Breast feeding and obesity: cross-sectional study. Br Med J 1999;319:147-150.
Ximenes da Sliva A, Lavialle F, Gendrot G, Guesnet P, Alessandri JM, Lavaille M. Glucose transport and utilization are altered in the brain of rats deficient in n-3 polyunsaturated fatty acids. J Neurochem 2002;81:1328-1337.
Zimmer L, Vancassel S, Contagrel S, Breton P, Delmanche S, Guilloteau D, Durand G. The dopamine mesocorticolimbic pathway is affected by deficiency in n-3 polyunsaturated fatty acids. Am J Clin Nutr 2002;75:662-777.

EPIDEMIOLOGY OF BREASTFEEDING

Advances and Multidisciplinary Applications

Rafael Pérez-Escamilla[1] and M. Lourdes Guerrero[2]

1. ABSTRACT

Advancing understanding of the importance of breastfeeding (BF) has required advances in application of epidemiologic methods to BF research. This chapter considers, in the context of BF epidemiology, how different research designs complement each other to establish firmer causal inferences, the need for multidisciplinary collaborations, and the application of powerful analytical methods to strengthen epidemiologic studies. A recent global meta-analysis of 47 studies documenting the inverse association between lifetime BF duration and breast cancer risk illustrates the value of longitudinal (cohort) studies to establish the temporal sequence of events and to rule out differential recall biases that can threaten the internal validity of case-control studies. The discovery of the transmission of human immunodeficiency virus (HIV) via human milk has led epidemiologists to provide important hypotheses to be tested at the molecular and cellular level and in turn test hypotheses generated in laboratory studies. Application of powerful statistical methods to BF epidemiology has helped strengthen causal inferences. A retrospective analysis of the 1976-1977 Malaysian Family Life Survey found interactive multivariate statistical models to better understand how different socioeconomic and cultural contexts modify the influence of BF on child health. Further, a study conducted in Cebu City, Philippines, demonstrated how structural equation models can be used to test the pathways through which proximate (e.g., BF) and distal (e.g., socioeconomic status) determinants affect child health after adjusting for reverse causality (i.e., child health influencing maternal BF choice). For ethical reasons, BF randomized controlled trials (RCTs) have seldom been conducted. Recent RCTs examining the link between BF peer counseling and BF outcomes in diverse settings provides a unique opportunity to firmly establish the causal inferences regarding BF and the prevention of diarrheal diseases. The value of rapid assessment anthropologic methods to guide development of peer counseling interventions subsequently tested through RCTs is presented. This chapter also illustrates how Cox regression and logistic regression can be applied to BF research.

[1]Department of Nutritional Sciences, University of Connecticut, Storrs, CT 06269
[2]Department of Infectious Diseases, National Institute of Medical Sciences & Nutrition, Mexico City, Mexico

Protecting Infants through Human Milk, edited by Pickering *et al.*
Kluwer Academic/Plenum Publishers, 2004

2. INTRODUCTION

Decades of research have shown that BF is linked causally with improved child and maternal health outcomes. This conclusion has been reached based on a continuum of studies using observational, quasi-experimental, and experimental epidemiologic research designs ranging from the population to the molecular level. Evidence indicates that human milk contains a remarkable array of bioactive substances that protect infants against disease through a variety of complementary mechanisms, including optimal nutrition, reduced exposure to enteropathogens (Pickering & Morrow 1993), enhanced growth of protective microflora (Benno et al. 1984) and various immunologic factors, including secretory antibody (Goldman 1994; Ishizaka et al. 1994) and glycoconjugated substances (Newburg & Neubauer 1995; Chaturvedi et al. 2001). Moreover, this complex of bioactive substances occurs uniquely in human milk.

While basic research provides our biologic understanding of the mechanisms by which an exposure causes or prevents disease, only epidemiology allows quantification of the magnitude of the exposure-disease relationship in humans and offers the possibility of altering the risk through intervention. If epidemiologic studies are well designed and conducted, and if data are properly analyzed and interpreted, they can provide strong and reliable evidence on which to base cost-effective public health policies and programs. Thus, the objectives of this paper are to: a) illustrate how different epidemiologic research designs complement each other and are needed to establish firm causal relationships, b) learn how different fields and disciplines have contributed to the development of research designs and/or analytical methods used in BF epidemiology, and consider the strength of multidisciplinary teams to understand links between a complex human behavior such as BF and biomedical outcomes of interest, and c) provide an update on innovative analytical approaches seldom applied in BF epidemiologic research.

3. THE UNIQUE CONTRIBUTION OF EPIDEMIOLOGY TO BREASTFEEDING RESEARCH

There is a natural progression in epidemiologic reasoning. The process begins with a suspicion concerning the possible influence of a particular factor on the occurrence of disease. This suspicion may arise from clinical practice, examination of disease patterns, observations from laboratory research, or even from theoretic speculation, and leads to the formulation of a specific hypothesis. This hypothesis is tested in epidemiologic studies of individuals that include an appropriate comparison group.

Recent years have witnessed rapid and systematic progress in the development of both principles and methods of epidemiologic research. The first major development was the design of studies and techniques for collecting and analyzing data to facilitate the evaluation of risk factors for acute and chronic diseases. One such strategy, developed specifically to address the problem of long latency periods, was to assemble a group of individuals with a particular disease as well as a comparable group of subjects without the disease and obtain information about previous medical history and health habits of people in the two groups (the case-control study). This approach allowed investigators to look backward in time to assess quickly the effect of a relevant exposure without having to wait many years for the disease to develop.

While the case-control study successfully addressed the problem of having to wait many years for an outcome to develop, other methods were required to address the need to obtain accurate and precise exposure information for a period of years prior to the disease event. The cohort study assembles a group of disease-free individuals, and monitors the subsequent development of the disease in exposed and nonexposed subjects over time. Defining the exact population at risk and choosing an appropriate comparison group is as important as considering whether other factors could affect or confound the results, such as age, duration of exposure, or general health status.

An analytical overview by The Collaborative Group on Hormonal Factors in Breast Cancer (2002) examining the link between BF and breast cancer illustrates how different epidemiologic studies are needed to draw firm inferences. This analytical overview used data from 47 studies conducted in 30 different countries (n=50,302 women with breast cancer and 96,973 women without breast cancer). Findings from these pooled analyses documented a 4.3% decrease in breast cancer risk for every 12 months of BF (95% Confidence Interval: 2.9, 5.8). Findings held across 15 key demographic, socioeconomic and biomedical confounders. Because 42 of the 47 studies followed a case-control design, a key question in interpretation of results is whether findings are explained by differential recall bias (i.e., women diagnosed with breast cancer understating and women without breast cancer overstating their BF duration). The availability of 5 cohort studies was crucial to rule out this bias as the magnitude in decreased breast cancer risk associate with 12 months of BF was comparable to that found with the case-control studies (4.1% vs. 4.6%, respectively). Thus, this study illustrates the power of combining in a single meta-analysis findings from case-control designs with more complex, time-intensive, and expensive longitudinal cohorts that are crucial to establish the temporal sequence of events and to rule out differential recall biases.

4. ESTABLISHING CAUSALITY IN EPIDEMIOLOGY RESEARCH

4.1. The Role of Multidisciplinary Teams

In his brief foreword to *Epidemiology in Medicine* (Henneken & Buring 1987), Sir Richard Doll made this insightful observation:

> Epidemiology is the simplest and most direct method of studying the causes of disease in humans, and many major contributions have been made by studies that have demanded nothing more than an ability to count, to think logically, and to have an imaginative idea. With the accumulation of knowledge, however, it has become harder for individuals working alone to make effective contributions, and epidemiological research is becoming increasingly a matter of teamwork, not only because of the large number of people that may have to be studied and the large amount of data that have to be collected and analyzed, but also because of the need to bring together for the design and conduct of the study, clinical experience, biological understanding, statistical expertise, and many other special skills that vary from one study to another.

Establishing causality in epidemiology research involves ruling out confounding and establishing biological plausibility. For this to be accomplished it is essential to work in multidisciplinary teams. This is illustrated by the group of researchers that have helped elucidate the causal link between BF and protection against gastrointestinal tract disorders in children. These studies have required collaborations between medical scientists, behavioral and other social scientists, nutritionists, microbiologists, and molecular and cell biologists. A case in point is the seminal longitudinal cohort study by Brown and co-workers in Peru (1989) in which they established the strong plausibility of a causal link between exclusive BF and a lower likelihood of infectious diseases in children. Even though this study had limited statistical power and variables to rule out socioeconomic confounding, the combination of a strong longitudinal design together with microbiologic evidence of the presence of gastrointestinal pathogens in fluids and utensils used to feed these infants, represented a major leap forward in establishing this causal relationship that subsequently was confirmed by others (Morrow & Pickering 1997).

Concern for transmission of microorganisms through human milk has been expressed for human immunodeficiency virus (HIV), human T-cell lymphotropic virus type 1 (HTLV-1), cytomegalovirus (CMV), herpes simplex virus, hepatitis B virus, hepatitis C virus, rubella virus, and bacteria. The cost of not engaging in multidisciplinary work is illustrated by the discovery of the vertical transmission of HIV through human milk. The first piece of evidence came in the mid 1980s from small case studies and the isolation of the viable HIV virus from human milk samples. These case studies were followed by case-control studies and confirmed by prospective studies with adequate sample sizes and eventually randomized controlled studies (Coutsoudis et al. 2002). It took scientists several years to choose the right paradigm for their work in this area. Despite considerable epidemiologic evidence, scientists were skeptical about this being a causal link as they began to isolate bioactive substances in human milk capable of inactivating HIV. Once the epidemiologic evidence became irrefutable, due to improvements in research designs and reproducibility of findings in different socioeconomic and cultural settings, basic scientists changed their paradigm to become: How is it that HIV is capable of circumventing the defense mechanisms present in human milk? Is there a threshold of viral load beyond which human milk defenses are overcome? A major gap in this area has been the lack of inclusion of social scientists. This has led to the biomedicalization of the research while paying little attention to crucial issues such as stigmatization of women who chose not to breastfeed in cultures where this infant-feeding behavior is the norm and where women lack the empowerment to decide by themselves (Coutsoudis et al. 2002; Pérez-Escamilla 2001).

4.2. The Problem of Reverse Causality in Breastfeeding Studies

Reverse causality is a serious threat to causal analysis in nutritional epidemiology. In the area of BF research this is illustrated with two examples: a) prolonged BF and child nutritional status, and b) BF and infectious diseases.

4.2.1. Prolonged Breastfeeding and Child Nutritional Status

Retrospective studies have shown that children who are breastfed beyond the first year of life are more likely to be stunted. This led researchers to conclude that prolonged BF may be detrimental to children's health perhaps as a result of displacement of higher energy dense foods by human milk from the child's diet. However, carefully designed longitudinal studies in diverse countries such as Peru (Marquis et al. 1997) and Senegal (Simondon et al. 2001) have shown that the temporal sequence of the relationship between prolonged BF and stunting is opposite to what others previously had concluded. These studies have documented that children who are "vulnerable" as indicated by poor growth are selected by their mothers, perhaps as a protective measure, to be breastfed for more prolonged periods of time (Marquis et al. 1997; Simondon et al. 2001; Habicht 2000).

4.2.2. Breastfeeding and Infectious Diseases: A Two-Way Street?

The scientific community has agreed that BF protects against gastrointestinal and respiratory tract diseases. However, the child's illness per se may affect infant-feeding choice or method (Habicht et al. 1986). An extreme situation that appeared in early cross-sectional mortality prevention estimates attributed to BF was the classification of children who died as nonbreastfed with the underlying assumption that the cause of death was lack of BF when in fact many of the children that had died were breastfed at the onset of the illness that resulted in death (Habicht et al. 1986). An important analytical tool that has applications to address the problem of reverse causality in BF research is structural equation modeling. The principles and BF research applications of this statistical model are illustrated in the following section.

4.2.3. Addressing Reverse Causality through Structural Equation Modeling

Structural equation modeling (SEM) is a statistical technique derived from the field of economics with strong input from the field of sociology (Raftery et al. 2002). This analytical model is based on solving a system of simultaneous equations to address a theoretical model being tested with empirical data (Bollen 1989), an approach based on a combination of path analysis and factor analysis. Path analysis is used to determine the regression coefficients of direct and indirect effects posited in the model. Factor analysis is used to determine the loading of indicators or variables with their respective constructs (so called "latent" variables). Structural equation modeling includes two broad categorization of variables included in models: endogenous and exogenous. Whereas endogenous variables are those determined by other variables in the model, exogenous variables are assumed to not be determined by other independent variables (exogenous variables are also referred to as "distal" or "underlying"). The application of structural equation modeling to BF research is highly attractive as it takes into account the possibility that health behaviors (e.g., infant-feeding choices, prenatal care-seeking behaviors) are affected themselves by health outcomes (e.g., child "vulnerability" or nutritional status) and not just the other way around. Secondly, structural equation modeling is useful for decomposing the paths through which exogenous variables affect health outcomes. For example, to simply document that higher levels of maternal education are associated with less incidence of childhood diarrhea is of little value for policy making. Rather, policy makers need to know the endogenous variables mediating this influence (e.g., health behaviors including feces disposal, child feeding methods, income-generating work opportunities) (Fig. 1).

Although structural equation modeling has been used in BF research with cross-sectional and retrospective data (Pérez-Escamilla et al. 1999), its most relevant application is with longitudinal study designs as illustrated in the Cebu City Study (CST 1991). This longitudinal cohort study involved 3,080 Filipino women with single live births who were recruited prenatally between 1983 and 1984. Women were interviewed during the third trimester of pregnancy, at birth, and at two-month intervals during the children's first two years of life. Researchers collected data on underlying or exogenous variables (e.g., education, assets), mediating or proximate variables (e.g., prenatal care, infant-feeding practices), and health outcomes (e.g., child growth and morbidity patterns). Researchers worked with two sets of structural equations. The first one dealt with predictors of health-seeking behaviors such as prenatal care and included

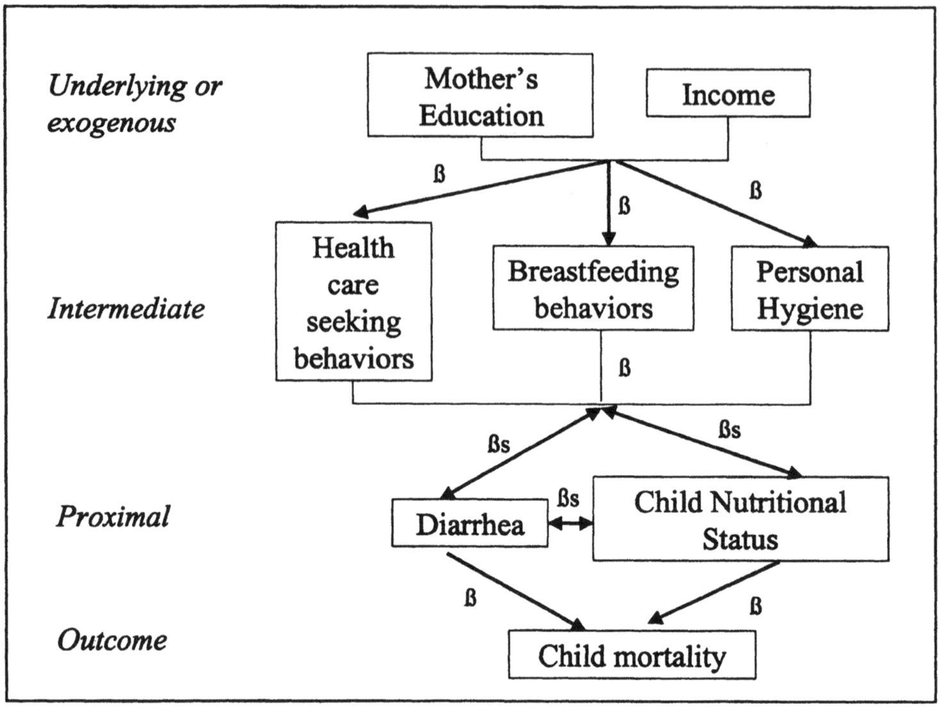

Figure 1. Child mortality theoretical model showing exogenous, intermediate, and proximal factors. Model can be tested through a system of simultaneous equations by applying structural equation modeling (SEM) to empirical data. As a result, the independent regression coefficients (ß) of each path are obtained. This allows for estimating the direct and indirect links among underlying, intermediate, and proximal determinants, and between each of the mediators and child mortality. Thus, the role played by modifiable intermediate, and proximal risk factors mediating the link between distal determinants (e.g., education) and child mortality can be assessed. Note that SEM based on longitudinal data can take into account bidirectional (or cyclical) relationships as denoted by the double arrows in diagram. Thus, SEM can adjust for the "reverse causality" confounding bias typically found in breastfeeding research (e.g., some children may have been weaned from the breast because they became quite ill rather than the other way around).

health (e.g., child growth and morbidity) during the previous time period as independent variables as well as underlying variables. The second structural equation dealt with predictors of health (e.g., child growth, morbidity or mortality) and included as independent variables underlying factors as well as health-seeking behaviors and child health during the previous time period. The authors solved the structural equation models for likelihood of diarrhea accounting for and ignoring endogeneity or reverse causality [i.e., the possibility that not only infant-feeding practices and health-seeking behaviors affect child health status, but also that child health status is a powerful determinant of choice of infant-feeding method (as demonstrated in the prolonged BF and stunting section of this chapter) and health-seeking behaviors]. For example, the predicted probability of having experienced diarrhea in the week preceding the survey associated with exclusive BF was 5.9 times lower when endogeneity was taken into account. Furthermore, the exclusive BF regression estimate was not statistically significant when endogeneity was ignored. Likewise, the estimate for preventive health care at preventing diarrhea was four times higher when taking endogeneity into account. As with exclusive

BF, the estimate ignoring endogeneity was not significantly different from zero. The interaction between poor excreta disposal and child age was in opposite directions and only significant when endogeneity was considered. This interaction suggested that the influence of adequate excreta disposal at preventing diarrhea was stronger during the first months of life. In short, ignoring endogeneity would have led us to conclude that exclusive BF, preventive care, and excreta disposal are unlikely to prevent diarrhea in a developing country setting! In this article, the authors also illustrated how an increase in one year of education has desired and undesired influences on intermediate behavioral variables. For example, more education was associated with more preventive health care and soap use and with a lower likelihood of BF. On balance, however, increased maternal education was associated with improved infant health. These findings derived from structural equation modeling are of enormous value for health policy makers.

5. ANALYTICAL ADVANCES IN BREASTFEEDING RESEARCH

Given the continued evolution of computer technology and large databases, many studies conducted today involve tens of thousands of individuals in which participants may provide data periodically over many years. In addition, because the etiologies of acute and chronic diseases are numerous and complex, obtaining information on a large number of variables may be necessary. In addition to the great potential that structural equation modeling has in BF and child health research, there are other analytical advances that deserve to be mentioned in this paper.

5.1. Time-Trend Logistic Regression Based on Repeated Cross Sectional Surveys

The Demographic and Health Surveys (DHS) program assists developing countries to conduct national population and health surveys. The program is funded primarily by the United States Agency for International Development (USAID) and is administered by Macro International Inc. in Calverton, Maryland (IRD/MI 1991) in collaboration with local governments. The DHS surveys target women of reproductive age (i.e., 15–49 years of age in most surveys) and are designed to generate nationally representative data on infant-feeding practices, population and family planning, and various maternal and child health outcomes (IRD/MI 1991). Sampling frameworks of DHS are based on complex stratified sampling designs. Strict training and quality control procedures are followed in all countries conducting DHS surveys (IRD/MI 1990). DHS replaced the World Fertility Surveys (WFS) as one of the most reliable sources to track infant feeding and family planning data worldwide.

Thus, DHS provides an opportunity to assess changes in BF behaviors across time based on repeated cross-sectional surveys. However, few attempts have been made to estimate adjusted changes in BF duration after adjusting for socioeconomic and demographic changes across time (Grummer-Strawn 1996), and none of these attempts have been based on single-step multivariate regression approaches. Pérez-Escamilla and Grajeda (2002) developed an analytical approach to estimate changes in BF duration after adjusting for key socioeconomic and demographic confounders. This approach will be illustrated with two DHS surveys conducted in Brazil in 1986 and 1996. Both data sets were downloaded as ASCII files from the DHS website www.measuredhs.com. The ASCII files were read as SPSS for Windows files using the syntax files downloaded from the same website. After creating a variable identifying the year of data collection

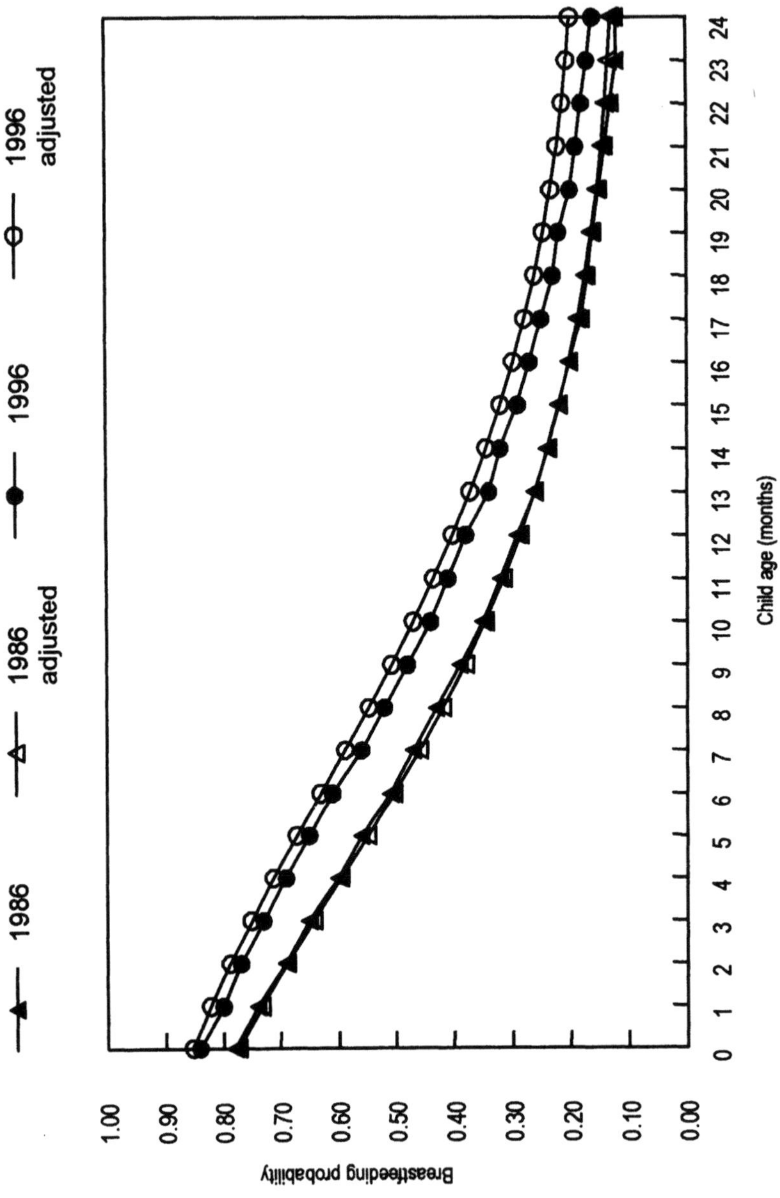

Figure 2. Secular changes in adjusted and unadjusted breastfeeding probabilities in Brazil

(i.e., the "survey wave") both data sets were then merged and subsequently analyzed using multivariate logistic regression. The dependent variable was breastfeeding at the time of the survey (yes/no), the key independent variable was "survey wave," and the covariates/confounders entered were: child age, child age^2, mother's education (none/primary/secondary/higher), mother's parity (primiparous/ multiparous), mother's age (years), employment status (employed/unemployed), and area of residence (urban/rural). Figure 2 shows the predicted BF probabilities with and without adjusting for confounders.

Unadjusted curves were generated by "survey wave" across child age with a logistic regression equation that included only the two child age terms as independent variables. Adjusted curves were generated by "survey wave" across child age at the mean values of covariates using the logistic regression equation:

$$PBF_{survey\ wave(child\ age)}=1/(1+exp(-(.947-.520*SURVEY-.227*CHAGE$$
$$+.004*CHAGE^2+.090*RESIDENCE-.163*MATEDUC-.203*EMPLOYED-$$
$$.289*PARITY+.030*MATAGE)))$$

Where: PBF=probability of breastfeeding, SURVEY=survey wave (1986=0.5, 1996=-0.5), CHAGE=child age in months, CHAGE^2=child age squared, RESIDENCE= area of residence (mean=1.27), MATEDUC=maternal education (mean=1.35), EMPLOYED= maternal employment (mean=0.35), PARITY=parity (mean=0.32), MATAGE=maternal age (mean=27.14).

Figure 2 shows that the difference in adjusted median BF duration increased from 6.1 to 9.3 months (i.e., a difference of 3.2 months) between 1986 and 1996, respectively. This increase would have been reported as lower had the adjustment for changes in socio-economic and demographic indicators in the 10 years of interest had not been made (from 6.2 to 8.5 months, a difference of 2.3 months). This is because most increasing trends in confounders (e.g., increase in proportion of population living in urban areas, higher levels of maternal employment outside the household) are associated with a lower likelihood of BF.

In summary, multivariate logistic regression is a powerful tool that can be applied by BF epidemiologists to estimate changes in adjusted BF duration across time based on national repeated cross-sectional surveys.

5.2. Cox Regression

Cox regression is a type of multivariate analysis based on survival analysis and the assumption of proportional hazards. It is a powerful technique because it can handle censored data often found in BF studies. For example, women may still be BF when they dropped out of the study or when the study ended. Thus, precise BF duration cannot be imputed if traditional regression methods are used. One approach that researchers have used to circumvent this problem is to conduct linear regression including only children beyond an age when an exact BF duration is known for the overwhelming majority of them. Two problems using this approach are: a) results would be biased towards older children, and b) a serious loss of statistical power. A key assumption of Cox regression is that hazards are proportional, (i.e., subgroup BF probability curves are not allowed to cross each other at any value of the independent variable, which is usually the age of the child). For example, if empirical data show that women with characteristic X are more likely to breastfeed than women without characteristic X when the children are less than 6 months of age but the opposite happens after six months of age, the Cox regression would not fit the data well (i.e., technique cannot model the interaction between characteristic X and child age on BF likelihood). When this happens, it is possible to still use Cox regression by conducting analyses by age subgroup (i.e., one Cox regression could compare women with and without condition X among children under 6 months of age, and a second regression could replicate the same model with children older than this age). Scientists have demonstrated the application of Cox regression to model BF behaviors based on cross-sectional (Pérez-Escamilla et al. 1996a) and longitudinal studies (Pérez-Escamilla et al. 1997; Lutter et al. 1997).

5.3. Interactive Models

The benefits of BF on preventing childhood diarrhea are more obvious and are easier to document in developing than in developed countries (i.e., the development level of a country modifies the strength of the association between BF and risk of diarrhea). This finding is likely to be the result of the much improved sanitary conditions in households in more developed nations. An important question is if household sanitation also modifies the association between BF and child mortality within developing countries. Habicht et al. (1998) used retrospective data from the 1976-1977 Malaysian Family Life Survey to answer this relevant public health question. Specifically, these researchers sought to find out if household sanitation level modified the association between BF and postperinatal infant mortality (i.e., 1 week to 1 year of age). The analytical sample consisted of 1,541 infants, including 165 who died during the postperinatal period. The analyses tested for the interaction between BF (yes/no) and household sanitation (piped water/toilet categories: a) neither toilet nor piped water, b) only toilet (flush or no flush), and c) both toilet and piped water. The authors validated one of the key independent variables by replicating the expected association between BF and lactational amenorrhea. They also documented the expected determinant of postperinatal mortality, thus also establishing the predictive validity of the outcome variable. The following key factors associated with postperinatal mortality were controlled for in the analyses: infant ethnicity, sex, year of birth, birth weight, and interpregnancy birth interval. Logistic regression results indicated that the relative risk (RR) of postperinatal mortality associated with not BF was twice as high (RR=5.20) in the absence of both toilet and piped water when compared with the mortality risk in households where a toilet and piped water were available (RR=2.51). Thus, lack of BF acts synergistically with lack of household sanitary conditions on postperinatal mortality. At the time, findings suggested that it was important to promote BF in households with adequate sanitation but where this infant-feeding behavior was not being practiced, at the same time that it was crucial to protect BF and promote improved sanitary services among households without them and with an already high prevalence of BF. These findings have major public health and policy implications and illustrate why in the area of BF epidemiology it is essential to have: a) a solid theoretical ground to guide the postulation of hypotheses involving statistical interactions, and b) the analytical capacity to formally test them.

6. DESIGN AND IMPLEMENTATION OF RANDOMIZED TRIALS

A major research design development has been the application of epidemiologic principles and methods to the design, conduct, and analysis of clinical trials—studies in which the investigators randomly allocate study participants to the exposure(s) being studied. One limitation in BF research is the difficulty in providing the ethical justification to conduct experimental studies that involve random assignment to breastfeed or not. Fortunately, BF promotion research has now contributed enormously to fill in this gap. Studies have been conducted in Belarus (Kramer et al. 2001), Bangladesh (Haider et al. 2000), and Mexico (Morrow et al. 1999) based on the randomized controlled study design to assess the effectiveness of hospital-based or community-based peer counseling.

The Belarus trial was a large-scale randomized trial evaluating the Baby Friendly Hospital Initiative in Belarus (Kramer et al. 2001). Although children were not assigned randomly to be breastfed their mothers were randomly assigned to be exposed or unexposed to the BF counseling intervention. Because the peer counseling interventions were successful at dramatically improving BF behaviors, the causal inferences that can be drawn with respect to the quasi-experimental analysis of infant-feeding mode and child morbidity is strong.

The Mexico study was the first randomized, controlled trial of peer-counseling or of any community-based intervention to promote exclusive BF, and the first experimental study to demonstrate a decreased incidence of infant diarrhea associated with BF promotion (Morrow et al. 1999). This randomized, community-based intervention trial included two intervention groups and a control group. Mother-infant pairs in the intervention groups received either six or three home visits from peer counselors in mid and late pregnancy and during the first eight weeks postpartum. Control group mothers with lactation problems were referred to their own physicians. No other sources of BF counseling were available in the community. Before the study started, the study community was mapped into 39 clusters with two or four city blocks each. A total of 13 clusters were allocated randomly to each study group and stratified by subdivision. This randomization schedule was generated by computer. Clusters rather than individuals were randomized to keep to a minimum the contamination of influences expected if relatives and close neighbors were assigned to different study groups. Because randomization was based on clusters, within-cluster correlation and design effects were assessed.

All data were collected through structured interviews of mothers residing in study households by two experienced staff other than the peer counselors. Although allocation concealment from staff and participants was not possible, bias was unlikely to explain the findings. Staff members were trained to administer all questions in a standard manner, and they undertook an equal proportion of interviews in each study group. The peer counselor training consisted of one week of classes and two months in lactation clinics and with mother-to-mother support groups. Finally, the peer counselors practiced in a neighborhood nearby the study community for six months before the intervention trial, during which the content of messages and problem-solving skills were refined. Although peer counselors taught intervention-group mothers that BF offers protection against diarrhea and respiratory tract infections, there were fewer reports of infant diarrhea in the intervention group than in the control group but no difference in non-specific respiratory signs and symptoms. Furthermore, most cases of infant diarrhea were confirmed by a visit to a physician. The Hawthorne effect (i.e., improved outcomes due to the mere presence of a home visitor) does not offer a plausible explanation of the results. Before this study, investigators undertook longitudinal studies that involved more intensive (i.e., weekly) home visits; however, exclusive BF remained uncommon.

The effect of the intervention on exclusive BF was analyzed by means of generalized estimating equation (GEE) models that accounted for within-individual correlation of outcomes measured at five time points from two weeks to three months postpartum. Maternal, infant and hospital factors were examined as risk factors, and for potential confounding and interaction effects relative to study outcomes. Interpretation of the dramatic increase in exclusive BF achieved in this trial should consider that the study community has a strong BF culture. Researchers speculated that BF counseling is likely to be most effective among women who possess a strong belief in the value of BF. By conducting a rapid ethnographic assessment prior to the intervention, researchers were able to use the information as marketing research and to develop messages and outreach methods tailored to the target population.

7. THE ROLE OF RAPID ASSESSMENT ANTHROPOLOGICAL METHODS IN BREASTFEEDING EPIDEMIOLOGY

A vast scientific literature demonstrates substantial health, social, and economic benefits associated with appropriate BF, including lower infant morbidity and mortality from diarrhea and other infectious diseases. Experts encourage exclusive BF of infants for six months, and continuation of BF, complemented by other sources of nutrition, well into the second year of life or beyond. Yet, even in countries with high BF rates, exclusive BF remains uncommon, with most mothers giving prelacteal feeds and supplementing BF within one to two months (Morrow & Guerrero 2001; Pérez-Escamilla et al. 1996b), often based on myths and misconceptions.

BF is a behavior that cannot be imposed, but must be chosen. Several factors facilitate or hamper BF and effective programs must examine and account for this variety of influences. Most interventions require the collaborative efforts of clinical researchers, epidemiologists, and social scientists. Community intervention programs are very difficult, and succeed only when they match the values and needs of the community. WHO has therefore advocated the use of focused ethnographic studies to provide essential data for designing communication messages, adapting communication training materials for health workers, and for aspects of program planning and problem solving (Scrimshaw et al. 1991). Rapid ethnographic assessment (REA) methods have been recommended as the basis of community-based intervention to reduce disease and promote community health (Gove & Pelto 1994; Stanton et al. 1992; Hundt & Forman 1993; O'Campo et al. 1993).

This section illustrates how REA was used to design the BF peer-counseling intervention in the Mexico City study described in the previous section. The project was designed to be conducted over a short period of time so that the findings would be used to plan and guide development and implementation of the community-based peer-counseling project to promote exclusive BF in Mexico City. During the preparation of the survey, free recall listing interviews were conducted. These consisted of open-ended questions in which five field workers and 15 mothers, randomly selected from the community, were asked to "list all the things you like about breastfeeding," "list all the things you don't like about breastfeeding," "list all the supplements that can be given to a breastfeeding baby," and "list the reasons why BF might be interrupted." A set of 29 items salient to the study population was obtained from these interviews. Project investigators summarized the responses and selected nine items for use in the systematic data collection phase. A 33-item, standardized questionnaire was developed. The questionnaire covered feeding practices relevant to the mother's experience with her youngest child and problems encountered by the mother that reduced the frequency of, or precluded, BF. In addition, respondents were asked to rank-order the following items in terms of their importance or relevance to her experience: the reasons to feed a child human milk or formula; perceived infant health status and infant-feeding choice; and sources of infant-feeding advice (Guerrero et al. 1999).

Results indicated a strong cultural consensus that BF is the ideal practice, and that the most important reason to choose an infant-feeding method is to meet infant health and growth needs. Cost, maternal comfort, and husbands' opinion were not primary considerations. At the same time, mothers indicated that BF should stop or be combined with supplementary liquids or foods under certain conditions such as: infant illness or when the infant is considered to be hot/thirsty; during maternal illness, especially folk illnesses (susto/coraje); when the mother has insufficient milk or bad quality milk; or a doctor's recommendation to cease BF. These findings from REA were instrumental in guiding the community intervention project that proved to be successful at increasing exclusive BF rates.

8. CONCLUSIONS

Epidemiology is based on two fundamental assumptions: first, that human disease does not occur at random; and second, that human disease has causal and preventive factors that can be identified through systematic investigation of different populations or subgroups of individuals within a population in different places or at different times (Hennekens & Buring 1987). The systematic collection and analysis of data involves the determination of whether a statistical association exists—in other words, whether the probability of developing a particular outcome in the presence of a given factor or exposure is different from the corresponding probability in its absence. It is then necessary to assess the validity of any observed statistical association by excluding possible alternative explanations, such as the luck of the draw (chance), systematic errors in collecting or interpreting data (bias), as well as the effects of additional variables that might be responsible for the observed association (confounding). Finally, a judgment is made as to whether that statistical association represents a cause-effect relationship between exposure and disease. Such a judgment requires inferences far beyond the data from any single study and involves consideration of criteria that include the magnitude of the association, the consistency of findings from all other studies, and biological plausibility. During the past decades, BF epidemiology has become essential for designing and evaluating sound child survival interventions. It is imperative that BF epidemiologists work in multidisciplinary teams and make use of the powerful analytical tools at their disposal, including ethnographic research (Sellen 2002).

9. ACKNOWLEDGMENTS

This is a contribution from the Storrs Agricultural Experiment Station; MLG supported by the National Institutes of Health (NICHHD grant HD13021).

10. REFERENCES

Benno Y, Sawada L, Mitsuoka T. The intestinal microflora of infants: composition of fecal flora in breastfed and bottlefed infants. Microbiol Immunol 1984;28:975-986.

Bollen KA. Structural Equations with Latent Variables. New York: Wiley, 1989.

Brown KH, Black RE, Lopez de Romaña G, Creed de Kanashiro H. Infant-feeding practices and their relationship with diarrheal and other diseases in Huascar (Lima), Peru. Pediatrics 1989;83:31-40.

Chaturvedi P, Warren CD, Altaye M, Morrow AL, Ruiz-Palacios GM, Pickering LK, Newburg DS. Fucosylated human milk oligosaccharides vary between individuals and over the course of lactation. Glycobiology 2001;11:365-372.

Collaborative Group on Hormonal Factors in Breast Cancer. Breast cancer and breastfeeding: collaborative reanalysis of individual data from 47 epidemiological studies in 30 countries, including 50302 women with breast cancer and 96973 women without the disease. Lancet 2002;360:187-195.

Coutsoudis A, Goga AE, Rollins N, Coovadia HM, The Child Health Group. Free formula milk for infants of HIV-infected women: blessing or curse? Health Policy Plan 2002;17:154-160.

[CST] The Cebu Study Team. Underlying and proximate determinants of child health: The Cebu Longitudinal Health and Nutrition Study. Am J Epidemiol 1991;133:185-201.

Goldman AS. The immune system of human milk: antimicrobial, anti-inflammatory and immunomodulating properties. Pediatr Infect Dis J 1994;12:664-671.

Gove S, Pelto GH. Focused ethnographic studies in the WHO Programme for the Control of Acute Respiratory Infections. Med Anthropol 1994;15:409-424.

Grummer-Strawn LM. The effect of changes in population characteristics on breastfeeding trends in fifteen developing countries. Int J Epidemiol 1996;25:94-102.

Guerrero ML, Morrow RC, Calva JJ, Ortega-Gallegos H, Weller SC, Ruiz-Palacios GM, Morrow AL. Rapid ethnographic assessment of breastfeeding practices in periurban Mexico City. Bull World Health Organ 1999;77:323-330.

Habicht JP, DaVanzo J, Butz WP. Does breastfeeding really save lives, or are apparent benefits due to biases? Am J Epidemiol 1986;123:279-290.

Habicht JP, DaVanzo J, Butz WP. Mother's milk and sewage: Their interactive effects on infant mortality. Pediatrics 1998;81:456-461.

Habicht JP. The association between prolonged breastfeeding and poor growth—what are the implications? Adv Exp Med Biol 2000;478:193-200.

Haider R, Ashworth A, Kabir I, Huttly SR. Effect of community-based peer counsellors on exclusive breastfeeding practices in Dhaka, Bangladesh: a randomised controlled trial. Lancet 2000;356:1643-1647.

Hennekens CH, Buring JE. Epidemiology in Medicine. Boston: Little Brown, 1987; pp 3-29.

Hundt GA, Forman MR. Interfacing anthropology and epidemiology: the Bedouin Arab infant feeding study. Soc Sci Med 1993;36:957-964.

[IRD/MI] Institute for Resource Development/Macro International. An Assessment of Demographic and Health Surveys-I: Data Quality. Calverton, MD; 1990.

[IRD/MI] Institute for Resource Development/Macro International. Proceedings of the Demographic and Health Surveys World Conference. Washington, DC; August 5-7, 1991.

Ishizaka S, Kimoto M, Tsujii T, Saito S. Antibody production system modulated by oral administration of human milk and TGF-β. Cell Immunol 1994;159:77-84.

Kramer MS, Chalmers B, Hodnett ED, Sevkovskaya Z, Dzikovich I, Shapiro S, Collet JP, Vanilovich I, Mezen I, Ducruet T, Shishko G, Zubovich V, Mknuik D, Gluchanina E, Dombrovskiy V, Ustinovitch A, Kot T, Bogdanovich N, Ovchinikova L, Helsing E; PROBIT Study Group. Promotion of Breastfeeding Intervention Trial (PROBIT): a randomized trial in the Republic of Belarus. JAMA 2001;285:413-420.

Lutter CK, Pérez-Escamilla R, Segall A, Teruya K, Sanghvi T, Fiedler J, Wickham C. Effectiveness of a hospital-based breastfeeding promotion program on exclusive breastfeeding among low-income women in Brazil. Am J Public Health 1997;87:659-663.

Marquis GS, Habicht JP, Lanata CF, Black RE, Rasmussen KM. Association of breastfeeding and stunting in Peruvian toddlers: an example of reverse causality. Int J Epidemiol 1997;26:349-356.

Morrow AL, Guerrero ML. From bioactive substances to research on breast-feeding promotion. Adv Exp Med Biol 2001;501:447-455.

Morrow AL, Pickering LK. Human milk and infectious diseases. In: Long S, Pickering LK, Prober CG, editors. Principles and Practice of Pediatric Infectious Diseases. New York: Churchill-Livingstone, 1997; pp 87-95.

Morrow AL, Guerrero ML, Shults J, Calva JJ, Lutter C, Bravo J, Ruiz-Palacios G, Morrow RC, Butterfoss FD. Efficacy of home-based peer counseling to promote exclusive breastfeeding: a randomised controlled trial. Lancet 1999;353:1226-1231.

Newburg DS, Neubauer SH. Carbohydrates in milks: analysis, quantities, and significance. In: Jensen RG, editor. Handbook of Milk Composition. Orlando: Academic Press, 1995; pp 273-349.
O'Campo P, Guyer B, Squires B, Weiss J, Sweitzer J, Coyle T. Needs assessment for reducing infant mortality in Baltimore City: the Healthy Start Program. South Med J 1993;86:1342-1349.
Pérez-Escamilla R. Promotion of breastfeeding in the AIDS era. Rev Panam Salud Pública 2001;9:357-361.
Pérez-Escamilla R, Maulén-Radován I, Dewey KG. Association between cesarean delivery and breastfeeding outcomes among Mexican women. Am J Public Health 1996a;86:832-836.
Pérez-Escamilla R, Segura-Millán S, Canahuati J, Allen, H. Prelacteal feeds are negatively associated with breastfeeding outcomes in Honduras. J Nutr 1996b;126:2765-2773.
Pérez-Escamilla R, Lutter C, Wickham C, Phillips M, Treviño-Siller S, Sanghvi T. Identification of risk factors for shorter breastfeeding durations in Mexico City through survival analysis. Ecol Food Nutr 1997;36:43-64.
Pérez-Escamilla R, Cobas JA, Balcazar H, Holland Benin M. Specifying the antecedents of breast-feeding duration in Peru through a structural equation model. Public Health Nutr 1999;2:461-467.
Pérez-Escamilla R, Grajeda R. Breastfeeding trends across time in Latin America: Results from the Demographic and Health Surveys. Experimental Biology Meetings, New Orleans, LA; April 20-24, 2002 (Abstract # 2752).
Pickering LK, Morrow AL. Factors in human milk that protect against diarrheal disease. Infection 1993;21:355-357.
Raftery AE, Tanner MA, Wells MT, editors. Statistics in the 21st Century. Boca Raton, FL: Chapman & Hall/CRC. Monographs on Statistics and Applied Probability no. 93, 2002.
Scrimshaw SC, Carballo M, Ramos L, Blair BA. The AIDS rapid anthropological assessment procedures: a tool for health education planning and evaluation. Health Edu Q 1991;18:111-123.
Sellen DW. Sub-optimal breast feeding practices: ethnographic approaches to building "baby friendly" communities. Adv Exp Med Biol 2002;503:223-232.
Simondon KB, Costes R, Delaunay V, Diallo A, Simondon F. Children's height, health and appetite influence mothers' weaning decisions in rural Senegal. Int J Epidemiol 2001;30:476-481.
Stanton B, Black R, Engle P, Pelto G. Theory-driven behavioural intervention research for the control of diarrheal diseases. Soc Sci Med 1992;35:1405-1420.

SECTION II

SCIENCE AND POLICY: OPTIMAL DURATION OF EXCLUSIVE BREASTFEEDING

THE OPTIMAL DURATION OF EXCLUSIVE BREASTFEEDING

A Systematic Review

Michael S. Kramer and Ritsuko Kakuma

1. ABSTRACT

Although the health benefits of breastfeeding are acknowledged widely, opinions and recommendations are divided on the optimal duration of exclusive breastfeeding. We systematically reviewed available evidence concerning the effects on child health, growth, and development and on maternal health of exclusive breastfeeding for 6 months vs. exclusive breastfeeding for 3-4 months followed by mixed breastfeeding (introduction of complementary liquid or solid foods with continued breastfeeding) to 6 months. Two independent literature searches were conducted, together comprising the following databases: MEDLINE (as of 1966), Index Medicus (prior to 1966), CINAHL, HealthSTAR, BIOSIS, CAB Abstracts, EMBASE-Medicine, EMBASE-Psychology, Econlit, Index Medicus for the WHO Eastern Mediterranean Region, African Index Medicus, Lilacs (Latin American and Carribean literature), EBM Reviews-Best Evidence, the Cochrane Database of Systematic Reviews, and the Cochrane Controlled Trials Register. No language restrictions were imposed. The two searches yielded a total of 2,668 unique citations. Contacts with experts in the field yielded additional published and unpublished studies. Studies were stratified according to study design (controlled trials vs. observational studies) and provenance (developing vs. developed countries).

The main outcome measures were weight and length gain, weight-for-age and length-for-age z-scores, head circumference, iron status, gastrointestinal and respiratory infectious morbidity, atopic eczema, asthma, neuromotor development, duration of lactational amenorrhea, and maternal postpartum weight loss.

Twenty independent studies meeting the selection criteria were identified by the literature search: 9 from developing countries (2 of which were controlled trials in Honduras) and 11 from developed countries (all observational studies). Neither the trials nor the observational studies suggest that infants who continue to be exclusively

---

Departments of Pediatrics and of Epidemiology and Biostatistics, McGill University Faculty of Medicine, 1020 Pine Avenue West, Montreal, Quebec, Canada H3A 1A2

Protecting Infants through Human Milk, edited by Pickering *et al.*
Kluwer Academic/Plenum Publishers, 2004

breastfed for 6 months show deficits in weight or length gain, although larger sample sizes would be required to rule out modest increases in the risk of undernutrition. The data are conflicting with respect to iron status but suggest that, at least in developing-country settings, where iron stores of newborn infants may be suboptimal, exclusive breastfeeding without iron supplementation through 6 months of age may compromise hematologic status. Based primarily on an observational analysis of a large randomized trial in Belarus, infants who continue exclusive breastfeeding for 6 months or more appear to have a significantly reduced risk of one or more episodes of gastrointestinal tract infection. No significant reduction in risk of atopic eczema, asthma, or other atopic outcomes has been demonstrated in studies from Finland, Australia, and Belarus. Data from the two Honduran trials suggest that exclusive breastfeeding through 6 months of age is associated with delayed resumption of menses and more rapid postpartum weight loss in the mother.

Infants who are breastfed exclusively for 6 months experience less morbidity from gastrointestinal tract infection than infants who were mixed breastfed as of 3 or 4 months of age. No deficits have been demonstrated in growth among infants from either developing or developed countries who are exclusively breastfed for 6 months or longer. Moreover, the mothers of such infants have more prolonged lactational amenorrhea and faster postpartum weight loss. Based on the results of this review, the World Health Assembly adopted a resolution to recommend exclusive breastfeeding for 6 months to its member countries. Large randomized trials are recommended in both developed and developing countries to ensure that exclusive breastfeeding for 6 months does not increase the risk of undernutrition (growth faltering), to confirm the health benefits reported thus far, and to investigate other potential effects on health and development, especially over the long term.

2. INTRODUCTION

The debate over the optimal duration of exclusive breastfeeding has had a long and checkered history. Growth faltering is a commonly observed phenomenon in developing countries after 3 months of age (Waterlow & Thomson 1979; Whitehead & Paul 1984). This growth faltering traditionally has been attributed to three factors: (1) inadequacy of energy intake from human milk alone after 3 or 4 months; (2) poor nutritional quality (i.e., low energy micronutrient content), of weaning foods commonly introduced in many developing countries; and (3) adverse effects of infection on energy intake and expenditure. The inadequacy of human milk for energy requirements beyond 3 or 4 months of age was based on calculations made by the Food and Agricultural Organization and World Health Organization (FAO/WHO 1973). More careful studies since the 1980s have shown that the earlier FAO/WHO figures substantially overestimate true energy requirements in infancy (Whitehead & Paul 1981; Garza & Butte 1990; Butte 1996; Brown et al. 1998).

The belief that human milk alone is nutritionally insufficient after 3 or 4 months of age, combined with the fact that weaning foods given in many developing countries are both nutritionally inadequate and contaminated, led to concern about the so-called "weanling's dilemma" (Rowland et al. 1978; Rowland 1986). Breastfeeding is a life-and-death issue in developing countries. A meta-analysis (WHO 2001a) reported markedly reduced infant mortality (especially due to infectious disease) with breastfeeding even into the second year of life.

The weanling's dilemma and the risk of mortality associated with early weaning are concerns primarily in developing countries. In most developed countries, uncontaminated, nutritionally adequate complementary foods are readily available, and growth faltering is uncommon. With the resurgence of breastfeeding in developed countries attention has turned to the importance of promoting breastfeeding duration and exclusivity. Epidemiologic evidence is now overwhelming that, even in developed countries, breastfeeding protects against gastrointestinal and respiratory tract infections, and that the protective effect is enhanced with greater duration and exclusivity of breastfeeding (Howie et al. 1990; Cunningham et al. 1991; Beaudry et al. 1995; Dewey et al. 1995a; Raisler et al. 1999).

Although growth faltering is uncommon in developed countries, available data indicate that infants who follow the then current WHO feeding recommendations (to exclusively breastfeed for 4 to 6 months of age and to continue breastfeeding with adequate complementary fluids up to 2 years of age) show a deceleration in both weight and length gain relative to the international WHO/CDC Growth Reference from around 3 to 12 months of age, with partial catch-up thereafter (WHO 1994; Dewey et al. 1995b; Nielsen et al. 1998; Hediger et al. 2000; Haschke & van't Hof 2000).

In recent years, a split had developed about recommendations for the optimal duration of exclusive breastfeeding. WHO recommended exclusive breastfeeding for 4 to 6 months, with the introduction of complementary foods thereafter (WHO 1995a), whereas UNICEF preferred the wording "about 6 months" (UNICEF 1993). This led to vigorous, and often acrimonious debate, not only between the two UN agencies but also in the larger infant nutrition and public health communities (Lutter 2000). The position of the American Academy of Pediatrics has been ambivalent; in two different sections of their 1998 Pediatric Nutrition Handbook (AAP 1998), they alternatively recommend human milk "as the exclusive nutrient source ... during the first 6 months" (p. 18) and "to delay introduction of solid foods until 4 to 6 months" (p. 38). Because of the ongoing controversy and polarization over this issue, the World Health Organization requested, in the spring of 2000, a systematic review of the available evidence before considering a revision or continuation of its current infant feeding recommendations. In the remainder of this report, we summarize the chapter, results, and conclusions of that review.

3. METHODS

3.1. Inclusion Criteria and Definitions

We selected controlled clinical trials and observational studies, published in all languages, examining whether or not exclusive breastfeeding (EBF) until 6 months of age has an impact on growth, development, morbidity, and survival of healthy, term infants and their mothers. Studies of (or including) low-birth-weight (<2500 g) infants were not excluded, provided that such infants were born at term (≥37 completed weeks). Only those studies with an internal comparison group were included in the review, i.e., we excluded studies based on external comparisons with reference data. The comparisons must have been based on one group of infants who received EBF for ≥3 but <6 months and mixed breastfeeding (MBF) until 6 months of age or later (i.e., infants were introduced to liquid or solid foods between 3 and 6 months of age), and another group of subjects who were breastfed exclusively for ≥6 months. This restriction was imposed to provide direct relevance to the clinical and public health decision context: whether infants who are breastfed exclusively for 3 to 4 months after birth should continue EBF or should receive complementary foods in addition to human milk (MBF). Thus studies comparing EBF and MBF from birth were excluded, as were studies that investigated the effects of age at introduction of nonhuman milk liquid or solid foods but did not ensure EBF ≥3 months prior to their introduction.

The "complementary" foods used in MBF included juices, formula, other milks, other liquids, or solid foods. Although WHO defines EBF as breastfeeding with no supplemental liquids or solid foods other than medications or vitamins (WHO 1991), few studies strictly adhered to the WHO definition. In some studies, so-called "EBF" included provision of water, teas, or juices (corresponding to WHO's definition of predominant breastfeeding [WHO 1991]) or even small amounts of infant formula.

3.2. Search Methods

In order to capture as many relevant studies as possible, two independent literature searches were conducted: one by staff at WHO's Department of Nutrition for Health and Development and one by the authors. The search details are shown below. The search by WHO was conducted on August 22, 2000, in the following databases: MEDLINE (1966 to August 2000), Pre-MEDLINE (Index Medicus previous to 1966), CINAHL (1982 to June 2000), HealthSTAR (1975 to August 2000), EBM Reviews-Best Evidence (1991 to July/August 2000), SocioFile (1974 to July 2000), Cochrane Database of Systematic Reviews (Issue 2, 2000), CAB Abstracts (1973 to July 2000), EMBASE-Psychology (1987 to 3rd Quarter, 2000), Econlit (1969 to August 2000), Index Medicus for the WHO Eastern Mediterranean (IMEMR), African Index Medicus (AIM), and Lilacs (Latin American and Caribbean literature). Where applicable, the medical subject heading (MeSH) "breast feeding," and otherwise the free language terms "breast-feeding," "breast feeding," or "breastfeeding" combined with "exclusive" or "exclusively" were used in the search strategy. Once duplicates were removed, 1,035 citations remained; these were then assessed for eligibility.

The authors' search was conducted on August 12, 2000, in the following databases: MEDLINE (1966 to wk 3 September, 2000), CINAHL (1982 to April 2000), HealthSTAR (1975 to August 2000), BIOSIS (1989 to 2000), CAB Abstracts (1973 to June 2000), Cochrane Database of Systematic Reviews (Issue 3, 2000), Cochrane Controlled Trials Register (Issue 3, 2000), and EMBASE-Medicine (1980 to present). The terms "breast feeding," "infant," and "growth," as MeSH headings and text words, were combined in the search strategy. Once duplicates among the databases were removed, 1,845 citations remained, 1,633 of which were different from the 1,035 identified by the WHO search. Thus 2,668 unique citations were identified by the two searches.

For both searches, every effort was made to identify relevant non-English language articles and abstracts. Given their own backgrounds, the reviewers themselves were able to determine the eligibility of articles in French, Spanish, and Japanese. For publications in other languages, two options were available. Many articles in languages other than English provided English abstracts. As such, all potentially relevant articles were obtained and checked for availability of English abstracts. If such abstracts were not available, or were available but did not provide enough information to determine their eligibility, then assistance was requested from WHO to determine their eligibility for inclusion. No article or abstract was excluded because of language of publication.

In addition to the studies found through the two electronic searches, reference lists of identified articles were checked, and contacts with experts in the field were made to identify other potentially relevant published or unpublished studies. Attempts were made to contact the authors of all studies that qualified for inclusion in the review to obtain methodologic details, clarify inconsistencies, and obtain unpublished data.

Many studies were identified that either compared outcomes in infants receiving EBF vs. MBF or investigated the effects of age at introduction of nonhuman-milk liquid or solid foods. The vast majority of these studies were ineligible for inclusion, however, because they did not ensure EBF ≥3 months prior to introducing these complementary foods in the MBF group and/or a comparison group with EBF ≥6 months.

We identified 38 unique citations (articles or abstracts) that met the selection criteria, comprising 19 separate studies. Of the 19 included studies, 8 were carried out in developing countries and the other 11 in developed countries. Ten of the 38 total citations were found by both electronic searches (Ahn & MacLean 1980; Åkeson et al. 1998a; Castillo et al. 1996; Cohen et al. 1994, 1995; Dewey et al. 1996, 1998a, 1998b, 1999; Khan 1984); 11 were identified only by the WHO search (Åkeson et al. 1998b; Duncan et al. 1993; Heiskanen et al. 1994; Kajosaari & Saarinen 1983; Kajosaari 1991, 1994; Kallio et al. 1992; Oddy et al. 1999; Pisacane et al. 1995; Rao & Kanade 1992; Savilahti et al. 1987); 6 were found only by the authors' search (Dewey 1995b; Heinig et al. 1993; Adair et al. 1993; Simondon & Simondon 1997; Åkeson et al. 1996; Frongillo et al. 1997). Eleven additional citations were located through contacts with experts and reference lists of relevant articles (Brown et al. 1998; WHO 1994; Kramer et al. 2000a 2000b, 2001, 2002; WHO 1995b, 2002; Gourbin & Masuy-Stroobant 1995; Dewey et al. 1997, 2001)

3.3. Data Extraction and Analysis

Studies were evaluated for methodologic quality and appropriateness for inclusion without consideration of the results. We used Cochrane criteria for assessing the adequacy of randomization and concealment of controlled clinical trials. The 5-point Jadad scale also was used to examine the quality of randomized control trials (Jadad et al. 1996). Observational studies (cohort, case-control, and cross-sectional) were assessed for control for confounding, losses to follow-up, and assessment of the outcome. Quality assessments of all the eligible studies were carried out independently by the two reviewers, with disagreements resolved by consensus. Attempts were made to contact authors of all included studies to obtain additional data, resolving consistencies, and obtain additional methodologic details.

The studies were stratified according to study design (controlled trials vs. observational studies) and provenance (developing vs. developed country). One study (Frongillo et al. 1997) based on a pooled analysis of 2 developed and 3 developing countries has been included with developed country studies because of the selection criteria (literate, educated, urban mothers) and the observed high infant growth rates. Analyses were carried out using the Review Manager 4.2 software for preparing Cochrane reviews. Effect measures are reported as the fixed-effect weighted mean difference (WMD) and its 95% confidence interval (CI) for continuous outcomes and the fixed-effect pooled relative risk (RR) and its 95% CI. For most continuous outcomes, a positive WMD denotes a higher (more favorable) value in the EBF group. All dichotomous outcomes are formulated as adverse; thus an RR <1 denotes that the EBF group had a lower risk of the outcome than the MBF group.

4. RESULTS

The stratification described in the Methods resulted in 3 separate strata for considering the results of the studies considered in this review: (1) controlled trials of exclusive vs. mixed breastfeeding for 4 to 6 months from developing countries, (2) observational studies of exclusive vs. mixed breastfeeding for 3 to 7 months from developing countries, and (3) observational studies of exclusive vs. mixed breastfeeding for 3 to 7 months from developed countries.

4.1. Stratum 1: Controlled Trials, Developing Countries

Two studies were found in this stratum, both from the same group of investigators and involving the same study setting (Honduras) (Cohen et al. 1994; Dewey et al. 1999). The first of these studies involved term infants unselected for birth weight but included 29 infants (20%) weighing <2500 g at birth. The second trial was restricted to term infants weighing <2500 g at birth. The quality ratings of these two trials were not high for several reasons: (1) allocation of treatment (continued EBF vs. MBF from 4–6 months) within clusters defined by calendar week, yet results analyzed with individual women and infants as units of analysis; (2) the first trial (Cohen et al. 1994) allocated the weeks by alternation, rather than by strict randomization; and (3) published results were not based on analysis by intention-to-treat. Nonetheless, the investigators made a considerable effort to ensure compliance with the assigned allocation and to standardize the training of the observers who performed the anthropometric measurements and other outcome assessments, and detailed comparisons between trial participants and eligible nonparticipants demonstrated no differences that would detract from the external validity of findings in the trials. For all analyses, the two mixed breastfeeding groups (one of which was intended to maintain frequency of breastfeeding) in the first trial were combined for the purposes of this review. Table 1 shows the results for weight gain and length gain from 4 to 6 months, for the two trials individually, and the pooled results. These outcomes were nearly identical in the two treatment groups, with reasonably narrow confidence intervals. The impact of the small sample size of the two Honduran trials is evident, however, when examining the risk of undernutrition, as represented by anthropometric z-scores ≤2, at 6 months of age. For weight-for-age, the proportions in the EBF vs. MBF groups were 2/50 vs. 0/91 in the first trial and 6/59 vs. 4/60 in the second trial, for a pooled relative risk (RR) of 2.14 (0.74–6.24). Corresponding results for low length-for-age were 4/50 vs. 6/91 in the first trial and 8/59 vs. 7/60 in the second trial, for a pooled RR of 1.18 (0.56–2.50).

The hematologic results are based on the first trial (Dewey et al. 1998b), since in the second trial (Cohen et al. 1994), infants with low hemoglobin concentration at 2 and 4 months of age were supplemented with iron. A nonsignificantly higher proportion of EBF vs. MBF infants (33/50 vs. 49/89, respectively) had a hemoglobin concentration <110 g/L at 6 months of age [RR=1.20 (0.91 to 1.58)]. The mean hemoglobin concentration was significantly lower at 6 months of age in the EBF group (104 g/L vs. 109 g/L), [difference = –5.0 (–8.5 to –1.5) g/L]. Similarly, mean plasma ferritin concentration was significantly lower at 6 months of age in the EBF group [difference = –18.9 (–37.3 to –0.50) μg/L] with a RR for a low (<15 μg/L) ferritin concentration of 2.93 (1.13–7.56).

In the pooled results from both Honduran trials, no significant difference was seen between the EBF and MBF group for the percentage of days of fever, cough, nasal congestion, nasal discharge, hoarseness, or diarrhea from 4 to 6 months of age.

Based on the pooled results from both trials (Dewey et al. 2001), mothers in the EBF group reported that their infants crawled at an average of 0.8 (0.3–1.3) months sooner. No difference was seen, however, in the mean age at which the infants were reported to have first sat from a lying position [WMD = –0.2 (–0.6 to +0.2) months]. The results from the two Honduras trials differed with respect to maternal reports of walking by 12 months of age, with a significantly lower proportion of EBF infants reported as not having walked by 12 months of age in the first trial [RR=0.66 (0.45–0.98)], but a nonsignificantly higher proportion not having done so in the second trial [RR=1.12 (0.90–1.38)], with significant (P<0.01) heterogeneity between the results of the two trials.

Mothers in the exclusively breastfed group, from the two trials combined (Dewey et al. 2001), had a significantly larger weight loss from 4 to 6 months [WMD = –0.42 (–0.82 to –0.02) kg] and were not significantly less likely to have resumed menses by 6 months postpartum [RR=0.58 (0.33–1.03)].

4.2. Stratum 2: Observational Studies, Developing Countries

Three cohort studies were identified in this category: one each from Peru (Brown 1991), the Philippines (Adair et al. 1993), and Senegal (Simondon & Simondon 1997). Table 2 shows the individual and pooled results for weight and length gain from 4 to 6 months of age from these three studies. The Senegal study also provided unpublished data on rates of low weight-for-age and length-for-age z-scores at 6 to 7 months of age: 19/154 vs. 29/216 in the EBF vs. MBF groups [RR=0.92 (0.54–1.58)] for low weight-for-age and 12/154 vs. 14/216 [RR=1.20 (0.57–2.53)] for low length-for-age.

Huffman et al. (1987) reported a longer median duration of lactational amenorrhea among women who practiced EBF for ≥7 months vs. MBF (16.1 vs. 15.3 months, respectively), but means and SD values were not reported. In a multivariate Cox regression model adjusting for maternal education, parity, religion, and weight, EBF for ≥6 months was associated with a significantly longer time to resumption of menses vs. EBF for <1 month, but no direct comparison was reported vs. MBF.

One large cross-sectional study from Chile (Castillo et al. 1996) reported a similar risk of weight-for-age z-score <–1 and height-for-age z-score <–1 among infants between 3 to 5 and 6 to 8 months of age in the two feeding groups, but the prevalences, confidence intervals, and standard errors for the reported prevalence ratios are not published, thus precluding any assessment of sampling variation.

4.3. Stratum 3: Observational Studies, Developed Countries

A pooled sample of breastfed infants from 6 developed countries (WHO 1994), a pooled analysis conducted by WHO of data from 5 countries (2 developed, 3 developing,

Table 1. Controlled trials conducted in developing countries: weight and length gains from 4 to 6 months of age

	EBF			MBF			
	n	Mean	SD	n	Mean	SD	WMD (95% CI)
Weight Gain (g/mo)							
Cohen et al. 1994	50	546	178	91	514	154	+32 (−27 to +91)
Dewey et al. 1999	63	512	173	61	504	182	+8 (−55 to +71)
Pooled	113			152			+21 (−22 to +64)
Length Gain (mm/mo)							
Cohen et al. 1994	50	19.5	6.0	91	19.0	5.5	+0.5 (−1.5 to +2.5)
Dewey et al. 1994	63	23.0	6.5	61	21.5	4.5	+1.5 (−0.5 to +3.5)
Pooled	113			152			+1.0 (−0.4 to +2.4)

EBF=exclusively breastfed; MBF=mixed breastfed; WMD=weighted mean difference; SD=standard deviation; CI=confidence interval

Table 2. Observational study conducted in developing countries: weight and length gains from 4 to 6 months of age

	EBF			MBF			
	n	Mean	SD	n	Mean	SD	WMD (95% CI)
Weight Gain (g/mo)							
Adair et al. 1993	370	336	157	834	350	167	−14 (−34 to +6)
Brown 1991	15	402	198	21	359	168	+43 (−80 to +166)
Simondon et al. 1997	154	323	250	216	289	286	+36 (−19 to +91)
Pooled	539			1071			−7 (−25 to +11)
Length Gain (mm/mo)							
Adair et al. 1993	370	16.0	8.0	834	16.0	7.5	0.0 (−1.0 to +1.0)
Brown 1991	15	16.3	2.7	21	15.7	4.4	+0.6 (−1.7 to +2.9)
Simondon et al. 1997	154	15.5	6.6	216	14.3	5.9	+1.2 (−0.1 to +2.5)
Pooled	539			1071			+0.4 (−0.3 to +1.2)

EBF=exclusively breastfed; MBF=mixed breastfed; WMD=weighted mean difference; SD=standard deviation; CI=confidence interval

Table 3. Observational studies conducted in developed countries: weight and length gains from 3 to 8 months of age

	EBF			MBF			
	n	Mean	SD	n	Mean	SD	WMD (95% CI)
Weight Gain (g/mo)							
Åkeson et al. 1998	10	498	118	9	438	127	+60 (−51 to +71)
Kramer et al. 2001	619	612	180	2836	641	186	−29 (−45 to −13)
WHO 1994	200	463	142	158	470	159	−7 (−39 to +25)
WHO 1997	179	419	100	377	414	100	+5 (−13 to +23)
Pooled	1008			3380			−12 (−23 to −1)
Length Gain (mm/mo)							
Åkeson et al. 1998	10	18.0	2.4	9	16.8	3.0	+1.2 (−1.3 to +3.7)
Kramer et al. 2001	618	19.3	6.4	2836	20.4	7.0	−1.1 (−1.7 to −0.5)
WHO 1994	200	17.2	4.3	156	17.6	4.8	−0.4 (−1.4 to +0.6)
WHO 1997	179	18.7	2.9	377	18.5	2.9	+0.2 (−0.3 to +0.7)
Pooled	1007			3378			−0.4 (−0.7 to 0.0)

EBF=exclusively breastfed; MBF=mixed breastfed; WMD=weighted mean difference; SD=standard deviation; CI=confidence interval

but in which study women were all literate and of middle to high socioeconomic status) (Frongillo et al. 1997), a large cohort study nested within a randomized trial in Belarus (Kramer et al. 2001), and a small study from Sweden (Åkeson et al. 1998a), reported on weight gain between 3 and 8 months of age. The WHO (Frongillo et al. 1997) and Belarus (Kramer et al. 2001) studies controlled for confounding by indication (size or growth in first 3-4 months) and other potential confounders using multilevel (mixed) regression analyses. The results are shown in Table 3. Statistically significant (P=0.02) heterogeneity was observed among the four studies, with considerably larger mean weight and length gains in both groups of infants in the Belarus study, and a slightly but significantly higher gain in the MBF group. Because of this heterogeneity, the WMDs shown in the table should be interpreted with caution; even the lower 95% confidence limits of these estimates, however, are compatible with differences of questionable clinical importance. Moreover, given the large weight gains in both groups in the Belarussian study, the higher gain of the MBF group is not necessarily a beneficial outcome.

Only the Belarussian study (Kramer et al. 2001) provided data on prevalence of low (< −2) z-scores, and the small number of infants with such low scores provided low statistical power to detect such differences. For low weight-for-age at 6 months, the proportions were 0/620 in the EBF group vs. 2/2841 in the MBF group [RR=0.92 (0.04–19.04)], while for length-for-age, the comparable proportions were 14/619 in the EBF group vs. 42/2841 in the MBF group [RR=1.53 (0.84–2.78)]. The Belarussian study also provided data on head circumference. No significant differences were observed at 6 months or 9 months, but the EBF group had a slightly but significantly larger circumference at 12 months (47.25 vs. 47.06 cm) [difference = +0.19 (0.06–0.32) cm].

Both the Belarussian (Kramer et al. 2001) and a Finnish cohort study (Kajosaari & Saarinen 1983) reported the occurrence of atopic eczema at 1 year of age. The two studies showed significant heterogeneity, with the Finnish study reporting a significantly reduced risk [10/70 vs. 23/65, RR=0.40 (0.21–0.78)], but the larger Belarussian study finding a much lower absolute risk in both feeding groups and no risk reduction with EBF [17/621 vs. 78/2865, RR=1.00 (0.60–1.69)]. Neither the Belarussian nor an Australian cohort study (Oddy et al. 1999) found a significant reduction in risk of recurrent (two or more episodes) wheezing during the first 12 months of life in the EBF group. No reduction in risk of atopic eczema at 5 years of age was observed in the Finnish study (Kajosaari 1994) (12/51 vs. 15/62) [RR=0.97 (0.50–1.89)]. Neither the Finnish (Kajosaari 1994) (4/51 vs. 9/62) nor Australian (Oddy 1999) (33/207 vs. 37/232) studies found a significant reduction in risk of asthma at 5 to 6 years of age; the pooled RR was 0.91 (0.61–1.36). Finally, the Australian study found no reduction in risk of a positive skin prick test at 6 years of age in the EBF group (53/160 vs. 57/171) [RR=0.99 (0.73–1.35)].

A small Italian study (Pisacane et al. 1995) of hematologic outcomes at 12 months of age reported a significantly higher hemoglobin concentration [117 vs. 109 g/L (95% CI for the difference = +4.0 to +12.0 g/L)], a nonsignificant reduction in anemia (hemoglobin <110 g/L) [RR=0.12 (0.01–1.80)], a nonsignificantly higher ferritin concentration [WMD = +4.7 (−6.3 to +15.7 μg/L)], and a nonsignificant reduction in the risk of low (<10 μg/L) ferritin concentration [RR=0.42 (0.12–1.54)] among infants in the exclusive breastfeeding group. Of note in this study is that the exclusive and mixed breastfeeding continued in both groups until at least 12 months of age (a criterion for selection into the study (Pisacane et al. 1995).

In the Belarussian study (Kramer et al. 2001) the EBF group had a significantly reduced risk of one or more episodes of gastrointestinal tract infection in the first 12 months of life (31/621 vs. 213/2862) [RR=0.67 (0.46–0.97)], which was maintained in a multivariate mixed model controlling for geographic origin, urban vs. rural location, maternal education, and number of siblings in the household [adjusted odds ratio = 0.61 (0.41–0.93)]. No significant reduction in risk was observed for hospitalization for gastrointestinal tract infection [11/621 vs. 64/2862 in the EBF vs. MBF groups, respectively; RR=0.79 (0.42–1.49)]. Neither the Australian (Oddy et al. 1999) nor the Belarussian study (Kramer et al. 2001) found reduced risks of either upper or lower respiratory tract infections (data not shown).

A study from Tucson, Arizona (Duncan et al. 1993), found no difference in the average number of episodes of acute otitis media in the first 12 months of life in the EBF vs. MBF groups [1.48 vs. 1.52 episodes, respectively (95% confidence interval for the difference = −0.49 to +0.41 episodes)]. The Tucson (Duncan et al. 1993) and Belarussian (Kramer et al. 2001) studies both found a slightly elevated risk for one or more episodes of otitis media [pooled RR=1.28 (1.04–1.57)], but the Tucson study found a nonsignificant reduction in risk for frequent otitis media [RR=0.81 (0.43–1.52)].

5. DISCUSSION

Neither the controlled clinical trials nor the predominantly cohort observational studies from either developing or developed countries suggest that infants who continue to be breastfed exclusively for 6 months show deficits in weight or length gain compared with infants who receive complementary feeding in addition to breastfeeding after 3 or 4 months. However, owing to the large sample sizes required to detect modest effects on the incidence of low (<−2) anthropometric z-scores, data are insufficient to rule out a modest increase in risk of undernutrition with exclusive breastfeeding for 6 months.

Consistent with the results of previous observational studies (WHO 2001a; Howie et al. 1990; Cunningham et al. 1991; Beaudry et al. 1995; Dewey et al. 1995a; Raisler et al. 1999), none of which met the selection criteria for this review, the large Belarussian study (Kramer et al. 2001) found a significant reduction in risk of one or more episodes of gastrointestinal tract infection. No other significant reduction in infectious morbidity has been demonstrated, and the combined data from Finland (Kajosaari & Saarinen 1983), Australia (Kajorsaari 1994), and Belarus (Kramer et al. 2001) do not suggest a protective effect against short- or long-term atopic outcomes.

The data are conflicting with respect to iron status, but controlled trials from Honduras (Cohen et al. 1994; Dewey et al. 1999) suggest that, at least in developing country settings where maternal iron status (and thus newborn iron stores) may be suboptimal, exclusive breastfeeding without iron supplementation may compromise hematologic status by 6 months of age. The reasons for the superior hematologic status reported in Italian infants (Pisacane et al. 1995) exclusively breastfed for ≥7 months are unclear.

Data from two Honduran trials (Cohen et al. 1994; Dewey et al. 1999) and the Bangladeshi cohort study (Huffman et al. 1987) suggest that exclusive breastfeeding through 6 months of age is associated with delayed resumption of menses, at least in settings with high breastfeeding frequency. The more prolonged lactational amenorrhea represents an additional advantage of continued exclusive breastfeeding in developing country settings.

The two Honduran trials also found prolonged exclusive breastfeeding to be associated with more rapid maternal postpartum weight loss (Dewey et al. 2001). Such an effect would be an additional benefit if it were generalizable to developed country settings where gestational weight gains and postpartum weight retention are high, but would be a disadvantage if it applied to undernourished women in developing countries.

In the two Honduran trials, mothers allocated to the prolonged exclusive breastfeeding group reported that their infants crawled at a significantly younger age (Dewey et al. 2001). No such difference was seen in the age at which the infants first sat from lying position, and the results for walking by 12 months of age differed in the two trials. The inconsistency of these results, coupled with the potential for biased maternal reporting due to nonblinding, suggest the need for cautious interpretation and further study.

In summary, we found no objective evidence of a "weanling's dilemma." Besides their reduced morbidity due to gastrointestinal tract infection, infants breastfed exclusively for 6 or more months had no observable deficits in growth, and their mothers were more likely to remain amenorrheic for 6 months postpartum. No benefits of introducing complementary foods between 4 and 6 months have been demonstrated, with the exception of improved iron status in one developing country setting (Honduras) (Dewey et al. 1998b). Since the latter benefit can be achieved more effectively by medicinal iron supplementation (e.g., vitamin drops), it does not appear to justify incurring the adverse effects of liquid or solid food supplementation on infectious morbidity, and lactational amenorrhea.

Thus, with the caveat that infants must be managed individually, so that insufficient growth or other adverse outcomes are not ignored and appropriate interventions are provided, the available evidence demonstrates no apparent risks in recommending, as a general policy, exclusive breastfeeding for the first 6 months of life in both developing and developed country settings. In fact, based on results of this systematic review, the World Health Organization and the World Health Assembly recently revised its infant feeding recommendations to recommend exclusive breastfeeding for 6 months (WHO 2001b). Large, rigorous cluster-randomized trials should help resolve residual uncertainties about the advantages and disadvantages of such a policy.

6. ACKNOWLEDGMENTS

Supported in part by the Canadian Cochrane Network and by the Department of Nutrition for Health and Development, World Health Organization, Geneva, Switzerland.

7. REFERENCES

[AAP] American Academy of Pediatrics, Committee on Nutrition. Pediatric Nutrition Handbook. 4th Edition. Elk Grove Village, Illinois: American Academy of Pediatrics, 1998.

Adair L, Popkin B, Vanderslice J, Akin J, Guilkey D, Black R, Briscoe J, Flieger W. Growth dynamics during the first two years of life: a prospective study in teh Phillipines. Eur J Clin Nutr 1993;47:42-51.

Ahn C, MacLean WJr. Growth of the exlusively breast-fed infant. Am J Clin Nutr 1980;33:183-192.

Åkeson P, Axelsson I, Raiha N. Human milk and standard infant formula together with high quality supplementary foods is sufficient for normal growth during infancy. Pediatr Res 1996;39 (Suppl):313A.

Åkeson P, Axelsson I, Raiha N. Growth and nutrient intake in three-to-twelve-month-old infants fed human milk or formulas with varying protein concentrations. J Pediatr Gastroenterol Nutr 1998a;26:1-8.

Åkeson P, Axelsson I, Raiha N. Protein and amino acid metabolism in three-to-twelve-month-old infants fed human milk or formulas with varying protein concentrations. J Pediatr Gastroenterol Nutr 1998b;26:297-304.

Beaudry M, Dufour R, Marcoux S. Relation between infant feeding and infections during the first six months of life. J Pediatr 1995;126:191-197.

Brown K. The relationship between diarrhoeal prevalence and growth of poor infants varies with their age and usual energy intake. FASEB J 1991;5:A1079.

Brown K, Dewey K, Allen L. Complementary Feeding of Young Children in Developing Countries: A Review of Current Scientific Knowledge. Geneva: WHO, 1998.

Butte N. Energy requirements of infants. Eur J Clin Nutr 1996;50(Suppl):24-36.

Castillo C, Atalah E, Riumallo J, Castro R. Breast-feeding and the nutritional status of nursing children in Chile. Bull PAHO 1996;30:125-133.

Cohen R, Brown K, Canahuati J, Rivera L, Dewey K. Effects of age of introduction of complementary foods on infant breast milk intake, total energy intake, and growth: a randomized intervention study in Honduras. Lancet 1994;344:288-293.

Cohen R, Brown K, Canahuati J, Rivera L, Dewey K. Determinants of growth from birth to 12 months among breast-fed Honduran infants in relation to age of introduction of complementary foods. Pediatrics 1995;96:504-510.

Cunningham A, Jelliffe D, Jelliffe E. Breast-feeding and health in the 1980's: a global epidemiologic review. J Pediatr 1991;118:659-666.

Dewey K, Heinig M, Nommsen-Rivers L. Differences in morbidity between breast-fed and formula fed infants. J Pediatr 1995a;126:696-702.

Dewey K, Peerson J, Brown K, Krebs N, Michaelsen K, Persson L, Salmenpera L, Whitehead RG, Yeung DL. Growth of breast-fed infants deviates from current reference data: a pooled analysis of US, Canadian, and European data sets. Pediatrics 1995b;96:495-503.

Dewey K, Cohen R, Rivera L, Canahuati J, Brown K. Do exclusively breast-fed infants require extra protein? Pediatr Res 1996;39:303-307.

Dewey K, Cohen R, Rivera L, Canahuati J, Brown K. Effects of age at introduction of complementary foods to breast-fed infants on duration of lactational amenorrhea in Honduran women. Am J Clin Nutr 1997;65:1403-1409.

Dewey K, Cohen R, Rivera L, Brown K. Effects of age of introduction of complementary foods on micronutrient status of term, low-birthweight, breastfed infants in Honduras. FASEB J 1998a;12:A648.

Dewey K, Cohen R, Rivera L, Brown K. Effects of age introduction of complementary foods on iron status of breast-fed infants in Honduras. Am J Clin Nutr 1998b;67:878-884.

Dewey K, Cohen R, Brown K, Rivera L. Age of introduction of complementary foods and growth of term, low-birthweight, breast-fed infants: a randomized intervention study in Honduras. Am J Clin Nutr 1999;69:679-686.

Dewey K, Cohen R, Brown K, Rivera L. Effects of exclusive breastfeeding for four versus six months on maternal nutritional status and infant motor development: results of two randomized trials in Honduras. J Nutr 2001;131:262-267.

Duncan B, Ey J, Holberg C, Wright A, Martinez F, Taussig L. Exclusive breast-feeding for at least 4 months protects against otitis media. Pediatrics 1993;91:867-872.

[FAO/WHO] Food and Agriculture Organization of the United Nations/World Health Organization. Energy and protein requirements. 52: FAO Nutrition meetings. Rome: FAO, 1973.

Frongillo EJ, de Onis M, Garza C. The World Health Organization Task Force on Methods for the Natural Regulation of Fertility. Effects of timing of complementary foods on post-natal growth. FASEB J 1997;11:A574.

Garza C, Butte N. Energy intakes of human milk-fed infants during the first year. J Pediatr 1990;117:S124-S131.

Gourbin C, Masuy-Stroobant G. Registration of vital data: are live births and stillbirths comparable all over Europe? Bull WHO 1995;73:449-460.

Haschke F, van't Hof M, Euro-growth study groups. Euro-Growth references for breast-fed boys and girls: influence of breast-feeding and solids on growth until 36 months of age. J Pediatr Gastroenterol Nutr 2000;31:S60-S71.

Hediger M, Overpeck M, Ruan W, Troendle J. Early infant feeding and growth status of US-born infants and children aged 4-71 mo: analyses from the third National Health and Nutrition Examination Survey, 1988-1994. Am J Clin Nutr 2000;72:159-167.

Heinig J, Nommsen L, Peerson J, Lonnerdal B, Dewey K. Intake and growth of breast-fed and formula-fed infants in relation to the timing of introduction of complementary foods: the DARLING study. Acta Paediatr Scand 1993;82:999-1006.

Heiskanen K, Salmenpera L, Perheentupa J, Siimes M. Infant vitamin B-6 status changes with age and with formula feeding. Am J Clin Nutr 1994;60:907-910.

Howie P, Forsyth J, Ogston S, Clark A, du V Florey C. Protective effect of breast feeding against infection. Br Med J 1990;300:11-16.

Huffman S, Ford K, Allen H, Streble P. Nutrition and fertility in Bangladesh: breastfeeding and post partum amenorrhoea. Popul Stud 1987;41:447-462.

Jadad AR, Moore RA, Carroll D, Jenkinson C, Reynolds DJ, Gavaghan DJ, McQuay HJ. Assessing the quality of reports of randomized clinical trials: is blinding necessary? Control Clin Trials 1996;17:1-12.

Kajosaari M. Atopy prophylaxis in high-risk infants. Prospective 5-year follow-up study of children with six months exclusive breastfeeding and solid food elimination. Adv Exp Med Biol 1991;310:453-458.

Kajosaari M. Atopy prevention in childhood: the role of diet: a prospective 5-year follow-up of high-risk infants with six months exclusive breastfeeding and solid food elimination. Pediatr Allerg Immunol 1994;5:26-28.

Kajosaari M, Saarinen U. Prophylaxis of atopic disease by six months' total solid food elimination. Evaluation of 135 exclusively breast-fed infants of atopic families. Acta Paediatr Scand 1983;72:411-414.

Kallio M, Salmenpera L, Siimes M, Perheentupa J, Miettinen T. Exclusive breast-feeding and weaning: effect on serum cholesterol and lipoprotein concentrations in infants during the first year of life. Pediatrics 1992;89:663-666.

Khan M. Breastfeeding, growth and diarrhoea in rural Bangladesh children. Hum Nutr Clin Nutr 1984;38:113-119.

Kramer MS, Chalmers B, Hodnett ED. Breastfeeding and infant growth: biology or bias? Pediatr Res 2000a;47:151A.

Kramer MS, Chalmers B, Hodnett ED, Sevkovs.kaya Z, Dzikovich I, Shapiro S, Collet JP, Vanilovich I, Mezen I, Ducruet T, Shishko G, Zubovich V, Mknuik D, Gluchanina E, Dombrovsky V, Ustinovitch A, Ko T, Bogdanovich N, Ovchinikova L, Helsing E. Promotion of breastfeeding intervention trial (PROBIT): A cluster-randomized trial in the Republic of Belarus. In: Koletzko B, Michaelsen KF, Hernell O, editors. Short and Long Term Effects of Breast Feeding on Child Health. New York: Kluwer Academic/Plenum Publishers, 2000b:327-345.

Kramer MS, Chalmers B, Hodnett ED, Sevkovs.kaya Z, Dzikovich I, Shapiro S, Collet JP, Vanilovich I, Mezen I, Ducruet T, Shishko G, Zubovich V, Mknuik D, Gluchanina E, Dombrovskiy V, Ustinovitch A, Kot T, Bogdanovich N, Ovchinikova L, Helsing E; PROBIT Study Group. Promotion of breastfeeding intervention trial (PROBIT): A randomized trial in the Republic of Belarus. JAMA 2001;285:413-420.

Kramer MS, Guo T, Platt RW, Shapiro S, Collet JP, Chalmers B, Hodnett E, Sevkovskaya Z, Dzikovich I, Vanilovich I; PROBIT Study Group. Breastfeeding and infant growth: biology or bias? Pediatrics 2002;110(2 Pt 1):343-347.

Lutter C. Length of exclusive breastfeeding: linking biology and scientific evidence to a public health recommendation. J Nutr 2000;130:1335-1338.

Nielsen G, Thomsen B, Michaelsen K. Influence of breastfeeding and complementary food on growth between 5 and 10 months. Acta Paediatr 1998;87:911-917.

Oddy W, Holt P, Sly P, Read A, Landau L, Stanley F, Kendall GE, Burton PR. Association between breast feeding and asthma in 6 year old children: findings of a prospective birth cohort study. BMJ 1999;319:815-819.

Pisacane A, De Vizia B, Valiante A, Vaccaro F, Russo M, Grillo G, Giustardi A. Iron status in breast-fed infants. J Pediatr 1995;127:429-431.

Raisler J, Alexander C, O'Campo P. Breast-feeding and infant illness: a dose-response relationship? Am J Public Health 1999;89:25-30.

Rao S, Kanade A. Prolonged breast-feeding and malnutrition among rural Indian children below 3 years of age. Eur J Clin Nutr 1992;46:187-195.

Rowland M. The weanling's dilemma: Are we making progress? Acta Paediatr Scand 1986;323(Suppl):33-42.

Rowland M, Barrell R, Whitehead R. Bacterial contamination in traditional Gambian weaning foods. Lancet 1978;i:136-138.

Savilahti E, Tainio V, Salmenpera L, Siimes M, Perheentupa J. Prolonged exclusive breast feeding and heredity as determinants in infantile atopy. Arch Dis Child 1987;62:269-273.

Simondon K, Simondon F. Age at introduction of complementary food and physical growth from 2 to 9 months in rural Senegal. Eur J Clin Nutr 1997;51:703-707.

[UNICEF] United Nations Children's Fund. Facts for Life. Wallingford: P&LA, 1993.

Waterlow J, Thomson A. Observations on the adequacy of breast-feeding. Lancet 1979;ii:238-241.

Whitehead R, Paul A. Infant growth and human milk requirements. Lancet 1981;161-163.

Whitehead R, Paul A. Growth charts and the assessment of infant feeding practices in the western world and in developing countries. Early Hum Dev 1984;9:187-207.

[WHO] World Health Organization. Indicators for Assessing Breast-Feeding Practices. Geneva: WHO Document WHO/CDD/SER 1991;91:14.

[WHO] World Health Organization. Working Group on Infant Growth. An evaluation of infant growth. Geneva: WHO, 1994.

[WHO] World Health Organization. Information and attitudes among health personnel about early feeding practices. WHO Wkly Epidemiol 1995a;117-120.

[WHO] World Health Organization. Working Group on Infant Growth. An evaluation of infant growth: the use and interpretation of anthropometry in infants. Bull WHO 1995b;73:165-174.

[WHO] World Health Organization. Collaborative Study Team on the Role of Breastfeeding on the Prevention of Infant Mortality. Effect of breastfeeding on infant and child mortality due to infectious diseases in less developed countries: a pooled analysis. Lancet 2001a;355:451-455.

[WHO] World Health Organization. Infant and young child nutrition. Fifty-fourth World Health Assembly. Geneva: WHO 54.2;2001b

[WHO] World Health Organization. Working Group on the Growth Reference Protocol and WHO Task Force on Methods for the Natural Regulation of Fertility. Growth of healthy infants and the timing, type, and frequency of complementary foods. Am J Clin Nutr 2002;76:620-627.

EXPERT CONSULTATION ON THE OPTIMAL DURATION OF EXCLUSIVE BREASTFEEDING

The Process, Recommendations, and Challenges for the Future

Jean-Pierre Habicht

1. ABSTRACT

In March, 2001 The World Health Organization (WHO) convened an Expert Consultation to recommend to WHO an optimal duration of exclusive breastfeeding. WHO formulated the specific questions to be addressed, selected the membership for the meeting, prepared background documents, and provided the venue for the meeting. After the meeting WHO formally accepted the recommendations and began to implement them.

The Consultation recommended that WHO change its recommendation on exclusive breastfeeding from four-to-six months to a recommendation to promote exclusive breastfeeding for six months. This recommendation was contingent upon WHO also accepting and implementing other recommendations to deal with possible detrimental side effects, and to support mothers who did not exclusively breastfeed for six months.

The amount of scientific evidence available was more than is often available for policy decisions in health, but much less than desirable to address issues of generalizability across and within populations. The evidence for the contingent recommendations was also less than desirable and raises a number of important research questions that now need to be addressed.

2. INTRODUCTION

The World Health Organization (WHO) was concerned that different United Nations agencies and different countries around the world were recommending two different durations of optimal exclusive breastfeeding. Some agencies recommended six months duration while WHO and other agencies recommended that complementary feeding be initiated between four and six months, thereby implying a duration of four months of

---

Division of Nutritional Sciences, Cornell University, Ithaca, NY 14853

Protecting Infants through Human Milk, edited by Pickering *et al.*
Kluwer Academic/Plenum Publishers, 2004

exclusive breastfeeding. WHO did not believe that either of these recommendations had been subjected to careful scientific review and hoped that such a review would resolve the controversy.

To that end, an Expert Consultation was convened on March 28-30, 2001, at the World Health Organization in Geneva, Switzerland. Organized under the direction of Mercedes de Onis, of the Nutrition Unit, with the help of Jose Martines from the Child and Adolescent Health Division, the purpose of the consultation was to decide which of the two recommendations for optimal duration of exclusive breastfeeding should be supported. The availability of two recommendations was a cause of confusion to health policy makers and providers.

Science is translated into public policy and action through various mechanisms. The mechanism of an expert consultation is one with which scientists tend to be comfortable, in part because it is more transparent and provides opportunities for significant input by scientists. This summary highlights features of the process, describes the conclusions, and considers the challenges that it presents for future research.

3. THE CONSULTATION PROCESS

The first step was to specify the issue in the form of a mandate for the consultation. This was formulated as follows:

(a) To review the scientific evidence on the optimal duration of exclusive breastfeeding

(b) To formulate recommendations for practice on optimal duration of exclusive breastfeeding

(c) To formulate recommendations for research needs in this area.

In preparation for the consultation a set of background papers was prepared, which included the following:

(a) The optimal duration of exclusive breastfeeding: a systematic review (Kramer & Kakuma 2002)

(b) Nutrient adequacy of exclusive breastfeeding for the term infant during the first six months of life (Butte et al. 2002)

(c) Description of worldwide exclusive breastfeeding practices by Mercedes De Onis (unpublished).

The first of these papers by Michael Kramer is included in this volume (Kramer & Kakuma 2004), although the annexes of the report are not. The information presented in the annexes (Kramer & Kakuma 2002) was particularly important in the deliberations of the consultation because the data are presented so fully that Kramer's conclusions in the report could be validated or challenged. Kramer's background paper went through a particularly exhaustive review process. It was sent widely to scientists who had been involved in research related to the duration of breastfeeding. Many of these scientists had strongly held views about the optimum duration of exclusive breastfeeding. Individuals submitted their reviews of the Kramer report, which were then shared with the participants to the consultation, and which he took into account in the final document.

An important step in the consultation process was the selection of the participants. The following people were invited and accepted: Maharaj K Bhan, India; Zulfiqar A Bhutta, Pakistan; Nancy F Butte, USA; Cutberto Garza, USA; Rosalind S Gibson, New Zealand; Jean-Pierre Habicht, USA (chair); Michael S Kramer, Canada; Anna Lartey, Ghana; James Neilson, UK; Kirsten Simondon, France; Cesar G Victora, Brazil; Narada Warnasuriya, Sri Lanka.The expertise of these individuals is fundamentally biological. Some are clinicians, and others are public health experts. A few have expertise in the more basic sciences. None have expertise in the social, economic, or political sciences. Most had contributed significantly to scientific knowledge about breastfeeding, and many had produced information relative to the optimum duration of breastfeeding. However, not all of the scientists who have made major contributions to knowledge about the optimum duration were members of the consultation.

Reviewing the participant list, my feeling is that before they were invited to the meeting most of them were generally in favor of retaining the WHO recommendation of exclusive breastfeeding from four to six months. Some of them became more favorably inclined to the six-month recommendation because of research that they undertook in the interim between the time of the invitation and the meeting. Before the meeting, my own view was one of ambivalence, based in part by the knowledge that a six-month duration of exclusive breastfeeding did not fit present majority practice in any society in the world today, and because I did not believe that the possible downsides of recommending longer breastfeeding had been properly examined (Frongillo & Habicht 1997). However, I understood that there were other legitimate reasons for the change, not least of which was the fact that the six-month recommendation was already in place, or rapidly moving into place, in many countries and in some international organizations.

WHO asked me to chair the consultation only a week before it took place, and I had not participated in its preparation. Therefore, I asked what flexibility the consultation would have in making recommendations that were likely to be followed up. I was assured that WHO would accept and follow up any recommendation made by the consultation, whether for maintaining the four- to six-month recommendation or for changing it to a six-month recommendation, or any other recommendation for a specific duration. However, a recommendation that more research was needed in order to make a recommendation would not be acceptable.

4. THE ORGANIZATION OF THE MEETING

The process that was used to conduct the consultation consisted of a series of plenary and drafting group sessions. The first substantive sessions were devoted to presentation and discussion of the background papers. This was followed by short presentations outlining the formulation of recommendations for practice and for research. Two drafting groups were then convened to draw up preliminary recommendations for practice and for research. The final sessions of the meeting were devoted to discussion of the recommendations from the two drafting groups in order to arrive at statements that constituted the recommendations of the Expert Consultation (WHO 2002).

Early in the meeting, a critical discussion about the criteria for evidence to arrive at a recommendation was held. The consultation participants considered the criteria presented in Kramer's background document (Kramer & Kakuma 2002) and decided that major weight should be given to randomized trials. In the case of breastfeeding, a randomized trial is one in which there is an intervention to increase breastfeeding to six months that is randomly provided to half the units in the study (individuals, villages, or hospitals.) The other half receives a control intervention.

Randomized trials have the advantage of transforming potential systematic biases into random error. This means that one may interpret the statistical probability (e.g., $P<0.05$), demonstrating a difference between the intervention and control group as due to the intervention and not due to some intrinsic extraneous difference between the comparison groups. This is the gold standard used in drug trials.

An important caveat in interpreting the results from a randomized trial is that a statistically significant result means only that the outcome is probably due to the intervention, not necessarily to the component of the intervention that one may think is the cause. For instance, biased measurements due to the measurers knowing which group received which intervention is certainly caused by the intervention, but is clearly not due to the presumed biological mechanism. Another potential problem in public health trials is that the test and control interventions may be dissimilar not only in the component of the intervention to be investigated, but also in other aspects, and one of these other aspects might be the reason for the results.

One member of the consultation felt strongly that only the results from randomized trials should be used in making policy decisions. We could not have arrived at a decision based solely on the results of the available randomized trials. I believe that the future will show that reliance only on randomized trials for public health and nutrition policy will lead to poorer decisions than using a more comprehensive approach (Victora et al., in press).

A second criterion discussed by the members of the consultation was that only studies that had been published in the peer-reviewed, scientific literature were considered. Only Kay Dewey, Rebecca Cohen, and their colleagues from the University of California at Davis had conducted randomized trials that addressed the optimal limits of exclusive breastfeeding. Without the results presented in their exhaustive publications (cited in Kramer & Kakuma 2002), the consultation could not have arrived at its unanimous conclusions. In addition, the results of a recently completed but not yet published randomized hospital trial in Belarus with findings in favor of a six-month recommendation (Kramer et al. 2003) also played an important role in the decision.

Another issue concerning criteria was the problem of generalizing results from a trial to other situations in which conditions are different. For instance, breastfeeding improves infant survival more in conditions where water and sanitation are poor (Habicht et al. 1988). Thus, a finding of little effect of breastfeeding on mortality in an economically advantaged population cannot be extrapolated to an economically disadvantaged population. The literature review did not address this issue, although it did differentiate between findings from economically developed and developing countries.

In the Systematic Review background paper, Kramer also reviewed other trials, which I call high "plausibility" trials (Habicht et al. 1999). These are studies in which, one can plausibly infer that the findings were caused by the intervention. This can be done by amassing evidence that the pathway from intervention to outcome was as expected, or by showing that the effects are modified by other factors as expected (Habicht et al. 1988), or by exclusion of other likely possible reasons (Habicht et al. 1986), or preferably by some combination of these approaches.

Early on in the meeting, some members felt that participants should declare their position about the duration of exclusive breastfeeding. I believed that a debate about that issue before we had explored all the ramifications of each of the possibilities would lock us into positions from which it would be difficult to move in seeking unanimity through compromise. Indeed, we all compromised from our initial positions on many issues, so that permitting ambiguity until we had to make a decision was useful. The recommendations reflect these compromises.

During the consultation, contrary opinions were strongly held and vigorously presented. It is noteworthy that none of the statistical results of the scientific studies discussed were called into question, nor were there disagreements that overall the statistical results in favor of a benefit were due to exclusive ingestion of human milk. The most important disagreements were about the unknown harm that could be done by a recommendation about which there was so little scientific information, and that no new drug would be released in the same circumstances. Another issue was that a proven benefit to most in a population does not preclude that some might suffer ill effects; a major concern to clinicians. My experience is that clinicians tend to be more concerned about harm to the few; public health tends to favor action that is beneficial to the many. In this case, the trade-off in favor of the proven benefits of exclusive breastfeeding in areas with poor sanitation and poor human milk substitutes overcame the clinicians' qualms.

The participants in the consultation also were concerned that the vast majority of mothers do not exclusively breastfeed for six months, and that efforts need to be made to establish policy about how to deal with this issue. This policy must include recommendations for the care and feeding of infants whose mothers do not extend exclusive breastfeeding to six months.

Another concern was about the societal infrastructure to support the recommendation. The consultation was not organized to deal with this issue, or any other behavioral or economic issues. In my opinion this reflects an implicit and mistaken view, also seen in many other health care settings, that only the biology of the situation is relevant. Fortunately, the participants were sensitive to the issue. These and other concerns are reflected in the recommendations.

5. THE RECOMMENDATIONS OF THE COMMITTEE

The major recommendations *for practice* in response to the mandate given to the consultation are as follows:

> **The Expert Consultation recommends exclusive breastfeeding for six months, with introduction of complementary foods and continued breastfeeding thereafter. This recommendation applies to populations. The Expert Consultation recognizes that some mothers will be unable to, or choose not to, follow this recommendation. These mothers should also be supported to optimize their infants' nutrition.**

It is notable that the main recommendation has two parts. The second part implies there will be no coercion to exclusively breastfeed.

There followed some ancillary considerations directed to fostering exclusive breastfeeding to six months, including promoting the health and nutrition of mother and child. Then came a sequence of recommendations in response to concerns that arose during the consultation.

> **The Expert Consultation also recognizes the need for complementary feeding at six months of age and recommends the introduction of nutritionally adequate, safe and appropriate complementary foods, in conjunction with continued breastfeeding.**

The Expert Consultation recognizes that exclusive breastfeeding to six months is still infrequent. However, it also notes that there have been substantial increases over time in several countries, particularly where lactation support is available. A prerequisite to the implementation of these recommendations is the provision of adequate social and nutritional support to lactating women.

6. CHALLENGES FOR FUTURE SCIENTIFIC WORK

The committee noted the paucity of data to address the questions raised by WHO and to address ancillary issues that arose during the consultation, and it issued the following recommendations for research:

The Expert Consultation recommends the following priority research areas:

(a) A comparison of exclusive breastfeeding/predominant breastfeeding and partial breastfeeding for four to six months on the following outcomes, to improve precision of estimates and their general applicability:

- **proportion with growth faltering and malnutrition at six and twelve months**
- **micronutrient status**
- **diarrhoeal morbidity**
- **neuromotor development**
- **changes in maternal weight**
- **lactational amenorrhoea**

Priority must be given to investigating these outcomes in infants born small-for-gestational-age or, alternatively, in those with low-weight-for-age at four months.

(b) Assess breast-milk production and composition from mothers with a body mass index <18.5 and the adequacy of breast milk for meeting infant requirements to six months.

(c) It is recognized that rates of exclusive breastfeeding decline substantially after four months. Identify biological and social constraints to exclusive breastfeeding to six months in different geographical and cultural settings, and develop appropriate and effective interventions to deal with these barriers and their consequences.

(d) Use available opportunities to gain greater insight into the impact on mortality of exclusive breastfeeding to six months. Example: incorporate additional variables in the Demographic and Health Surveys.

(e) Develop and evaluate interventions for micronutrient supplementation and for complementary foods in different areas of the world. This would include formative studies to identify processing and preparation methods, and local ingredients required to prepare nutritionally adequate, safe and appropriate complementary foods.

(f) Assess the role of care during pregnancy in relation to the adequacy of lactation in the first six months.

Another way to conceptualize the research recommendations is to describe them in terms of the challenges that the "recommendations for practice" imply. I have made a list of issues that I think are important and formulated them as questions toward which research should be directed. Some of these questions are biological, but many require other types of expertise, including economics, anthropology, organizational psychology, political science. This expertise currently is not being applied to these challenges.

Challenge 1

- How do we support mothers to exclusively breastfeed for six months?
- How do we motivate societies to provide mothers with the incentives (remove disincentives) for six months of exclusive breastfeeding?

Challenge 2

- How to identify mothers who **cannot** produce enough milk for six months of exclusive breastfeeding?
    - How many are in this category? To date the conventional wisdom is that this is rare, but data are so scarce that we have no idea about prevalence.
    - What are determinants of biologic failure to exclusively breastfeed to six months, and how can these determinants be influenced? One determinant appears to be severe maternal malnutrition (Gonzalez-Cossio et al. 1998). The solution is not to curtail breastfeeding, but to feed the mother. This solution often is not obvious to policy makers and program officers in the field. Promoting such insights require research not just into the biology, but also into human and institutional behavior.

Challenge 3

- How to conceptualize and model trade-offs between six months of exclusive breastfeeding and other uses of resources, including maternal time?

Challenge 4

- How do we develop an integrated strategy to make human milk substitutes and complementary feeding available to mothers who do not wish to or cannot effectively breastfeed for six months?

Challenge 5

- How do we harmonize the findings that children who exclusively breastfeed to six months typically are sufficiently depleted in iron and zinc that no readily available complementary foods can meet their requirements thereafter? (To date, the only solution proposed is micronutrient supplementation during exclusive breastfeeding and thereafter. How does this fit with the fact that our species evolved without such supplementation?

Challenge 6

- What motivation is there to do the research necessary to elucidate the benefits and disbenefits of exclusive breastfeeding between four to six months now that "everybody knows" that exclusive breastfeeding to six months is best?
- Is there any serious interest in the question of "optimal for what"?

I am concerned that addressing these questions will be regarded as unnecessary now that the recommendation has been made in favor of six months.

Challenge 7

- How long should we promote breastfeeding after six months? Present WHO recommendations are two years. How do we promote it?
- How do we proceed to assure appropriate food to complement continued breastfeeding after six months? Historically efforts have concentrated on local self-sufficiency and public action. This is not enough. To meet this challenge and the other challenges cited above that involve infant foods, it is certain that some solutions will be provided by the private sector. How, in this context, are we to develop a constructive relationship with the private sector to promote the best nutrition for infants?

7. CONCLUSIONS

While the main thrust of this commentary has been on the recommendations and future research needs, I also have reviewed the consultation process in order to highlight particular features. Aside from historic importance, the consultation was noteworthy for its process. The consultation was organized to permit differing points of view, at the same time as ensuring that the process did not degenerate into bickering without being able to come to a consensus. This consultation was notable for its lack of bickering, a major mark of the quality of its preparation.

The extensive investment in preparing for the consultation was, in my view, an important element in being able to achieve the goal that was set for it. A major innovation was the wide circulation of the background paper before the meeting, the circulation of the reviewers' comments to the future participants of the consultation, and the circulation of the second draft to all involved. An author rarely can satisfy all reviewers. I also would have found it useful to have had available at the consultation the views of reviewers who were not satisfied. This would have provided the opportunity to address their concerns explicitly in the consultation.

When similar types of consultations are required in the future, an additional feature to consider would be the use of a preparatory meeting that would include persons who can fairly represent the views of important stakeholders in the final decision. The purposes of this meeting would be to review the question for which the organization requires an answer and further develop the framework for addressing it. This framework would permit the identification of questions not envisaged by the organization, but which will have to be dealt with by the consultation. As the Expert Consultation on the Optimal Duration of Exclusive Breastfeeding did not have the benefit of that process, the ancillary recommendations were not supported by the background documents and the expertise needed to make firm recommendations on these subjects. Such a preparatory meeting would have added expense and time to the whole process—but I would encourage future consultations to make this investment.

The Expert Consultation on the Optimal Duration of Exclusive Breastfeeding fulfilled the mandate it was given. It offered WHO recommendations for practice that have helped to reduce policy and programmatic conflicts within and between agencies. This has not only permitted a clearer focus within breastfeeding promotion programs, but also helped to remove barriers to program and research activities on complementary feeding. At the same time, as outlined in the previous sections, the consultation identified important research needs on breastfeeding that also need serious attention, particularly now that a global recommendation is in place. It would be an unfortunate, even tragic, outcome for public health and for the welfare of mothers and children if these issues are not addressed with the same rigor and care that produced the data on which the recommendations were made.

8. ACKNOWLEDGMENT

I thank Gretel Pelto for a critical review of this paper leading to major changes.

9. REFERENCES

Butte NF, Lopez-Alarcon MG, Garza C, Nutrient adequacy of exclusive breastfeeding for the term infant during the first six months of life. Geneva: World Health Organization, 2002. Available in hard copy from WHO or on the web at www.who.int/nut/documents/nut_adequacy_of_exc_bfeeding_eng.pdf; or http://www.who.int/nut/documents/nut_adequacy_of_exc_bfeeding_eng.pdf.

Frongillo EA Jr, Habicht J-P. Investigating the weanling's dilemma: Lessons from Honduras. Nutr Rev 1997;55:390-395.

Gonzalez-Cossio T, Habicht J-P, Rasmussen K, Delgado HL. Impact of food supplementation during lactation on infant breast-milk intake and on the proportion of infants exclusively breast-fed. J Nutr1998;128:1692-1702.

Habicht J-P, DaVanzo J, Butz WP. Does breastfeeding really save lives, or are apparent benefits due to biases? Am J Epidemiol 1986;123:279-290.

Habicht J-P, DaVanzo J, Butz WP. Mother's milk and sewage: Their interactive effects on infant mortality. Pediatrics 1988;81:456-461.

Habicht J-P, Victora CG, Vaughan JP. Evaluation designs for adequacy, plausibility and probability of public health programme performance and impact. Int J Epidemiol 1999;28:10-18.

Kramer MS, Kakuma R. The optimal duration of exclusive breastfeeding: A systematic review. Geneva: World Health Organization, 2002. Available with the annexes from WHO in hard copy or on the web at www.who.int/nut/documents/optimal_duration_of_exc_bfeeding_review_eng.pdf; or http://www.who.int/nut/documents/optimal_duration_of_exc_bfeeding_review_eng.pdf.

Kramer MS, Kakuma R. The optimal duration of exclusive breastfeeding: a systematic review. In: Pickering LK, Morrow AL, Ruiz-Palacios GM, Schanler RJ. Protecting Infants through Human Milk: Advancing the Scientific Evidence. Advances in Experimental Medicine and Biology Series. New York: Kluwer Academic/Plenum Publishers, 2004; this volume.

Kramer MS, Guo T, Platt RW, Sevkovskaya Z, Dzikovich I, Collet JP, Shapiro S, Chalmers B, Hodnett E, Vanilovich I, Mezen I, Ducruet T, Shishko G, Bogdanovich N. Infant growth and health outcomes associated with 3 compared with 6 mo of exclusive breastfeeding. Am J Clin Nutr 2003;78:291-295.

Victora CG, Habicht J-P, Bryce J. Evidence-based public health: Moving beyond randomized trials. Am J Public Health (in press).

[WHO] World Health Organization. The Optimal Duration of Exclusive Breastfeeding: Report of an Expert Consultation, 28-30 March 2001. Geneva: World Health Organization, 2002. Available in hard copy from WHO or on the web at: www.who.int/nut/documents/optimal_duration_of_exc_bfeeding_report_eng.pdf; or www.who.int/nut/documents/optimal_duration_of_exc_bfeeding_report_eng.pdf.

SECTION III

BREASTFEEDING FROM THE MOTHER'S PERSPECTIVE

IMPACT OF BREASTFEEDING ON MATERNAL NUTRITIONAL STATUS

Kathryn G. Dewey

1. ABSTRACT

This review covers the impact of breastfeeding on maternal postpartum weight loss and micronutrient status. Results regarding the impact on weight loss have been conflicting. This may be due to differences in study quality. Of six observational studies in which postpartum weight change was *estimated* (rather than measured directly), only one showed an association with breastfeeding. By contrast, six of the seven studies in which postpartum weight change was *measured* showed greater weight or fat loss in women who breastfed longer, particularly at 3 to 6 months postpartum. The results of the higher quality studies are consistent with two experimental studies conducted in Honduras, which demonstrated that the degree of breastfeeding affects the rate of weight loss. Thus, it appears that breastfeeding does enhance the rate of weight loss postpartum, but the effect is relatively small and may not be detectable in studies that lack adequate statistical power, have imprecise data on postpartum weight change, or do not account for the exclusivity and/or duration of breastfeeding. There is very little information with regard to micronutrient status during lactation. Nutrient requirements for vitamins A, B_6, and C, and for iodine and zinc are increased by more than 50%, but lactation may actually be protective against maternal iron deficiency. More research is needed on the effects of lactation on maternal nutritional status and on strategies for optimizing nutrient intake to meet the needs of both the mother and her infant.

2. INTRODUCTION

There has been considerable debate regarding the influence of lactation on changes in maternal weight and body composition postpartum (Butte & Hopkinson 1998; Winkvist & Rasmussen 1999). Although it is generally acknowledged that, on average, women lose weight and body fat during lactation (Winkvist & Rasmussen 1999), it has been pointed out that there is a great deal of individual variation (Butte & Hopkinson 1998). Results have been mixed with regard to the question of whether lactating women

---

Department of Nutrition, One Shields Avenue, University of California, Davis, CA 95616-8669

Protecting Infants through Human Milk, edited by Pickering *et al.*
Kluwer Academic/Plenum Publishers, 2004

lose more weight than nonlactating women. In view of the variable quality of the studies on this issue, it is worthwhile to revisit this question.

Body composition is but one aspect of maternal nutritional status. To adequately assess the impact of lactation, one would need extensive biochemical data reflecting the mother's vitamin and mineral nutriture, as well as indicators of protein and fatty acid status. Because of the paucity of such data, previous reviews have generally focused solely on anthropometric outcomes.

In this chapter, an attempt is made to address both issues: the impact of lactation on weight loss postpartum and on maternal micronutrient status. In the first section, the focus is on studies that meet predefined minimum quality criteria and directly compare weight loss of lactating and nonlactating women. In the second section, a discussion of the theoretical micronutrient burden imposed by lactation is followed by a brief review of relevant studies. In both sections, only data for generally healthy women are considered (e.g., studies of HIV-positive women are not included).

3. EFFECT OF LACTATION ON MATERNAL WEIGHT LOSS POSTPARTUM

3.1. Theoretical Considerations

If there were no increase in maternal energy intake during lactation, relative to the nonpregnant, nonlactating state, the energy cost of lactation would result in substantial weight loss. The energy cost of milk production can be estimated based on average milk volume, the energy content of milk, and the energy required for milk synthesis. For exclusively breastfeeding women, the total energy cost is estimated to be 595 kcal/day at 0 to 2 months postpartum and 670 kcal/day at 3 to 6 months postpartum (Dewey 1997). Over the first 6 months of lactation, this would represent a total of 117,390 kcal. Assuming no other changes in energy metabolism, this would require the mobilization of approximately 13 kg of body fat in a 6-month period. This rate of weight loss is rare, so there must be alterations in energy expenditure and/or energy intake during lactation that compensate for the increased energy demand. There is little evidence for energy-sparing adaptations in energy expenditure during lactation, with the possible exception of reductions in physical activity (Prentice et al. 1996). Thus, increased energy intake remains as the principal explanation for why breastfeeding women do not lose as much weight as would be predicted by the amount of energy secreted in milk. The question is whether the increase in food intake, given no constraints on food availability, compensates *completely* for the energy cost of lactation.

There are several hormonal changes during lactation that may affect body composition or metabolism, many of which favor lipolysis (Butte & Hopkinson 1998). For example, lipoprotein lipase activity decreases and lipid mobilization increases in the femoral region (Rebuffe et al. 1985). On the other hand, the high levels of prolactin that occur during lactation are associated with increased appetite and food intake in animal studies (Grattan 2002). Prolactin receptors are up-regulated during lactation, and this phenomenon appears to play a long-term role in body weight regulation. Thus, on balance it is difficult to predict whether there should be a net loss in body weight among lactating women who are eating *ad libitum*.

3.2. Methodological Challenges

Evaluating the effect of breastfeeding on postpartum weight change in humans presents several methodological difficulties. Given that it is not ethical (or feasible) to randomly assign women to breastfeeding and nonbreastfeeding groups, the next best source of unbiased data are experimental studies in which the duration or exclusivity of breastfeeding have been altered by an intervention. There have been few intervention studies to date, however, so most of the information on this issue has come from observational studies. Potential confounding variables in observational studies are numerous and include maternal age, ethnicity, education, income, prepregnancy body mass index (BMI), pregnancy weight gain, parity, interbirth interval, physical activity, and dietary practices. Of particular importance is the intentional restriction of energy intake. Because it was long believed that breastfeeding women should not "diet," energy restriction is likely to be less common among lactating than among nonlactating women in industrialized countries. Studies that do not control for this possibility run the risk of not detecting a greater rate of weight loss associated with lactation.

A second methodological challenge is assessment of the outcome variable, in this case weight change postpartum. The ideal design is a longitudinal study, with a "baseline" weight measured within the first few weeks postpartum and subsequent weights measured during a follow-up period of a year or more. The timing of the first postpartum assessment is important because there is substantial fluid retention during the early postpartum period. It is desirable to wait until hydration status and short-term fluctuations in body composition have stabilized. The length of follow-up is also critical because weight loss associated with lactation may only be evident after some minimal duration of breastfeeding. Unfortunately, many observational studies are based on data that do not meet these ideal criteria. In some cases, weight data were based on self-reported weights, which often are biased. In others, postpartum weight was estimated by subtracting infant birth weight from a measured weight in late pregnancy, which does not account for the weight of the placenta and other tissues lost during childbirth. In many studies, the outcome variable was actually weight *retention* at some point postpartum, relative to prepregnancy weight, rather than weight *change* postpartum. Weight retention is the result of both weight gain during pregnancy and weight change postpartum. Women who gain more weight during pregnancy are likely to lose more weight postpartum (Butte & Hopkinson 1998). If the statistical analysis controls for pregnancy weight gain, then it is possible to examine factors associated with weight change postpartum. Otherwise, the risk of confounding is too great to draw conclusions about the relationship between breastfeeding and postpartum weight change.

Finally, the definition of "breastfeeding" varies greatly among studies. Ideally, data are collected on both the duration and the exclusivity of breastfeeding at several time points postpartum. Several investigators have developed a lactation "score" that is based on these two dimensions. Without actually measuring human milk intake, it is difficult to assess the exclusivity dimension. One approach is to measure the infant's intake of formula, other milks, and/or other nonhuman milk foods, as an inverse "proxy" of human milk intake. Another is to base the estimate on breastfeeding frequency (although the relationship between breastfeeding frequency and human milk intake is modest at best), or on the relative frequency of breastfeeds to feedings of formula or other milks. Many studies, however, lack any information on exclusivity of breastfeeding. Some are based solely on whether the infant was ever breastfed, regardless of whether this was for only a few days. Imprecise indicators for the degree of breastfeeding would make it more difficult to detect an association with weight change postpartum.

3.3. Experimental Studies

As mentioned, the best way to evaluate the effect of breastfeeding on maternal weight change is to compare groups for whom the degree of breastfeeding was randomly assigned. The only published data of this nature come from two studies in Honduras in which mothers were randomly assigned to breastfeed exclusively for six months (EBF), or to breastfeed exclusively for four months and to feed their infants complementary foods (while continuing to breastfeed) from four to six months (Dewey et al. 2001). Data on maternal weight change are available from 141 primiparous mothers in the first study and 119 mothers of term, low-birth-weight infants in the second study. In both studies, the EBF and complementary feeding groups were similar in weight and BMI at four months, before the intervention phase. Maternal weight loss from 4 to 6 months was significantly greater in the EBF than in the complementary feeding group in the first study, which reported a between-group difference of 0.6 kg, but not in the second study, which reported a between-group difference of 0.2 kg. The differing results of these two studies is attributable to the fact that the difference in milk energy output between the EBF and complementary feeding groups was much greater in the first study (a between-group difference of 5520 kcal during the 2-month interval) than in the second (a between-group difference of 2700 kcal). Assuming that nearly all of the weight lost was fat (9 kcal/g), these values are in close agreement with the between-group differences in maternal weight loss. Thus, the results support the conclusion that the degree of breastfeeding affects the rate of maternal weight loss during this time interval post-partum. It should be noted that only about 10% of the mothers in the Honduras studies had a low-body-mass index (<19 kg/m^2), so weight loss was not necessarily disadvantageous for most of the women.

3.4. Observational Studies

For this review, observational studies had to meet two quality criteria to be included: 1) sample size of >20 women per feeding group (e.g., lactating vs. nonlactating); and 2) assessment of postpartum weight change, or assessment of weight retention relative to prepregnancy status if the analysis controlled for pregnancy weight gain. Thirteen studies met these minimum criteria. Table 1 shows the seven studies in which postpartum weight change was actually measured, and Table 2 shows the six studies in which it was based on estimated weights or weight retention controlling for pregnancy weight gain. Except for one study in the Philippines (Adair & Popkin 1992), all of the studies were conducted in industrialized countries. There was considerable variability in sample size, the definition of breastfeeding, and the duration of follow-up postpartum. Of the seven studies with measured weight change (Table 1), six showed a significant association between greater breastfeeding and greater loss in weight or body fat, at least during certain time intervals (e.g., 3–6 months postpartum). Of these seven studies, the only study that did not report a significant association between greater breastfeeding and weight loss was a study that did not account for the exclusivity of breastfeeding (Dugdale & Eaton 1989). By contrast, of the six studies in which postpartum weight change was estimated (Table 2), only one (the largest) observed a significant relationship between breastfeeding and greater weight loss (Greene et al. 1988). Of these six studies, only two were able to

Table 1. Studies with *measured* postpartum weight change[a]

Study[b]	No.	BF definition	Outcome	BF associated with greater wt loss?
Adair 1992, Philippines	1620	Pred BF – no nutr. food or liquid	Weight change 2–24 mo	Yes
Butte 1998, USA	40 BF, 36 FF	EBF ≥4 mo	Change in fat mass 0–12 mo	Yes (FM 3–6 mo)
Dewey 1993, USA	46 BF, 39 FF	Full BF ≥12 mo	Weight change 1–24 mo	Yes
Dugdale 1988, Australia	151	Any BF: 0–3, 3–6, or >6 mo	Weight change 1–12 mo	No
Janney 1997, USA	110	Duration full or partial BF	Weight retention 0–20 mo	Yes
McKeown 1957, UK	1118	Full BF <3, 3–6, or 6+ mo	Weight change 3–24 mo	Yes
Ohlin 1990, Sweden	1423	Lactation score	Weight change 2.5–12 mo	Yes

[a]Abbreviations: BF=breastfed, FF=formula fed, Pred BF=predominantly BF, EBF=exclusively breastfed, FM=fat mass
[b]First author, date, country

Table 2. Studies with *estimated* postpartum weight change[a]

Study[b]	No.	BF Definition	Outcome	BF associated with greater wt loss?
Boardley 1995, USA	345	Any BF >1wk	Weight retention	No
Green 1998; USA	7116	Any BF	Weight retention	Yes
Haieck 2001, Canada	236	Pred BF, Mixed-fed, Pred FF	Weight change 0–9 mo	No
Harris 1997, USA	243	Any BF	Weight retention	No
Parker 1993, USA	2119	Duration–intensity score	Weight retention, ≥20 lb	No
Potter 1991, USA	411	Any BF ≥6 wk	Weight change 0–12 mo	No

[a]Abbreviations: BF=breastfed, FF=formula fed, Pred BF=predominantly BF, EBF=exclusively breastfed, FM=fat mass
[b]First author, date, country

account for the exclusivity of breastfeeding (Haiek et al. 2001; Parker & Abrams 1993) and three based the feeding groups solely on "any" breastfeeding since birth (Greene et al. 1988; Harris et al. 1997) or for ≥1 week postpartum (Boardley et al. 1995).

Five of the studies in Table 1 are of special interest because they used a precise definition of breastfeeding and categorized the groups in such a way that allows for evaluation of differences by degree of breastfeeding or the time interval when differences are most apparent. Butte and Hopkinson (1998) compared body composition changes in 40 women who breastfed exclusively for at least 4 months with those of 36 women who did not breastfeed at all. Weight loss from 0 to 12 months was not significantly different between groups (–4.9 vs. –3.6 kg in lactating vs. nonlactating women), but between 3 and 6 months postpartum loss in body fat was significantly greater in the lactating group than in the nonlactating group. Dewey et al. (1993) compared weight change of 46 women who breastfed exclusively for at least 4 months and continued to breastfeed as the sole source of milk for at least 12 months with that of 39 formula-feeding women matched to the breastfeeding group for initial anthropometric status and other characteristics. Excluding women who intentionally altered their diet to lose weight, weight loss was significantly greater in the former group than in the latter (–4.4 vs. –2.4 kg, 1–12 months), particularly from 3 to 6 months postpartum (–2.2 vs. –0.3 kg). Janney et al. (1997) categorized 110 women by the duration and degree of breastfeeding and found a significant dose-response relationship with weight retention postpartum, controlling for several potentially confounding variables such as pregnancy weight gain, age, education, parity, dietary fat, and physical activity. There was a difference of about –2 kg by 18 months postpartum between women who breastfed the longest and those who did not breastfeed. McKeown and Record (1957) evaluated weight change from 3 to 24 months postpartum in 1,118 women who fully breastfed for <3 months, 3–6 months, or ≥6 months. Statistical analyses of the data were not presented, but the weight loss patterns reveal that women who breastfed the longest lost about 1.1 kg more by 12 months than those who breastfed the least, with the middle group being intermediate. Ohlin and Rossner (1990) compared weight change from 2.5 to 12 months postpartum among 1,423 Swedish women divided into five groups based on a lactation score calculated from the duration and degree of breastfeeding. Weight loss over the entire interval did not differ significantly among groups (although women in the group with the highest lactation scores lost 0.6 kg more than the other groups). However, weight loss from 2.5 to 6 months postpartum was significantly greater in the three groups with higher lactation scores than in the two groups with lower lactation scores.

Three tentative conclusions can be drawn from these five studies. First, there is evidence for a dose-response relationship between the degree of breastfeeding and the degree of weight loss, from the studies by Janney et al. (1997), McKeown and Record (1957), and Ohlin and Rossner (1990). Second, the interval during which differences in weight change between lactating and nonlactating women are most evident is 3 to 6 months postpartum. This is consistent with the hypothesis that the appetite-enhancing effects of prolactin influence the likelihood of weight loss. In the first few months of lactation, maternal serum prolactin concentrations are high, which would be expected to lead to high energy intakes that would balance the high energy demands of milk production. After the first few months, prolactin levels normally decline even though energy output in milk is still considerable. This would result in reduced appetite relative to energy demands and thus greater weight loss. After 6 months, energy output in milk decreases as the infant consumes other foods, resulting in less lactation-associated weight loss. Third, although breastfeeding appears to enhance the rate of weight loss, at least during certain time intervals, the magnitude of this effect is modest. Among these five studies, the difference in weight loss during the first year postpartum between the nonlactating group and the group who lactated the longest ranged from 0.6 to 2.0 kg.

4. EFFECT OF LACTATION ON MATERNAL MICRONUTRIENT STATUS

There has been very little research on the effect of lactation on maternal micronutrient status. There are some data on the micronutrient status of lactating women (mostly in developing countries), but almost no comparisons of lactating and nonlactating women. Hypothetically, one can estimate the micronutrient "burden" of lactation by calculating the increase in nutrient requirements during lactation, compared with the nonpregnant, nonlactating state. Table 3 shows these values for several vitamins and minerals, based on the most recent Recommended Dietary Allowances (RDA) published by the U.S. Institute of Medicine (1997, 1998, 2000, 2001). Of the vitamins, the percentage increase in the RDA during lactation ranges from 17% for vitamin B_{12} to 86% for vitamin A. Of the minerals, there is a net decrease in the RDA for iron (–50%), and no net increase in the RDA for calcium, magnesium, or phosphorus. The RDA is increased by 27–93% for selenium, copper, zinc, and iodine. Of the 17 nutrients listed, the increased demand during lactation exceeds 50% for vitamins A, B_6, and C, and for zinc and iodine. Thus, one could hypothesize that these five nutrients would be the most likely to differ in comparisons of micronutrient status between lactating and nonlactating women. However, data are lacking to evaluate this hypothesis.

There is some evidence that lactation is protective against maternal iron deficiency. The decrease in iron needs during lactation is due to the fact that lactating women are usually amenorrheic for at least six months (if they are exclusively breastfeeding), which eliminates iron losses in menstrual blood (about 0.5 mg Fe/day). There is relatively little iron secreted in human milk (about 0.24 mg/day), so the net iron loss is lower than

Table 3. Micronutrient needs during lactation

Vitamins	% Increase over RDA[a]	Minerals	% Increase over RDA
Vitamin A	86	Calcium	0
Vitamin C	60	Copper	44
Vitamin E	27	Iodine	93
Thiamin	27	Iron	–50
Riboflavin	45	Magnesium	0
Niacin	21	Phosphorus	0
Vitamin B_6	54	Selenium	27
Folate	25	Zinc	50
Vitamin B_{12}	17		

[a]Percent increase over the Recommended Dietary Allowances (Institute of Medicine 1997, 1998, 2000, 2001) for nonpregnant, nonlactating women

for nonlactating women. In an analysis of data for 59,428 U.S. women, Bodnar et al. (2001) demonstrated that the percentage of women who were anemic at 4 to 26 weeks postpartum was significantly lower among those who breastfed for at least four weeks than among those who did not breastfeed or did so for less than four weeks (adjusted odds ratios of 0.76 for 7 or more weeks of breastfeeding and 0.82 for 4 to 6 weeks of breastfeeding, compared to no breastfeeding). They controlled for maternal ethnicity, age, time of assessment postpartum, time of entry to prenatal care, participation in the Women, Infants and Children nutrition program, education, marital status, prenatal anemia, prepregnancy body mass index, and infant birth order. They did not, however, have data on the use of iron supplements, which may be a confounding variable (e.g., breastfeeding women may be more likely to use iron supplements postpartum). Kalkwarf and Harrast (1998) found that lactating women had greater serum ferritin concentrations (reflective of iron stores) than nonlactating women, even after controlling for prior iron supplement use. However, there were no significant differences in hemoglobin between groups.

Lactation may pose a significant burden with regard to certain fatty acids. For example, it has been shown that the docosahexaenoic acid content of human milk and maternal blood decreases during lactation (Lauritzen et al. 2001), which may reflect a relative depletion in the mother in order to provide the infant with adequate amounts of this key nutrient. There is inadequate information directly comparing fatty acid status of lactating and nonlactating women, however.

5. SUMMARY

The studies reviewed herein suggest that breastfeeding enhances the rate of weight loss postpartum, but the effect is relatively small and often not detectable in studies that lack adequate statistical power, have imprecise data on postpartum weight change, or do not account for the exclusivity and/or duration of breastfeeding. Of the six observational studies in which postpartum weight change was estimated (rather than measured directly), only one showed an association with breastfeeding. By contrast, six of the seven studies in which postpartum weight change was measured showed greater weight or fat loss in women who breastfed longer, at least during certain time intervals. The only one of these seven studies that did not show such an association was the one that did not account for the exclusivity of breastfeeding. The results of these seven observational studies are consistent with the two experimental studies conducted in Honduras, which demonstrated that the degree of breastfeeding affects the rate of weight loss. The interval during which the effect of lactation is most evident is 3 to 6 months postpartum.

The role of breastfeeding is small compared with other factors such as pregnancy weight gain, dietary practices, and physical activity. In fact, some women gain weight while breastfeeding, perhaps because of increased appetite and/or reduced physical activity. The average difference in weight loss by 12 months postpartum between lactating and nonlactating women is about 0.6–2.0 kg. Although the magnitude of this difference is not large, it may have important implications with regard to adult-onset obesity associated with childbirth. On the other hand, increased weight loss postpartum may be a disadvantage for thin women, particularly those in developing countries who lack access to adequate food. However, for populations with low rates of contraception use, this potential risk needs to be evaluated in the context of the risk of a subsequent pregnancy if breastfeeding duration or exclusivity is decreased in an effort to reduce maternal "depletion."

With regard to micronutrient status, it is well known that nutrient needs during lactation are substantial. The increase in nutrient requirements exceeds 50% (relative to the values for nonpregnant, nonlactating women) for vitamins A, B_6, and C, and for iodine and zinc. By contrast, lactation may be protective against iron deficiency. There is an urgent need for more research on the effects of lactation on maternal micronutrient status, and on strategies for optimizing nutrient intake to meet the needs of both the mother and her infant.

6. ACKNOWLEDGMENTS

The author greatly appreciates the assistance of Roberta J. Cohen in preparing this paper.

7. REFERENCES

Adair LS, Popkin BM. Prolonged lactation contributes to depletion of maternal energy reserves in Filipino woman. J Nutr 1992;122:1643-1655.

Boardley DJ, Sargent RG, Coker AL, Hussey JR, Sharpe PA. The relationship between diet, activity, and other factors, and postpartum weight change by race. Obstet Gynecol 1995;86:834-838.

Bodnar LM, Scanlon KS, Freedman DS, Siega-Riz AM, Cogswell ME. High prevalence of postpartum anemia among low-income women in the United States. Am J Obstet Gynecol 2001;185:438-443.

Butte NF, Hopkinson JM. Body composition changes during lactation are highly variable among woman. J Nutr 1998;128:318S-385S.

Dewey KG, Heinig MJ, Nommsen LA. Maternal weight-loss patterns during prolonged lactation. Am J Clin Nutr 1993;58:162-166.

Dewey KG. Energy and protein requirements during lactation. Annu Rev Nutr 1997;17:19-36.

Dewey KG, Cohen RJ, Brown KH, Rivera LL. Effects of exclusive breastfeeding for four versus six months on maternal nutritional status and infant motor development: results of two randomized trials in Honduras. J Nutr 2001;131:262-267.

Dugdale AE, Eaton EJ. The effect of lactation and other factors on postpartum changes in body weight and triceps skinfold thickness. Br J Nutr 1989;61:149-153.

Grattan DR. Behavioural significance of prolactin signalling in the central nervous system during pregnancy and lactation. Reproduction 2002;123:497-506.

Greene GW, Wright HS, Scholl TO, Karp RJ. Postpartum weight change: how much of the weight gained in pregnancy will be lost after delivery? Obstet Gynecol 1988;71:701-707.

Haiek LN, Kramer MS, Ciampi A, Tirado R. Postpartum weight loss and infant feeding. J Am Board Fam Pract 2001;14:85-94.

Harris HE, Ellison GTH, Holliday M, Lucassin E. The impact of pregnancy on the long-term weight gain of primiparous women in England. Int J Obes 1997;21:747-755.

Institute of Medicine. Dietary reference intakes for calcium, phosphorus, magnesium, vitamin D and fluoride. Washington, DC: National Academy Press; 1997.

Institute of Medicine. Dietary reference intakes for thiamin, riboflavin, niacin, vitamin B_6, folate, vitamin B_{12}, pantothenic acid, biotin, and choline. Washington, DC: National Academy Press; 1998.

Institute of Medicine. Dietary reference intakes for vitamin A, vitamin K, arsenic, boron, chromium, copper, iodine, iron, manganese, molybdenum, nickel, silicon, vanadium, and zinc. Washington, DC: National Academy Press; 2001.

Institute of Medicine. Dietary reference intakes for vitamin C, vitamin E, selenium, and carotenoids. Washington, DC: National Academy Press; 2000.

Janney CA, Zhang D, Sowers MF. Lactation and weight retention. Am J Clin Nutr 1997;66:1116-1124.

Kalkwarf HJ, Harrast SD. Effects of calcium supplementation and lactation on iron status. Am J Clin Nutr 1998;67:1244-1249.

Lauritzen L, Hansen HS, Jorgensen MH, Michaelsen KF. The essentiality of long chain n-3 fatty acids in relation to development and function of the brain and retina. Prog Lipid Res 2001;40:1-94.

McKeown T, Record RG. The influence of reproduction on body weight in women. J Endocrinol 1957;15:393-409.

Ohlin A, S. Rossner S. Maternal body weight development after pregnancy. Int J Obes 1990;14:159-173.

Parker JD, Abrams B. Differences in postpartum weight retention between black and white mothers. Obstet Gynecol 1993;81:768-774.

Potter S, Hannum S, McFarlin B, Essex SD, Campbell E, Trupin S. Does infant feeding method influence maternal postpartum weight loss? J Am Diet Assoc 1991;91:441-446.

Prentice AM, Spaaij CJK, Goldberg GR, Poppitt SD, Van Raaij JMA, Totton M, Swann D, Black AE. Energy requirements of pregnant and lactating women. Eur J Clin Nutr 1996;50:S82-S111.

Rebuffe SM, Enk L, Crona N, Lonnroth P, Abrahamsson L, Smith U, Bjorntorp P. Fat cell metabolism in different regions in woman. Effect of menstrual cycle, pregnancy, and lactation. J Clin Invest 1985;75:1973-1976.

Winkvist A, Rasmussen KM. Impact of lactation on maternal body weight and body composition. J Mammary Gland Biol Neoplasia 1999;4:309-318.

LACTATION AND MATERNAL BONE HEALTH

Heidi J. Kalkwarf

1. ABSTRACT

Women lose bone during lactation, and this is an important mechanism to provide calcium for human milk. Bone loss during lactation occurs even in women with high calcium intakes. Lactation-induced bone loss is transient because bone density increases rapidly after weaning. Bone loss during lactation and recovery after weaning are related to ovarian function and the length of postpartum amenorrhea. The recovery of bone after weaning can occur with shortly spaced pregnancies. Women who have breastfed several infants do not have reduced bone density after menopause. Overall, the transient bone loss during lactation does not seem to increase a woman's risk of osteoporotic fracture in her elder years. Further research is needed on special subgroups of women, such as adolescents, women who are vitamin D deficient or have extremely low calcium intakes, and women who have simultaneously breastfed multiple infants to determine whether these women are able to regain sufficient bone mass after lactation to preserve their bone health.

2. INTRODUCTION

There has been concern about the long-term effects of lactation on maternal bone health and future risk osteoporotic fracture. This concern has been prompted by two physiologic changes during lactation that may potentially result in loss of maternal bone: 1) a significant loss of calcium from the mother to her milk, and 2) a prolonged period of postpartum amenorrhea. A permanent loss of bone mass during lactation potentially could adversely affect bone health as low bone mass and density are associated with increased risk of osteoporotic fracture later in life. This is an important public health concern since the risk of osteoporotic fracture among elderly women increases 2.6-fold for a 1 standard deviation decrease (≈10–13% reduction) in bone density (Marshall et al. 1996).

Division of General and Community Pediatrics, Children's Hospital Medical Center, 3333 Burnet Avenue, Cincinnati, OH 45229

The maternal loss of calcium in human milk is substantial. The average daily calcium loss in human milk is about 250 mg/day, but some women lose up to 450 mg/day (Laskey et al. 1998; Ritchie et al. 1998). The maternal skeleton contains about 800 g to 900 g of calcium, which constitutes about 30% to 40% of the total skeletal mass (Recker et al. 1992; Ellis et al. 1996). Assuming there were no compensations to conserve calcium, a woman who breastfeeds for 6 months, theoretically, could lose 38 g of calcium or 4% of her total skeletal calcium content, and a woman who breastfeeds for 1 year could lose 76 g of calcium or 9% of her skeletal calcium content. Prior to the release of the 1997 Dietary Reference Intakes for calcium, the prevailing belief was that lactating women needed to consume extra calcium to compensate for calcium lost in human milk, maintain her bone calcium reserves, and preserve her future bone health (Standing Committee on the Scientific Evaluation of Dietary Reference Intakes 1997).

Endocrinologic changes associated with the prolonged postpartum amenorrhea in lactating women theoretically also could reduce maternal bone mass and have an adverse effect on maternal bone health. Estrogen has physiologically and biomechanically important effects on bone. The effects of estrogen on bone are mediated through multiple pathways involving osteoblasts, the cells responsible for bone formation, and osteoclasts, the cells responsible for bone resorption (Riggs et al. 2002). Bone mass and density reflect the net balance of bone formation and bone resorption. Bone mass and density are reduced in all experimental and clinical models of hypoestrogenemia. Lactation results in suppression of the hypothalmic-pituitary-gonadal axis, reduced ovarian estrogen production, and a prolonged period of postpartum amenorrhea (McNeilly et al. 1994). Nonlactating women usually resume menses between six to eight weeks postpartum, whereas fully lactating women resume menses at an average of 8 to 10 months postpartum (Howie et al. 1982a; Lewis et al. 1991). The length of postpartum amenorrhea and hypoestrogenemia vary considerably among women and are influenced by duration and intensity of breastfeeding (Howie et al. 1982a, 1982b). Thus, we could anticipate that reduced estrogen concentrations in addition to the loss of calcium in human milk would result in reduced bone mass and density among lactating women.

3. ADAPTATIONS IN THE CALCIUM ECONOMY DURING LACTATION

Adaptations in the maternal calcium economy during lactation are necessary to provide calcium for human milk production while maintaining maternal serum calcium concentrations within the narrow range necessary for other metabolic functions. There are three physiologic adaptations that may occur to secure calcium in times of high calcium demand: increased efficiency of intestinal absorption, decreased urinary excretion, and mobilization of calcium from bone—the body's major reservoir of calcium. In contrast to pregnancy when intestinal calcium absorption is increased markedly (Kent et al. 1991; Ritchie et al. 1998), there is no increase in intestinal calcium absorption during lactation (Kent et al. 1991; Fairweather-Tait et al. 1995; Kalkwarf et al. 1996; Ritchie et al. 1998; Moser-Veillon et al. 2001). Several studies have documented alterations in renal calcium handling and a reduction in urinary calcium excretion in lactating women (Kent et al. 1990; Klein et al. 1995; Donangelo et al. 1996; Ritchie et al. 1998). However, part of this calcium conservation may be due to the postpartum state, and studies that have used postpartum controls have not found differences in urinary calcium excretion between lactating and nonlactating postpartum women (Affinito et al. 1996; Krebs et al. 1997;

Kalkwarf et al. 1999; Moser-Veillon et al. 2001). The majority of calcium needed for human milk presumably comes from demineralization of bone.

4. MEASUREMENT OF BONE DENSITY

Several methods have been used to measure bone mineral content and bone mineral density in studies of human lactation. The magnitude of bone loss reported is affected by the imaging modality used to measure bone mass and density and the skeletal site measured. Studies of lactation in the early 1980s used single photon absorptiometry (SPA). This technology was restricted to measurements at the forearm because there is a limited amount of soft tissue at this site. The advent of dual photon absorptiometry (DPA) enabled measurement of bone density at skeletal sites surrounded by larger amounts of soft tissue, such as the lumbar spine. Currently, the most commonly used method for measuring bone mass and density in studies of lactation is dual energy x-ray absorptiometry (DXA). DXA has replaced DPA due to its shorter scanning time, better precision, and lower radiation exposure. Quantitative computed tomography (QCT) has been used in one study of lactating women to measure bone density at the lumbar spine, but QCT is not used commonly because of its higher radiation exposure.

Bone density measurements typically are obtained at the lumbar spine, proximal femur (hip), and forearm because these are the skeletal sites where osteoporotic fractures are common. The advantage of measuring different skeletal sites is that they contain different amounts of trabecular and cortical bone and may respond differently to lactation. Trabecular bone has a higher turnover rate due to its greater surface area-to-volume ratio and responds more quickly to metabolic perturbations and hormonal changes than does cortical bone. As a consequence, quicker and more dramatic changes in bone density in response to lactation have been reported for skeletal sites that have a large amount of trabecular bone. Skeletal sites containing predominantly trabecular bone include the lumbar spine and the ultra-distal radius. The majority of the skeleton is made up of cortical bone, and cortical bone provides most of the structural resistance to fracture (Mazess 1990). Skeletal sites that contain mostly cortical bone are the femoral and radial shafts. The femoral neck contains both trabecular and cortical bone (Eastell et al. 1990; Lundeen et al. 2001). Spinal QCT measures just the trabecular bone in the interior of the vertebral body and, consequently, demonstrates the largest changes in bone density due to lactation.

5. BONE DENSITY DURING LACTATION

There have been over 20 longitudinal studies that have examined changes in bone mass and density over the course of lactation (Table 1). Despite variations, all measurement techniques have found bone loss at one or more skeletal sites. Bone loss at the lumbar spine and femoral neck has been a consistent finding across all studies that have measured these sites. Reported decreases in bone density at the lumbar spine as measured by DXA have ranged from 3% to 7% (Table 1). A larger decrease in lumbar spine bone density (9.9%) was reported in one study that used QCT owing to its selective measurement of trabecular bone (Ritchie et al. 1998). Decreases in bone density at the femoral neck have ranged from 2% to 7%. The decreases in bone density of the spine and hip occur rapidly within the first three to 6 months of lactation, and bone density remains lower with continued lactation (Sowers et al. 1993; Laskey & Prentice 1999). The rate of bone loss at these sites in the first 6 months of lactation is noteworthy as it is approaches 1% per month. In comparison, menopausal and early postmenopausal women lose bone at the rate of 1% to 2% per year (Nordin et al. 1990).

Results of studies that have measured changes in bone density of the forearm at the ultra-distal site (primarily trabecular bone) and the radial shaft site (cortical bone) have been inconsistent. Reported changes in bone density at the ultra-distal radius during lactation have ranged from losses of 5% to gains of 3%. Large decreases in bone density (10–14%) at the radial shaft were reported in early studies (Chan et al. 1982; 1987), but more recent studies have found no change, a small decrease (1.1%), or even an increase in bone density at this site during lactation. Thus it is difficult to make conclusions about the effects of lactation on bone mass or density of the forearm at either trabecular-rich or cortical bone sites. It is not clear why bone loss at the forearm has been an inconsistent finding in contrast to the consistency of findings at the lumbar spine and hip. Possible reasons include precision in measurement or true differences in responsiveness of various parts of the skeleton.

6. FACTORS AFFECTING BONE LOSS DURING LACTATION

The amount of bone lost at the lumbar spine and femoral neck during lactation is highly variable among women. This large variation has motivated investigation of factors that may predict the amount of bone lost during lactation. The amount of bone lost is related to the length of lactation: women who breastfeed for 1 to 3 months experience less bone loss than women who breastfeed for 6 months or longer (Table 1) (Sowers et al. 1993; Kolthoff et al. 1998; Karlsson et al. 2001; More et al. 2001). Intuitively, one would predict that the daily amount of human milk produced and the daily calcium loss would be related to the amount of bone loss. This hypothesis has received limited attention, however, as few studies have quantified the amount of human milk produced and its calcium content. Lasky et al. (1998) investigated predictors of bone loss among women who had been breastfeeding for 3 months. They found that human milk volume and total milk calcium output were significant predictors of bone loss at the lumbar spine. Likewise, Little and Clapp (1998) found that human milk calcium loss was associated with change in femoral neck bone density by 3 months of lactation. It is likely that the amount of bone lost during lactation is affected not only by the duration of breastfeeding, but also by the amount of milk produced and the total amount of calcium lost in human milk.

Dietary calcium intake initially was hypothesized to affect bone loss during lactation, with women consuming high amounts of calcium hypothesized to have no or little bone loss. However, several lines of evidence do not support this hypothesis. Observational studies have documented bone loss at the lumber spine and femoral neck in women with high dietary intakes of calcium (>1500 mg/day) (Hayslip et al. 1989; Sowers et al. 1993; Affinito et al. 1996; Kolthoff et al. 1998). Furthermore, dietary calcium intake does not predict the magnitude of bone loss during lactation (Sowers et al. 1993; Krebs et al. 1997; Laskey 1998; Little & Clapp 1998).

Table 1. Longitudinal studies examining bone loss during lactation and recovery after weaning

First author, year	Bone measurement technology	No. subjects, lactation status, age	% Change in bone density during lactation by skeletal site[a] Lumbar spine (LS)	Femoral neck (FN)	Ultradistal radius (UD)	Radial shaft (RS)	Sites with complete recovery after weaning[b]
Chan, 1982	SPA	12 L, ≤18 y	--	--	--	–14*	--
		36 L, >18 y	--	--	--	1	--
Chan, 1987	SPA	15 L, <18 y	--	--	--	–10*	--
		21 L, <18 y w/Ca	--	--	--	–3	--
		12 L, >18 y	--	--	--	5	--
Hayslip, 1988	DPA, SPA	12 L	–6.5*	--	–2.0	0.0	--
		7 L	1.6	--	2.0	1.4	--
Sowers, 1993	DXA	20 L 0-1 mo	0.2	–1.4	--	--	--
		26 L 2-5 mo	0.1	0.1	--	--	--
		64 L ≥6 mo	–5.1*	–4.8*	--	--	LS
Prentice, 1995	SPA	60 L	--	--	–0.5	–1.1*	RS
Cross, 1995	DXA	15 L	–4.9*	--	3.1*	3.1*	none
Matsumoto, 1995	DXA	11 L	--	--	–8.3*	--	none
		11 NL	--	--	1.4	--	--
Affinito, 1996	DPA	18 L	–7.5*	--	–5.0	--	none
		18 L	0	--	0	--	--
Lopez, 1996	DXA	30 L	–1.1	–3.1	--	--	LS, FN
		26 controls	–0.4	0.2	--	--	--
Krebs, 1997	DPA, DXA, SPA	26 L	–5*	--	--	nc	LS
		8 NL	0	--	--	nc	--
Kalkwarf, 1997	DXA	87 L	–4.6*	--	0.0	–0.2	LS[c]
		81 NL	1.3	--	0.2	–0.3	--
Ritchie, 1998	QCT, DXA	14 L	–9.9*	--	--	--	LS

Laskey, 1998	DXA	47 L	–4.0*	–2.4*	–0.3	–0.1	--
		11 NL	–1.0	–0.4	1.1	0.6	--
Kolthoff, 1998	DXA	16 L 4.8 mo	–3.6*	4*	nc	nc	LS
		26 L 8.8 mo	–5.5*	–5*	nc	nc	LS
		17 L 12.2 mo	–7*	–7*	nc	nc	none
Little, 1998	DXA	20 L	–4.7*	–2.9*	--	--	--
Honda, 1998	DXA	69 L	–5.9*	--	--	--	--
		42 NL	0.2	--	--	--	--
Yasumiza, 1998	DXA	13 L <3 mo	–3.3*	--	--	--	LS
		14 L >6-12 mo	–2.9*	--	--	--	none
Polatti, 1999	DXA	135 L w/o Ca	–4.4*	--	–2.2*	--	LS, UD
		139 L w/Ca	–4.0*	--	–2.0*	--	LS, UD
		153 NL	1.4*	--	0.9*	--	--
Laskey, 1999	DXA	59 L	–5*	–5*	–2*	nc	LS
		11 NL	nc	nc	nc	nc	--
Holmberg-Marttila, 1999	DXA	76 L	–5.0*	–4.3*	--	--	LS
Hopkinson, 2000	DXA	40 L	–3.1*	--	--	--	LS
		36 NL	--	nc	--	--	--
More, 2001	DXA	7 L 0-1 mo	1.4	--	4.6*	1.4	--
		11 L 1-6 mo	–4.9*	--	–4.1	0.5	UD
		20 L >6 mo	–7.4*	--	–4.5*	1.1	UD
Karlsson, 2001	DXA	14 L 0-1 mo	0.0	–2.1	--	--	--
		26 L 1-6 mo	–3.3	–2.0*	--	--	LS
		25 L >6 mo	–4.1*	–5.7*	--	--	LS

[a]Maximum % change reported irrespective of time postpartum; *P<0.05
[b]Recovery of bone density at skeletal sites that experienced a statistically significant bone loss during lactation
[c]Recovery measured in a separate group of previously lactating women
SPA=single photon absorptiometry; DPA=dual photon absorptiometry; DXA=dual energy x-ray absorptiometry;
QCT=quantitative computed tomography; L=lactating; NL=nonlactating; nc=no change, numeric value not reported;
LS=lumbar spine; FN=femoral neck; UD=ultradistal radius; RS=radial shaft

In keeping with results from observational studies, randomized intervention studies conducted in women of various racial/ethnic backgrounds and dietary habits have demonstrated that provision of supplemental calcium (i.e., such that total calcium intake exceeds 1000–1800 mg/day) does not prevent bone loss during lactation (Prentice et al. 1995; Kalkwarf et al. 1997; Polatti et al. 1999). Kalkwarf et al. (1997) randomized 83 lactating women and 81 nonlactating postpartum women in the U.S. whose dietary calcium intake averaged 735 mg/day to receive a calcium supplement (1 g/day) or placebo for 6 months. There was no effect of calcium supplementation or lactation on bone density of the ultra-distal radius or the radial shaft. At the lumbar spine there was a small effect of calcium supplementation on bone density (+1.2%) as measured by DXA when considering all women. However, bone loss at the lumbar spine did not significantly differ between lactating women who received the calcium supplement and women that received the placebo (4.2 vs. 4.9%, $P>0.05$). Nonlactating women appeared to benefit from supplemental calcium as much as lactating women. Polatti et al. (1999) conducted a randomized calcium supplementation trial in Italian women who breastfed for 6 months; 139 women received a calcium supplement of 1 g/day during lactation, and 135 women did not receive a supplement. There was no difference in the amount of bone loss at the lumbar spine (4.0 vs. 4.4%) or ultra-distal radius (2.0 vs. 2.2%) over the 6-month study period between calcium supplemented and unsupplemented women ($P=0.16$). The calcium intake from the diet in these women was not reported. These studies showed that provision of additional calcium does not prevent bone loss during lactation, and does not appear to benefit lactating women more than nonlactating women. It currently is recommended that lactating women consume 1000 mg/day of calcium, the same amount as for nonlactating women (Standing Committee on the Scientific Evaluation of Dietary Reference Intakes 1997).

If dietary calcium is important in modifying bone loss during lactation, any beneficial effect of calcium supplementation should be most evident in women with low dietary calcium intakes. Prentice et al. (1995) conducted a randomized calcium supplementation trial in The Gambia in lactating women (n=60) whose average dietary calcium intake was only 283 mg/day. Women received a supplement that provided an average of 714 mg/day of calcium or a placebo for 12 months. There was a significant decrease in bone mass at the radial shaft as measured by SPA by 13 weeks of lactation, but there was no difference in bone loss between mothers who received the calcium supplement and those who received the placebo. Failure to find an effect of calcium supplementation in this population is important as it provides evidence that dietary calcium intake may not be effective in reducing bone loss during lactation in women with extremely low calcium intakes. However, bone density of the spine and hip, which typically show larger changes due to lactation than the radial shaft, were not measured. Thus the benefit of calcium supplementation in women with extremely low calcium intakes is unknown.

With the exception of ovarian function (reviewed below) there has been limited investigation of other maternal factors that may be associated with the amount of bone lost during lactation. Little and Clapp (1998) found that the amount of bone loss during the first 3 months of lactation did not differ between women who engaged in regular physical activity (n=11) and women who did not (n=9). Maternal age has not been found to be a significant predictor of bone loss during lactation, either (Sowers et al. 1993; Kolthoff et al. 1998). An important exception to this may be lactating adolescents who are still accreting bone mass. There have been only a few investigations of lactating adolescents. Early studies found large decreases (i.e., 14%) in bone mineral at the radial shaft among lactating adolescents, but no decrease in bone mineral content among lactating adult women (Chan et al. 1982). These findings were followed up with an intervention trial in lactating adolescents. The 21 lactating adolescents who were counseled to consume a higher calcium intake (1850 mg/day) had no significant bone loss at the radial shaft, whereas the 15 adolescents who only consumed 900 mg/day of calcium had a 10% decrease in bone mineral at this skeletal site (Chan et al. 1987). The beneficial effects of increased calcium intake on bone mass in this study contrasts with the larger calcium intervention studies in adult women that found no effect of calcium supplementation on changes in bone density during lactation. It is unknown whether these contradictory findings reflect the true differences in response to lactation of the adolescent vs. adult skeleton, differences due to increasing calcium intake by foods vs. a supplement, or a small sample size. More research is needed on the relation between calcium intake and bone loss among lactating adolescents to better understand their calcium needs and preserve their future bone health.

7. RECOVERY OF BONE AFTER WEANING

Several studies have documented that the bone loss that occurs during lactation is transient, because there is a rapid increase in bone density after weaning (Table 1). Much of the bone is recovered within 6 months of weaning, but the time course for recovery varies among skeletal sites. Increases in bone density occur earlier in the spine than the femoral neck, probably due to the greater amount of trabecular bone in the spine (Sowers et al. 1993; Kolthoff et al. 1998; Laskey & Prentice 1999; Polatti et al. 1999; Karlsson et al. 2001). Whether bone density fully recovers after weaning, or if a small deficit in bone density remains, has important implications for future risk of osteoporotic fracture. Although most studies show some increase in bone density after weaning, in several studies a deficit in bone density, particularly at the femoral neck, was still evident at the end of the follow-up period (Table 1). It is unknown whether these deficits in bone density after weaning reflect a permanent loss of bone density or the need for a longer follow-up period in order to adequately document the recovery of bone mass after weaning. The fact that bone density is recovered after weaning is why many cross-sectional studies of bone density in postmenopausal women have found that lactation history is not a significant predictor of bone density (Kritz-Silverstein et al. 1992; Fox et al. 1993; Melton et al. 1993; Grainge et al. 2001). Henderson et al. (2000) found that bone density of 30 grand multiparous women who breastfed at least 6 children for greater than 6 months each had the same bone density as nulliparous women.

Ovarian function and the length of postpartum amenorrhea are important determinants of the amount of bone lost during lactation and the recovery of bone after weaning. The length of postpartum amenorrhea has been found to be as strong of a predictor as the length of lactation in predicting bone density (Kolthoff et al. 1998; Laskey & Prentice 1999; Polatti et al. 1999). Although women who breastfeed longer tend to have a longer length of postpartum amenorrhea, the durations of postpartum amenorrhea and lactation are not perfectly correlated. Some women who breastfeed for a long time have a short period of postpartum amenorrhea, whereas some women who breastfeed for a short time have a long period of postpartum amenorrhea. The discordance between these two factors has allowed investigation of their independent effects on bone turnover during and after lactation. The importance of ovarian function in modulating bone loss and recovery during lactation is illustrated by the fact that lactating women who resume menses when still fully breastfeeding start to recover some of the bone loss that occurred earlier in lactation (Kalkwarf & Specker 1995; Polatti et al. 1999). Kalkwarf & Specker (1995) found that the net change in bone density at the lumbar spine at 6 months postpartum was only –1.8% in women who had resumed menses, whereas it was –4.4% in women who had not resumed menses despite the fact that both groups were breastfeeding 5 to 6 times per day. Polatti et al. (1999) also found earlier recovery of bone density in lactating women who resumed menses by 5 months postpartum, but by 18 months postpartum (12 months after weaning) there was no difference in bone density of the lumbar spine and radius between lactating women who resumed menses early (≤5 months postpartum) vs. those who resumed menses late (>5 months postpartum).

An increase in bone density after weaning or the resumption of menses occurs in women across a wide range of dietary calcium intakes. Some evidence suggests that the rate of recovery of bone density after weaning may be faster in women who received 1 g/day of supplemental calcium (Kalkwarf et al. 1997; Polatti et al. 1999). By 12 months after weaning, however, there is no difference in bone density between women who receive a calcium supplement and those who do not (Polatti et al. 1999). It appears that both earlier return of ovarian functioning and supplemental calcium may speed the process of bone recovery after weaning, but ultimately do not result in a greater bone density.

Although bone recovery appears to occur after weaning for most women, it is conceivable that there may be subgroups of women for whom this process is compromised. For instance, it is unknown whether women can adequately recover bone mass after lactation when they are vitamin D deficient. It is also unknown whether women who breastfeed multiple infants have a greater bone deficit during lactation due to increased demand, and, if so, whether there are limits on the amount of bone that can be regained. Furthermore, women who bear children in their mid-40s may not have sufficient opportunity to regain bone after lactation prior to the onset of menopause. There has been particular concern about the bone health of women who have long lactations and shortly spaced pregnancies. However, recovery of lactation-induced bone loss occurs with closely spaced pregnancies, and part of the bone gain may possibly occur during a subsequent pregnancy (Sowers et al. 1995; Laskey & Prentice 1997; Matsushita et al. 2002).

8. LACTATION AND FRACTURE RISK

Whether or not bone lost during lactation is sufficiently recovered after weaning is important in terms of the long-term effects of lactation on risk of osteoporotic fracture. Two epidemiologic studies of postmenopausal women found no association between lactation history and fractures of the forearm (Alderman et al. 1986; Kelsey et al. 1992). In a case-control study of postmenopausal women with spinal crush fractures (n=58), breastfeeding was associated with a slightly lower risk of fracture ($P<0.05$) (Aloia et al. 1985). These findings are consistent with longitudinal studies of lactating women, which show little bone loss of the forearm and that bone loss at the lumbar spine is recovered rapidly after weaning and appears to be complete (Sowers et al. 1993; Lopez et al. 1996; Kalkwarf et al. 1997; Kolthoff et al. 1998; Ritchie et al. 1998).

Most of the epidemiologic studies that have examined the effects of lactation on risk of fracture have focused hip fracture. Hip fracture represents a major public health concern as the mortality rate after hip fracture is approximately 20% (Cooper et al. 1993). Furthermore, results from longitudinal studies of lactating women show that recovery of bone at the femoral neck occurs more slowly than at the spine, and it is not clear whether recovery of bone density at the femoral neck is complete. Table 2 lists studies that have investigated the relation between lactation history and risk of hip fracture later in life. Although studies have varied in terms of their design and the way in which they have quantified lactation history, overall it does not appear that lactation increases a woman's risk of hip fracture. In fact, the odds ratios or relative risk estimates in all studies tended to be less than 1.0, but this was statistically significant in only one study (Kreiger et al. 1982).

In order to adequately evaluate the effects of lactation per se on risk of osteoprotic fracture, it is first necessary to consider the effects of pregnancy on risk of fracture. Parity or ever being pregnant have been shown to be associated with a lower risk of hip fracture in several (Cummings et al. 1995; Nguyen et al. 1995; Jacobsen et al. 1998; Michaelsson et al. 2001) but not all studies (Parazzini et al. 1996). This may be due to the high circulating estrogen concentrations and increased body weight during and after pregnancy, which may have positive effects on bone. Alternatively, it may be reflective of the fact that some nulliparous women have a compromised steroid hormone production, which ultimately affects their ability to become pregnant as well as their bone density. Infertility and nulliparity have been found to be associated with increased risk of hip fracture (Tuppurainen et al. 1993; Nguyen et al. 1995; Hesdorffer et al. 1999; Petersen et al. 2002). Interestingly, one study found that Danish men, as well as women, who had no biologic children also had higher hip fracture rates (Petersen et al. 2002). This could be due to the effects of male infertility on bone density, or it could be that having children affects life style in a way that benefits long-term bone health.

In order to assess the true effects of lactation on risk of hip fracture it is necessary to examine this relation only among parous women. None of the four studies that restricted their analyses to parous women found an association, positive or negative, between lactation history and risk of hip fracture. Most notable is the case-control study by Michaelsson et al. (2001) who studied 664 elderly women with hip fracture and 1,848 controls. The odds ratios (95% confidence intervals) associated with breastfeeding for 6–10 months, 11–16 months, and >16 months were 0.9 (0.70, 1.15), 0.95 (0.72, 1.26), and 1.01 (0.75, 1.15), none of which were significantly different from 1.0. The tight confidence intervals around these risk estimates diminish the likelihood of failing to detect a small increased risk or even a small benefit due to lack of statistical power. Based on the evidence to date, lactation history does not appear to affect risk of osteoporotic fracture later in life.

Table 2. Studies of lactation and risk of postmenopausal hip fracture

First author, year	Study design	Study size: Fracture cases	Study size: Controls	Breastfeeding history	Odds ratio[a] (95% CI)	Accounted for parity[b]	Exclude nulliparous
Kreiger, 1982	case-control	98	801	per 12 mo	0.6 (0.3, 1.0)	yes	no
			trauma 80	per 12 mo	0.5 (0.2, 0.9)[c]	yes	no
Alderman, 1986	case-control	164	318	0 mo	1.0	yes	no
				1-12 mo	1.6 (0.9, 2.9)	yes	no
				13-24 mo	0.4 (0.2, 1.1)		
Cumming, 1993	case-control	166	137	ever/never	0.64 (0.30, 1.38)	yes	no
		131	107	ever/never	0.55 (0.10, 2.90)	yes	yes
				all/no children	0.53 (0.14, 2.00)		
Hoffman, 1993	case-control	170	173	ever/never	0.66 (0.41, 1.05)	no	no
		103	125	ever/never	0.87 (0.47, 1.61)	yes	yes
Cummings, 1995	cohort	192	9324	per child	0.9 (0.8, 1.0)	yes	no
Jacobsen, 1998[d]	cohort	465	62,625	0 mo	1.00	yes	no
				1-9 mo	0.70 (0.45, 1.10)		
				10-19 mo	0.76 (0.40, 1.19)		
				20-29 mo	0.78 (0.48, 1.28)		
				≥30 mo	0.80 (0.48, 1.35)		
Michaelsson, 2001	case-control	664	1,848	0-5 mo	1.00	yes	yes
				6-10 mo	0.90 (0.70, 1.15)		
				11-16 mo	0.95 (0.72, 1.26)		
				>16 mo	1.01 (0.75, 1.28)		

[a]Relative risk estimate for cohort studies
[b]Accounted for parity in the statistical analysis or by demonstrating no relation between parity and hip fracture
[c]95% confidence interval excludes 1.0
[d]Cases were deaths associated with hip fracture

9. REFERENCES

Affinito P, Tommaselli GA, di Carlo C, Guida F, Nappi C. Changes in bone mineral density and calcium metabolism in breastfeeding women: a one year follow-up study. J Clin Endocrinol Metab 1996;81:2314-2318.

Alderman BW, Weiss NS, Daling JR, Ure CL, Ballard JH. Reproductive history and postmenopausal risk of hip and forearm fracture. Am J Epidemiol 1986;124:262-267.

Aloia JF, Cohn SH, Vaswani A, Yeh JK, Yuen K, Ellis K. Risk factors for postmenopausal osteoporosis. Am J Med 1985;78:95-100.

Chan GM, Ronald N, Slater P, Hollis J, Thomas MR. Decreased bone mineral status in lactating adolescent mothers. J Pediatr 1982;101:767-770.

Chan GM, McMurry M, Westover K, Engelbert-Fenton K, Thomas MR. Effects of increased dietary calcium intake upon the calcium and bone mineral status of lactating adolescent and adult women. Am J Clin Nutr 1987;46:319-323.

Cooper C, Atkinson EJ, Jacobsen SJ, O'Fallon WM, Melton LJ, 3rd. Population-based study of survival after osteoporotic fractures. Am J Epidemiol 1993;137:1001-1005.

Cross NA, Hillman LS, Allen SH, Krause GF. Changes in bone mineral density and markers of bone remodeling during lactation and postweaning in women consuming high amounts of calcium. J Bone Miner Res 1995;10:1312-1320.

Cumming RG, Klineberg RJ. Breastfeeding and other reproductive factors and the risk of hip fractures in elderly women. Int J Epidemiol 1993;22:684-691.

Cummings SR, Nevitt MC, Browner WS, Stone K, Fox KM, Ensrud KE, Cauley J, Black D, Vogt TM. Risk factors for hip fracture in white women. Study of Osteoporotic Fractures Research Group. N Engl J Med 1995;332:767-773.

Donangelo CM, Trugo NM, Melo GJO, Gomes DD, Henriques C. Calcium homeostasis during pregnancy and lactation in primiparous and multiparous women with sub-adequate calcium intakes. Nutr Res 1996;16:1631-1640.

Eastell R, Mosekilde L, Hodgson SF, Riggs BL. Proportion of human vertebral body bone that is cancellous. J Bone Miner Res 1990;5:1237-1241.

Ellis KJ, Shypailo RJ, Hergenroeder A, Perez M, Abrams S. Total body calcium and bone mineral content: comparison of dual-energy X-ray absorptiometry with neutron activation analysis. J Bone Miner Res 1996;11:843-848.

Fairweather-Tait S, Prentice A, Heumann KG, Jarjou LM, Stirling DM, Wharf SG, Turnlund JR. Effect of calcium supplements and stage of lactation on the calcium absorption efficiency of lactating women accustomed to low calcium intakes. Am J Clin Nutr 1995;62:1188-1192.

Fox KM, Magaziner J, Sherwin R, Scott JC, Plato CC, Nevitt M, Cummings S. Reproductive correlates of bone mass in elderly women. Study of Osteoporotic Fractures Research Group. J Bone Miner Res 1993;8:901-908.

Grainge MJ, Coupland CA, Cliffe SJ, Chilvers CE, Hosking DJ. Reproductive, menstrual and menopausal factors: which are associated with bone mineral density in early postmenopausal women? Osteoporos Int 2001;12:777-787.

Hayslip CC, Klein TA, Wray HL, Duncan WE. The effects of lactation on bone mineral content in healthy postpartum women. Obstet Gynecol 1989;73:588-592.

Henderson PH, 3rd, Sowers M, Kutzko KE, Jannausch ML. Bone mineral density in grand multiparous women with extended lactation. Am J Obstet Gynecol 2000;182:1371-1377.

Hesdorffer DC, Melton LJ, 3rd, Malkasian GD, Atkinson EJ, Brinton LA, O'Fallon WM. Hip fractures among infertile women. Am J Epidemiol 1999;149:810-813.

Hoffman S, Grisso JA, Kelsey JL, Gammon MD, O'Brien LA. Parity, lactation and hip fracture. Osteoporos Int 1993;3:171-176.

Holmberg-Marttila D, Sievanen H. Prevalence of bone mineral changes during postpartum amenorrhea and after resumption of menstruation. Am J Obstet Gynecol 1999;180:537-538.

Honda A, Kurabayashi T, Yahata T, Tomita M, Takakuwa K, Tanaka K. Lumbar bone mineral density changes during pregnancy and lactation. Int J Gynaecol Obstet 1998;63:253-258.

Hopkinson JM, Butte NF, Ellis K, Smith EO. Lactation delays postpartum bone mineral accretion and temporarily alters its regional distribution in women. J Nutr 2000;130:777-783.

Howie PW, McNeilly AS, Houston MJ, Cook A, Boyle H. Fertility after childbirth: post-partum ovulation and menstruation in bottle and breast feeding mothers. Clin Endocrinol (Oxf) 1982a;17:323-332.

Howie PW, McNeilly AS, Houston MJ, Cook A, Boyle H. Fertility after childbirth: infant feeding patterns, basal PRL levels and post-partum ovulation. Clin Endocrinol (Oxf) 1982b;17:315-322.

Jacobsen BK, Nilssen S, Heuch I, Kvale G. Reproductive factors and fatal hip fractures. A Norwegian prospective study of 63,000 women. J Epidemiol Community Health 1998;52:645-650.

Kalkwarf HJ, Specker BL. Bone mineral loss during lactation and recovery after weaning. Obstet Gynecol 1995;86:26-32.
Kalkwarf HJ, Specker BL, Heubi JE, Vieira NE, Yergey AL. Intestinal calcium absorption of women during lactation and after weaning. Am J Clin Nutr 1996;63:526-531.
Kalkwarf HJ, Specker BL, Ho M. Effects of calcium supplementation on calcium homeostasis and bone turnover in lactating women. J Clin Endocrinol Metab 1999;84:464-470.
Karlsson C, Obrant KJ, Karlsson M. Pregnancy and lactation confer reversible bone loss in humans. Osteoporos Int 2001;12:828-834.
Kelsey JL, Browner WS, Seeley DG, Nevitt MC, Cummings SR. Risk factors for fractures of the distal forearm and proximal humerus. The Study of Osteoporotic Fractures Research Group. Am J Epidemiol 1992;135:477-489.
Kent GN, Price RI, Gutteridge DH, Smith M, Allen JR, Bhagat CI, Barnes MP, Hickling CJ, Retallack RW, Wilson SG, et al. Human lactation: forearm trabecular bone loss, increased bone turnover, and renal conservation of calcium and inorganic phosphate with recovery of bone mass following weaning. J Bone Miner Res 1990;5:361-369.
Kent GN, Price RI, Gutteridge DH, Rosman KJ, Smith M, Allen JR, Hickling CJ, Blakeman SL. The efficiency of intestinal calcium absorption is increased in late pregnancy but not in established lactation. Calcif Tissue Int 1991;48:293-295.
Klein CJ, Moser-Veillon PB, Douglass LW, Ruben KA, Trocki O. A longitudinal study of urinary calcium, magnesium, and zinc excretion in lactating and nonlactating postpartum women. Am J Clin Nutr 1995;61:779-786.
Kolthoff N, Eiken P, Kristensen B, Nielsen SP. Bone mineral changes during pregnancy and lactation: a longitudinal cohort study. Clin Sci (Lond) 1998;94:405-412.
Krebs NF, Reidinger CJ, Robertson AD, Brenner M. Bone mineral density changes during lactation: maternal, dietary, and biochemical correlates. Am J Clin Nutr 1997;65:1738-1746.
Kreiger N, Kelsey JL, Holford TR, O'Connor T. An epidemiologic study of hip fracture in postmenopausal women. Am J Epidemiol 1982;116:141-148.
Kritz-Silverstein D, Barrett-Connor E, Hollenbach KA. Pregnancy and lactation as determinants of bone mineral density in postmenopausal women. Am J Epidemiol 1992;136:1052-1059.
Laskey MA, Prentice A. Effect of pregnancy on recovery of lactational bone loss. Lancet 1997;349:1518-1519.
Laskey MA, Prentice A. Bone mineral changes during and after lactation. Obstet Gynecol 1999;94:608-615.
Laskey MA, Prentice A, Hanratty LA, Jarjou LM, Dibba B, Beavan SR, Cole TJ. Bone changes after 3 mo of lactation: influence of calcium intake, breast-milk output, and vitamin D-receptor genotype. Am J Clin Nutr 1998;67:685-692.
Lewis PR, Brown JB, Renfree MB, Short RV. The resumption of ovulation and menstruation in a well-nourished population of women breastfeeding for an extended period of time. Fertil Steril 1991;55:529-536.
Little KD, Clapp JF, 3rd. Self-selected recreational exercise has no impact on early postpartum lactation-induced bone loss. Med Sci Sports Exerc 1998;30:831-836.
Lopez JM, Gonzalez G, Reyes V, Campino C, Diaz S. Bone turnover and density in healthy women during breastfeeding and after weaning. Osteoporos Int 1996;6:153-159.
Lundeen GA, Knecht SL, Vajda EG, Bloebaum RD, Hofmann AA. The contribution of cortical and cancellous bone to dual-energy X-ray absorptiometry measurements in the female proximal femur. Osteoporos Int 2001;12:192-198.
Marshall D, Johnell O, Wedel H. Meta-analysis of how well measures of bone mineral density predict occurrence of osteoporotic fractures. BMJ 1996;312:1254-1259.
Matsumoto I, Kosha S, Noguchi S, Kojima N, Oki T, Douchi T, Nagata Y. Changes of bone mineral density in pregnant and postpartum women. J Obstet Gynaecol 1995;21:419-425.
Matsushita H, Kurabayashi T, Tomita M, Honda A, Takakuwa K, Tanaka K. The effect of multiple pregnancies on lumbar bone mineral density in Japanese women. Calcif Tissue Int 2002;71:10-13.
Mazess RB. Fracture risk: a role for compact bone. Calcif Tissue Int 1990;47:191-193.
McNeilly AS, Tay CC, Glasier A. Physiological mechanisms underlying lactational amenorrhea. Ann N Y Acad Sci 1994;709:145-155.
Melton LJ, 3rd, Bryant SC, Wahner HW, O'Fallon WM, Malkasian GD, Judd HL, Riggs BL. Influence of breastfeeding and other reproductive factors on bone mass later in life. Osteoporos Int 1993;3:76-83.
Michaelsson K, Baron JA, Farahmand BY, Ljunghall S. Influence of parity and lactation on hip fracture risk. Am J Epidemiol 2001;153:1166-1172.
More C, Bettembuk P, Bhattoa HP, Balogh A. The effects of pregnancy and lactation on bone mineral density. Osteoporos Int 2001;12:732-737.

Moser-Veillon PB, Mangels AR, Vieira NE, Yergey AL, Patterson KY, Hill AD, Veillon C. Calcium fractional absorption and metabolism assessed using stable isotopes differ between postpartum and never pregnant women. J Nutr 2001;131:2295-2299.

Nguyen TV, Jones G, Sambrook PN, White CP, Kelly PJ, Eisman JA. Effects of estrogen exposure and reproductive factors on bone mineral density and osteoporotic fractures. J Clin Endocrinol Metab 1995;80:2709-2714.

Nordin BE, Need AG, Chatterton BE, Horowitz M, Morris HA. The relative contributions of age and years since menopause to postmenopausal bone loss. J Clin Endocrinol Metab 1990;70:83-88.

Parazzini F, Tavani A, Ricci E, La Vecchia C. Menstrual and reproductive factors and hip fractures in post menopausal women. Maturitas 1996;24:191-196.

Petersen HC, Jeune B, Vaupel JW, Christensen K. Reproduction life history and hip fractures. Ann Epidemiol 2002;12:257-263.

Polatti F, Capuzzo E, Viazzo F, Colleoni R, Klersy C. Bone mineral changes during and after lactation. Obstet Gynecol 1999;94:52-56.

Prentice A, Jarjou LM, Cole TJ, Stirling DM, Dibba B, Fairweather-Tait S. Calcium requirements of lactating Gambian mothers: effects of a calcium supplement on breast-milk calcium concentration, maternal bone mineral content, and urinary calcium excretion. Am J Clin Nutr 1995;62:58-67.

Recker RR, Davies KM, Hinders SM, Heaney RP, Stegman MR, Kimmel DB. Bone gain in young adult women. JAMA 1992;268:2403-2408.

Riggs BL, Khosla S, Melton LJ, 3rd. Sex steroids and the construction and conservation of the adult skeleton. Endocr Rev 2002;23:279-302.

Ritchie LD, Fung EB, Halloran BP, Turnlund JR, Van Loan MD, Cann CE, King JC. A longitudinal study of calcium homeostasis during human pregnancy and lactation and after resumption of menses. Am J Clin Nutr 1998;67:693-701.

Standing Committee on the Scientific Evaluation of Dietary Reference Intakes. Dietary Reference Intakes for Calcium, Phosphorus, Magnesium, Vitamin D, and Fluoride. Washington: National Academy Press, 1997.

Sowers M, Corton G, Shapiro B, Jannausch ML, Crutchfield M, Smith ML, Randolph JF, Hollis B. Changes in bone density with lactation. JAMA 1993;269:3130-3135.

Sowers M, Randolph J, Shapiro B, Jannausch M. A prospective study of bone density and pregnancy after an extended period of lactation with bone loss. Obstet Gynecol 1995;85:285-289.

Tuppurainen M, Honkanen R, Kroger H, Saarikoski S, Alhava E. Osteoporosis risk factors, gynaecological history and fractures in perimenopausal women--the results of the baseline postal enquiry of the Kuopio Osteoporosis Risk Factor and Prevention Study. Maturitas 1993;17:89-100.

Yasumizu T, Nakamura Y, Hoshi K, Iijima S, Asaka A. Bone metabolism after human parturition and the effect of lactation: longitudinal analysis of serum bone-related proteins and bone mineral content of the lumbar spine. Endocr J 1998;45:679-686.

THE IMPACT OF ENERGY RESTRICTION AND EXERCISE IN LACTATING WOMEN

Cheryl A. Lovelady

1. ABSTRACT

Exercise improves cardiovascular fitness, plasma lipids, and insulin response in lactating women. However, exercise alone, without caloric restriction, does not promote weight loss. Once lactation is established, over-weight women may restrict their energy intake by 500 kcal/day to promote a weight loss of 0.5 kg/week without affecting the growth of their infants. Moderate exercise does not affect maternal immune status or levels of sIgA, lactoferrin, and lysozyme in human milk. Further research is needed to determine the effect of exercise and energy restriction on maternal bone health and immune status and composition of human milk.

2. INTRODUCTION

The prevalence of obesity among women is increasing at an alarming rate (Flegal et al. 2002). The percent of obese women [body mass index (BMI) equal to or greater than 30] aged 20 to 39 increased from 21% in 1988-94 to 28% in 1999-2000. In addition, 54% of women in this age group were overweight (BMI equal to or greater than 25). Excess weight gain during pregnancy and changes in lifestyle during the postpartum period are likely important contributors to obesity among women (Gunderson et al. 2000; Williamson et al. 1994; Wolfe et al. 1997). While many epidemiologic studies report that the average weight retained from pregnancy is only 0.5 to 3.0 kg; between 14% and 20% of women are 5 kg heavier at 6 to 18 months postpartum than they were before pregnancy (Gunderson et al. 2000).

During the postpartum period, many women desire to lose excess weight gained during pregnancy. Rossner and Ohlin (1995) reported that 40% to 50% of their female patients requested professional support to lose weight after the birth of their infants. Contrary to popular belief, breastfeeding is not always associated with return to pre-pregnancy weight. In fact, some women report gaining weight during lactation (Butte & Hopkinson 1998), possibly due to changes in lifestyle during the postpartum period that may be an ideal time to implement an exercise and diet program to prevent obesity. How-

Department of Nutrition, University of North Carolina, PO Box 26170, Greensboro, NC 27402-6170

Protecting Infants through Human Milk, edited by Pickering *et al.*
Kluwer Academic/Plenum Publishers, 2004

Table 1. Effect of exercise by lactating women on maternal health and milk composition

Variable	Outcomes in lactating women who did and did not exercise	References
Lactation performance	No difference in milk volume, macronutrient composition, or infant growth	Lovelady et al. 1990, 1995, 2000 Dewey et al. 1994 McCrory et al. 1999
Maternal health	Exercise group more fit, leaner, consumed more energy[a]	Lovelady et al. 1990, 1995 Dewey et al. 1994
Maternal bone health	Exercise had minimal effect on bone density	Drinkwater & Chesnut 1991 Little & Clapp 1998
Maternal immune status and immunological factors in milk	Exercise had no effect	Lovelady et al. 2003 Phipps et al. 2000

[a]Exercise alone without caloric restriction does not promote weight loss.

ever, while exercise and energy restriction may improve maternal health during lactation, their effect on milk volume and composition and, consequently, infant growth and health, must be considered. Table 1 summarizes the effects of exercise by lactating women on maternal health and milk composition.

3. EFFECT OF EXERCISE ON LACTATION PERFORMANCE AND MATERNAL HEALTH

One of the early studies to investigate the impact of exercise on lactation performance was a cross-sectional study of exclusively breastfeeding women with infants aged 9 to 24 weeks. This study reported no difference in the macronutrient composition or volume of milk produced between exercising and sedentary women (Lovelady et al. 1990). Women who exercised were more fit (vO_2 max: 46.4±2.4 vs. 30.3±4.7 mL O_2/kg), leaner (21.7±3.5 vs. 27.9±4.7 % body fat), and consumed more energy (2739±309 vs. 2051±335 kcal/day) than the sedentary women. The majority of exercising women had been competitive athletes at some time in their lives, and they reported exercising (mainly swimming and running) an average of 88 minutes/day during lactation. They expended significantly more energy than the sedentary women (3169±273 vs. 2398±214 kcal/day, including the calories in human milk produced).

The results of this study suggest that physically fit women can exercise for long periods of time without affecting human milk production or macronutrient composition, given that their caloric intake is adequate to meet increased energy needs. Dewey et al. (1994) evaluated women who were not physically fit, but wanted to begin an exercise program in the postpartum period, by studying sedentary lactating women. At six to eight weeks postpartum, the subjects were assigned randomly to an exercise or control group.

The exercise program consisted of aerobic exercise (walking, jogging, or cycling), at 60% to 70% of maximum heart rate, 5 days/week for 12 weeks. The sessions were initially 20 minutes long, with increases of 5 minutes every 3 days until 45 minutes/day was achieved. Women in the control group did not engage in aerobic exercise more than once per week during the same period. Both groups were instructed to not restrict their dietary intake.

Women in the exercise group significantly increased their cardiovascular fitness level more than sedentary women (25% vs. 5% increase). Plasma triglycerides, total cholesterol, and LDL-cholesterol decreased significantly in both groups over time (Lovelady et al. 1995). There was a trend for HDL-cholesterol to increase in the exercise group and decrease in the control group. Insulin response to a test meal decreased significantly in the exercise group, but not in the control women. Both groups lost an average of 1.6 kg (which was predominantly fat loss) during the 12-week period. There were no differences in the changes of the macronutrient composition or the volume of human milk produced between groups. Infant weight gain was also similar between groups. This study demonstrated that sedentary women can begin an exercise program without affecting their milk macronutrient composition or volume. However, exercise without energy restriction did not promote weight loss.

4. EFFECT OF EXERCISE AND ENERGY RESTRICTION ON LACTATION PERFORMANCE

McCrory and colleagues (1999) examined the effects of exercise and dieting for 11 days on milk volume and composition. Exclusively breastfeeding women were assigned randomly to one of three groups at approximately 12 weeks postpartum: 1) diet group, which had an energy deficit of 35% by restricting energy intake by approximately 1000 kcal/day; 2) diet plus exercise group, which had an energy deficit of 35% by decreasing energy intake by approximately 720 kcal/day and exercising for 86 minutes/day for 9 of the 11 days; or, 3) control group, which had no energy deficit, but exercised an average of 40 minutes/day, 3 days/week. Women in the diet group lost 1.9±0.7 kg, while the diet and exercise group lost 1.6±0.5 kg, and the control group lost 0.2±0.6 kg. It is interesting to note that almost half of the weight loss in the diet group was fat-free mass, while the diet and exercise group lost no fat-free mass, on the average. This short-term energy deficit did not affect infant growth or milk volume and macronutrient composition. However, there was a relationship between the change in milk energy output and maternal percent body fat in the diet group (r=0.48), but not in the other two groups. That is, fatter women tended to increase the milk energy output, while the leaner women decreased milk energy output during caloric restriction. Only three women actually had a decrease in the energy content of their milk of more than 50 kcal/day. This study suggested that the effect of energy deficit on milk energy output might depend on the duration of the deficit, as well as maternal energy reserves (fat stores).

Lovelady et al. (2000) investigated the effects of longer (10 weeks) energy restriction and exercise on infant growth. Overweight (BMI equaled 25 to 30), sedentary, exclusively breastfeeding women were assigned randomly to one of two groups at four weeks postpartum. The diet and exercise group restricted their energy intake by 500 kcal/day and exercised for 4 days/week at 65% to 80% of their maximum heart rate. Their reported energy intake averaged approximately 2200 kcal/day prior to the intervention. The exercise sessions initially were 15 minutes, then were increased by 2 minutes every day until the women were exercising (walking, jogging, or aerobic dancing) for 45 minutes/day. Women in the control group were instructed not to restrict their energy intake and not to perform vigorous exercise more than once per week.

Women in the diet and exercise group lost significantly more weight (4.8±1.7 kg vs. 0.8±2.3 kg) and fat mass (4.0±2.0 kg vs. 0.3±1.8 kg) than mothers in the control group. Cardiovascular fitness increased significantly more in the diet and exercise group compared with the control group (13% vs. 2% increase). The gains in infant weight and length were similar in both groups. The results of this study suggest that overweight women may begin a program of moderate exercise and energy restriction at four weeks postpartum and that a weight loss of 0.5 kg/week will not affect infant growth.

5. EFFECT OF EXERCISE ON MATERNAL BONE HEALTH

There is a paucity of studies regarding the effect of exercise on bone density during lactation. Drinkwater and Chestnut (1991) measured changes in bone density before pregnancy and during lactation (one and six months postpartum) in six active women. Subjects walked, ran, or swam for 1 hour/day, 5 to 6 days/week. During lactation, women reported consuming an average of 1622±164 mg of calcium per day. After six months of lactation, bone density of the radial shaft returned to the prepregnancy level and there were no changes in the tibial density. The femoral neck density declined during pregnancy and continued to decline during lactation. The density of the lumbar spine decreased during pregnancy and increased during lactation; however, these changes were not significant. There were no significant changes in the density of the femoral shaft, fibula, or distal radius during pregnancy or lactation. A major limitation of this study is the small sample size and the lack of a comparison group of nonexercising lactating women. The decrease observed in the femoral neck is similar to that observed in other studies of nonexercising lactating women (Sowers et al. 1993). However, the increase in the lumbar spine density is in contrast to the decline usually reported among sedentary lactating women (Sowers et al. 1993; Cross et al. 1995; Hayslip et al. 1989; Kalkwarf & Specker 1995). This suggests there may be some beneficial effects of exercise during lactation on maternal bone health.

Little and Clapp (1998) reported the results of a case-control study of exercising and sedentary lactating women's bone density changes at 2 weeks and 12 to 14 weeks postpartum. Women exercised (mainly walking, running, aerobics, or stair machines) 3 to 6 days/week at 55% to 75% of vO_2 max for 25 to 70 minutes per session. Women in the control group exercised less than this or not at all. Both groups lost density in the lumbar spine and the femur neck; however, total bone density did not change. These authors concluded that regular recreational exercise had no effect on the normal decline in bone density during lactation. They suggested that high impact, site-specific exercise may be needed to counterbalance the negative effects of low estrogen levels and daily calcium secretion in human milk on bone density.

6. EFFECT OF EXERCISE ON MATERNAL IMMUNE STATUS AND IMMUNOLOGICAL PROPERTIES OF HUMAN MILK

The effect of exercise on the immune system is dependent on the degree of intensity and duration of exercise, as well as the fitness level of individuals. The "Inverted J Hypothesis" suggests that moderate exercise enhances resistance to infection, while heavy exertion may result in lower resistance and increased risk of upper respiratory tract infections (Nieman 1994).

There are few published studies on maternal immune status during lactation. Lovelady and colleagues compared the cellular immunologic profile and immune function of exercising and sedentary women at three months postpartum. Women in the exercise group reported exercising aerobically at least 30 minutes/day, 3 days/week. Sedentary women exercised only once a week or not at all.

The characteristics of the groups were similar except that exercising women had significantly higher levels of cardiovascular fitness (vO_2 max: 39.5±1.0 vs. 32.4±1.0 mL O_2/kg). There were no significant differences between groups in their complete blood cell counts, the differential white cell counts, or their cellular immunological profile (helper T cells, CD3+CD4+; cytotoxic T cells, CD3+CD8+; B cells, CD19+ and natural killer cells, CD56+) (Phipps et al. 2000). The values were similar to those reported for lactating women (Zimmer et al. 1996, 1998; Hyung et al. 1997). Immune function was determined by neutrophil bacterial killing and oxidative burst activities, and mitogenic-induced proliferation of lymphocytes. There were no differences between groups in the results of these functional assays as well. Early morning samples of human milk were collected and secretory immunoglobulin A (sIgA), lactoferrin, and lysozyme concentrations were measured. There were no significant differences between groups in these immunologic components of human milk.

A subsample of women from the exercise group participated in a study to determine the acute effects of moderate exercise on the concentrations of sIgA, lactoferrin, and lysozyme in human milk (Lovelady et al. 2003). These women came to the laboratory two additional times for either a 30-minute sitting rest session or a 30-minute exercise session on the treadmill at 75% of their predicted maximum heart rate. The order of these sessions was randomized. Human milk samples were collected before and at 10 and 60 minutes after each session. There were no differences in concentrations of sIgA, lactoferrin, or lysozyme after exercise compared with sitting rest. These results are in contrast to those reported by Gregory and colleagues (1997). They reported that sIgA concentrations were lower 10 and 30 minutes after women had completed a graded maximal exercise test compared with samples at 10 and 30 minutes after sitting rest. By 60 minutes after exercise, the concentrations of sIgA were similar to those after 60 minutes of rest. Their different results may be due to the fact that women were exercising until exhaustion, versus exercising for 30 minutes at moderate intensity. While moderate exercise may enhance or have no effect on immune status, exhaustive exercise may be detrimental to immune function.

7. REFERENCES

Butte NF, Hopkinson JM. Body composition changes during lactation are highly variable among women. J Nutr 1998;128:381S-385S.

Cross NA, Hillman LS, Allen SH, Krause GF. Changes in bone mineral density and markers of bone remodeling during lactation and postweaning in women consuming high amounts of calcium. J Bone Miner Res 1995;10:1312-1320.

Dewey KG, Lovelady CA, Nommsen-Rivers LA, McCrory MA, Lonnerdal B. A randomized study of the effects of aerobic exercise by lactating women on breast-milk volume and composition. N Engl J Med 1994;330:449-453.

Drinkwater BL, Chesnut CH. Bone density changes during pregnancy and lactation in active women: a longitudinal study. Bone Miner 1991;14:153-160.

Flegal KM, Carroll MD, Ogden CL, Johnson CL. Prevalence and trends in obesity among US adults, 1999-2000. JAMA 2002;288:1723-1727.

Gregory RL, Wallace JP, Gfell LE, Marks J, King BA. Effect of exercise on milk immunoglobulin A. Med Sci Sports Exerc 1997;29:1596-1601.

Gunderson EP, Abrams B, Selvin S. The relative importance of gestational gain and maternal characteristics associated with the risk of becoming overweight after pregnancy. Int J Obes 2000;24:1660-1668.

Hayslip CC, Klein TA, Wray HL, Duncan WE. The effects of lactation on bone mineral content in healthy postpartum women. Obstet Gynecol 1989;73:588-592.

Hyung RN, Daniels LC, Seelig LL. Preliminary study of how alcohol consumption during pregnancy affects immune components in breast milk and blood of postpartum women. Alcohol Alcohol 1997;32:581-589.

Kalkwarf HJ, Specker BL. Bone mineral loss during lactation and recovery after weaning. Obstet Gynecol 1995;86:26-32.

Little KD, Clapp JF. Self-selected recreational exercise has no impact on early postpartum lactation-induced bone loss. Med Sci Sports Exerc 1998;30:831-836.

Lovelady CA, Lonnerdal B, Dewey KG. Lactation performance of exercising women. Am J Clin Nutr 1990;52:103-109.

Lovelady CA, Nommsen-Rivers LA, McCrory MA, Dewey KG. Effects of exercise on plasma lipids and metabolism of lactating women. Med Sci Sports Exerc 1995;27:22-28.

Lovelady CA, Garner KE, Moreno KL, Williams JP. The effect of weight loss in overweight, lactating women on the growth of their infants. N Eng J Med 2000;342:449-453.

Lovelady CA, Hunter CP, Geigerman C. Effect of exercise on immunological factors in breast milk. Pediatrics 2003;111:e148-e152.

McCrory MA, Nommsen-Rivers LA, Mole PA, Lonnerdal B, Dewey KG. A randomized trial of the short-term effects of dieting vs dieting with aerobic exercise on lactation performance. Am J Clin Nutr 1999;69:959-967.

Nieman DC. The effect of exercise on immune function. Bull Rheumatic Dis 1994;43:5-8.

Phipps CL, Lovelady CA, Fuller CJ, Failla ML, Geigerman CM, Ham T, Kinsella T, Reavis CL, Synnott K. Immune status of exercising, lactating women. FASEB J 2000;14:A508.

Rossner S, Ohlin A. Pregnancy as a risk factor for obesity: lessons from the Stockholm pregnancy and weight development study. Obes Res 1995;3:267s-275s.

Sowers MF, Corton G, Shapiro B, Jannausch ML, Crutchfield M, Smith ML, Randolph JF, Hollis B. Changes in bone density with lactation. JAMA 1993;269:3130-3135.

Williamson DF, Madans J, Pamuk E, Flegal KM, Kendrick JS, Serdula MK. A prospective study of childbearing and 10-year weight gain in US white women 25 to 45 years of age. Int J Obes Relat Metab Disord 1994;18:561-569.

Wolfe WS, Sobal J, Olson CM, Frongillo EA, Williamson DF. Parity-associated weight gain and its modification by sociodemographic and behavioral factors: a prospective analysis in US women. Int J Obes 1997;21:802-810.

Zimmer JP, Garza C, Heller ME, Butte N, Goldman AS. Relationship between serum prolactin, lactation and changes in maternal blood B-cell (CD19+) percents during the first 8 months post-partum. J Reprod Immunol 1996;30:81-95.

Zimmer JP, Garza C, Heller ME, Butte N, Goldman AS. Postpartum maternal blood helper T (CD3+CD4+) and cytotoxic T (CD3+CD8+) cells: correlations with iron status, parity, supplement use, and lactation status. Am J Clin Nutr 1998;67:897-904.

PROTECTING, PROMOTING, AND SUPPORTING BREASTFEEDING AMONG WOMEN IN THE LABOR FORCE

Marina Ferreira Rea[1] and Ardythe L. Morrow[2]

1. ABSTRACT

The need to protect, promote, and support breastfeeding among women in the labor force is an important global issue that requires greater attention. An increasing proportion of women of child-bearing age are employed outside the home. Women who resume full-time work outside the home when their infants are young tend to have shorter durations of breastfeeding and less exclusive breastfeeding. However, evidence indicates that appropriate breastfeeding policy and support programs can help sustain breastfeeding among employed women. Effective strategies include delayed return to work, working part-time, improved conditions at work for breastfeeding, breastfeeding breaks during work hours, milk expression and storage, and access to breastfeeding counseling. In this chapter, we consider the special needs of women working outside the home; provide a brief overview of the literature; and address international policy regarding the protection, promotion, and support of breastfeeding among women who work outside the home.

2. INTRODUCTION

Women in modern society need protection, information, and encouragement to breastfeed successfully. Unlike ancient times, when the view of a woman breastfeeding was familiar, society has changed in ways that discourage breastfeeding. The presence of women in the labor force has increased; consumerism is the rule; health systems typically are focused on disease treatment rather than healthy behaviors; and many mothers lack the role models, experience, and social support for breastfeeding. When a woman is employed outside the home, challenges to successful breastfeeding increase. Unfortunately, the special needs of breastfeeding women who work outside the home typically are overlooked. The objective of this paper is to discuss the rationale for, and studies and policies related to breastfeeding by women who work outside the home.

[1]Instituto de Saude, Coordination of Institutes of Research, Secretaria de Estado da Saude de São Paulo, Brazil
[2]Center for Epidemiology and Biostatistics, Cincinnati Children's Hospital Medical Center, Cincinnati, OH

3. LITERATURE REVIEW

In this section, we provide a brief review of published studies relevant to working women and breastfeeding (Table 1). This literature review is not exhaustive but identifies a few key points as background.

When a mother resumes work outside the home, optimal breastfeeding can be sustained. However, if the mother returns to work outside the home when the infant is young, exclusive breastfeeding often becomes more challenging because of the geographic separation of the mother and infant and, in many cases, greater maternal time constraints. As a result, maternal work outside the home in the first few months postpartum has been associated with shortened duration of breastfeeding or lower rates of exclusive breastfeeding in many areas of the world (Ashworth et al. 2000; Dearden et al. 2002; Valdes et al. 2000). Fein and Roe (1998) showed that working part-time does not interfere with the likelihood of breastfeeding, but that working full-time does; working full time at three months postpartum decreased breastfeeding duration by 8.6 weeks ($P<0.001$) compared with not working. Other researchers have shown that among mothers in the United States in paid jobs, earlier resumption of employment is associated with earlier weaning (Auerbach & Guss 1984).

Breastfeeding support programs can help contribute to the success of employed mothers (O'Gara et al. 1994). Yilmaz et al. (2002) conducted a study in Turkey and found that support for breastfeeding women who work outside the home should involve longer leave from work and improved breastfeeding conditions at work. Rea and others (1999) reported that the duration of exclusive breastfeeding in Sao Paulo, Brazil, was longer among factory workers who had support for breastfeeding at work, did not do shift work, and did not work on weekends. Valdés et al. (2000) conducted a prospective, controlled intervention trial among working mothers in Santiago, Chile. Breastfeeding support that included anticipatory counseling combined with monthly postpartum clinical follow-up visits significantly increased the proportion of working women who exclusively breastfed their infants to 6 months of age, from 6% of women in the control group to 53% of women in the intervention group. Most of the working women who maintained exclusive breastfeeding expressed and stored their milk.

Unfortunately, available studies on breastfeeding and work (Table 1) provide a limited evidence base for this important area. The studies typically do not describe job patterns (part-time, full-time, seasonal, domestic, or per piece). Thus, the studies are often not comparable. Given the variation in job circumstances, working mothers may confront very different issues, and the solutions from one circumstance may not apply to other circumstances. There also are many questions that are not addressed in the literature on working women and breastfeeding. What legislation is effective and available to support working breastfeeding mothers? When women are first time mothers and are likely to have little empowerment, are they able to negotiate breastfeeding needs? While wages for women are lower than wages for men, more women are now heads of households. Does this inequity in wages interfere with mothering and breastfeeding decisions? The majority of working women are informal workers, and consequently have no legal benefits and unsafe job positions, which may be a reason for early weaning. How can migrant women who live alone be protected and supported so they can breastfeed? Do working women need greater or different support to breastfeed than other women? If summary, is there a need for different information on lactation management? The topic of breastfeeding among women who work outside the home needs much more study.

Table 1. Summary of relevant studies on working women and breastfeeding

Author, Country, Year	Study / Design	Sample	Results	Conclusions	Comments
Cohen et al., USA, 1995a	Cohort	Participants self-selected: 2 corporations with 2400 and 1200 female employees 55 BF 42 ff	Infants with no illness: 86% BF 14% ff Absences of at least 1 day: 25% in BF 75% in ff	Fewer and less severe infant illness and less absenteeism among breastfeeding mothers	Breastfeeding support can benefit businesses by reduced health care costs and reduced absenteeism.
Cohen et al., Honduras, 1995b	Cohort	140 women: compared working women with mothers not employed	Breastfeeding time was similar (75 min/12 hr)	Time constraints are not a barrier to exclusive breastfeeding in this population	Needs of working women may differ between populations.
Rea et al., Brazil, 1999	Cross-sectional	69 formally employed	Median EBF: 10 days PBF: 7 days BF: 150 days	EBF longer among working women with a nursery on site for milk extraction at the workplace	All women had 120 days of maternity leave, but needed stronger health care support.
Haider et al., Bangladesh, 1995	Cross-sectional	238 working women with children below 30 months of age	Complementary feeding – 41days 99% unaware of their entitlements 20% break for breastfeeding	Duration of BF was shorter in mothers who started other feeds before 41 days postpartum	Provision of facilities to support BF in the workplace also must be encouraged so that maternal employment does not hamper BF.
Kurinij et al., USA, 1989	Survey	668 black women 511 white women	Women BF more often when in professional vs. sales or technical occupations. Black women who returned to work BF less.	Women in professional occupations had a longer duration of BF than women in sales or technical positions	If the maternity policy discourages BF, the recommended 6 months of BF will not be followed. National maternity policy needs to support working women to BF to 6 months.

BF=breastfeeding; ff=formula-feeding; EBF=exclusive breastfeeding; PBF=partial breastfeeding; full-time=f-t; part-time=p-t

Table 1. Summary of relevant studies on working women and breastfeeding (continued)

Author, Country, Year	Study / Design	Sample	Results	Conclusions	Comments
Valdés et al., Chile, 2000	Intervention trial	Control group vs. Intervention group: Monthly counseling	CG: 6% EBF: 6 mo LG: 53% EBF: 6mo CG: 23% milk express LG: 66% milk express	BF support with counseling increased BF among working women	All counseled women would advise a friend to combine EBF and work.
Auerbach & Guss, USA, 1984	Survey	567 women who report employment and breastfeeding	Timing of return to work had a more negative effect than the number of hours worked	Breastfeeding is possible following maternal return to employment	Early return to work can negatively impact breastfeeding
Fein & Roe, USA, 1998	Cohort	Working women in part time (p-t) or full-time (f-t)	Expecting to work p-t neither decreased nor increased BF, but f-t decreased (OR =0.47, $P<0.001$)	Working full time at 3 months postpartum decreased BF duration by average of 8.6 weeks	Part-time work is an effective strategy to help mothers combine BF and employment
Visness & Kennedy, USA, 1997	Cohort	9,087 U.S. women	BF initiation (53%) was not associated with maternal employment, but among breastfeeders returning to work within a year of delivery was associated with a shorter duration of BF when other factors were controlled	The low rates of BF are not attributable to maternal employment, but returning to work is associated with earlier weaning among women who breastfeed	Duration of maternity leave was associated positively with duration of breastfeeding
Arlotti et al., USA, 1998	Controlled trial	18 peer counselor group 18 without counselor	Women who return to work breastfed 6–9 weeks less than women that stay home	Factors discouraged BF: returning to work, school, or both and use of milk supplement	Peer support is one important component of social support to enhance BF success in this population

Bridges et al., USA, 1997	Descriptive exploratory	69 male and female employers in rural community	Business variables appeared to be better predictors of a positive level of support toward BF in the work place than personal attributes	The health care provider needs to become instrumental in promoting BF in the workplace.	Approaches to partnership with business regarding breastfeeding need to consider the business perspective.
Zanon et al., Italy, 1997	Cross-sectional	963 rural women were interviewed (85.6%) from 1978 to 1993	PBF: 61% in 1978 and 81% in 1993 Mean duration: 4–6.3 months PBF in working women: 66% PBF in housewives: 79%	The factor that most strongly influenced BF was a mother's working	The authors emphasize the need to carry out concrete new initiatives in favor of working mothers
Yimyam & Morrow Thailand, 1999	Cross-sectional	313 working women	Site of working % BF at 6 months: Home: 80% Public sector: 37% Private: 39%	Women work outside the home for long periods	There is a need for multisectorial policies on working women and BF
Miller et al., USA, 1996	Cross-sectional	450 female residents in medical schools; 60 had a child	80% initiated BF 15% BF 6 months of 24 BF- 83% pumped 79% insufficient time 42% No place for pumping	To modify medical resident's workplaces is necessary to BF	Maternity leave for medical residents is 7 weeks (mean) and all used it for BF
Yilmaz et al., Turkey, 2002	Descriptive	301 working women	77% BF 4 months Factors important for weaning: work conditions Maternal leave Smoking Breast pump	Maternity leave must be increased and work conditions should be improved	

BF=breastfeeding; ff=formula-feeding; EBF=exclusive breastfeeding; PBF=partial breastfeeding; full-time=f-t; part-time=p-t

4. BREASTFEEDING PROTECTION, PROMOTION, AND SUPPORT

In 1989, the World Health Organization (WHO) and UNICEF launched a powerful joint statement that begins with the phrase, "Protecting, Promoting and Supporting Breastfeeding" (WHO-UNICEF 1989). However, this document did not address the special needs of employed mothers. Thus, we propose the following thoughts on the meaning of protecting, promoting, and supporting in relation to women in the labor force.

Protection should come from society, community, nations, and international bodies that recognize the importance of lactation and enact laws and policies to benefit mothers and their children. Women should be entitled to the benefits of maternity protection as soon as they obtain paid employment.

Promotion of breastfeeding is always important to continue in general; however, promotion should be elaborated to account for the situation of working women who may otherwise disregard the messages as irrelevant to their needs and circumstances. The WHO/UNICEF strategic document "Global Strategy for Infant and Young Child Feeding," encourages breastfeeding promotion to not be limited to the health sector. Rather, the strategy document encourages involvement by the private sector, families, community groups, employers, unions, and others related to job activities—those who have power to facilitate and encourage working mothers to breastfeed.

Support is necessary for all nursing women, to include information about the benefits of breastfeeding, lactation management and the best way to introduce complementary feeding, while sustaining breastfeeding. However, when working outside the home and distant from their infants for certain hours, women must have the skills needed to adequately express and store milk safely, as well as to overcome lactation problems that sometimes occur due to ongoing mother-infant separation.

5. PROTECTING BREASTFEEDING FOR WORKING WOMEN

There are different policies that can be used to protect working women as mothers. *The Innocenti Declaration*, adopted in 1990 by 31 countries and many intergovernmental organizations, UNICEF, and WHO, established that, "All governments should enact imaginative legislation to protect the rights of working women and establish means for its enforcement." While this seminal document advanced the protection of breastfeeding, enacting "imaginative legislation" has not been easily defined or accomplished.

Countries that are members of the UN and its organization for employment recommendations and international treaties, the International Labor Organization (ILO), must follow ILO conventions as a minimum standard and adapt it to their own national laws and culture. ILO Convention 103, revised in 1952, contains provisions related to lactating women, including 12 weeks of maternity leave and two breastfeeding breaks each day during working hours. According to one assessment conducted in 1998 by the UN, only 30 countries have ratified that convention. However, approximately 80 countries were found to have better policies than those stated in the ILO Conventions, and, among those 31 countries who signed the Innocenti Declaration, 18 had made progress on maternity benefits, including Brazil, China, Chile, India, Italy, Mexico, Zimbabwe, and others. In 2000, ILO Convention 183 on maternity protection of working women was voted in plenary session after two years of discussions. To date, this new convention has been ratified by only five countries.

When thinking about the need of the majority of women, we must recognize that, according to the ILO (1996), women are concentrated in low-wage and informal employment, including "temporary or casual work, multiple part-time jobs, domestic, subcontracting or 'putting-out' systems, and self-employment in micro-enterprises and small firms in the informal sector." In industrialized countries, women represent 65% to 90% of all part-time workers, while in developing countries they are mostly in the informal sector, including self-employment, small trading enterprises, short-term and fixed term contracts, many small family owned and operated businesses, self-employed craftspeople and market women (ILO 1996).

The ILO is concerned with enacting labor legislation that is accepted and subsequently ratified by the majority of member states, particularly with support of the United States. In 1997 the ILO decided to review legislation protecting maternity. As a result, a new revised document was approved in June 2000, in the 88th Session (Convention 183). Countries were consulted about their positions, among Ministers of Labor, trade unions and employers' organizations, and a synthesis report was submitted for discussion. According to some observers, only limited progress resulted from this review, due to the general decrease in social benefits and the increase in global unemployment. An important achievement of Convention 183 was the universal coverage achieved, meaning that all employed women were included independent of job categories, whether informally or formally employed.

Regarding the special needs of working mothers in relation to breastfeeding, we note that to establish successful lactation, it is necessary for the mother to stay with her infant after delivery. A period of maternity leave is therefore essential to the working breastfeeding mother. According to the ILO, maternity leave is defined as *leave whose purpose is to safeguard the health of a woman employee and that of her child during the perinatal period, whether immediately before or after the birth.*

ILO Convention 183 approved 14 weeks of maternity leave. Research suggests that with respect to the condition of the mother, a longer maternity leave is advisable (Treffers 2000), but determination of the optimal duration from the standpoint of a woman's health is difficult. With respect to infant health more data are available, if the optimal period of breastfeeding is considered to be adequate duration of leave consistent with the need to practice exclusive breastfeeding for six months.

Another essential component to protection of working women's ability to breastfeed is to require employers to provide for working mothers to either breastfeed or express her own milk, i.e., *breastfeeding breaks*. The ILO states that breastfeeding breaks, defined as interruptions of work for the purpose of nursing, are to be counted as working hours. Special breaks for nursing mothers are well established in legislation worldwide and were approved in Convention 183. Regulations of one hour of nursing per day, often divided into two 30-minute periods can be found in many countries, and in some countries, the breaks may be extended. Nursing facilities in the workplace including a quiet, dedicated room with seats, safe water, and refrigerator are required in a few countries. Such facilities provide a place for mothers to either breastfeed or express and store milk. In ILO Convention 183, space in the workplace for nursing facilities was not approved, but providing space subsequently was voted as a recommendation (Recommendation 191). This ILO Recommendation also included 17 weeks of maternity leave. Conventions, if ratified, must be followed, while Recommendations are merely guidelines for countries to follow or not follow.

While some countries have reasonable legal protection for breastfeeding, serious difficulties remain in the combination of employment, especially full-time employment, and breastfeeding. The practice of breastfeeding in the workplace and/or maintaining lactation while working outside the home is an enormous effort.

Like other countries, breastfeeding is more prevalent in the United States now than previously. In the United States, at the federal level, maternity leave consists of a 12-week unpaid period. However, in November 1999, the President proposed labor regulations that would allow individual states to decide about funding family and medical leave. Considering the global leadership position of the United States, it is important to know how working women in the United States combine their roles of workers and mothers, and the possible potential policies to protect them.

Examples of employers in the United States offering workplaces that provide spaces designated for pumping and storage of human milk during working hours are increasing, as is the case of the Los Angeles Department of Water and Power and of the Hewlett Packard company, in the same city. In the first example, the cost of a sick day of leave for one woman employee was calculated and compared with the cost of lost productive time used for milk extraction with an electric pump. The result showed that a company providing the space to express and store mother's milk was cost effective.

Research questions continue to need to be addressed to clarify policy about support of breastfeeding by mothers in the working environment. For example, during working hours, how long should a woman expect to spend pumping her milk in order to keep adequate milk production? Is it better (more effective and safe) to use hands or breast pumps in milk expression in work environments? If women elect to use breast pumps, is it better to use single or double pumps? Are two breastfeeding breaks during working hours replaceable by one extra hour at the end of the workday to sustain effective lactation?

Another important general policy to protect breastfeeding is the *International Code of Marketing of Breast Milk Substitutes* (Sokol 1997) and subsequent WHO-related resolutions. This code could be translated into legislation within countries to become more effective. Issues concerning unethical advertisement of infant formula, bottles, and teats, as well as the attitudes and practices of health care workers are all regulated by the Code and should be monitored to protect breastfeeding from commercial interest.

To protect breastfeeding in modern society with the increasing participation of women in the labor force, legal protective measures are important, but social mobilization also is important to ensure that all sectors, especially employers, understand and cooperate with mothers' needs during lactation.

6. PROMOTING BREASTFEEDING AMONG WORKING MOTHERS

Although effective breastfeeding promotional campaigns have been designed and executed, there are problems that must be considered, particularly when the target audience is working mothers. Unfortunately, there are gaps in research pertaining to evaluation of breastfeeding promotion; in the few studies found, description and analysis of each component of the campaign is lacking.

Since the 1980s, the best methods of conducting breastfeeding campaigns have been discussed with the participation of media experts (Jelliffe & Jelliffe, 1988). Since circumstances vary, the first step needed is a situation analysis of infant feeding and working women in the country. Not everywhere do women work in places distant from their homes and take their infants with them to the work place, as they do in some rural areas of Africa, for instance. Not everywhere do women have only one child, delay

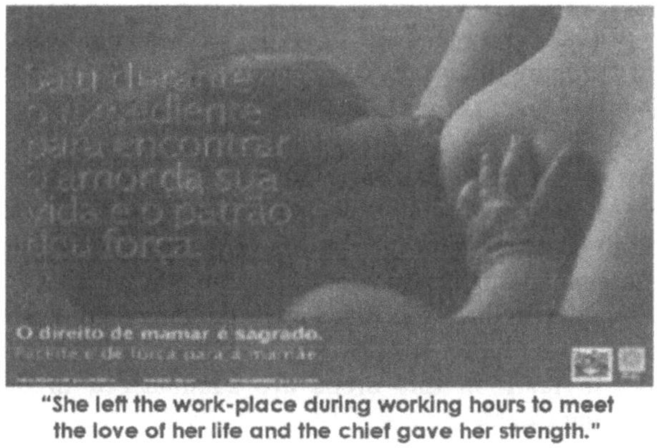

Figure 1. Promotion-Brazilian Breastfeeding Programme: Poster

pregnancy, and give primacy to their careers, as some women in urban areas of North America or Europe may do. Therefore, when planning a breastfeeding promotional campaign targeted to working women, we should consider the needs of the specific populations being considered. Secondary target audiences also should be identified, such as employers, landowners, housewives, trade unions, bosses or chiefs, and ministers of labor. Health professionals should always be considered to be a target audience. Messages to the health professionals also should be a result of a situation analysis regarding working women and breastfeeding.

After conducting the analysis of barriers to breastfeeding and defining audiences, the next step is to design appropriate messages. A study performed before starting the campaign should include qualitative research to indicate cultural values of the community, including language, taboos, job relations, and responses to problems with infant feeding that matter to mobilizing and provoking the desired changes in breastfeeding. The message must be a simple and clear concept, including the constraints identified in the qualitative research, arguments and solutions (Manoff 1988). The third step is to select the media for message delivery. Working women may not have time to listen to the radio and, therefore, radio may not be a good medium for communication of target audiences in many places. If television is chosen, it is important to consider the time of exposure to optimize the period of time when working women may watch television. For example, in our experience, we have learned to always include media specialists in our strategic planning process, while providing them with the goals and specific aims of targeting working mothers, and familiarizing them with the breastfeeding circumstances and outcomes we seek to improve.

There are other aspects of planning a media campaign, but here we have attempted to suggest only a few key points. Figure 1 illustrates a component of a successful breastfeeding promotion campaign conducted in Brazil that focuses on working women.

7. SUPPORTING BREASTFEEDING BY WORKING MOTHERS

Lactating mothers who plan to resume work outside the home after delivery often express the need to "prepare" the baby either by cessation of breastfeeding or by complementing with another food. Many pediatricians or nurses also encourage this attitude. However, is it necessary to wean when the mother goes back to work? And is it really necessary to "prepare" the baby? Of course, the answers depend on when the mother is obliged to go back to work and the time and support given to sustaining breastfeeding.

All women, during the first weeks after delivery should be taught to hand-express milk, because this skill prepares lactating women to address any situation in which they may suddenly need to be away from their infant (e.g., going shopping or working part-time). Confidence in maintaining lactation after returning to work will occur if healthcare providers or peers help the mother. The first step in building confidence is listening to the woman and paying attention to her specific needs. The skills the health care provider or the counselor have to learn in this arena are summarized in the WHO/UNICEF Breastfeeding Counseling Course:

- **How to listen to and learn with a mother:**
  - Establish a nonverbal communication
  - Ask open questions and avoid judging
  - Respond showing interest and showing you can realize or feel what she feels (empathize)
- **How to give a mother confidence and support:**
  - Accept what the mother says, praising what she is doing right
  - Give practical help and few suggestions, not orders
  - Give relevant information in simple language

It is more likely that advice given to a working mother will be accepted and followed if the counselor understands the woman's specific circumstances and, together, they consider the different possibilities of combining work and breastfeeding. The single most relevant piece of information for a mother who must return to work and who wants to continue breastfeeding is to reassure her that *this is possible.* Lactation can be adapted successfully to the new situation of separation from her infant. Lactating women who return to work need to know the following information:

- Milk production is a demand – supply system. More suckling makes more milk; in the absence of suckling, it is imperative to extract milk.
- Prolactin, the hormone responsible for milk production, is produced more at night. Thus, breastfeeding at night helps to maintain milk supply. Prolactin also may make the mother feel relaxed and sleep better.
- If another food or fluid is offered to the baby, it is important not to use a bottle to avoid nipple confusion. It is easy to feed a baby with a cup or spoon.
- How to express milk by hand or pump and information on appropriate storage.
- The volume of mother's milk per feed and per day that an infant needs by month of age.

It is important that the mother is not made to feel guilty if she concludes that none of the solutions offered to her are possible and she therefore reduces breastfeeding.

8. CONCLUSIONS

Although there are many important aspects of breastfeeding that policy makers need to consider to protect, promote, and support working women to enable breastfeeding, it also is advisable to conduct studies to identify and prioritize which components are cost effective in different countries and circumstances. Proper messages should be designed to reach working mothers, taking into account their needs to practice breastfeeding while they work outside the home.

9. ACKNOWLEDGMENT

We appreciate the contribution to the literature review of Patricia Crucello, a postgraduate student with a fellowship of the CNPq (National Research Council), Brazil. Partial support was provided by HD13021.

10. REFERENCES

Arlotti JP, Cottrell BH, Lee SH, Curtin JJ. Breastfeeding among low-income women with and without peer support. J Community Health Nurs 1998;15:163-178.

Ashworth A, Awang H, Salleh AL. Determinants of breastfeeding duration in Peninsular Malaysia. Asia Pac J Public Health 2000;12:102-106.

Auerbach KG, Guss E. Maternal employment and breastfeeding: a study of 567 women's experiences. Am J Dis Child 1984;138:958-960.

Bridges CB, Frank DI, Curtin J. Employer attitudes toward breastfeeding in the workplace. J Hum Lact. 1997;13:215-219.

Cohen R, Mrtek MB. The impact of two corporate lactation programs on the incidence and duration of breast-feeding by employed mothers. Am J Health Promot 1994;8:436-441.

Cohen R, Mrtek MB, Mrtek RG. Comparison of maternal absenteeism and infant illness rates among breast-feeding and formula-feeding women in two corporations. Am J Health Promot 1995a;10:148-153.

Cohen, RJ, Haddix, K, Hurtado, E, Dewey KG. Maternal activity budgets: feasibility of exclusive breastfeeding for six months among urban women in Honduras. Soc Sci Med 1995b;41:527-536.

Dearden K, Altaye M, de Maza I, de Oliva M, Stone-Jimenez M, Morrow AL, Burkhalter BR. Determinants of optimal breast-feeding in peri-urban Guatemala City, Guatemala. Rev Panam Salud Publica 2002;12:185-192.

Fein SB, Roe B. The effect of work status on initiation and duration of breast-feeding. Am J Public Health 1998;88:1042-1046.

Gielen AC, Faden RR, O'Campo P, Brown CH, Paige DM. Maternal employment during the early postpartum period: effects on initiation and continuation of breast-feeding. Pediatrics 1991;87:298-305.

Haider R, Begum S. Working women, maternity entitlements, and breastfeeding: a report from Bangladesh. J Hum Lact 1995;11:273-277.

Hills-Bonczyk SG, Avery MD, Savik K, Potter S, Duckett LJ. Women's experiences with combining breast-feeding and employment. J Nurse Midwifery 1993;38:257-266.

Innocenti Declaration on the Protection, Promotion and Support of Breastfeeding. Breastfeeding in the 1990s: A Global Initiative. WHO/UNICEF, Florence, Italy, 1990.

International Labour Conference. Provisional Record 20. Eighty-seventh Session, Geneva, 1999.

International Labour Organization. Report of the Committee on Maternity Protection. Committee report/ Proposed Conclusions/ Resolution; 1999.

Katcher A, Lanese M. Breastfeeding by employed mothers: a reasonable accommodation in the work place. Pediatrics 1985;75:644-647.

Kearney MH, Cronenwett L. Breastfeeding and employment. J Obstet Gynecol Neonatal Nurs 1991;20:471-480.
Kurinij N, Shiono PH, Ezrine SF, Rhoads GG. Does maternal employment affect breast-feeding? Am J Public Health 1989;79:1247-1250.
Kvale JK. To wean or not: Help from the workplace. J Hum Lact 1993;94:220-221.
Manoff RK. Social marketing: new imperative for public health. New York: Praeger, 1985.
Manoff RK. Mass media and breastfeeding promotion. In: Jelliffe DB, Jelliffe EFP, editors. Programmes to Promote Breastfeeding. New York: Oxford University Press, 1988.
Miller NH, Miller DJ, Chism M. Breastfeeding practices among resident physicians. Pediatrics 1996;98:434-437.
O'Gara C, Canahuati J, Martin AM. Every mother is a working mother: Breastfeeding and women's work. Int J Gynaecol Obstet 1994; 47:S33-38.
Rea MF. The Brazilian National Breastfeeding Promotion Program: A Success Story. Int J Gynaecol Obstet 1990;31:79-82.
Rea MF, Venancio SI, Batista LE, Greiner T. Determinants of the breastfeeding pattern among working women in sao paulo. journal of human lactation. 1999;15:233-239.
Rea MF. Reflexões sobre a amamentação no Brasil: de como passamos a 10 meses de duração. Cadernos de Saúde Pública, Rio de Janeiro 2003;19:109-118.
Renfrew M, Fisher C, Arms S. Best Feeding: Getting Breastfeeding Right For You. Berkeley, CA: Celestial Arts, 1990; 225 pp.
Roe B, Whittington LA, Fein SB, Teisl MF. Is there competition between breast-feeding and maternal employment? Demography 1999;36:157-171.
Sokol EJ. The Code Handbook. Penang, Malaysia: International Baby Food Action Network (IBFAN), 1997; 361 pp.
The Innocenti Declaration: Progress and Achievements, Part I. Geneva: World Health Organization. Wkly Epidemiol Rec 1998;73:25-30
Treffers PE. "Health aspects of maternity protection," paper prepared for WHO, as a review of literature about Maternity Protection, 2000; mimeo, 8 pp.
Valdes V, Pugin E, Schooley J, Catalan S, Aravena R. Clinical support can make the difference in exclusive breastfeeding success among working women. J Trop Pediatr 2000;46:149-154.
Visness CM, Kennedy KI. Maternal employment and breast-feeding: findings from the 1988 National Maternal and Infant Health Survey. Am J Public Health 1997;87:945-950.
WHO/UNICEF Breastfeeding Counselling: a training course, 1993.
Yee V, Ranutunga D. The clearinghouse on infant feeding and maternal nutrition. Women's rights to maternity protection. Am Public Health Assoc. 6, 10-11, 17-18, 24. 1996.
Yilmaz G, Gurakan B, Akgun S, Ozbek N. Factors influencing breastfeeding for working mothers. Turk J Pediatr 2002;44:30-34.
Yimyam S, Morrow M. Breastfeeding practices among employed Thai women in Chiang Mai. J Hum Lact 1999;15:225-232.
Zanon A, Formentin P, Bolesani C, Lago F, Errico G, Mastroprimiano S, Toffanin R, Sorgato R, De Giorgi G. [Breast feeding in the province of Padua from 1978 to 1993.] Minerva Pediatr 1997;49:39-48.

SECTION IV

INNATE AND ACQUIRED IMMUNE SYSTEMS OF HUMAN MILK

HISTO-BLOOD GROUP ANTIGEN AND HUMAN MILK OLIGOSACCHARIDES

Genetic Polymorphism and Risk of Infectious Diseases

Jacques Le Pendu

1. ABSTRACT

ABH and Lewis antigens are carbohydrates present on gut epithelial cells. These antigens provide diversity within the human population. Their biosynthesis largely is controlled by the enzyme products of alleles at the *ABO*, *FUT2* and *FUT3* loci. We have shown that Norwalk virus (NV) uses structures based on H type 1 as its primary receptor. Norwalk virus is the prototype of human caliciviruses, which collectively are responsible for the majority of gastroenteritis outbreaks in people of all ages. Individuals with two mutated *FUT2* alleles, and therefore devoid of H type 1 epitopes on their gut epithelial cells, are called nonsecretors and are resistant to infection by NV. This genetically controlled mechanism of resistance to NV also might be important in the protection of infants by human milk, yet in an inverse manner since, unlike milk from secretors, the milk from nonsecretor mothers does not inhibit attachment of recombinant NV particles to their primary receptor. This suggests that breastfeeding by a secretor mother should protect a secretor child from NV infection, whereas breastfeeding by a nonsecretor mother should not.

2. INTRODUCTION

ABO antigens were discovered a century ago on erythrocytes. Subsequently, similar molecules were identified in body fluids such as saliva and milk, as well as on various cell types. These molecules are carbohydrates that represent the terminal part of glycan chains of glycolipids or glycoproteins (Watkins 1999). They also may be present as free oligosaccharides in milk and have been found in many animal species, although their presence on red blood cells is restricted to humans and some anthropoid apes (Blancher & Socha 1997). ABO antigens also are expressed in relatively large quantities in the intestine and respiratory tracts, and they may play a role in the attachment of microorganisms (Marionneau et al. 2001). Furthermore, data support the fact that cell

Inserm U419, Institut de Biologie, 9 Quai Moncousu, F-44093, Nantes, France

Protecting Infants through Human Milk, edited by Pickering *et al.*
Kluwer Academic/Plenum Publishers, 2004

surface carbohydrates serve as initial receptors for numerous pathogens and toxins. For example, uropathogenic strains of *Escherichia coli* bind to the glycolipid Galβ3GalNAcβ3Galα4Galβ4Glcβ-Cer through type I or type II adhesins, strains of *Helicobacter pylori* equipped with the BabA adhesin bind to the Le^b antigen Fucα2Galβ3[Fucα4]GlcNAc, and some strains of *Staphylococcus saprophyticus* or *Pseudomonas aeruginosa* have been reported to attach to the histo-blood group A antigen GalNAcα3[Fucα2]Gal. Similarly, the cholera toxin (CT) and *Escherichia coli* labile toxin (LT) bind to the GM1 glycolipid Galβ3GalNAcβ4[NeuAcα2,3]Galβ4Glc-Cer, and Shiga and Shiga-like toxins from *E. coli* bind to the Gb_3 glycolipid Galα4Galβ4Glc-Cer. Toxin A from *Clostridium difficile* strains infecting rabbits bind to Galα3Galβ4GlcNAcβ3Galβ4GlcNAc. *Bacillus thuringiensis* toxin binds to glycans terminated with a β3-linked galactose residue (Moulds et al. 1996; Zopf & Roth 1996; Dai et al. 2000). *B. thuringiensis* toxin has been used in agriculture to control plant parasites such as caterpillars and beetles. However, this toxin also is lethal to the worm *Caenorhabditis elegans*. Most interestingly, a mutation that inactivates β3-galactosyltransferase from *C. elegans* was found to confer resistance to the toxin, indicating that the genetic polymorphism of expression of a glycan structure can confer protection against a pathogen (Griffitts et al. 2001).

Many viruses also are known to attach to glycans. This most often involves recognition of a sialic acid residue as in the case of influenza virus, rotavirus, coronavirus, or polyomavirus. Until recently, the only virus known to attach to a neutral glycan was parvovirus B19, which uses GalNAcβ3Galα4Galβ4Glc-Cer, the P histo-blood group antigen, as receptor (Brown et al. 1993).

The biosynthesis of ABO and related antigens proceeds from precursors by stepwise addition of monosaccharide units through the action of a set of glycosyltransferases. There are five types of precursors that have disaccharides sharing a galactose in β-linkage to the subjacent sugar unit: Type 1, **Galβ3**GlcNAcβ-R; Type 2, **Galβ4**GlcNAcβ-R; Type 3, Galβ3**GalNAcα**-R; Type 4, Galβ3**GalNAcβ**-R; and Type 5, Galβ4**Glcβ**-R. Type 1 and 2 precursors can be part of O- or N-glycoproteins, as well as of glycolipids of the lacto series (represented by the R letter). Type 3 is found exclusively on O-glycans, where it corresponds to core 1. Type 4, is only found on glycolipids of the globo and ganglio series, and Type 5 corresponds to the glycolipid lactosylceramide or to free lactose. In milk, all types of precursor structures can be present since this biologic fluid contains large amounts of glycoproteins with N-linked and O-linked glycans, glycolipids as well as free oligosaccharides. The major biosynthesis pathways of these antigens from the type 1 precursor is presented in Figure 1.

Addition onto precursors of a fucose in α1,2 linkage gives the H antigens. This step is catalyzed by an α1,2-fucosyltransferase. In humans, two α1,2-fucosyltransferases able to participate in the synthesis of these antigens are known. They are encoded by two distinct genes, *FUT1* and *FUT2*. There exists a third α1,2-fucosyltransferase gene called *Sec1* which is inactivated by insertion of a nucleotide leading to a frameshift in the coding sequence. *Sec1* is therefore a pseudogene. Fully or partially inactivating mutations of *FUT1* and *FUT2* define a genetic polymorphism at each of these two loci. Lack of a functional *FUT1* allele leads to the Bombay phenotype characterized by an absence of ABH antigens on erythrocytes. This phenotype is rare with a frequency in the 10^{-5} to 10^{-6} range. The lack of a functional *FUT2* allele is responsible for the nonsecretor phenotype, as opposed to the secretor phenotype, characterized by the absence of ABH antigens in

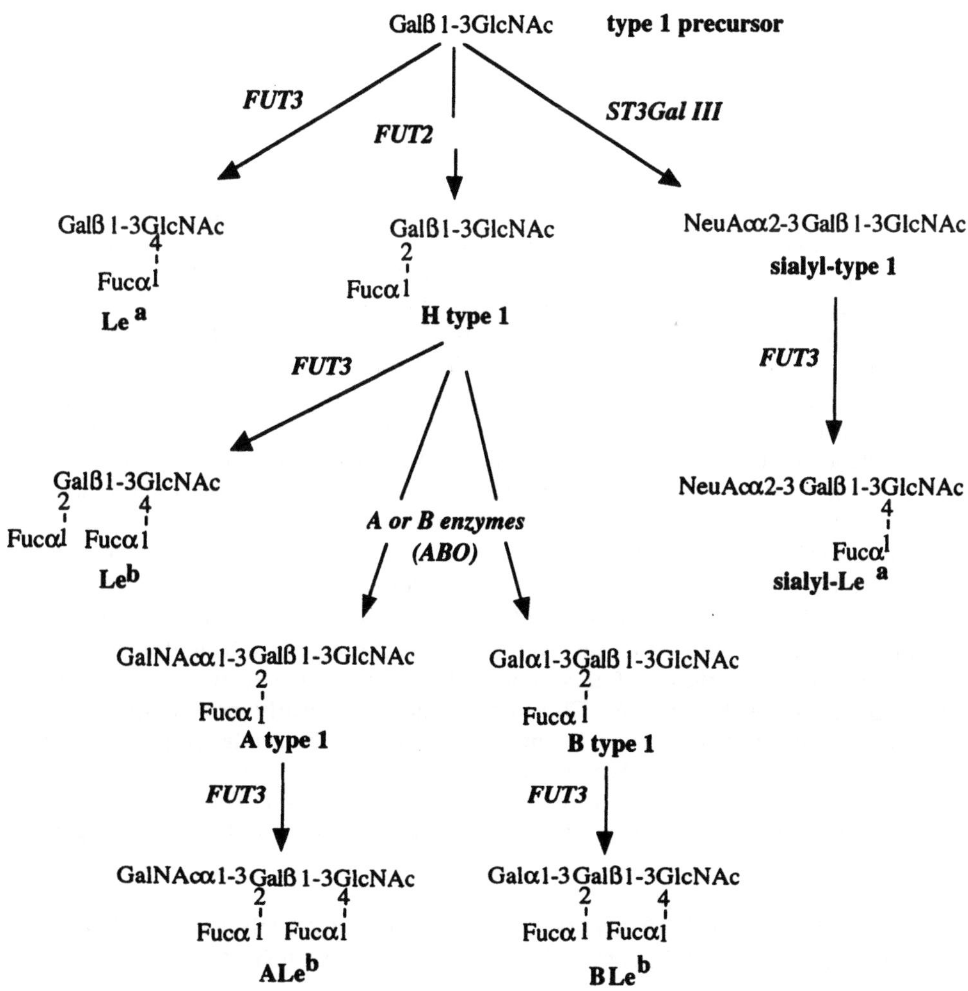

Figure 1. Major biosynthetic pathways of the ABH and Lewis antigens based on the type 1 precursor disaccharide. The name of the antigens are in bold, and the enzymes acting at each catalytic step are marked in italics.

saliva and on various epithelial cell types. Unlike the Bombay phenotype, nonsecretor phenotype is not rare since it is found in about 20% of Europeans and white Americans.

Once the H antigens are formed, biosynthesis can proceed by addition of either an *N*-acetylgalactosamine or a galactose in α1,3 linkage to give the A or B antigens, respectively. This step is catalysed by the A or B enzymes, which are encoded by different alleles at the *ABO* locus. A large series of alleles at this locus has been described: some alleles code for variants of A and B enzymes, others are inactivated by various mutations corresponding to O alleles (Hakomori 1999).

In the case of antigens derived from types 1 and 2 precursors, a fucose can be added in α1,4 or α1,3 of the *N*-acetylglucosamine residue of the precursor giving the Le^a or Le^x antigens, respectively. Addition of a fucose in the same position of the H types 1 and 2 antigens will give the Le^b and Le^y antigens, respectively. The A or BLe^b and A or BLe^y are obtained by addition of a fucose residue on the A/B type 1 or A/B type 2 antigens.

Six fucosyltransferases able to catalyze the addition of fucose in α1,3 or α1,4 position are known in humans. The FUT3 and FUT5 enzymes can use both type 1 and type 2 precursors as substrates, FUT3 having a marked preference for type 1 and FUT5 for type 2. The FUT4, FUT6, FUT7, and FUT9 enzymes catalyze addition of a fucose exclusively onto the type 2 precursor (Cailleau-Thomas et al. 2000). Like the *FUT1* and *FUT2* genes, polymorphisms have been described for *FUT3*, *FUT5*, *FUT6*, and more recently for *FUT7* (Bengston et al. 2001; Mollicone et al. 1994a, 1994b). Individuals lacking a functional *FUT3* allele are called "Lewis negative" and are characterized by the red cell phenotype Le^{a-b-}. They represent nearly 10% of the European population. People with a "Lewis positive" phenotype, either Le^{a-b+} or Le^{a+b-}, possess at least one functional *FUT3* allele and are, respectively, secretors or nonsecretors. The frequency of individuals deficient in FUT5, FUT6 or FUT7 enzymes is not well known as yet, but is low in the case of FUT6 (Mollicone et al. 1994a). The sialyl-Le^a and sialyl-Le^x antigens are obtained by addition of a sialic acid in α2,3 linkage followed by addition of a fucose in α1,4 or α1,3 linkage onto either the type 1 or type 2 precursors. Therefore, the genes involved in the biosynthesis of this group of carbohydrate structures can be either polymorphic, such as the *ABO*, *FUT2*, and *FUT3* genes, or nearly monomorphic such as the *FUT1*, *FUT4*, and *FUT7* genes. In epithelia, most of the biosynthesis is performed by the enzyme products of the polymorphic genes *ABO*, *FUT2*, and *FUT3*, which act in concert to generate a diversity of glycans at the population level. This diversity may be expected to be related with distinct individual susceptibility to a spectrum of pathogens.

3. HISTO-BLOOD GROUP ANTIGENS WITH AN α1,2-LINKED FUCOSE CONSTITUTE THE PRIMARY RECEPTOR FOR NORWALK VIRUS

The Caliciviridae constitute a family of small, positive strand RNA viruses that include animal and human pathogens. They are divided in four genera, two of them, the norovirus and sapovirus, causing acute gastroenteritis in humans (Thiel & König 1999). Epidemiologic studies indicate that noroviruses are responsible for the majority of outbreaks in developed countries, affecting people of all ages including very young children (Glass et al. 2001). Noroviruses are spread by the fecal-oral route from person to person or from contaminated water or food items.

Our group recently observed that another member of the calicivirus family, the lagovirus RHDV (rabbit haemorrhagic virus), binds to the histo-blood group antigen H

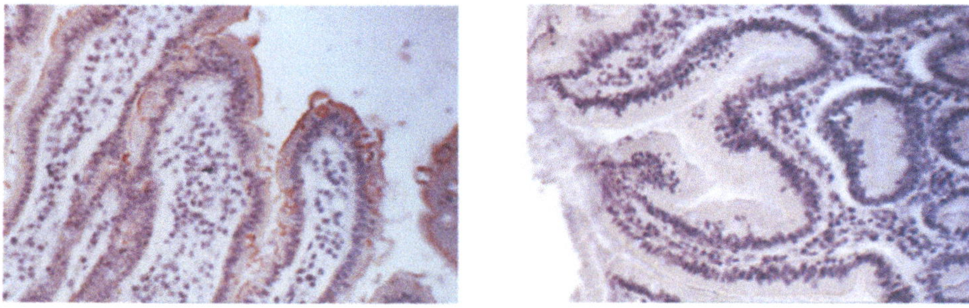

Figure 2. Binding of rNV VLPs to human duodenum tissue sections from a secretor and a nonsecretor individual. Sections were incubated with rNV VLPs, then with an anti-VLP followed by a peroxidase-labeled mouse anti-IgG detection system.

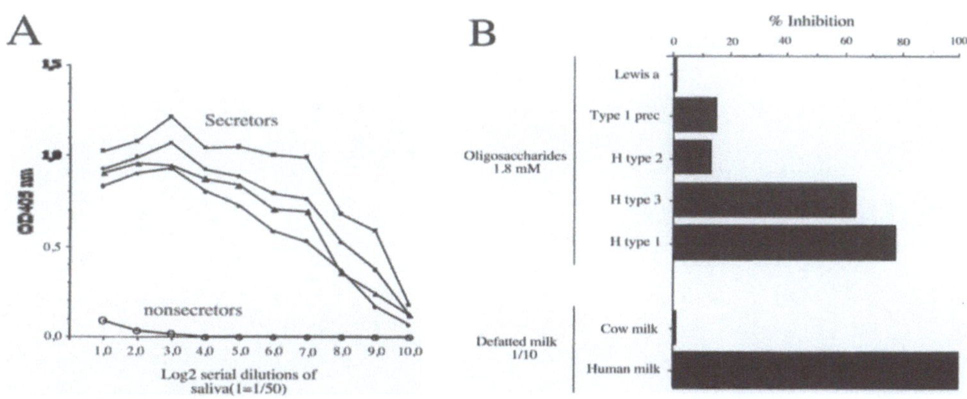

Figure 3. (A) Binding of rNV VLPs to serially diluted saliva samples from either secretors or nonsecretors coated to an EIA plate. (B) Inhibition of rNV VLPs binding to saliva from a secretor individual with synthetic oligosaccharides, cow milk or human milk from a secretor mother. Milk from nonsecretor mothers is not inhibitory (not shown).

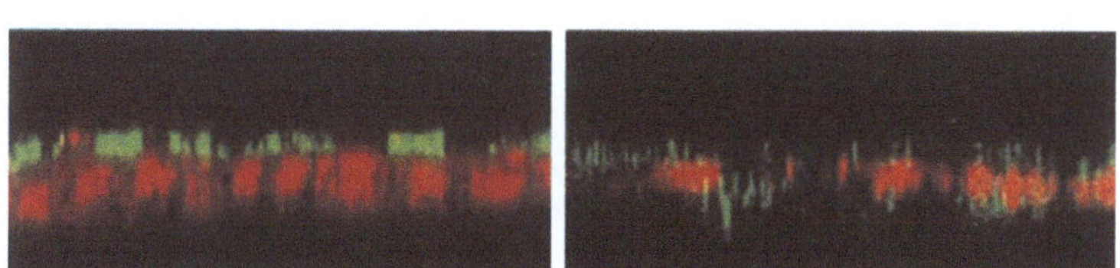

Figure 4. Confocal microscopy experiment showing internalization of rNV VLPs in Caco-2 cells. Caco-2 cells were maintained in culture on filters for 15 days postconfluency to obtain differentiation. The cells were then incubated with rNV VLPs at 4°C or 37°C. After incubation, cells were fixed and permeabilized. The localization of the rNV VLPs was visualized using an antibody against the capsid protein (green fluorescence) and the cell nuclei were stained with iodide propidium (red fluorescence).

type 2 (Fucα2Galβ4GlcNAc) present at the cell surface of the rabbit upper respiratory and digestive epithelial cells (Ruvoën-Clouet et al. 2000). This finding prompted us to determine if human caliciviruses could share this property of attachment to fucosylated glycans. For this aim, we used virus-like particles (VLPs) prepared from recombinant capsid protein of Norwalk virus (NV) by Jiang and colleagues (1992). NV is the prototype of the norovirus genera, discovered in 1972 by electron microscopy (Kapikian 2000). To study interaction of NV with digestive epithelial cells, we used an approach that we developed with RHDV where the VLPs are incubated with tissue sections and their attachment is detected with antibodies directed against the capsid protein by classical immunohistochemistry. Using this technique on human tissue sections from the stomach and duodenum, we observed a clear binding of rNV VLPs on the surface epithelial cells from all secretor individuals, but not from nonsecretors. This was the first indication that a functional *FUT2* allele, and therefore the presence of an α2-linked fucose residue, was necessary for attachment of rNV VLPs to the tissue sections (Fig. 2).

This finding was confirmed by treating tissue sections with a fucosidase that specifically cleaves α2-linked fucose residues, completely abolishing the binding of rNV VLPs. Since α2-fucosylated antigens also are present in the saliva under control of the *FUT2* genetic polymorphism, we developed an assay using boiled saliva samples coated on wells of microtiter plates. A strong binding of rNV VLPs to saliva samples from secretor individuals was observed. In contrast, no binding was obtained using saliva from nonsecretors (Fig. 3A). The binding of rNV VLPs to these saliva samples from secretors could be inhibited by synthetic oligosaccharides with an aliphatic tail. The best inhibition was obtained with the H type 1 trisaccharide, while the H type 3 trisaccharide also proved inhibitory. Other related oligosaccharides such as Le^a or the type 1 precursor were not inhibitory (Fig. 3B). Since then, others have shown that rNV VLPs bind to the H type 1, H type 3, and Le^b synthetic oligosaccharides coupled to polyacrylamide (Hutson et al. 2003; Harrington et al. 2002). These results indicate that these α2-fucosylated antigens are sufficient to mediate attachment of the recombinant virus particles. Using an anti-H type 1 specific antibody, we could inhibit binding of the rNV VLPs to duodenum tissue sections. An antibody specific to H type 3 and H type 4 antigens gave a partial inhibition whereas an anti-H type 2 specific antibody did not inhibit at all, showing that the H type 1 epitope of the digestive surface epithelial cells is recognized by the virus particles. In order to confirm the importance of the α2-linked fucose residue, CHO cells were transfected with a *FUT2* cDNA, allowing cell surface expression of H type 3 and H type 2 epitopes. This was sufficient to mediate attachment of rNV VLPs.

These data indicate that the α2-linked fucose residue under control of the *FUT2* gene is necessary and sufficient to mediate attachment of rNV VLPs. To further support the role of α2-linked fucose residues on the attachment of noroviruses to epithelial cells, we first performed confocal microscopy experiments in order to monitor the possible internalization of rNV VLPs following their attachment to cells expressing the α2-fucosylated ligand. At 4°C, rNV VLPs bound to the surface of either FUT2 transfected CHO cells or of differentiated Caco-2 cells. The latter cells originate from a human colon carcinoma and have the property to spontaneously differentiate in culture when maintained two weeks postconfluency. Additionally, these differentiated Caco-2 cells are the only cultivable cells known to express the H type 1 antigen. For this reason, Caco-2 cells are able to bind rNV VLPs. Upon incubation at 37°C, we could visualize internalization of the recombinant viral particles in both the transfected CHO cells and the differentiated Caco-2 cells (Fig. 4). This result provided the first indication that the attachment of rNV VLPs to the α2-fucosylated antigens could be of functional relevance (Marionneau et al. 2002). However, it did not prove that native virions would behave similarly and that the carbohydrate recognition was absolutely required for infection.

At that stage we had the chance to collaborate with Christine Moe and her colleagues Ralph Baric and Lisa Lindensmith who had just performed a challenge study where 77 healthy volunteers had received an NV inoculum. Of these volunteers, 64% presented signs of infection. When their secretor status was determined, it appeared that all of these infected individuals were in the secretor group. None of the 22 nonsecretors presented signs of infection defined by clinical evidence of gastroenteritis, RT-PCR detectable virus particles in stool, or a 4-fold increase in anti-NV serum IgG (Lindesmith et al. 2003). This result clearly proved that the H type 1, or a closely related antigen requiring an active FUT2 enzyme for its synthesis, is not only sufficient to mediate attachment of the virus but also that it is necessary for infection. Therefore, it can be concluded that the α1,2 epitope constitutes the Norwalk virus primary receptor and that a genetically defined absence of this receptor confers full protection from NV infection.

Since the FUT2 enzyme collaborates with the *FUT3* and *ABO* gene products to synthesize A, B, H type 1, and Le^b antigens, it is quite possible that Norwalk virus will show different affinities for these carbohydrate structures and, therefore, that the polymorphisms at the *FUT3* and *ABO* loci will have some influence on the ability of the virus to infect people. As a first approach to test this possibility, we used the saliva binding assay and noticed an influence of the *ABO* polymorphism on rNV VLPs binding to saliva samples from secretor individuals. The strongest binding was obtained on saliva samples from blood group A individuals. A somewhat lower binding was obtained on saliva samples from blood group O individuals, and a much lower binding was detected on saliva samples from blood group B individuals (Fig. 5).

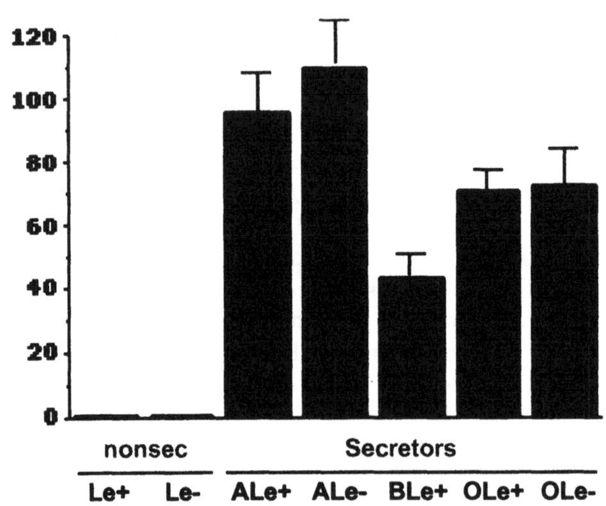

Figure 5. Influence of the ABO and secretor and Lewis phenotypes on the attachment of rNV VLPs particles to saliva samples. The binding of rNV VLPs to saliva samples, diluted 1/800, phenotyped for ABO, secretor and Lewis was determined by EIA. Values are normalized against a set of positive control saliva samples used on each plate.

Interestingly, a study published in 2002 reported that blood group B individuals had a lower risk of being infected by NV, indicating that besides the *FUT2* polymorphism, the *ABO* polymorphism can modulate the susceptibility to Norwalk virus (Hutson et al.). In contrast, no difference was observed between Lewis positive and Lewis negative saliva samples, that is, saliva specimens from individuals with at least a functional *FUT3* allele or with two mutated *FUT3* alleles, respectively. This result is not surprising since NV can attach equally well to H type 1 and to Le^b, which are the two major histo-blood group antigens present in saliva samples from the two subgroups. It is therefore unlikely that the *FUT3* polymorphism should influence infection by NV.

4. PROTECTION FROM NORWALK VIRUS INFECTION BY HUMAN MILK AND THE HISTO-BLOOD GROUP POLYMORPHISM—WHAT SHOULD WE EXPECT?

Human milk is well known to contain histo-blood group antigens either as free oligosaccharides, as glycolipids, and as glycoproteins. It is thus expected that some of these components could inhibit the attachment of NV to its cellular receptor and therefore participate in the protection of infants from NV-mediated gastroenteritis. When human milk samples were used in an inhibition assay of the binding of rNV VLPs to α2-fucosylated ligands, all samples from secretor mothers were strongly inhibitory whereas the samples from nonsecretor mothers were not, indicating that the *FUT2* polymorphism determines not only the attachment of the virus to its primary receptor but also controls the presence of potential protective molecules in human milk. We then tested the ability of the purified milk pentasaccharide Fucα2Galβ3GlcNAcβ3Galβ4Glc to inhibit rNV VLPs binding to immobilized H type 1 complexed to polyacrylamide. Despite the presence of the H type 1 trisaccharide as the terminal portion of this milk oligosaccharide, no inhibition could be obtained, even at a 10 mM concentration. This negative result tends to indicate that the specific inhibitory components from human milk are not the simple free oligosaccharides. Instead, they could be either the complex highly branched oligosaccharides or the multimeric glycans carried by proteins. For this reason we are now trying to characterize and purify the glycoproteins from the milk of secretor mothers that carry α2-fucosylated epitopes and potentially could inhibit the virus attachment to the infant's gut epithelial cells.

As shown in Figure 6, some children can be expected to be genetically resistant to NV since they are nonsecretors. Among the susceptible children, those who are breastfed by a secretor-positive mother could be protected by decoy receptors from the milk. Unfortunately, susceptible children whose mothers are nonsecretors would not be protected since the milk does not contain the appropriate decoy receptor. It is also important to remember that cow milk does not contain histo-blood group structures either as free oligosaccharides or on glycoproteins. Therefore, cow milk does not inhibit the binding of rNV VLPs to immobilized H type 1 (Fig. 3B). Thus, formula-fed infants do not benefit from the protection potentially conferred by the soluble histo-blood group antigens contained in human milk.

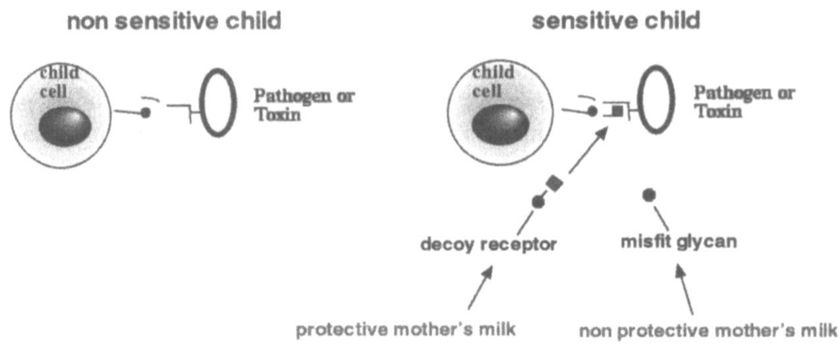

Figure 6. Hypothetical influence of the mother/infant combined histo-blood group polymorphism on the protection of infants from histo-blood group binding pathogens such as NV.

5. ACKNOWLEDGMENT

This work was supported in part by a program project grant from the National Institute of Child Health and Human Development (HD13021).

6. REFERENCES

Bengston P, Larson C, Lundblad A, Larson G, Pahlsson P. Identification of a missense mutation (G329A; Arg(110)>GLN) in the human FUT7 gene. J Biol Chem 2001:276;31575-31582.

Blancher A, Socha WW. ABO, Hh and Lewis blood groups in humans and nonhuman primates. In: Blancher A, Klein J, Socha WW, editors. Molecular Biology and Evolution of Blood Group and MHC Antigens in Primates. Berlin: Springer-Verlag, 1997; pp 30-92.

Brown KE, Anderson SM, Young NS. Erythrocyte P antigen: cellular receptor for B19 parvovirus. Science 1993;262:114-116.

Cailleau-Thomas A, Coullin P, Candelier JJ, Balanzino L, Mennesson B, Oriol R, Mollicone R. *FUT4* and *FUT9* genes are expressed early in human embryogenesis. Glycobiology 2000;10:789-802.

Dai D, Nanthakumar NN, Newburg DS, Walker AM. Role of oligosaccharides and glycoconjugates in intestinal host defense. J Pediatr Gastroenterol Nutr 2000;30:S23-S33.

Glass RI, Bresee JS, Jiang B, Gentsch JR, Ando T, Fankhauser R, Noel J, Parashar UD, Rosen B, Monroe SS. Gastroenteritis viruses: an overview. Novartis Foundation Symposium 2001;238:5-19.

Griffitts JS, Whitacre JL, Stevens DE, Aroian RV. Bt toxin resistance from loss of a putative carbohydrate-modifying enzyme. Science 2001:293;860-864.

Hakomori S. Antigen structure and genetic basis of histo-blood groups A, B and O: their changes associated with human cancer. Biochim Biophys Acta 1999:1473;247-266.

Harrington PR, Lindensmith L, Yount B, Moe CL, Baric RS. Binding of Norwalk virus-like particles to ABH histo-blood group antigens is blocked by antisera from infected human volunteers or experimentally vaccinated mice. J Virol 2002:76;12325-12343.

Hutson AM, Atmar RL, Graham DY, Estes MK. Norwalk virus infection and disease is associated with ABO histo-blood group type. J Infect Dis 2002:185;1335-1337.

Hutson AM, Atmar RL, Marcus DM, Estes MK. Norwalk virus-like particles hemagglutination by binding to H histo-blood group antigens. J Virol 2003:77;405-415.

Jiang X, Wang M, Graham DY, Estes MK. Expresion, self-assembly, and antigenicity of the Norwalk virus capsid protein. J Virol 1992:66;6527-6532.

Kapikian AZ. The discovery of the 27-nm Norwalk virus: an historic perspective. J Infect Dis 2000:181;S295-S296.

Lindesmith L, Moe C, Marionneau S, Ruvoen N, Jiang X, Lindblad L, Stewart P, LePendu J, Baric R. Human susceptibility and resistance to Norwalk virus infection. Nat Med 2003;9:548-553.

Marionneau S, Cailleau-Thomas A, Rocher J, Le Moullac-Vaidye B, Ruvoën-Clouet N, Clément M, Le Pendu J. ABH and Lewis histo-blood group antigens, a model for the meaning of oligosaccharide diversity in the face of a changing world. Biochimie 2001:83;565-573.

Marionneau S, Ruvöen-Clouet N, Le Moullac-Vaidye B, Clement M, Cailleau-Thomas A, Ruiz-Palacios G, Huang PW, Jiang X, Le Pendu J. Norwalk virus binds to H types 1/3 histo-blood group antigens on gastro-duodenal epithelial cells of "secretor" individuals. Gastroenterology 2002:122;1967-1977.

Mollicone R, Reguigne I, Fletcher A, Aziz A, Rustam M, Weston BW, Kelly RJ, Lowe JB, Oriol R. Molecular basis for plasma alpha(1,3)-fucosyltransferase gene deficiency (FUT6). J Biol Chem 1994a:269;12662-12671.

Mollicone R, Reguigne I, Kelly RJ, Fletcher A, Watt J, Chatfield S, Aziz A, Cameron HS, Weston BW, Lowe JB. Molecular basis for Lewis alpha(1,3/1,4)-fucosyltransferase gene deficiency (FUT3) found in Lewis-negative Indonesian pedigrees. J Biol Chem 1994b:269;20987-20994.

Moulds JM, Nowicki S, Moulds JJ, Nowicki BJ. Human blood groups: incidental receptors for viruses and bacteria. Transfusion 1996:36;362-374.

Ruvoën-Clouet N, Ganière JP, André-Fontaine G, Blanchard D, Le Pendu J. Binding of rabbit hemorrhagic disease virus to antigens of the ABH histo-blood group family. J Virol 2000:74;11950-11954.

Thiel HJ, König M. Caliciviruses: an overview. Vet Microbiol 1999:69;55-62.

Watkins WM. A half century of blood-group antigen research. Some personal recollections. Trends Glycosci Glycotechnol 1999:11;391-411.

Zopf D, Roth S. Oligosaccharide anti-infective agents. Lancet 1996:347;1017-1021.

HUMAN MILK PROTECTIVE MECHANISMS

Thomas G. Cleary

1. ABSTRACT

The survival of a nonimmune infant faced with a new pathogen depends in part on an array of specific and nonspecific human milk factors. Human milk protects via multiple redundant strategies. It targets shared virulence mechanisms to provide cross protection. By interfering with fundamental processes such as attachment to glycoconjugates, human milk anticipates new mutations and new pathogens that utilize carbohydrates as receptors. Furthermore, human milk IgA present appears to reflect long-term maternal immunologic memory. These overlapping protective strategies endow human milk with the unique ability to protect infants from organisms that mutate rapidly and are present in vast numbers.

2. INTRODUCTION

Human milk protects infants from illness both during breastfeeding and long after the infant is no longer breastfed. The illnesses that are prevented during breastfeeding are primarily acute infections including diarrheal diseases, upper respiratory tract infections, otitis media, urinary tract infection, meningitis, and neonatal sepsis. Premature infants are protected from acute necrotizing enterocolitis, an illness of uncertain etiology. In addition, epidemiologic data suggest that breastfeeding provides long-term protection against Crohn's disease, ulcerative colitis, type I diabetes mellitus, multiple sclerosis, rheumatoid arthritis, hypertension, obesity, and celiac disease. The studies that suggest long-term effects are more controversial than those showing protection during breastfeeding. The mechanism responsible for many of the long-term effects is not understood fully. In contrast, the mechanism underlying short-term anti-infective properties of human milk, particularly as related to amelioration of gastrointestinal tract infections, are understood at least in part. Several epidemiologic studies have demonstrated the protective effect of breastfeeding against several pathogens, including *Shigella* (and presumably the closely related enteroinvasive *Escherichia coli* [EIEC] that

---

University of Texas Medical School at Houston, Department of Pediatrics, Division of Infectious Diseases, 6431 Fannin, Houston, TX 77030

Protecting Infants through Human Milk, edited by Pickering *et al.*
Kluwer Academic/Plenum Publishers, 2004

have an identical mechanism of virulence) (Hayani et al. 1992), *Vibrio cholerae* (Glass et al. 1983), *Campylobacter* (Ruiz-Palacios et al. 1990), enterotoxigenic *E. coli* [ETEC] (Cruz et al. 1988), rotavirus (Newburg et al. 1998), and *Giardia duodenalis* (Walterspiel et al. 1994). There are factors in human milk that may protect against other infectious agents, including Shiga toxin-producing *E. coli* [STEC], enteropathogenic *E. coli* [EPEC], *Clostridium difficile*, and caliciviruses. In these latter agents the data are primarily from in vitro rather than epidemiologic studies.

There is now a plethora of descriptive information regarding potentially protective factors found in human milk. Still the central question regarding protection from gut infections is the underlying mechanism(s). The fundamental paradox involves two key differences between bacteria and mammals. First, bacterial enteropathogens have the ability to change their DNA by introducing new mutations approximately every 20 minutes when they divide. Organisms that have new mutations that give them a selective advantage in the human gut should have a survival advantage over organisms that lack such mutations. Humans, on the other hand, recombine DNA during the process of making new individuals much less frequently. Mutations that might be useful for protection are introduced infrequently. Second, bacteria can produce millions of copies of themselves in a short time, while humans produce small numbers of individuals comparatively infrequently. With a potentially infinite variety of pathogens in the environment, the human faces a task that should be nearly impossible. Obviously, mutations can be introduced into some mammalian tissues without making a whole new individual (i.e., less than a generation time); B lymphocytes can be selected with somatic mutations in their immunoglobulin genes that allow high affinity antibodies to be produced. However, these antibodies are produced after a relatively long lag time (days to weeks) when compared with the more versatile and numerous pathogens (minutes to hours). The problem for the infant is surviving infection with an enteropathogen long enough to develop pathogen-specific humoral and cellular immunity. The outcome of an encounter with a pathogen depends on an array of specific and nonspecific factors that increase the odds of survival in the face of a new challenge. Human milk provides that protection in fundamentally unique ways. Three principles involved in human milk protection of the nonimmune infant who is faced with a new pathogen are discussed below.

3. FUNDAMENTAL PRINCIPLES OF HUMAN MILK PROTECTION

3.1. Human Milk Targets Shared Virulence Mechanisms

The first principle is that human milk targets mechanisms shared by multiple pathogens. Such targeting is a parsimonious strategy. A given milk factor has the capacity to neutralize or impair the function of many bacteria at the same time because enteropathogens found in the gut have freely exchanged useful genes. Even bacteria of different species appear over time to have transferred genes to one another when those genes have given the bacteria a survival advantage (Table 1). Thus, for example, Shiga toxin is made by the STEC, such as the *E. coli* 0157:H7, 026:H11, O111:NM, and roughly 200 other *E. coli* serotypes; the same toxin (or a very closely related variant) also is made by *Shigella dysenteriae* serotype 1 and occasionally other *Shigella* spp. Likewise, heat-stable enterotoxin of ETEC is related closely to guanylate cyclase-stimulating

Table 1. Bacterial promiscuity: Examples of virulence proteins shared by multiple enteropathogens[a]

Pathogen[b]	Type III secretion system	Shiga toxin	Guanylate cyclase-stimulating heat-stable enterotoxin[c]	Adenylate cyclase-stimulating heat labile enterotoxin	Invasion antigens[d]	Needle complex mechanism
STEC	++	++ (2 major variants share ~55% amino acids)	+ (EAST1)			++
EPEC	++		+ (EAST1)			++
EIEC	++				++ (IpaBCDA)	++ (likely present)
EAEC			+ (EAST1)			
ETEC			+ (STa and EAST1)	+		
Shigella spp	++	+			++ (IpaBCDA)	++
Salmonella spp	++			+	++ (SipBCDA)	++
Yersinia enterocolitica	++		+		++ (YspBCDA)	++ (likely present)
Vibrio cholerae			+ (clinical relevance uncertain)	++		

[a]++=always present; +=sometimes present

[b]STEC=Shiga toxin-producing *E. coli*; EPEC=enteropathogenic *E. coli*; EIEC=enteroinvasive *E. coli*; ETEC=enterotoxigenic *E. coli*

[c]EAST1=an enterotoxin first recognized in enteroadherent *E. coli* [EAggEC]; Sta=heat-stable enterotoxin; all guanylate cyclase-stimulating, heat-stable toxins share a key motif CE(I/V/L)CCNPAC

[d]The four secreted invasion antigens (BCDA) of *Shigella* (Ipas), *Salmonella* (Sips), and *Yersinia* (Ysps) are related closely enough that they can sometimes cross complement between species to replace the homologous protein when it has been deleted artificially.

proteins made by multiple bacteria that cause watery diarrhea; all share a key motif with guanylin, a peptide secreted by intestinal epithelium. The same is true for the adenylate cyclase-stimulating, heat-labile enterotoxin of ETEC; this protein is related to cholera toxin made by classic O1 as well as O139 *V. cholerae.* A similar toxin is produced by approximately 60% of *Salmonella* spp. The genes that allow a *Shigella* to be invasive are found in EIEC and in *Salmonella* spp. The mechanism for colonizing the intestinal epithelium found in EPEC is nearly identical to that of STEC.

Not only are virulence proteins related among the various enteropathogens; the mechanism for secreting these factors is highly conserved. Bacterial proteins are secreted by several pathways. One of these pathways is used by multiple organisms as machinery for secretion of virulence proteins. This machinery (the Type III Secretion System) is closely related in the EPEC, STEC, EIEC, *Shigella* spp, *Salmonella* spp, and *Yersinia* spp (Fig. 1). The unusual feature of this pathway is that the secretory system is induced when the pathogens sense that they are in the presence of their target. This system is incredibly complex; for example, in EPEC and STEC there are five operons involving over 30 different genes. Electron microscopic studies have demonstrated that a needle complex is made that can be used by the bacteria to directly inject virulence proteins into the host cell cytoplasm. The Type III Secretion System allows the bacteria to transiently express virulence antigens. Transient expression of virulence factors has major advantages for the pathogens. The brief expression and exposure may result in suboptimal stimulation of the immune system. Even when plasma cells in the lamina propria are programmed to make IgA specific to the pathogen, up-regulation of the response may be far too sluggish to effectively clear the infection. The needle complex injection system has further advan-

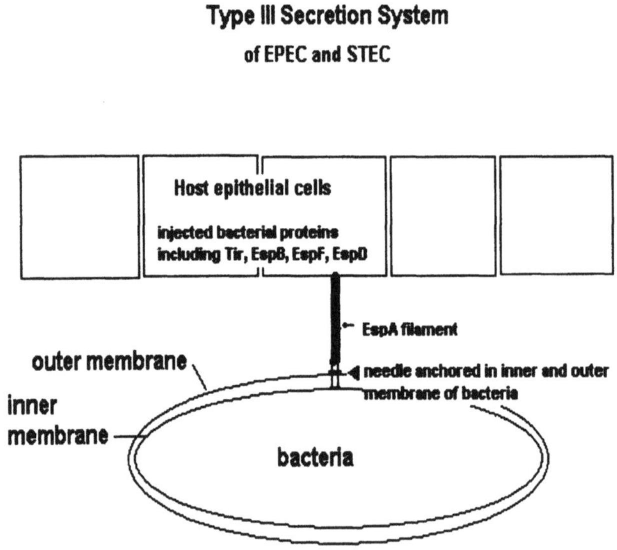

Figure 1. The interaction of the needle complex with host epithelial cells. This mechanism is identical in Shiga toxin-producing *E. coli* [STEC] and enteropathogenic *E. coli* [EPEC] and similar in other enteropathogens using a Type III Secretion System. The needle and its extension (made of EspA multimers) serve as a conduit for bacterial virulence proteins to be injected into host cells. The nearly thirty proteins involved in moving the virulence proteins from the bacterial cytoplasm into the needle are not shown.

tages for the pathogen. Virulence proteins are delivered directly into host cells where they act rather than into the gut lumen; this mechanism evades digestive enzymes and IgA that might limit their uptake. However, the complexity of the Type III Secretion System comes at a price. The bacteria lose flexibility to deal with the protective mechanisms developed by their target host. It may be difficult to change a single protein in such a complex, delicately balanced machine.

3.1.1. Process Rather Than Just Product

Implicit in the concept of targeting is the notion that human milk factors are focused on *process rather than just product*. For example, EspA, a multimeric protein secreted by a Type III Secretion System of EPEC and STEC, forms tubes that bridge the space between bacterial and host cells. Human milk secretory IgA that has been affinity purified to EPEC EspA prevents the triggering of actin polymerization of epithelial cells not only in EPEC but also in STEC in in vitro infection [M. Noguera-Obenza, personal communication]. The ability of a single antibody to block a key virulence step in different classes of diarrheagenic *E. coli* provides a unique advantage to the breastfed infant. Even if the infant's mother has never been infected with an STEC, she may provide protective secretory antibody if she has been infected with an EPEC that shares a closely related colonization mechanism.

Oligosaccharides in human milk also represent examples of the *process rather than product* concept. There is a vast number of complex oligosaccharides present in human milk. Enteropathogens usually target glycoconjugates both for attachment of adhesins and uptake of toxins and other virulence proteins. Presumably the hydrophilic nature of complex carbohydrates makes them ideal for interacting with virulence factors that must work in an aqueous environment. By flooding the gut with a complex mixture of receptor analog oligosaccharides (perhaps representing all or most of the complex carbohydrates the mother is capable of making), human milk blocks groups of pathogens that share related carbohydrate receptors. Examples of pathogens for which the oligosaccharides are likely to be critically important include the heat-stable enterotoxin of ETEC (Newburg et al. 1990; Cleary et al. 1983), invasin of *Campylobacter jejuni* (Ruiz-Palacios et al. 2003), adhesins of *Haemophilus* and *Streptococcus pneumoniae* (Andersson et al. 1986), and the caliciviruses [X. Jiang, personal communication].

A non-enteropathogen provides the most dramatic example of milk targeting process. HIV apparently has not existed throughout human evolution until quite recently. Nonetheless, the *process of carbohydrate-focused pathogen attachment* is common to many unrelated organisms. Because milk contains receptor analogs to potential targets that organisms might recognize and bind to, it is therefore not surprising that human milk contains a glycosaminoglycan that inhibits binding of gp120 to CD4, the first step in HIV pathogenesis (Newburg et al. 1995).

3.1.2. Bacterial Virulence Is the Result of Acquisition of Multiple Weapons

Bacterial promiscuity has resulted in selection of pathogens that typically have a mix of virulence traits (Table 1). For the bacterium this may mean multiple mechanisms to promote its proliferation and survival. For the breastfed infant the complexity of the pathogens is both a challenge and an opportunity. An organism that can cause illness in multiple ways has versatility, but if a key process can be attacked, all of the pathogen's arsenal may be rendered inoperative. In particular, strategies that block attachment steps may make downstream virulence proteins irrelevant. If, for example, anti-EspA prevents an STEC from attaching intimately to gut epithelium, the organism may not be able to deliver Shiga toxins to the epithelial surface for uptake.

Lactoferrin represents another example of process rather than product targeting and also is an example of targeting at a point that blocks the ability of pathogens to utilize their full arsenal of virulence factors. Lactoferrin is known to have multiple activities that might be relevant to protection from infection. These include growth inhibition, iron sequestration, binding to lipopolysaccharide and causing its release, as well as anti-viral, anti-fungal, and anti-inflammatory effects. However, the ability of lactoferrin to interfere with the Type III secretion system may be critical. Lactoferrin interferes with proteins that associate with the outer membrane during their function. Two different organisms (*Shigella flexneri* and EPEC) that express Type III Secretion Systems show dysfunction of that system in the presence of lactoferrin.

S. flexneri serotype 5 strain M90T has been found to be less invasive after incubation in recombinant human lactoferrin at the concentration present in colostrum; this decrease in invasion occurs without a change in bacterial viability (Gomez et al. 2001). The decrease in invasiveness has been found to be due to loss and degradation of invasion plasmid antigens, IpaB and IpaC, that normally form a complex that induces uptake by human cells. This complex is degraded in the presence of lactoferrin. Degradation is not affected by iron saturation. Studies using synthetic peptides (N-terminal amino acids 1-33) suggest that there may be two separate activities induced by different parts of lactoferrin. This small lipid A-binding peptide induced increased release of virulence antigens IpaB/IpaC but not their breakdown. The proteolytic activity appears to reside elsewhere in the lactoferrin molecule. Protease inhibitor studies suggest that lactoferrin may have a serine protease activity (Gomez et al. 2003). The in vitro observations appear to be relevant in vivo because in the rabbit *Shigella*-infection model, lactoferrin blocks the development of severe inflammatory enteritis (Gomez et al. 2002).

EPEC O127:H6 strain E2348/69 when grown in the presence of recombinant human lactoferrin (at concentrations present in colostrum) secretes little or no EspA and EspB, proteins normally secreted by the EPEC Type III Secretion System. The intracellular levels of these proteins within the bacteria are decreased in parallel with the low levels of proteins secreted into the growth medium. Brief incubation of the secreted proteins with lactoferrin (either recombinant or purified from milk) leads to rapid degradation of these virulence antigens (T. Ochoa, personal communication). EspA is essential for construction of the tube that connects the bacteria with host cells and EspB is necessary for making a hole in the host cell to allow injection of virulence proteins into the host. Thus, lactoferrin blocks the initial Type III Secretion System dependent attachment step of EPEC.

Whether these observations have relevance for all *Shigella*, all EPEC, or all organisms that possess a Type III Secretion System, remains to be determined. Such broad targeting of a fundamental virulence mechanism has major advantages to the infant who may encounter pathogens his or her mother has by chance failed to previously meet.

3.2. Mammary Secretory IgA Reflects Stimulation in the Distant Past

The second concept regarding the ability of human milk to survive the onslaught of rapidly changing enteropathogens is that the system appears to have been designed to endow the infant with much, perhaps all, of his or her mother's previous experience with enteropathogens. As such, human milk IgA appears to be produced in a very different way than IgA at mucosal surfaces. Typically IgA made in response to a respiratory or intestinal tract infection is made for a relatively brief period of time, usually weeks to months. After this brief period of production the levels of IgA to a specific antigen decrease to low levels, or even levels that are undetectable. For example, in monkeys infected with *Shigella* the gut IgA response peaks in two weeks and is no longer detectable by one month (Dinari et al. 1987). Rabbits infected with *Shigella* have likewise returned their gut IgA levels to baseline by one month after infection (Keren 1987). The trafficking of lymphocytes from the Peyer's patches in the intestine to the mammary glands assures that IgA produced in milk will reflect the antigenic experience of the common mucosal immune system of the mother. However, the array of antibodies found in human milk suggests that the cells that have been recruited to the breast during lactation reflect antigenic stimulation in the distant past.

Unlike the transiently expressed gut IgA found in the months after infection, milk IgA seems to reflect experiences with infections many years before. For example, human milk antibodies to *S. flexneri* serotype 5 and *Shigella sonnei* lipopolysacchorides are present even in women who live in an area where these infections are relatively infrequent. Fifty nine percent of women living in Houston have antibodies to *S. flexneri* in their milk; 26% have antibodies to *S. sonnei* (Hayani et al. 1991). It is extremely unlikely that 75% of women in Houston have recently been infected with *Shigella* species given that most individuals have less than four episodes of diarrhea each year and less than 5% of episodes are due to *Shigella* spp. Some of these antibodies could represent cross reactive antibodies stimulated by another organism. *S. flexneri* serotype 5 cross reacts with *Shigella* serotypes 1, 2, 3, 4, X and Y. These cross reactions undoubtedly reflect the [rhamnose α 1,2-rhamnose α 1,3-rhamnose *N*-acetylglucosamine β 1,2] repeat unit of the O antigens that all of these serotypes share (Carlin & Lindberg 1987).

The lack of cross reactions with *E. coli* makes it unlikely that infections with organisms other than *Shigella* have elicited these antibodies. The O antigen of *S. sonnei* is even more restricted since this antigen is shared only with *Pleisomonas shigelloides* (Batta et al. 1997). The rarity of the *S. sonnei* O antigen sugars 2,4,6-trideoxy-2-acetamino-4-amino-D-galactose and 2-acetamido-2-deoxy-L-altruronic acid that are connected through 1,2-*trans* interglycosidic linkages (Kontrohr 1977) makes it difficult to explain the presence of milk antibodies to these antigens as "cross reactive." Likewise the high frequency of human milk antibodies to EPEC virulence antigens in women from North America (Noguera-Obenza et al. 2003) (e.g., 90% have α EspA in their milk) is explained most easily as reflecting long-term memory of the cells recruited to the breast. We hypothesize that the cells recruited to the breast during lactation reflect the mother's prior experience with pathogens years before her pregnancy. The antibodies produced may well represent her whole life experience with enteropathogens.

A benefit of mammary gland IgA secretion with long memory is that the infant can receive antibodies even against organisms that transiently express virulence antigens via a Type III Secretion System. The result is that passive mucosal immunity may protect the breastfeeding infant better than active mucosal immunity does in the older child or adult. For example, protection from *Shigella* spp in the adult is serotype (lipopolysaccharide) specific. Although antibodies to virulence protein antigens develop during infection, they do not provide protection on subsequent challenge with a different serotype. Presumably, the virulence plasmid antigen-specific antibodies rapidly decrease to baseline. In contrast, the infant receives milk antibodies that are directed against these virulence plasmid antigens (Cleary et al. 1989, 1991) and is protected in a nonserotype specific manner. In prospective studies in which we evaluated weekly stool cultures of Mexican infants and collected monthly human milk samples, we were able to identify infants who were infected with *Shigella* spp. Some of these infants were sick with diarrhea and others were well. The amount of antibody to virulence antigens found in the human milk sample from the month prior to first *Shigella* spp infection was predictive of development of illness. If the infants were consuming human milk with high titers against the virulence plasmid antigens they were protected, while if the milk had low titers, the infants developed symptomatic infection (Hayani et al. 1992).

3.3. Human Milk Protective Mechanisms Are Redundant

A third principle explaining the ability of human milk to protect infants from organisms that have the capacity to change rapidly is that *human milk typically provides multiple factors aimed at a given pathogen or mechanism.* The factors that contribute to protection against a pathogen may include secretory IgA, oligosaccharides, glycoproteins, glycolipids, mucins, lactoferrin, lysozyme, lipases and other enzymes, fatty acids, lactadherin, and other factors. Redundancy is a major reason that breastfeeding manages to remain protective despite the vast numbers and rapid mutations of enteropathogens. Redundancy is manifest in several ways.

There is *targeting of complex systems* by several factors. For example, the virulence plasmid antigens of *Shigella* spp are targeted by both nonspecific/innate immune factors, such as lactoferrin, that interfere with Type III Secretion System function, and by adaptive immunity by specific secretory IgA that interferes with bacterial invasion. Likewise, lactoferrin impairs function of the EPEC Type III Secretion System in a fashion similar to that identified with *Shigella* spp and blocks attachment by specific secretory IgA (anti-EspA, anti-EspB, anti-EspD) directed toward the attachment organelle. Fucosylated oligosaccharides in human milk also may block the Type III Secretion System-mediated attachment of EPEC (Cravioto et al. 1991).

There also is *targeting of specific virulence antigens* such as toxins by receptor analogs and secretory antibodies. For example, Shiga toxin is made by both *S. dysenteriae* serotype 1 and STEC including *E. coli* O157:H7, O26:H11, O111:NM. Antibodies are present in human milk that recognize the surface exposed amino acid residues of the receptor binding B subunit of the toxin (Gomez et al. 1995). However, in addition, the receptor, a neutral glycolipid called Gb3, is present in human milk unattached to cells so that toxin binding receptor may never escape the gut (Herrera-Insua et al. 2001).

It is often difficult to identify which factor is the key one. The correct answer is sometimes inconsistent with long held opinions. For example, in the case of rotavirus data surprisingly show that lactadherin, a 46 kDa mucin-associated glycoprotein, is the major protective factor. In one study the amount of antirotaviral secretory IgA present in milk did not determine symptom status (Newburg et al. 1998). The vast array of protective factors and the difficulty and complexity of doing the required epidemiologic studies make it difficult to fully understand the relative importance of all the putative protective factors found in human milk.

The advantage of redundancy can be seen when considering spontaneous mutation rates that occur in DNA-based microbes such as *E. coli*. For a variety of proteins the spontaneous mutation rate is in the range of 10^{-6} to 10^{-7} and the rate per base pair is in the order of 10^{-10} (Drake 1991). If mutations needed to be in specific base pairs to circumvent two milk protective factors (likely a common requirement), the frequency of spontaneous mutations in both targets would occur approximately 10^{-20}. Given that human milk often contains many factors directed to a given pathogen, it becomes clear why the task of developing resistance becomes insurmountable for the enteropathogens.

Efforts of modern medicine to treat enteropathogens have led to rapid emergence of antimicrobial resistance. We have targeted single mechanisms that have allowed rapidly mutating organisms to produce vast numbers of bacteria containing resistance genes that have resulted in resistance of many of these bacteria to antimicrobial agents. In contrast, human milk has stood the test of time. Human milk has targeted virulence mechanisms that are widely shared among many enteropathogens. The milk machinery has often focused on the first steps (adhesins) that the pathogen uses before subsequent virulence proteins can act. The whole redundant repertoire of human milk factors has the ability to overwhelm pathogens. In addition, development of resistance to these milk factors generally does not occur. By using multiple strategies, each of which is nontoxic, human milk has limited opportunity for mutant organisms to be selected.

4. ACKNOWLEDGMENT

This work was supported by a program project grant from the National Institute of Child Health and Human Development (HD13021).

5. REFERENCES

Anderson B, Porras O, Hanson LA, Lagergard T, Svanborg-Eden C. Inhibition of attachment of Streptococcus pneumoniae and Haemophilus influenzae by human milk and receptor oligosaccharides. J Infect Dis 1986;153:232-237.

Batta G, Liptak A, Schneerson R, Pozsgay V. Conformational stabilization of the altruronic acid residue in the O-specific polysaccharide of Shigella sonnei/Plesiomonas shigelloides. Carbohydr Res 1997;305:93-99.

Carlin NI, Lindberg AA. Monoclonal antibodies specific for Shigella flexneri lipopolysaccharides: clones binding to type IV, V, and VI antigens group 3,4 antigen, and an epitope common to all Shigella flexneri and Shigella dysenteriae type 1 strains. Infect Immun 1987;55:1412-1420.

Cleary TG, Chambers JP, Pickering LK. Protection of suckling mice from the heat-stable enterotoxin of Escherichia coli by human milk. J Infect Dis 1983;48:1114-1119.

Cleary TG, Winsor DK, Reich D, Ruiz-Palacios G, Calva JJ. Human milk immunoglobulin A antibodies to Shigella virulence determinants. Infect Immun 1989;57:1675-1679.

Cleary TG, West MS, Ruiz-Palacios G, Winsor DK, Calva JJ, Guerrero ML, Van R. Human milk secretory immunoglobulin A to Shigella virulence plasmid-coded antigens. J Pediatr 1991;118:34-38.

Cravioto A, Tello A, Villafan H, Ruiz J, del Vedovo S, Neeser JR. Inhibition of localized adhesion of enteropathogenic Escherichia coli to HEp-2 cells by immunoglobulin and oligosaccharide fractions of human colostrum and breast milk. J Infect Dis 1991;163:1247-1255.

Cruz JR, Gil L, Cano F, Caceres P, Pareja G. Breast milk anti-Escherichia coli heat-labile toxin IgA antibodies protect against toxin-induced infantile diarrhea. Acta Paediatr Scand 1988;77:658-662.

Dinari G, Hale TL, Austin SW, Formal SB. Local and systemic antibody responses to Shigella infection in rhesus monkeys. J Infect Dis 1987;155:1065-1069.

Drake JW. A constant rate of spontaneous mutation in DNA-based microbes. Proc Natl Acad Sci USA 1991;88:7160-7164.

Glass RI, Svennerholm AM, Stoll BJ, Khan MR, Hossain KM, Huq MI, Holmgren J. Protection against cholera in breast-fed children by antibodies in breast milk. N Engl J Med 1983;308:1389-1392.

Gomez HF, Ho H, Shah S, Lopez EL, Cleary TG. Mapping epitopic regions of shiga toxin b-subunit using milk secretory immunoglobulin A (sIgA). In: Karmali MA, Goglio AG, editors. Recent Advances in Verocytotoxin-producing *Escherichia coli* Infections. New York: Elsevier Science B.V., 1995; pp 345-347.

Gomez HF, Herrera-Insua I, Siddiqui MM, Diaz-Gonzalez VA, Caceres E, Newburg DS, Cleary TG. Protective role of human lactoferrin against invasion of Shigella flexneri M90T. Adv Exp Med Biol 2001;501:457-467.

Gomez HF, Ochoa TJ, Herrera-Insua I, Carlin LG, Cleary TG. Lactoferrin protects rabbits from Shigella flexneri-induced inflammatory enteritis. Infect Immun 2002;70:7050-7053.

Gomez HF, Ochoa TJ, Carlin LG, Cleary TG. Human lactoferrin impairs virulence of Shigella flexneri. J Infect Dis 2003;187:87-95.

Hayani KC, Guerrero ML, Ruiz-Palacios GM, Gomez HF, Cleary TG. Evidence for long-term memory of the mucosal immune system: milk secretory immunoglobulin A against Shigella lipopolysaccharides. J Clin Microbiol 1991;29:2599-603.

Hayani KC, Guerrero ML, Morrow AL, Gomez HF, Winsor DK, Ruiz-Palacios GM, Cleary TG. Concentration of milk secretory immunoglobulin A against *Shigella* virulence plasmid-associated antigens as a predictor of symptom status in *Shigella*-infected breast-fed infants. J Pediatr 1992;121:852-856.

Herrera-Insua I, Gomez HF, Diaz-Gonzalez VA, Chaturvedi P, Newburg DS, Cleary TG. Human milk lipids bind SLT-I. Adv Exp Biol Med 2001:501;333-340.

Keren DF. Models to follow secretory IgA response to mucosal infections. Pathol Immunopathol Res 1987;6:128-136.

Kontrohr T. The identification of 2-amino-2-deoxy-L-altruronic acid as a constituent of Shigella sonnei phase I lipopolysaccharide. Carbohydr Res 1977;58:498-500.

Newburg DS, Pickering LK, McCluer RH, Cleary TG. Fucosylated oligosaccharides of human milk protect suckling mice from heat-stabile enterotoxin of Escherichia coli. J Infect Dis 1990;162:1075-1080.

Newburg DS, Linhardt RJ, Ampofo SA, Yolken RH. Human milk glycosaminoglycans inhibit HIV glycoprotein gp 120 binding to its host cell CD4 receptor. J Nutr 1995;125:419-424.

Newburg D, Peterson J, Ruiz-Palacios G, Matson D, Morrow A, Shults J, Guerrero M, Chaturvedi P, Newburg S, Scallan C, Taylor M, Ceriani R, Pickering L. Role of human-milk lactadherin in protection against symptomatic rotavirus infection. Lancet 1998;351:1160-1164.

Noguera-Obenza M, Ochoa TJ, Gomez HF, Guerrero ML, Herrera-Insua I, Morrow AL, Ruiz-Palacios G, Pickering LK, Guzman CA, Cleary TG. Human milk secretory antibodies against attaching and effacing Escherichia coli antigens. Emerg Infect Dis 2003;9:545-551.

Ruiz-Palacios G, Calva JJ, Pickering LK, Lopez-Vidal Y, Volkow P, Pezzarossi H, West MS. Protection of breast-fed infants against *Campylobacter* diarrhea by antibodies in human milk. J Pediatr 1990;116:707-713.

Ruiz-Palacios GM, Cervantes LE, Ramos P, Chavez-Munguia B, Newburg DS. Campylobacter jejuni binds intestinal H(O) antigen (Fucα1,2Gal β1,4GlcNAc), and fucosyloligosaccharides of human milk inhibit its binding and infection. J Biol Chem 2003;278:14112-14120.

Walterspiel JN, Morrow AL, Guerrero ML, Ruiz-Palacios GM, Pickering LK. Secretory anti-Giardia lamblia antibodies in human milk: protective effect against diarrhea. Pediatrics 1994;93:28-31.

THE DYNAMIC EFFECTS OF BREASTFEEDING ON INTESTINAL DEVELOPMENT AND HOST DEFENSE

W. Allan Walker

1. ABSTRACT

In this review, evidence is provided to support the hypothesis that human milk provides a link between the mother and her newborn infant in the extrauterine environment in a manner similar to the placental link between mother and fetus in utero. In addition, breastfeeding helps prevent age-related diseases affecting the gastrointestinal tract during the newborn period. To provide evidence to support this hypothesis, anecdotal clinical studies are sited to suggest that human milk contains factors that may be missing in inherited diseases of inborn errors in metabolism and provide passive protective factors that lessen the expression of neonatal allergic and infectious diseases. In some instances, by providing the missing factor in an inherited disease, the newborn may be protected from serious damage to its developing brain. A second line of evidence to support this hypothesis is the observation that the composition of human milk varies with the infant's needs. To illustrate this principal, the composition of milk from mothers delivering prematurely and milk of mothers of full-term infants were compared, and the differences in trophic and protective factors in colostrum versus mature milk from mothers delivering full-term are cited. Finally, using observations from the laboratory that define the immaturities in neonatal and premature human intestinal defenses as the neonate's host defense deficiency, the specific effect that anti-inflammatory and maturational factors in human milk has on these immaturities is discussed. The active stimulus of maternal milk on the rapid development of host defenses is underscored. These cited examples of human milk effects in the newborn help support the stated hypothesis. Additional studies of human immature gut function along with translational and clinical studies are necessary to provide further objective evidence in support of breastfeeding for all neonates, particularly premature neonates.

Departments of Nutrition and Pediatrics, Harvard Medical School, and Developmental Gastroenterology Laboratory, Massachusetts General Hospital, 114 16th Street (114-3503), Charlestown, MA 02129

Protecting Infants through Human Milk, edited by Pickering *et al.*
Kluwer Academic/Plenum Publishers, 2004

2. INTRODUCTION

For the past twenty years, this author has actively studied human milk immunology. As a result of research studies done in our laboratory as well as published observations from the literature, an overall theme regarding the importance of human milk in the newborn infant's adjustment to the birth process has evolved. We hypothesize that ***human milk provides a protective link from mother to newborn in the extrauterine environment and as such helps to prevent the expression of age-related diseases during that period.*** In utero, the developing fetus exists in an idyllic environment for optimal growth and development. Nutrients, hormones, growth factors, and protective substances are shunted preferentially from mother to the fetus via the placenta and its circulation. Factors in amniotic fluid are swallowed in later stages of gestation and bathe the developing gut to directly interact with the intestinal epithelium to assure its appropriate preparation for existence in the extrauterine environment. During the period of gestation, the fetal environment is virtually pathogen-free to allow the infant to direct its energy and its exposure to trophic factor sources from mother to growth, development, and maturation. As a result, at term, the neonate is prepared for an independent existence.

However, several aspects of gastrointestinal tract maturation require "fine turning" to be fully independent as an organ system in the extrauterine environment. For example, although the components of mucosal host defense are developed fully after forty weeks of gestation, "efferent" protective immune responses (e.g., polymeric IgA in intestinal secretions, etc.) require initial appropriate colonization of the gastrointestinal tract by microorganisms to provide adjuvant and antigen stimulation for activation of these mucosal defenses (Fig. 1) (Insoft et al. 1996). Since the major maturation of gut absorptive and protective function occurs at the end of the gestational period, a premature infant's gut capacity to function independently remains precarious, resulting in a high incidence of infectious disease and less than optimal adjustment to the extrauterine environment. From a variety of publications (Bernt et al. 1999, 2001; Chandra 1979), there is evidence that human milk is an important link between mother and her newborn infant in the extrauterine environment in the same manner that the placenta provides the link to mother in the intrauterine environment. Components of human milk provide an optimal nutrition for the newborn, including nutrients that can be digested and absorbed by the still immature gastrointestinal tract. In like manner, inadequacies in the newborn's mucosal defenses are provided passively by protective substances in human milk or by an active, accelerated stimulation of the infant's defenses by trophic factors and cytokines secreted into human milk. Since the premature's extrauterine survival is more precarious than that of the full-term newborn, the importance of ingesting its mother's own milk is more apparent (Schanler et al. 1986). In fact, with regard to the composition of human milk from mothers delivering premature infants compared with full-term infants, the composition differs (Groer et al. 1996) and contains substances that are uniquely needed by the premature compared with the full-term newborn for its postdelivery survival.

In this review, evidence will be provided to support the hypothesis that previously has been stated. The role of human milk in the prevention of the expression of a variety of age-related neonatal disease states will be considered. Human milk composition in mothers who deliver prematurely compared with that of mothers of full-term infants with regard to the infant's needs will be reviewed, as well as a difference in the composition of human milk at early versus later stages of gestation. The presence of factors in human milk, which provide passive protection for the vulnerable newborn, also will be considered. Finally, experimental evidence from the author's laboratory, as well as other

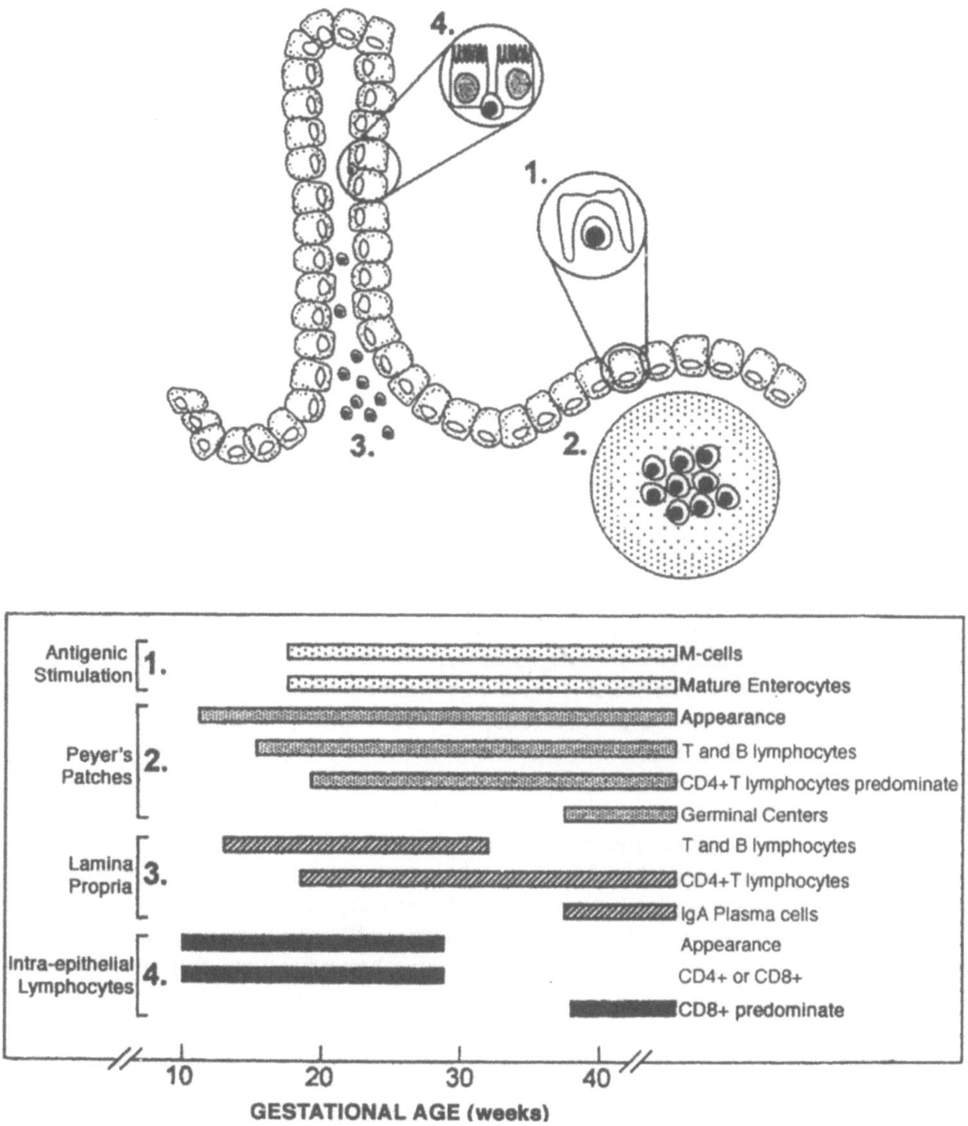

Figure 1. Ontogeny of the human mucosal immune system. The major components of the mucosal immune system are shown. The respective developmental time points for key components are highlighted. Note germinal centers in Peyer's patches. IgA plasma cells in the lamina propria and predominant CD8+ intraepithelial lymphocytes do not appear until the perinatal and neonatal periods. Reprinted from Pediatr Clin North Am, Vol. 43, Insoft et al., The development of immune function within the human intestine and its role in neonatal diseases, pp 551-571, Copyright (1996), with permission from Elsevier.

laboratories, will be considered to support the notion that hormones/cytokines/trophic factors in human milk, particularly colostrum, can actively accelerate the development of the infant's own host defenses. In conclusion, the evidence that supports the hypothesis will be used to make recommendations for support of exclusive breastfeeding during the transition to independence in the extrauterine environment.

3. PROTECTION AGAINST CLINICAL DISEASE

Several disease states are more common during the newborn period than at other times in the life of an infant or child. This increased incidence of disease could be due to an inborn error of organ function that is not manifest in utero because the defect is not apparent due to the infant's mother providing the defective substance or clearing a potentially toxic substance that results from the inherited defect. Alternatively, the newborn infant, particularly the premature infant, is not capable of protecting itself from harmful stimuli in the extrauterine environment, e.g., microorganisms and foreign antigens, and thus is likely to react to these environmental factors by expression of disease. There is strong clinical and experimental evidence that human milk may overcome the increased susceptibility to these diseases during the newborn period by providing the missing factor or by passively/actively protecting against an immature reaction to harmful environmental exposure. In this section of the review, clinical evidence will be presented to suggest that human milk can prevent disease, particularly a disease due to an inborn error in metabolism.

3.1. Congenital Hypothyroidism

The importance of thyroid hormone in the development of the newborn has been documented extensively in the literature. Infants born with a defect in the production of thyroxine not only manifest clinical signs of hypothyroidism (constipation, altered skin texture, etc.) but are defective in brain development leading to retardation. The importance of thyroid hormone in brain function is most critcal during the period of rapid brain growth after birth. Because manifestations of hypothyroidism are subtle in infancy, the diagnosis of congenital hypothyroidism usually occurs after irreversible brain damage has developed. A seminal study (Bode et al. 1978) showed that infants with congenital hypothyroidism are protected from the severe associated brain damage if breastfed during the critical postpartum period. After weaning, symptoms referable to hypothyroidism result in the diagnosis and treatment with thyroid replacement therapy. Bode and colleagues reported that thyroxin levels in human milk, particularly colostrum, were sufficiently high to lessen the damage to developing brain function, thereby preventing the concomitant brain damage (cretinism) that occurs with congenital hypothyroidism.

3.2. Acrodermatitis Enteropathica

Acrodermatitis enteropathica is a rare condition that is associated with a defect in the zinc transporter on the surface of the small intestine, a surface molecule that is necessary for absorption of the trace element zinc from the newborn intestine (Lonnerdal et al. 1982). The condition is manifest by severe diarrhea and a desquamating rash (Hurley et al. 1979). It is frequently confused with cow's milk allergy associated with "weeping eczema." When the diagnosis is made, the condition can be corrected with excessive doses of oral zinc or periodic infusion of zinc parenterally (Shaw et al. 1979). Infants with this condition who are breastfed are free of symptoms until weaning. Initially, an explanation for protection against acrodermatitis enteropathica by breastfeeding was an enigma since the levels of zinc in human milk were not considered sufficient to overcome the transport defect. However, more recently it has been shown (Eckhert et al. 1997) that human milk not only contains zinc, but also contains the soluble transporter for zinc, which when bound to zinc can function as if the transporter existed on the intestine. This report explained the facilitated uptake of low levels of human milk zinc by the nursing infant (Lonnerdal et al. 1980). This observation also suggests that human milk can overcome this congenital defect and prevent expression of disease.

3.3. Premature Sepsis and Diarrhea

As stated, gastrointestinal tract host defenses are not completely operational at birth, particularly in premature infants. Accordingly, these infants have an increased susceptibility to sepsis and infectious diseases. Sepsis in these patients generally occurs because of increased permeability of the gut and a lack of fully developed intestinal defenses against pathogens causing these infants to develop a variety of infectious diarrheas. Several studies (Groer et al. 1996) have shown a protective effect of giving premature infants their mother's expressed milk. Since human milk expressed from the infant's own mother contains the protective factors that are most needed by the premature infant, protection resulting from the recently expressed milk from mothers delivering premature infants is better than human milk bank supplementation (Goldman et al. 1982). Human milk bank samples are either frozen or pasteurized to prevent transmission of infection from an unrelated donor to the infant and therefore contain less protective factors since antibodies, cytokines, and other factors are inactivated by these procedures (Xanthou et al. 1995). Furthermore, samples in human milk banks are from women nursing term infants during the mature milk phase of nursing and, as such, contain fewer protective factors. Accordingly, expressed human milk from the premature infant's mother is more effective in protection against sepsis and infectious diarrhea.

3.4. Necrotizing Enterocolitis

The most common premature intensive care nursery gastrointestinal tract emergency is necrotizing enterocolitis (NEC) (Kurscheid et al. 1993). Depending on the nursery, up to 7% of infants born with a birth weight of less than 1500 g can develop this condition. Risk factors are prematurity and the introduction of enteric feedings (formula) (Caplan et al. 2001). This laboratory has had a longstanding interest in the pathophysiology of NEC. We suggest that a component of this inflammatory intestinal condition is an inappropriate and accentuated inflammatory response to bacteria colonizing the intestine (Claud 2001). These data will be considered in detail later in this review. Suffice it to say there is good evidence to suggest that the ingestion of expressed human milk from the premature infant's mother may prevent or lessen the severity of NEC in these patients (Lucas et al. 1990a). As with sepsis and infectious diarrheal prevention, expressed fresh milk from the premature infant's own mother is more effective in protection than human milk obtained from human milk banks (Kliegman 1979).

3.5. Cow's Milk Allergy

Cow's milk allergy is usually manifested during infancy. This condition appears to be multifactorial and includes a genetic predisposition, e.g., increased incidence if parents and siblings are allergic, as well as environmental factors. Breastfeeding in IgE-mediated allergy manifested as dermatitis or asthma is less effective than in non-IgE-mediated, e.g., gastrointestinal symptoms of allergic disease, in part because exposure to allergens other than cow's milk or other ingested proteins, e.g., pollens, dust, and animal dander, can sustain and prolong IgE-mediated reactions to cow's milk after infancy, thus prolonging allergic conditions. In contrast, non-IgE-mediated gastrointestinal tract allergic disease is related to the developmental delay in expression of intestinal host defenses and therefore generally abates in time with maturation of host defenses (Chandra 1997). Accordingly, studies of allergy-prone (genetically predisposed) infants to exclusive breastfeeding have resulted in a mixed result (Lucas 1990b). A meta-analysis of studies done (Kramer 1988) has suggested an improvement in expression of allergic symptoms or a delay in the expression of allergic symptoms in exclusively breastfed infants (Saarinen et al. 1995), a better result in breastfed infants with non-IgE, gastrointestinal cow's milk allergy, and variable results in allergy-prone infants breastfed by symptomatic atopic mothers. More recent studies suggest that probiotic-fed (*Lactobacillus* GG) (Majamaa et al. 1997) allergy-prone mothers during the third trimester of infancy and while breastfeeding may result in the best preventative effects in this area of disease prevention.

4. COMPOSITION OF HUMAN MILK

This section will review the composition of human milk at various times during lactation and the composition from mothers expressing their milk after premature delivery compared with colostrum and transitional milk from mothers of full-term infants. As mentioned, the development of intestinal defenses at birth requires help from maternal milk to provide factors that passively protect the neonate and to actively stimulate an accelerated maturation of the infant's own mucosal defenses to prevent adverse infectious reactions and reduce intestinal inflammation. Over time postpartum, in part due to the stimulus of active trophic human milk factors, nonspecific and immunologic host defenses in the intestine mature and allow the mucosal surface to protect itself from hostile forces in the luminal environment, e.g., pathologic microorganisms, bacterial toxins, and food antigens that can result in systemic or local disease (Insoft et al. 1996). Figure 2 depicts the various mucosal barriers of the mature gastrointestinal tract that are available to protect the mucosal surface from penetration by these hostile luminal forces.

At birth, full-term infants, although their mucosal immune defenses are intact, lack the capacity to mount a mucosal immune response. For example, polymeric IgA (pIgA), the unique antibody that coats mucosal surfaces, reaches protective levels in the gut several months after birth (Selner et al. 1968). Colonization of the gut and stimulus from human milk trophic factors are necessary to activate the secretion of protective levels of the infant's pIgA. During this period of relative pIgA deficiency, human milk supplies adequate protective levels of pIgA. In fact, in previous studies from this laboratory, we have shown that human milk during the colostral phase of lactation preferentially supplies a disproportionate amount of pIgA relative to total human milk protein content (Hyslop et al. 1974). Over time and with an increase of endogenous pIgA, the need for human milk contributions becomes less and the relative concentrations of human milk IgA decrease. In like manner, early-phase human milk compared with late-phase human milk actively stimulates enterocyte turnover as an added protection against damage (Fig. 3) (Tapper et al. 1979; Berseth 1990).

Another aspect of human milk pIgA is the "enteromammary system" of producing specific IgA antibodies against antigens in the maternal environment. Under the stimulus of prolactin, lactating mothers produce specific IgA antibodies against microflora and other antigens in the maternal gut. These same pIgA antibodies are transferred rapidly to human milk as an added specific protection for the newborn. Since the principal enteric

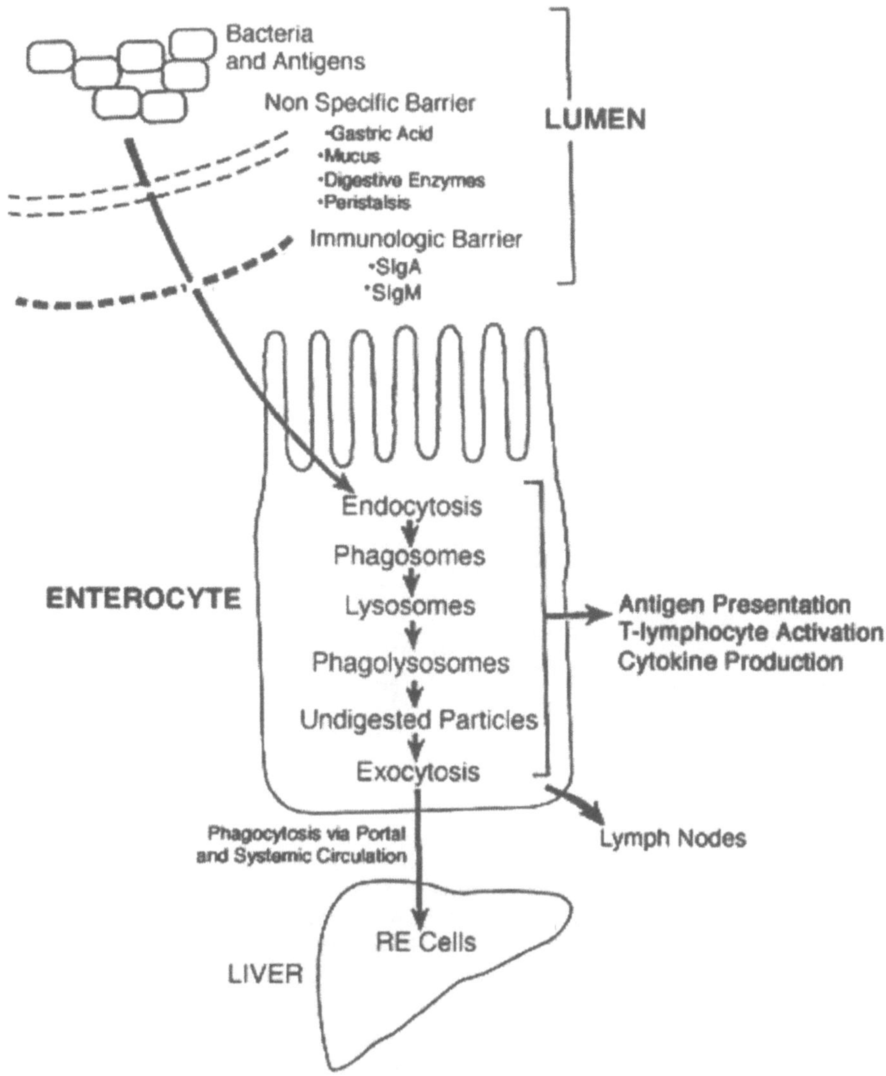

Figure 2. Barriers to antigenic absorption in the intestine. Antigen entry is limited by nonimmunologic and immunologic mechanisms and by the structure of the epithelium. If potential antigens cross into the enterocyte, as they are being degraded and presented as antigens, signals are produced, causing T-lymphocyte activation and subsequent additional cytokine production and release. Reprinted from Pediatr Clin North Am, Vol. 43, Insoft et al., The development of immune function within the human intestine and its role in neonatal diseases, pp 551-571, Copyright (1996), with permission from Elsevier.

environment of the newborn is influenced by the baby's close maternal contact, these specific pIgA antibodies in human milk provide an added protection to the vulnerable neonatal environment. Figure 4 depicts the concept of the enteromammary system (Kleinman et al. 1979). A study from 2002 has shown that newborns at risk for specific infectious diseases, e.g., pneumococal meningitis, can be protected by immunizing

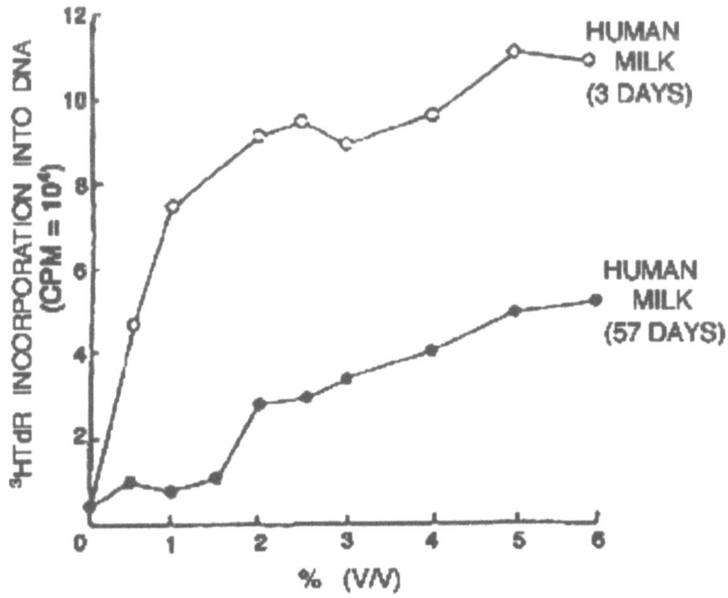

Figure 3. Stimulation of DNA synthesis by human milk as a function of time in the lactation period. Mitogenic activity is present at 6 months, but its ability to stimulate DNA synthesis decreases as time in the lactation period increases. Reprinted from J Pediatr Surg, Vol. 14, Tapper et al., Growth factors in early and late lactation, pp 803-807, Copyright (1979), with permission from Elsevier.

mothers against the infectious agent. Antibodies to this organism are secreted into human milk and can provide passive protection during the period of risk (Munoz et al. 2002).

In addition to the differential amounts of protective substances in colostrum compared with mature milk of mothers of full-term neonates, there is evidence that different quantities of protective substances and other needed ingredients exist in the milk of mothers delivering prematurely compared with mothers delivering full-term neonates (Read et al. 1995; Gross et al. 1980). Several years ago, we compared the content of expressed milk from mothers who delivered prematurely with milk from mothers of full-term infants (Groer et al. 1996). We noted that the concentration of many needed substances was greater in the milk of the mothers delivering prematurely than in that of mothers delivering full-term infants. Subsequently, a similar study has shown that pIgA levels in milk from mothers delivering premature infants compared with mothers delivering full-term infants is significantly higher (Fig. 5) (Gross et al. 1981). These examples of a different milk composition under different nursing conditions provide compelling evidence that human milk gives the newborn infant whatever its underdeveloped gut is lacking, and that composition varies with time postpartum and with circumstances of the neonate's birth (premature or full-term).

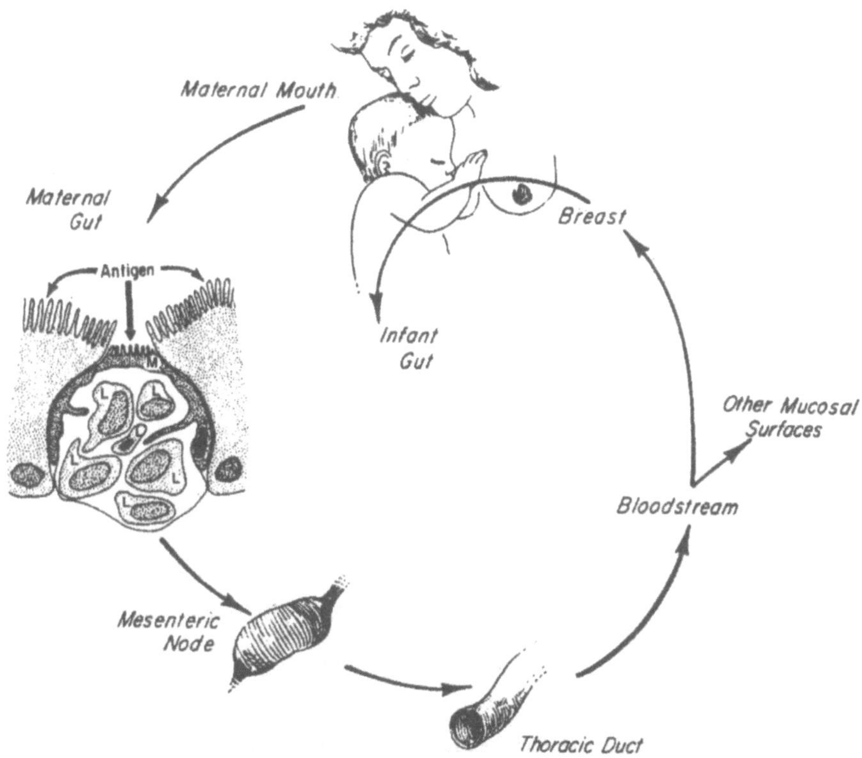

Figure 4. Antigen presented to maternal gut is brought into proximity to lymphoid follicles by specialized transport cells (M). The presence of antigen commits the lymphoblasts (L) to specific IgA production, and they then migrate via mesenteric nodes and thoracic duct into the systemic circulation. During periods of proper hormonal stimulation, these cells populate the human and secrete sIgA, which is ingested by the infant and functions in the infant gut much as endogenous IgA. T cells, B cells, and macrophages also are extruded into human milk and are immunologically active. Reprinted from Digest Dis Sci, Vol. 24, Kleinman & Walker, The enteromammary immune system, pp 876-882, Copyright (1979), with permission from Kluwer Academic/ Plenum Publishers.

5. ACTIVATION OF NEONATAL INTESTINAL DEFENSES

Not only does human milk provide passive protective factors in quantities commensurate with the infant's needs, it also provides factors that can accelerate the maturation of the infant's own defenses. In this section several examples of these active stimulating factors will be provided to underscore the maternal influence on the infant's own adjustment to survival in the extrauterine environment. Some examples are observations from studies in our laboratory to determine the specific mechanism by which human milk components affect active protection by the infant against inflammatory agents.

5.1. Prebiotic (Bifidofactor) Effect

The full-term newborn has mature intestinal defenses capable of responding to noxious stimuli at birth. However, for an "active efferent immune response" to occur, the

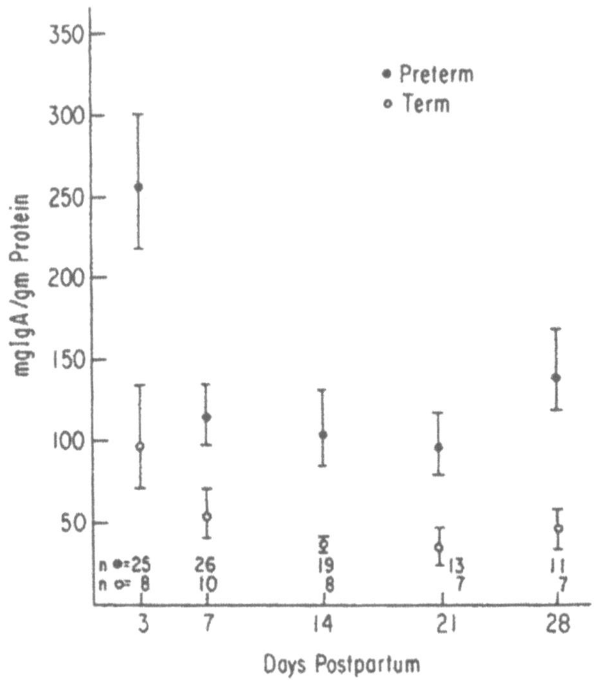

Figure 5. Geometric means ±1 SEM of IgA concentrations in morning milk samples from mothers in the preterm and term groups. Linear regression analysis demonstrated significantly higher IgA concentrations in milk from mothers who delivered preterm infants (P<0.01). Reprinted from J Peditr, Vol. 99, Gross et al., Elevated IgA concentration in milk produced by mothers delivered of preterm infants, pp 389-393, Copyright (1981), with permission from Elsevier.

gut must first be colonized with appropriate microorganisms. The initial colonization provides the needed adjuvant and antigen stimulus to promote an immune response (Bernt et al. 2001). Factors in human milk, e.g., nondigestible oligosaccharides, can enter the colon and are fermented by bacteria. This fermentation can create the appropriate luminal milieu (acidic pH, increased lactic acid, etc.) to facilitate the proliferation of bifidobacteria and lactobacillus organisms (Rubaltelli et al. 1993; Adlerberth et al. 1999), organisms termed "probiotics" for their health-promoting effect. These human milk oligosaccharides promote an appropriate bacterial proliferation through fermentation by colonic bacteria leading to the production of organic acids, particularly lactic acid, which act to establish an acidic colonic content. In such a colonic environment, immuno-enhancing (probiotic) bacteria, such as bifidobacteria and lactobacilli, thrive. In addition to being substrate for fermentation, human milk oligosaccharides inhibit the adherence of pathogens to intestinal glycoconjugates, a necessary first step in bacterial translocation and stimulation of inflammation, and thereby help protect the newborn gut from intestinal bacterial infection. The oligosaccharides in human milk have been termed "prebiotics" because their fermentation facilitates the growth of health-promoting probiotic organisms. Formula companies are trying to simulate this human milk effect on gut bacteria by adding fructose oligosaccharides to their formulas (Dai et al. 2000). Another recently identified "bifidio" factor, or prebiotic, in human milk is peptide fragments of partially digested human milk proteins, which also promote the growth of bifidobacteria in the colon of breastfed infants (Wold et al. 2000; Munoz et al. 2002).

5.2. Influence of Initial Colonization on Gut Protection

In studies from this laboratory (Nanthakumar et al. 2002), we have shown how the initial bacterial colonization of the gut can influence glycosyltransferase enzymes on enterocytes, which determine the structure of terminal sugars on microvillus membrane glycoprotiens and glycolipids, e.g., glycoconjugates. Since surface adherence and colonization is determined by the nature of terminal sugars on microvillus glycoconjugates (e.g., *E. coli* binds to mannose, *Vibrio cholera* binds to fructose, etc.), the function of these enzymes is critical to bacterial colonization and to host defense of the gut. The pattern of glycoconjugate expression is developmentally regulated (e.g., the sialic acid/fucose ratio is high in the immature and is low in the mature gut). As a result, an appropriate initial colonization of the newborn gut with bacteria that can stimulate maturation of these enzymes that result in a mature glycoconjugate pattern on the microvillus surface of enterocytes is a critical deterrent against pathologic colonization of the gut and infectious gastroenteritis. In a publication from this laboratory (Nanthakumar et al. 2002), we have shown that colonization of the newborn gut with the micro-organisms stimulated by prebiotics in human milk has a maturation effect on microvillus enzymes and glycoconjugate expression. In previous studies, we have shown that pathologic microorganisms interacting with the immature gut would adhere and trans-locate more readily than those interacting with the mature gut (Schiffrin et al. 1993). We conclude that the maturational effect of prebiotics in human milk, and the concomitant stimulation of probiotic organisms that initially colonize the gut, is an important active stimulation by human milk to maturation of the newborn's host defense against pathologic colonization of the gut and possible development of infectious gastroenteritis (McClelland et al. 1978).

5.3. Inflammation in the Neonatal Gastrointestinal Tract

A major factor in the expression of NEC in premature infants is the immature interaction of the gut with colonizing bacteria after birth (Claud & Walker 2001). The immature surface of the gut facilitates adherence and translocation of pathogens compared with the mature gut. This helps explain the increased sepsis and intestinal inflammation that occurs in this age group. In addition, immunoprotective factors, such as pIgA, and protective cytokines are underexpressed at birth leading to an increased inflammatory response to bacteria and their endo/exotoxins. This collective enhanced susceptibility to bacterial inflammation helps explain the increased incidence of NEC in this age group (Claud & Walker, 2001). In addition, Goldman et al. (1988) have shown that human milk, particularly colostrum, contains high concentrations of anti-inflammatory factors.

In the last five years, this laboratory has demonstrated an additional immaturity of bacterial/gut interaction in human prematures. We have shown that the inflammatory response to bacteria and their endotoxins (lipopolysaccharide [LPS]) is accentuated in the immature compared with mature enterocyte. In immature vs. mature human enterocytes (H4, a primary human fetal small intestinal crypt cell line; and Caco-2, a transformed mature human colonic cell line) the response to LPS and an endogenous inflammatory cytokine, IL-1α, is 20-fold higher as measured by IL-8 levels. This same difference in

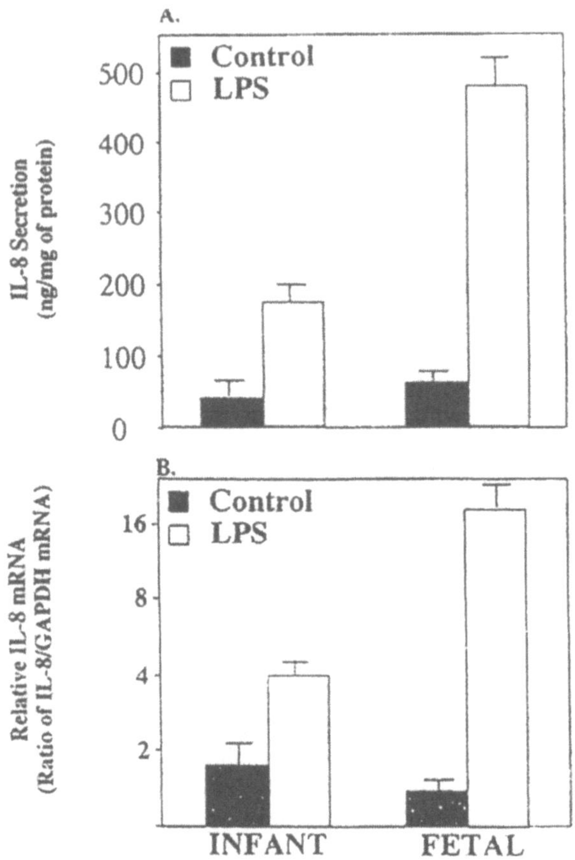

Figure 6. Depiction of IL-8 (A) and IL-8 mRNA induction (B) in infant and fetal intestinal organ culture in response to lipopolysaccharide (LPS) (50 μg/mL) or media alone as a control. Secreted IL-8 is expressed as ng/mg of total tissue protein. IL-8 mRNA was quatitated by densitometry and normalized to the relative level of GAPDH mRNA. The results are given as means ±SEM. The number of independent experiments for each data point ranged from three to four. Reprinted from PNAS, Vol. 97, Nanthakumar et al., Inflammation in the developing human intestine: a possible pathophysiologic basis for necrotizing enterocolitis, pp 6043-6048, Copyright (2000), with permission from the National Academy of Sciences U.S.A.

response to LPS and IL-1α was also noted in fetal vs. child biopsy organ cultures (Fig. 6) (Nanthakumar et al. 2000).

We and others (Mattsby-Balzer et al. 1996) have begun to determine the mechanism of action of the anti-inflammatory factors in human milk on gut inflammation during this period of immaturity. We know from clinical studies that ingestion of their mothers' expressed milk by premature infants prevents or lessens the severity of NEC (Lucas & Cole 1990). In these studies, we specifically examined the effect of known human milk anti-inflammatory factors on the IL-8 response to endogenous inflammatory cytokines using H4 and Caco-2 or T84 cells as examples of immature and mature enterocytes, respectively. The following factors were examined: interleukin 10 (IL-10), transforming growth factor beta, (TGF-β), erythropoietin, and epidermal growth factor (EGF). These studies suggest that these factors down-regulate the IL-8 response to TNF-α, suggesting

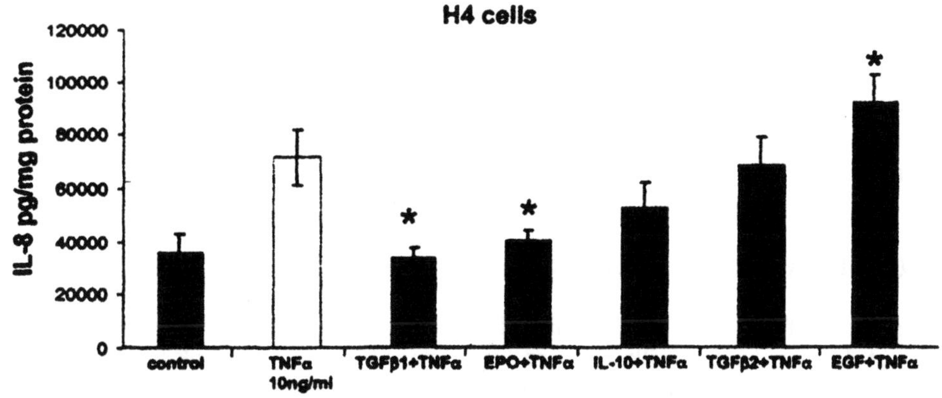

Figure 7. Effect of the human milk factors on TNF-α-stimulated IL-8 secretion by human IEC. Cells were pretreated with one of five human milk factors for 24 h before stimulation with TNF-α (10 ng/mL for 6 h). IL-8 was measured by EIA and compared with measured protein concentrations from cell lysates. Findings are presented ±SEM; n≥4. Results in the nontransformed fetal small IEC line, H4. *Statistical significance at $P<0.05$ for inhibition by TGF-β1 and Epo and accentuated stimulation by EGF of TNF-α-induced IL-8 secretion compared with stimulation with TNF-α alone, without a human milk factor pretreatment. Reprinted from Pediatr Res, Vol. 53, Claud et al., Modulation of human intestinal epithelial cell interleukin-8 secretion by human milk factors, pp 419-425, Copyright (2003), with permission from Lippincott Williams & Wilkins.

a specific mechanism for human milk anti-inflammation as part of the immature inflammatory response of the premature infant (Fig. 7) (Claud et al. 2003). These experimental studies of inflammation in the immature human gut and role of human milk anti-inflammatory factors support the premise that human milk provides the protection lacking in the newborn, particularly the premature, gut until the infant can develop protective mucosal defenses.

5.4. Bacterial Exotoxins

In addition to studying the immaturity of the newborn infant's response to microbacteria and their endotoxins, we have examined the developmental effect of bacterial exotoxins, particularly cholera toxin (CT), on the immature human gut. In a series of publications during the last decade using pre- and postweaned rats as an animal model for development, we showed that the chloride secretory response to CT was enhanced in immature vs. mature intestine (Chu et al. 1993). We further demonstrated that the enhanced immature response was due to an accentuated postreceptor reaction (Seo et al. 1989) and to an immature handling of electrolytes by preweaned intestine (Zemelman et al. 1992). Finally, we reported that pre-exposure of preweaned small intestine to a human milk trophic factor, cortisone, could accelerate the maturation of the secretary response to CT (Chu et al. 1989).

More recently, we have established models for the study of human small intestine [an H4 fetal human small intestinal primary cell line (Sanderson et al. 1996), fetal human intestinal organ cultures (He et al. 1994), microUssing chambers (Pratha et al. 1998), and a fetal human intestinal xenograph transplant model (Savidge et al. 2001)]. Using these techniques, we have begun to study the human immature enterocyte response to exotoxins. In recent experiments, we demonstrate that the postreceptor, cyclic adenosine monophosphate (cAMP), response to CT in H4 cells and in fetal organ culture is significantly higher than the CT cAMP response in T84 and Caco-2 cells (Lu et al. 2003). It is our intent to determine if the known trophic factors in human milk (cortisone, thyroxin, TGF-β, EGF, etc.) can cause a maturation of this accentuated immature response. Based on the animal model data, we would predict that pre-exposure to a human milk trophic factor would cause maturation of the fetal human enterocyte's signal transduction response to CT stimulation.

6. SUMMARY AND CONCLUSIONS

In this brief review of the dynamic effects of breastfeeding on intestinal development and host defense, human milk has been hypothesized to provide a link between mother and her newborn infant in the extrauterine environment and to protect the newborn, particularly the premature newborn, from age-related gastrointestinal diseases due in part to the immature development of intestinal host defenses. To support the stated hypothesis, we provide examples of human milk mitigating the clinical expression of inherited disease by providing the missing factor that causes the disease. In some instances, the provision of a lacking host defense factor, e.g., pIgA, cytokines, etc., may prevent the expression of an age-related infectious/inflammatory disease state. After comparing components of human milk from mothers delivering prematurely with mothers delivering full-term infants, and comparing the composition of early human milk (colostrum) with later milk (mature milk), we also suggest that human milk uniquely provides factors for the newborn that are lacking during a transient period of newborn existence. Finally, we review experimental data from our laboratory and others that the newborn infant responds inappropriately to microorganisms and their endo- and exotoxins. We further show that factors in human milk can actively stimulate the maturation of enterocyte function to appropriately respond to the initial bacterial colonization of the gut and to protect against pathogens and their toxins.

We strongly believe that these examples of the effect of human milk on the newborn's intestinal environment and defenses provides compelling evidence to support our hypothesis and to strongly support breastfeeding as the principal source of nutrition for newborns and as an essential supplemental enteric source for feeding the premature infant. It is important that ongoing research be conducted on the subtle effects of human milk on the adjustment of the neonate to the external environment. Observations made in basic research laboratories regarding the mechanism of human milk action on the newborn's gut function must be quickly translated into clinical trials and multicenter studies in order to more aggressively recommend and support breastfeeding in our society.

7. REFERENCES

Adlerberth I, Hanson LA, Wold AE. The ontogeny of the intestinal flora. In: Sanderson IR, Walker WA, editors. Development of the Gastrointestinal Tract. Hamilton, Ontario: BC Decker, 1999.

Bernt KM, Walker WA. Human milk as a carrier of biochemical messages. Acta Paediatr 1999;430(Suppl):27-41.

Bernt KM, Walker WA. Human milk and the response of intestinal epithelium to infection. In: Newburg DS, editor. Bioactive Components of Human Milk. New York: Kluwer Academic/Plenum Publishers. Adv Exp Med Biol 2001;501:11-30.

Berseth CL, Michener SR, Nordyke CK, Go VL. Postpartum changes in pattern of gastrointestinal regulatory peptides in human milk. Am J Clin Nutr 1990;51:985-990.

Bode HH, Vanjonack WJ, Crawford JD. Mitigation of cretinism by breast-feeding. Pediatrics 1978;62:13-16.

Caplan MS, Jilling T. New concepts in necrotizing enterocolitis. Curr Opin Pediatr 2001;13:111-115.

Chandra RK. Prospective studies of the effect of breastfeeding on incidence of infection and allergy. Acta Paediatr Scand 1979;68:691-694.

Chandra RK. Five year follow-up of high risk infants with family history of allergy who were exclusively breast-fed or fed partial whey hydrolysate, soy, and conventional cow's milk formulas. J Pediatr Gastroenterol Nutr 1997;24:380-388.

Chu SW, Walker WA. Bacterial toxin interaction with the developing intestine. A possible explanation for toxigenic diarrhea of infancy. Gastroenterology 1993;104:916-925.

Chu WS, Ely IG, Walker WA. Age and cortisol alter host responsiveness to cholera toxin in the developing gut. Am J Physiol 1989;256:G220-G226.

Claud EC, Walker WA. Hypothesis: inappropriate colonization of the premature intestine can cause neonatal necrotizing enterocolitis. FASEB J 2001;15:1398-1403.

Claud EC, Savidge T, Walker WA. Modulation of human intestinal epithelial cell interleukin-8 secretion by human milk factors. Pediatr Res 2003;53:419-425.

Dai D, Nanthkumar NN, Newburg DS, Walker WA. Role of oligosaccharides and glycoconjugates in intestinal host defense. Proceedings of the Sino-American Symposium, Shanghai. J Pediatr Gastroenterol Nutr 2000;30:S23-33.

Eckhert CD, Sloan MV, Hurley DL. Zinc binding: A difference between human and bovine milk. Science 1997;195:789-790.

Groer M, Walker WA. What is the role of preterm human milk supplement in the host defenses of the preterm infant? Science vs. Fiction. Adv Pediatr 1996;43:335-358.

Gross SJ, David RJ, Bauman L, Tomarelli RM. Nutritional composition of milk produced by mothers delivering preterm. J Pediatr 1980;96:641-644.

Gross SJ, Buckley RH, Wakil SS, McAllister DC, David RJ, Faix RG. Elevated IgA concentration in milk produced by mothers delivered of preterm infants. J Pediatr 1981;99:389-393.

He Y, Sanderson IR, Walker WA. Uptake, transport and metabolism of exogenous nucleosides in intestinal epithelial cell cultures. J Nutr 1994;124:1942-1949.

Hurley LS, Lonnerdal B, Stanislowski AG. Zinc citrate, human milk and actodermatitis enteropathica. Lancet 1979;1:677-678.

Hyslop NE, Kern KC, Walker WA. Lysozyme in human colostrums and human milk. In: Osserman EF, Canfield RE, Boyshok S, editors. Lysozyme. New York: Academic Press, 1974; pp 449-462.

Insoft RM, Sanderson IS, Walker WA. The development of immune function within the human intestine and its role in neonatal diseases. Pediatr Clin North Am 1996;43:551-571.

Kleinman RE, Walker WA. The enteromammary immune system. Digest Dis Sci 1979;24:876-882.

Kliegman RM, Pittard WV, Fanaroff AA. Necrotizing enterocolitis in neonates fed human milk. J Pediatr 1979;95:450-453.

Kramer MS. Does breast-feeding help protect against atopic disease? Biology, methodology, and a golden jubilee of controversy. J Pediatr 1988;112:181-190.

Kurscheid T, Holschneider AM. Necrotizing enterocolitis (NEC)—mortality and long-term results. Eur J Pediatr Surg 1993;3:139-143.

Lonnerdal B, Stanislowski AF, Hurley LS. Isolation of a low molecular weight zinc binding ligand from human milk. J Inorg Biochem 1980;12:71-78.

Lonnerdal B, Hoffman BS, Hurley LS. Zinc and copper binding proteins in human milk. Am J Clin Nutr 1982:36:1170-1176.

Lu L, Baldeon ME, Savidge T, Pothoulakis C, Walker WA. Development of microbial-human enterocyte interaction: Cholera toxin. Pediatr Res 2003;54:212-8.

Lucas A, Brooke OG, Morley R, Cole TJ, Bamford MF. Early diet of preterm infants and development of allergic or atopic disease: randomised prospective study. Br Med J 1990a;300:837-840.

Lucas A, Cole TJ. Human milk and neonatal necrotizing enterocolitis. Lancet 1990b;336:1519.

Majamaa H, Isolauri E. Probiotics: a novel approach in the management of food allergy. J Allergy Clin Immunol 1997;99:179-185.

Mattsby-Baltzer I, Roseanu A, Motas C, Elverfors J, Engberg I, Hanson LA. Lactoferrin or a fragment thereof inhibits the endotoxin-induced interleukin-6 response in human monocytic cells. Pediatr Res 1996;40:257-262.

McClelland DBL, McGrath J, Samson RR. Antimicrobial factors in human milk. Studies of concentration and transfer to the infant during the early stages of lactation. Acta Paediatr Scand 1978;271(Suppl):1-20.

Munoz FM, Englund JA, Cheesman CC, Maccato ML, Pinell PM, Nahm MH, Mason EO, Kozinetz CA, Thompson RA, Glezen WP. Maternal immunization with pneumococcal polysaccharide vaccine in the third trimester of gestation. Vaccine 2002:20:826-837.

Nanthakumar NN, Fusunyan RD, Sanderson I, Walker WA. Inflammation in the developing human intestine: A possible pathophysiologic basis for necrotizing enterocolitis. Proc Natl Acad Sci USA 2000;97:6043-6048.

Nanthakumar NN, Dai D, Newburg DS, Walker AW. The role of indigenous microflora in the development of murine intestinal fucosyl- and sialyltransferases. FASEB J Express 10.1096/fj.02-0031fje, November 15, 2002.

Pratha VS, Thompson SM, Hogan DL, Paulus P, Dreilinger AD, Barrett KE, Isenberg JI. Utility of endoscopic biopsy samples to quantitate human duodenal ion transport. J Lab Clin Med 1998;132:512-518.

Read LC, Francis GL, Wallace JC, Ballard FJ. Growth factor concentrations and growth-promoting activity in human milk following premature birth. J Dev Physiol 1985;7:135-145.

Rubaltelli FF, Biadaioli R, Pecile P, Nicoletti P. Intestinal flora in breast- and bottle-fed infants. J Perinat Med 1998;26:186-191.

Sanderson IR, Ezzell RM, Kedinger M, Erlanger M, Xu ZX, Pringault E, Leon-Robine S, Louvard D, Walker WA. Human fetal enterocytes in vitro: modulation of the phenotype by extracellular matrix. Proc Natl Acad Sci USA 1996;93:7717-7722.

Saarinen UM, Kajosaari M. Breastfeeding as prophylaxis against atopic disease: prospective follow-up study until 17 years old. Lancet 1995;346:1065-1069.

Savidge TC, Lowe DC, Walker WA. Developmental regulation of intestinal epithelial hydrolyase activity in human jejunal xenografts maintained in severe-combined immunodeficient mice. Pediatr Res 2001;50:196-202.

Schanler RJ, Goldblum RM, Garza C, Goldman AS. Enhanced fecal excretion of selected immune factors in very low birth weight infants fed fortified human milk. Pediatr Res 1986;20:711-715.

Schiffrin EJ, Carter EA, Walker WA, Frieberg E, Benjamin J, Israel EJ. Influence of prenatal corticosteroids on bacterial colonization in the newborn rat. J Pediatr Gastroenterol Nutr 1993;17:271-275.

Selner JC, Merrill DA, Claman HN. Salivary immuno-globulin and albumin: development during the newborn period. J Pediatr 1968;72:685-689.

Seo JK, Chu SW, Walker WA. Development of intestinal host defense: An increased sensitivity in the adenylate cyclase response to cholera toxin in suckling rats. Pediatr Res 189;25:225-227.

Shaw JCL. Trace elements in the fetus and young infant. I. Zinc. Am J Dis Child 1979;133:1260-1268.

Tapper D, Klagsburn M, Newman J. Growth factors in early and late lactation. J Pediatr Surg 1979;14:803-807.

Wold AE, Adlerberth I. Breast feeding and the intestinal microflora of the infant—implications for protection against infectious diseases. In: Koletzko B, Michaelsen K, Hernell O, editors. Short and Long Term Effects of Breast Feeding on Child Health. New York: Kluwer Academic/Plenum Publishers. Adv Exp Med Biol. 2000;478:77-93.

Xanthou M, Bines J, Walker WA. Human milk and intestinal host defense in newborns. Adv Pediatr 1995;42:171-208.

Zemelman BW, Walker WA, Chu SW. Expression and developmental regulation of Na^+, K^+ adenosine triphosphatase in the rat small intestine. J Clin Invest 1992; 90:1016-1022.

UNDERSTANDING THE ORIGIN OF ASTHMA AND ITS RELATIONSHIP TO BREASTFEEDING

Marsha Wills-Karp[1], Dominique Brandt[2], and Ardythe L. Morrow[2]

1. ABSTRACT

Asthma is a chronic disease of the lung that has been increasing at an alarming rate in industrialized countries around the world over the last few decades. Although considerable progress has been made in our understanding of the underlying pathogenesis of the disease, the exact causes of the increasing prevalence are unknown. Studies suggest that most asthma develops in early childhood and that environmental factors present early in life may be crucial in the development of disease. One potential explanation for the recent epidemic referred to as the "hygiene hypothesis" postulates that factors that have resulted in a reduction in exposure to microbial products and/or infections in the western world may be contributing to this rise in disease prevalence. As early life influences are known to play an important role in establishment of asthma, studies have focused on the interface between mother and child that occurs during gestation and through breastfeeding. In this regard, the body of evidence regarding the relationship between breastfeeding and asthma indicates benefit but with the potential for risk. While providing population-level protection from infections and atopy in infancy and early childhood, breastfeeding might also pose an increased risk of atopic asthma among children with asthmatic mothers. In order to put this controversy in context, we discuss our current understanding of asthma pathogenesis, current theories on the factors driving the rising prevalence of asthma, and then discuss the potential influence of breastfeeding on asthma pathogenesis.

2. INTRODUCTION

Breastfeeding is a complex biosystem involving the mother, her infant, and the environment, which has been shaped by evolutionary biology to maximize infant survival. The rapid environmental and behavioral changes of modern society, however,

[1]Division of Immunobiology, Human Milk Research Program, Cincinnati Children's Hospital Research Foundation, 3333 Burnet Avenue, Cincinnati, OH 45229
[2]Center for Epidemiology and Biostatistics, Human Milk Research Program, Cincinnati Children's Hospital Research Foundation, Cincinnati, OH

affect the equilibrium of this triad. In industrialized countries compared to traditional societies, asthma prevalence is generally higher, hygiene standards are generally higher, and breastfeeding initiation and duration is typically shorter. There is evidence that increased prevalence of immunologic disorders and changes in gastrointestinal tract flora in mothers have introduced changes in the immunoregulatory cytokine profile found in maternal milk. Further, human milk samples collected worldwide reflect exposure to environmental chemicals associated with modern life-style.

Asthma prevalence is increasing worldwide. Evidence that asthma has early life origins suggests that breastfeeding or its lack may play an important role in its development. The relationship between breastfeeding and asthma appears to be developmentally important but complex—potentially dependent on maternal genetics, immune phenotype, and environmental exposures. Clarification of this relationship depends on understanding the origins of asthma as an allergic disease and defining the role of differing bioactive factors in maternal milk, endogenous and exogenous, on development of asthma in childhood.

3. ASTHMA

3.1. Definition and Natural History

Asthma is a chronic inflammatory disorder of the lungs that manifests as recurrent episodes of wheezing, breathlessness, chest tightness, and coughing (Kay 2001). These episodes can be triggered by exposures to a variety of environmental stimuli, such as: allergens (i.e., molds, house dust mites, plant and animal debris), pharmacologic agents (i.e., aspirin), infectious stimuli (particularly viruses), airborne pollutants (ozone, diesel) and irritants (tobacco smoke).

Asthma is a heterogeneous condition with patients exhibiting different signs and symptoms, as well as variability in the age of onset, persistence, and severity of disease. Although asthma can develop at any stage of life, the majority of individuals develop asthma in early childhood. Clearly the strongest identifiable predisposing factor for development of asthma is atopy, the genetic predisposition for the development of an IgE-mediated response to common environmental inhalant allergens. Although development of asthma as an adult generally is not associated with identifiable allergic sensitivities, most childhood asthma is atopic in nature. In support of this contention, recent longitudinal studies in children suggests that wheezing illnesses in early childhood may have different origins and may not be associated with the presence of asthma in later life. Three distinct clinical phenotypes have emerged to explain the diversity in wheezing illness in children [Fig. 1] (Martinez 2002). The first group is designated as "early transient wheezers." Generally, transient wheezing in infants is not associated with a family history of asthma. The primary risk factor seems to be reduced pulmonary function due to a variety of factors including prematurity and maternal smoking during pregnancy. The symptoms usually resolve because of an increase in airway size as the child matures. The second phenotype is referred to as "non-atopic wheezers." This phenotype includes infants who have had viral respiratory illness with wheezing in the first year of life. Most of these infants do not have positive skin test reactivity to allergens and do not have asthma in later life. The last clinical phenotype is characterized by development of wheezing illnesses in early childhood, which persists into adulthood ("IgE-mediated wheezers/asthma"). The prevalence of asthma in this group of children is

Natural History of Asthma

Although asthma can develop at any stage of life, the majority of individuals develop asthma in early childhood

90% of childhood asthma is allergic in nature

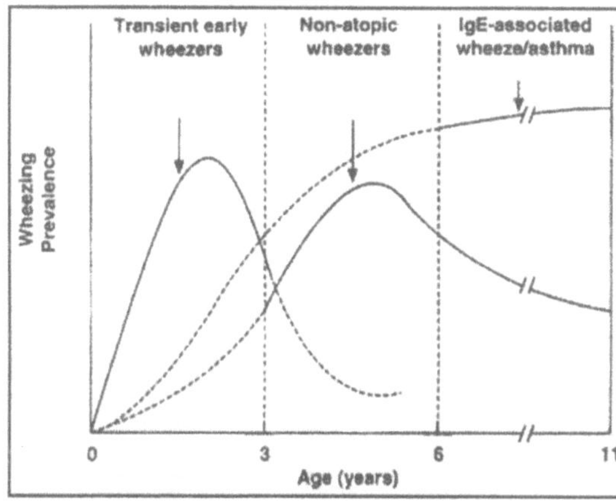

Figure 1. Hypothetical yearly peak prevalence of wheezing according to phenotype in childhood. Asthma phenotypes reflect a heterogeneous group of conditions characterized by recurrent airway obstruction. Three of these phenotypes are shown. Dashed lines suggest that wheezing can be represented by different curve shapes resulting from many different factors, including overlap of groups. Adapted from Stein et al. (Thorax 1997;52:946-952) with permission from the BMJ Publishing Group.

strongly correlated with serum IgE levels and with skin-test reactivity to allergens. Thus although other wheezing illnesses in childhood may masquerade as asthma, wheezing in association with atopy is the most reliable predictor of persistent asthma.

3.2. Prevalence

The incidence, morbidity, and mortality of asthma have been increasing at an alarming rate in industrialized countries around the world over the last few decades [Fig. 2] (Mannino et al. 1998; ISAAC 1998; Beasley 2002). In such countries, 30% of the population manifest some form of allergic disease at some time in their lives (ISAAC 1998). In the United States alone, the self-reported prevalence rate for asthma increased 75% between 1980 and 1994, with an increase of 160% among children younger than 4 years of age and 74% among children 5 to 14 years of age (Mannino et al. 1998). Currently, asthma is thought to afflict 6.4% of Americans (Mannino et al. 1998). Despite better diagnosis and treatment strategies, there was a 40% increase in the number of asthma deaths between 1982 and 1992 according to the Centers for Disease Control and Prevention (MMWR 1995). The economic burden of asthma in the United States, including health care costs and lost productivity, was estimated at $12.7 billion in 1998 alone. In marked contrast to the dramatic increases in asthma prevalence in westernized nations, the low baseline prevalence of asthma has not changed appreciably in countries such as Indonesia, Eastern Europe, China, India, Mexico, and parts of Africa [Fig. 2] (Beasley 2002). The reasons for the differential expression of disease between developed and nondeveloped countries are not well understood.

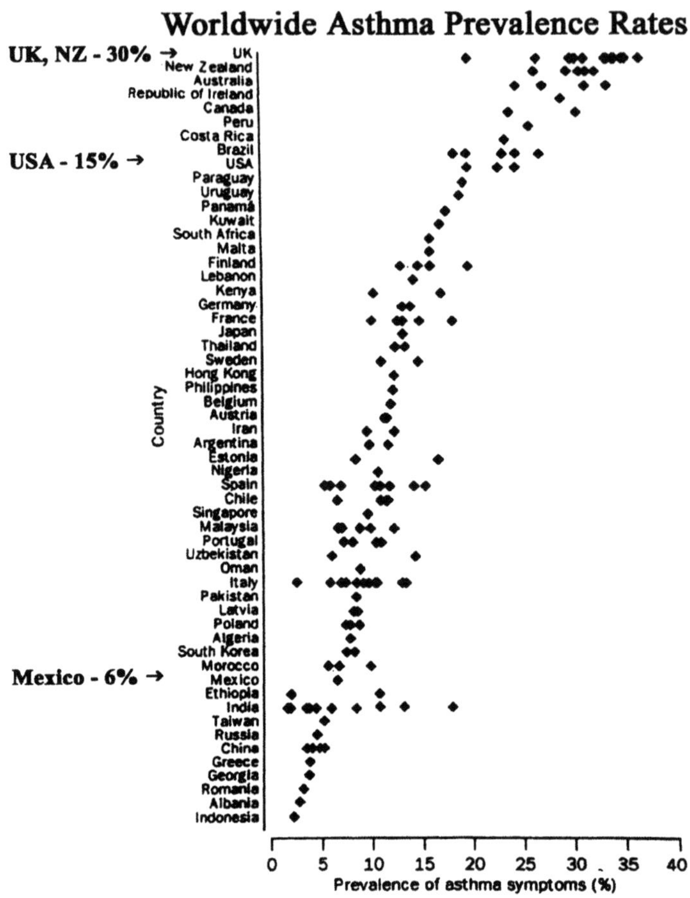

Figure 2. Twelve-month prevalence of self-reported asthma symptoms in 13- to 14-year old children. Reprinted from ISAAC Steering Committee: Worldwide variation in prevalence of symptoms of asthma, allergic rhinoconjunctivitis, and atopic eczema (Lancet 1998;351:1225-1232) with permission from Elsevier.

3.3. Asthma Pathophysiology, Pathogenesis

The primary pathophysiologic characteristics of asthma are airflow obstruction, airway hyperresponsiveness, and airway inflammation. Structurally the airways of asthmatics are characterized by the presence of lymphocytes, eosinophils, and mast cells, along with epithelial desquamation, goblet cell hyperplasia, and thickening of the submucosa (Kay 2001; Wills-Karp 1999). These cellular findings consistently have been associated with the main physiologic abnormalities of the disease, namely airway obstruction and airway hyperresponsiveness. Although asthma is multifactorial in origin, the inflammatory process in the most common form of the disease (allergic) is believed to be a result of inappropriate immune responses to a variety of ubiquitous, and otherwise innocuous, antigens in genetically susceptible individuals. Such IgE production is a tightly regulated process, part of a complex network of cellular and molecular events necessary for development of the allergic response. Initiation of this response appears to occur with presentation of the allergen by antigen presenting cells to CD4+ T-lymphocytes (a process referred to as sensitization). As the primary orchestrator of the specific immune response, the T-lymphocyte has been implicated in the pathogenesis of allergic airway disease. As has long been appreciated, CD4 T-lymphocytes are subdivided functionally into two distinct populations based on the distinct pattern of cytokines they produce. Namely, T-helper type1 (Th1) cells produce IL-2, IFN-γ, and TNF-α and are important in cell-mediated immune responses (Mosmann et al. 1986; Street & Mosmann 1991). T-helper type2 (Th2) cells, on the other hand, produce IL-4, IL-5, and IL-13 and regulate humoral immune responses. Numerous studies have established that T-cells from the lungs of asthmatics express a pattern of cytokines consistent with a Th2 pattern (Azzawi et al. 1990; Corrigan & Kay 1990; Wilkinson et al. 1991). Further, it has also been shown that successful therapeutic treatment is associated with shifting of the cytokine phenotype from a Th2 to a Th1 pattern (Wilkinson et al. 1991). An immunopathogenic role for Th2 cytokines in asthma has been postulated based on the role that these cytokines play in orchestrating the complex series of events leading to IgE production, and development, recruitment, and activation of the primary effector cells of the allergic response, the mast cell and the eosinophil (Wills-Karp 1999). Data from experimental murine models of disease have underscored the absolute requirement for T-lymphocytes in development of allergic airway symptoms (Mosmann et al. 1986). The quintessential question that remains is—what drives the skewed Th2 response to otherwise harmless antigens in people with asthma?

3.4. Factors Influencing Th2 Skewing in Asthmatic Individuals

T-cell differentiation is known to be influenced by several factors including the genetic background of the host, the nature and dose of the antigen, and the cytokine milieu present at the time of initial antigen presentation [Fig. 3]. Many intracellular pathogens such as bacterial and viral pathogens elicit Th1-mediated immune responses, while soluble and extracellular organisms such as parasites elicit strong Th2 responses. By far the most important determinant of CD4+ T-cell polarization is the cytokine milieu during T-cell priming (Hsieh 1993). In this regard, IL-12 is indispensable for development of most Th1 responses, and IL-4 has a similar role for Th2 responses. Thus one may postulate that the skewed Th2 immune responses in asthma may be due to either genetic or environmental influences resulting in either overzealous Th2 immune responses or impaired Th1 responses as a result of either an inability to generate a Th1 response or a lack of exposure to Th1 promoting agents.

3.4.1. Genetic Influences on Antigen Sensitization

The production of a Th2 pattern of cytokines appears to be genetically determined and established early during childhood. In an elegant longitudinal study of children, Martinez and colleagues (1995a) show that the propensity to develop allergic asthma is associated with low stimulated levels of IFN-γ in children at 9 months of age, which suggests that a type-1 response is a protective factor [Fig. 3]. Furthermore, low stimulated levels of IL-2 and IFN-γ at 9 months of age were correlated positively with parental immediate skin test reactivity. In this regard, familial aggregation and twin studies have confirmed a fundamental contribution of genetic factors to the development of asthma and specific clinical asthma phenotypes (Sandford et al. 1996; Ober 2001). Specifically,

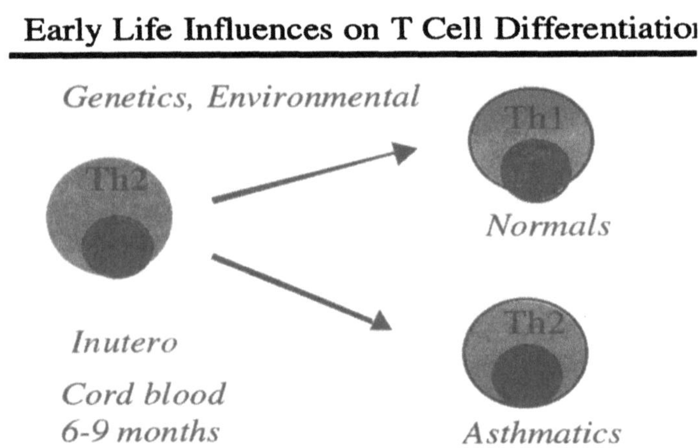

Figure 3. Early life influences on allergic sensitization

individuals with a first degree relative with asthma are at a significantly greater risk of developing asthma. Moreover, individuals with two asthmatic parents are at a greater risk of developing an allergic disease than those with only one asthmatic parent. Further support for a genetic underpinning for asthma is the fact that there is a greater concordance for asthma between monozygotic twins compared with dizygotic twins (Sandford et al. 1996; Ober 2001; Falliers et al. 1971). The concordance is not 100% suggesting that asthma is a polygenic disorder with strong environmental influences. Nonetheless, several groups have provided evidence for linkage of asthma-related traits with multiple broad chromosomal regions (Postma et al. 1995; Cookson et al. 1989). Candidate genes identified in these studies include those encoding Th2 cytokines [IL-4, IL-13] (Marsh et al. 1994; Heinzmann et al. 2000) and their signaling pathways [IL-4Ra] (Hershey et al. 1997; Bottini et al. 2002).

3.4.2. Environmental Influences on Allergen Sensitization

It is likely that multiple environmental factors influence development of allergic diseases, and that there may be complex interactions between these individual factors. The spectrum of antigens to which a person with asthma is sensitized is dependent on their environment in early life. This tenet is based on the positive correlations observed between allergen exposures present during the month of birth and the development of sensitization to the same allergens later in childhood [e.g., birch, grass, and dust mite allergens] (Bjorksten et al. 1980; Carosso et al. 1986). For example, Scandinavian infants born in late winter or early spring are more likely to develop IgE antibody to birch pollen, which is prevalent during the spring, than infants born at other times of the year (Bjorksten et al. 1980). In addition, withholding certain allergenic foods during the first few months of life tends to prevent sensitization and subsequent allergic responses to these particular foods.

Numerous studies have demonstrated the relationship between sensitization risk and the level of allergen exposure (Wahn et al. 1997; NHLBI/WHO 1995). This has been best studied in relationship to dust mite and cat antigens in early life. When both parents are atopic, dust mite sensitization occurred with <1% prevalence when infants were exposed to <0.1 mcg of house dust mite allergen per gram of dust, but this value increased to 6% with allergen levels over 10 mcg per gram of dust (Wahn et al. 1997). Although antigen dose is correlated positively with sensitization, studies suggest that the relationship may be more complex. Specifically, high exposure to animal dander early in life has been shown to be protective against manifestations of asthma (Remes et al. 2001). Whether this represents immune tolerance as a result of high antigen dose or concomitant exposure to other factors such as endotoxin as a result of living in proximity to a pet is unknown.

More important than the actual dose of allergen is the age at which exposure occurs. The immune system of neonates is thought to have a Th2 bias (Prescott et al. 1998a; Barrios et al. 1996) as a result of skewing of immune responses in the in utero environment. Th2 skewing is thought to occur in order to suppress IFN-γ production, which is toxic to the fetus. Studies of human infants indicate that this Th2 skew gradually diminishes during the first two years of life in nonallergic individuals (Prescott et al. 1998b, 1999). In allergic infants, the reverse occurs, with the strength of neonatal Th2 responses increasing over a similar period. The persistence of this neonatal bias and the failure to produce Th1 type responses may be an important feature of the asthmatic disease state (Prescott et al. 1999). The redirection of Th2 responses is thought to occur simultaneously with exposures to a variety of environmental antigens such as bacterial or viral infections and food antigens.

Exposure to other environmental agents such as diesel particles, ozone, second hand tobacco smoke, and rhinoviruses can also enhance sensitization to allergens in young children (Bjorksten 1999). Numerous epidemiologic studies illustrate clear associations between exposure to these agents and enhanced antigenic sensitization and worsening of disease. Ozone can alter both immediate and late-phase responses of asthmatics to inhaled allergen. Nasal challenge with diesel alone increased IgE production in both atopic and non-atopic individuals suggesting that indeed diesel may be a sensitizer (Diaz-Sanchez et al. 1999). When evaluated together with allergen, diesel exposure of ragweed sensitive subjects resulted in a significant increase in allergen-specific IgE with an increase in Th2 cytokine production. In summary, the complex interplay between genetic and environmental factors in early childhood likely governs susceptibility to development of asthma.

4. POTENTIAL EXPLANATIONS FOR THE ASTHMA EPIDEMIC

Despite the clearly heritable component of asthma, the rate at which the incidence is rising suggests a recent change in environmental influences. The aspects of the westernized lifestyle that are responsible have not been defined clearly: changes in air pollution, indoor exposure to allergens, changes in diet, and general living standards have all been suspected. Although there is an association between certain types of air pollution (particulates, diesel) and asthma exacerbation, overall air quality has improved throughout this epidemic of allergy. Indeed, careful comparison of asthma prevalence in former East Germany (low asthma prevalence, high levels of air pollution) and West Germany (the reverse) failed to support an important role for pollution (Nicolai & von Mutius 1997). Furthermore, although exposure to indoor allergens does increase with a sedentary lifestyle and the provision of energy-efficient housing, a strong correlation between the intensity of exposure to such allergens and development of allergic disease has yet to be found (Crater & Platts-Mills 1998).

The hypothesis that has gained the most attention is derived from the observation by Strachan in the 1960s that the risk of hay fever is related inversely to family size (Strachan 1989). This relationship has been capsulated in the "hygiene hypothesis," which argues that early childhood infections inhibit the tendency to develop allergic disease. Several epidemiologic studies have provided support for this hypothesis (Weiland et al. 1999; Bodner et al. 1998; Matricardi et al. 1998). One such study compared allergic sensitization and atopy in children from West and East Germany (Weiland et al. 1999), and noted that the frequency of atopy was considerably higher in West German children (37%) than in their peers in East Germany (18%). The authors attributed the increase in allergy to the "Western Lifestyle," with decreased family size, improved housing, and prevention of infectious diseases in early childhood. Further epidemiologic support for this hypothesis comes from studies demonstrating an inverse relationship between farm living (Kilpelainen et al. 2000), pet ownership (Remes et al. 2001), childcare attendance (Ball et al. 2000) in early life and atopy. Although the general implication of these studies is that increased risk from allergy seems to be associated with a decrease in microbial exposure, the link has remained fairly indirect.

4.1. Pathogens and Commensal Organisms

Although epidemiologic studies provide strong support for a relationship between childhood infectious syndromes and allergy, few studies have documented a direct relationship between a specific pathogen and protection from asthma. One study that has addressed the relationship between asthma and a specific pathogen is a cross-sectional study of Italian military recruits (Matricardi 1998). The authors found a significant, inverse association between the presence of antibodies to hepatitis A and various measures of atopy. In all likelihood, such evidence of previous infection with hepatitis A merely provides evidence of a risk of exposure to fecal-oral pathogens. At a population level, Shirakawa et al. (1997) found that among Japanese schoolchildren there was a strong inverse association between delayed-type hypersensitivity (Th1-mediated immune response) to Bacillus Calmette-Guerin (BCG) and atopy. Positive tuberculin responses predicted a lower incidence of asthma, lower serum IgE levels, and cytokine profile biases toward a type-1 profile. These results suggest that exposure and response to bacteria such as BCG may, by modification of immune cytokine profiles, inhibit atopic disorders. In a study of defined infectious exposures, Aaby and co-workers (2000) documented that vaccination with *Mycobacterium bovis* BCG was associated with a reduction in the prevalence of allergy in Guinea-Bissau. However, such protection was not observed in a similar retrospective study of BCG vaccination in Swedish children with a family history of allergy (Alm 1997).

The complex interface with the microbial world provided by the GI tract might well be important to the interrelationship between infection and allergy. The endogenous flora of the gut provides a wealth of stimuli for the developing immune system at birth. There seem to be both quantitative and qualitative differences in early childhood patterns of bacterial colonization between the developed and developing world. For example, a study of Swedish and Pakistani infants indicates that intestinal colonization with aerobic Gram-negative bacteria tends to occur later in westernized than in developing countries (Adlerberth et al. 1991). Once they are colonized, infants in developed countries tend to carry the same enterobacterial strains, whereas infants in developing countries are often colonized serially with different strains (Adlerberth et al. 1998). Differences in intestinal flora also have been found between allergic and nonallergic children in Europe (Böttcher et al. 2000a; Kalliomaki et al. 2001). Allergic 2-year-old children seem to be colonized less often with lactobacilli in Sweden and Estonia than nonallergic controls (Bjorksten et al. 1999). The intestine has been shown to affect immune response at other mucosal surfaces including the bronchial and genital tract, lacrimal, salivary, and mammary glands, through secretory IgA antibodies (Pabst 1987; Brandtzaeg 2002).

Another factor, which may have contributed to the change in infectious stimuli in infants from westernized cultures, is the widespread use of broad-spectrum antimicrobial agents. Although there are some discrepancies between studies examining the influence of use of antimicrobial agents on asthma, several studies have shown that antibiotic use during the first two years of life is associated with a pronounced, dose-dependant increase in the risk of developing allergic disease. Use of antimicrobial agents may have a profound impact on the balance of gut-associated immunity by depleting important Th1-promoting elements at a crucial age leading to a shift towards the development of Th2 immunity (Farooqi & Hopkin 1998; Wickens et al. 1999).

4.2. Counter-Regulatory Hypothesis

Mechanistic explanations for the hygiene hypothesis have typically evoked the Th1-Th2 model. The current thought is that the developing immune system needs a Th1 stimulus from the environment to redirect the immune response and avoid development of asthma. Consistent with this assumption, many bacterial infections, including mycobacteria, can provide just such a stimulus. Indeed, bacterial exposures have been shown to reduce sensitization to inhaled antigens in mice. Specifically, sensitization to ovalbumin can be inhibited by previous or concurrent infection with *Mycobacterium vaccae* or *M. bovis* (Erb et al. 1999) or by simultaneous administration of LPS and bacterial unmethylated CpG motifs (Kline et al. 1998).

Although Th2 immune responses are important in development of allergic disease, several lines of evidence suggest that interpretation of the "hygiene hypothesis" in the context of the Th1/Th2 paradigm may be overly simplistic. First, Th1 immune responses do not always protect against allergic disease, as most Th1-mediated respiratory tract viral infections (i.e., rhinoviruses, RSV) do not provide protection, and might be associated positively with development of allergic disease (Martinez 1995; Busse 1989). In addition, many viruses including measles leave a profound type 2 cytokine bias associated with suppression of IL-12 production in its wake (Atabani et al. 2001). In addition, recent epidemiologic studies suggest that the incidence of several Th1-mediated diseases such as type I diabetes also have increased in prevalence in the westernized world during the same time period (Stene & Nafstad 2001). The biggest paradox is the fact that parasitism with helminths in the developing world protects from asthma. Helminth infections such as *Schistosoma mansoni* are strong inducers of Th2 immune responses. Helminth-related protection from allergic disease, observed in mouse models (Wang et al. 2001) as well as in humans (Lynch et al. 1993), is therefore clearly not due to a remedial provision of an absent Th1 stimulus.

Although several postulates have been put forth to explain this paradox, a recent study of schistosome-parasitized children in Gabon suggests an entirely plausible mechanism for the helminth-related protection from asthma, and provides a potentially unifying explanation for many of the phenomenon that fall under the rubric of the "hygiene hypothesis." Specifically, van den Biggelaar and colleagues (2000) found evidence that parasite-driven IL-10 production was associated with a lower risk of developing skin-test reactivity to aeroallergens. Interestingly, most bacteria, Gram-negative and Gram-positive directly induce IL-10 secretion by a variety of immune cells. IL-10 provides, in many ways, an all purpose "anti-danger" signal. IL-10 has been shown to have multiple immunoregulatory effects, especially dampening down most immune responses, whether such responses result from activation of the innate or the adaptive immune system. In terms of the hygiene hypothesis, chronic (or serial) infection or colonization with various microbial agents (whether a Th1 stimulus or a Th2 stimulus or neither) leads to up-regulation of IL-10 production, secondarily suppressing an underlying predisposition to allergy [Fig. 4] (Wills-Karp et al. 2001). The decreased infectious and antigenic pressure of the westernized lifestyle has deprived us of this important counter-regulatory feedback, leading to an increased incidence of asthma and allergy.

Several lines of evidence support the validity of the counter-regulatory explanation for the hygiene hypothesis. First, it has been shown that IL-10 protein levels in the bronchoalveolar lavage fluids of asthmatics are lower than those observed in people without asthma (Borish et al. 1996). Furthermore, a generalized defect in IL-10 production seems to be present in patients with allergic asthma. Secondly, chronic tissue parasitism with helminths leads to an increase in IL-10 production. Most bacteria are also powerful inducers of IL-10 from antigen-presenting cells in vitro. It is therefore not surprising that there are clear data on in vivo up-regulation of IL-10 during infection with

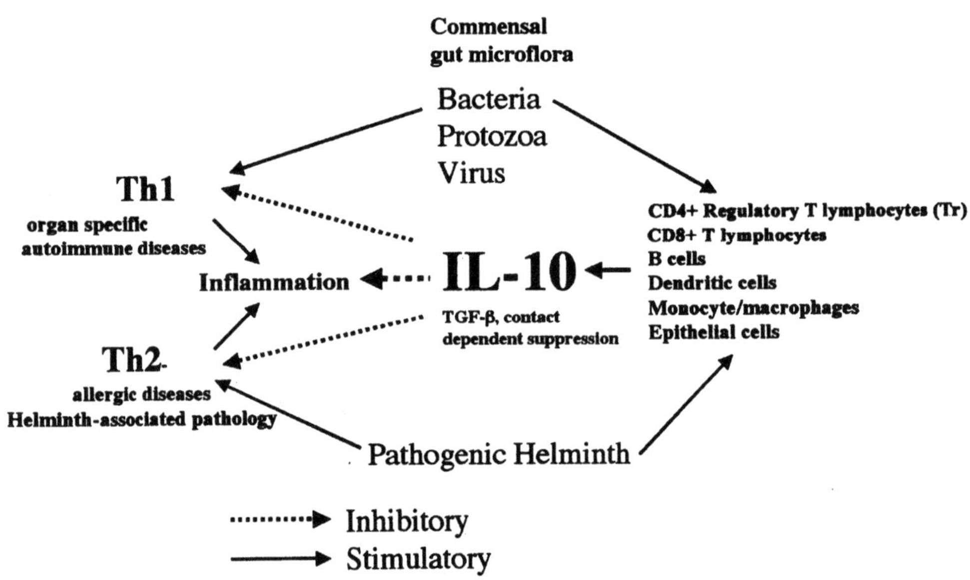

Figure 4. Schematic view of the counter-regulation hypothesis. Production by cells of both innate and adaptive immune systems, interleukin-10 has a key homeostatic role in the control of inflammatory processes. Most exposures that lead to immune activation leave IL-10 in their wake. Chronic infection or colonization with various microbial agents leads to up regulation of IL-10 production, secondarily suppressing underlying allergic and autoimmune diathesis. Immunologic "negotiations" in the intestinal tract may be of vital importance to this process of feedback inhibition. The decreased infectious and antigenic pressure of the westernized lifestyle weakens this important counter-regulatory input to the developing immune system, leading to an increased incidence of allergy and organ-specific autoimmune diseases. Note that IL-10 functions in this scheme as a marker of counter-regulatory processes, but various complementary and redundant mechanisms are likely to be involved. TGF-β, transforming growth factor β.

bacterial agents that have been implicated in the hygiene hypothesis, including BCG and *Mycobacterium tuberculosis* (Kaufmann et al. 1995; Barnes et al. 1993). As for diarrheal diseases, that are so important in early childhood mortality in the developing world, both viral [rotavirus] (Azim et al. 1999) and bacterial [shigella] (Raqib et al. 1995) diarrheal diseases lead to IL-10 production. Lastly, the gut may be an especially important site of counter-regulation as the gastrointestinal tract is normally an IL-10 dominant environment. Notably, IL-10 knockout mice develop spontaneous inflammatory bowel disease in response to normal gut flora (Kuhn et al. 1993). Studies suggest that priming for allergy to aeroallergens may occur in the gut (Wilson et al. 1973; Sudo et al. 1997). It is notable that oral tolerance is difficult to achieve in germ-free mice, and that administration of endotoxin together with food antigens increases the tolerizing effect of feeding in mouse models (Kim & Ohsawa 1995). Interestingly, Lactobacillus administration to children with atopic dermatitis, a strategy shown to have some preventative and therapeutic efficacy, induces IL-10 up-regulation in vivo (Pessi et al. 2000).

It should be noted that IL-10 is unlikely to carry out this homeostatic counter-regulatory role alone. Other mediators such as TGF-β are likely to be important as well. The role of IL-10 in immunoregulation is also likely to be indirect. Recent studies suggest that CD4+CD25+ T-regulatory lymphocytes produce predominantly IL-10 in vitro and in vivo. These cells have been shown to be important in providing protection against many inflammatory conditions (Shevach et al. 2001). With the counter-regulatory hypothesis in mind, we might surmise that factors in the environment in early childhood that disturb or alter production of immunoregulatory factors such as IL-10 and TGF-β either directly or indirectly via alteration of microbial exposures may contribute to the rising incidence in allergic disease.

4.3. Maternal Influences

Epidemiologic studies have reported that maternal, more than paternal, asthma is a significant risk factor for development of asthma (Martinez et al. 1995b). Mechanistic explanations have been proposed for gender specific inheritance patterns that relate to processes of gene imprinting (Reik & Walter 1998) and/or transfer of mitochondrial DNA (Johns 1996). However, other maternal influences independent of shared genetic material are implicated. The exclusive maternal effects observed in asthma might occur as a result of factors present during gestation and/or breastfeeding.

4.3.1. In Utero Influences on Asthma

The origins of asthma in early life suggest that prenatal events may influence susceptibility to allergic airway disease. Several independent studies have provided support for this postulate. For example, cord blood mononuclear cells have been shown to respond to inhalant and food allergens suggesting that initial priming of allergen-specific T-cell responses may occur before birth (Prescott et al. 1998a; Warner et al. 1994). Prescott et al. demonstrated that the responding cord blood T-cells were indeed of fetal origin, since they did not respond to common vaccine antigens such as tetanus toxoid, against which the majority of adults in the study population expressed active immunity. These findings suggest that transfer of substances from mother to child (e.g., allergens, antibodies, toxins, hormones, or other immune mediators via the placenta), may occur during gestation, which might prime or sensitize the developing infant for increased susceptibility to asthma. Indeed, Loibichler and colleagues (2002) have observed transplacental transfer of several allergens including beta-lactoglobulin, ovalbumin, and birch pollen allergen.

In addition, as discussed above, factors present in the uterine environment may influence the nature of the immune response of the fetus to allergens crossing the placenta. For example, exogenous antigens that leak across the placenta are likely to be presented to the fetal immune system within a milieu conducive to selection for Th2 immunity. This contention is supported by studies showing that cord blood cells from both allergic and nonallergic infants produce high levels of Th2 cytokines and low IFN-γ levels (Böttcher et al. 2003a). Although these studies demonstrate that initial allergen priming may occur in utero, they also suggest that the Th2 cell phenotype is determined to a substantial degree after birth as only a minority of the infants who exhibit allergen specific Th2 responses at birth, go on to develop disease.

4.3.2. Intrapartum and Postpartum Influences on Asthma

Another change in behavior in the westernized world that may alter risk of asthma due to early life exposures relates to changes in the mode of child delivery. There has been a clear increase in caesarean sections over vaginal deliveries in many westernized countries (Usha Kiran & Jayawickrama 2002). It is proposed that an increase in caesarean sections may reduce initial microbial exposure and thereby alter Th1/Th2 cell development and affect the risk of developing atopy. Kero et al. (2002) reported a significantly higher incidence of asthma among children at age 7 who were born by caesarean section compared with children of the same age who were born vaginally (4.2% vs. 3.3%). Although this association may be due to factors associated with caesarean birth other than microbial exposure, this study suggests that early life encounters with microbes may be relevant to protection against the development of asthma.

The transfer of immunological information from mother to child continues to occur postpartum via breastfeeding. Human milk contains a variety of bioactive constituents including antibodies, oligosaccharides, cells, lactoferrin, and cytokines, which extend maternal protection against infectious diseases as the infant immature immune system develops (Hanson et al. 2002; Morrow et al. 1999; Xanthou 1998). Some of these protective factors provide specific immunity, e.g., antibodies and lymphocytes (Buescher 2001). Human milk contains also nonspecific and multifunctional protective factors, such as lactoferrin, lysozyme, and oligosaccharides (Coppa et al. 2001), and is rich in anti-inflammatory factors, including omega-3-fatty acids (Hamosh 2002). Decades of epidemiologic and laboratory studies have established that human milk protects against infectious diseases in the breastfed infant; a growing body of literature indicates that breastfeeding protects against wheezing symptoms in infancy and early childhood, but may have a different relationship with later-onset asthma.

5. RELATIONSHIP BETWEEN BREASTFEEDING AND ASTHMA

While breastfeeding is known to protect against infectious diseases, the relationship between breastfeeding and development of childhood allergy is controversial. Protection by breastfeeding has been demonstrated convincingly against wheezing and atopic eczema in infants and children up to 6 years of age (Oddy et al. 1999; Dell & To 2001;

Kramer et al. 2001; Chulada et al. 2003; Oddy et al. 2003a). Breastfeeding protection against wheezing has been shown from longitudinal and cross-sectional studies conducted in a variety of populations; the strongest protection has been shown against recurrent wheezing in infancy (Chulada et al. 2003; Oddy et al. 2003a; Wright et al. 1989). While the mechanism of protection has not been established, it may be due to prevention of respiratory infections and/or delays in allergic sensitization (Chulada et al. 2003). There is increasing evidence that this breastfeeding protection is related to bioactive immune factors in human milk, e.g., T-regulatory cytokines (Oddy et al. 2003b; Böttcher et al. 2000b, 2000c; Hawkes et al. 1999; Kalliomaki et al. 1999) as described further below.

In contrast, several studies have reported increased risk of asthma and atopy at older ages associated with a history of breastfeeding. Sears et al. (2002), in a longitudinal study of 1,037 New Zealand children greater than 9 years of age, found that a history of breastfeeding was a risk factor for atopy and asthma. Allergic status was determined through questionnaire and skin prick to common allergens in study children. Wright et al. (2001a) studied a cohort of 1,246 normal infants in Tucson, Arizona, from birth to 13 years of age and found that children of asthmatic mothers were significantly more likely to have asthma the greater the dose exposure to their mother's milk. In the Tucson study, the asthma status in the study child was obtained through questionnaire, medical examination, and skin prick to common allergens. The relationship between breastfeeding history and asthma in the child was stratified by the presence of maternal and paternal asthma.

Inconsistencies in the literature regarding the relationship between breastfeeding and development of asthma may arise from methodologic issues such as misclassification of exposures and outcomes and measuring different aspects of atopy/asthma in children at different ages. Although wheezing frequently is used as a predictor of subsequent asthma later in life, it is a heterogeneous disorder in children (Fig. 2). According to the Tucson study, about half of all children ever experience wheezing: 20%, transient wheezing (wheezing before the age of 3); 15%, persistent wheezing; and 14%, late-onset asthma (Taussig et al. 2003). The causes of wheeze at different ages appear to differ; the observed association between increased breastfeeding and reduced risk of asthma symptoms in the first years of life is likely to be mediated by protection against respiratory tract illnesses, which may be different than the breastfeeding relationship with later-onset asthma.

The primary outcomes of asthma and atopy are subject to serious potential misclassification. Since there is no clear and general definition of asthma, doctor's diagnosis may differ, and a questionnaire alone may not be an adequate screening tool for asthma (Gruchalla et al. 2003). Few studies report asthma and allergy symptoms using more objective markers such as IgE measurements, skin prick tests, bronchial responsiveness, or lung function measurements (Wieringa et al. 2001). The measurement of human milk exposure is also subject to error, particularly when assessed retrospectively. Breastfeeding should be assessed in terms of duration and exclusivity, but often breastfeeding is characterized inadequately (Becquet et al. 2003; van Odijk et al. 2003). Further, heredity plays an important role but has not been characterized adequately in most studies.

Progress in understanding the relationship between breastfeeding and asthma depends on carefully designed clinical studies that also characterize the bioactive components of human milk that may provide the mechanism of protection against, or risk of, asthma in the child.

5.1. Immunoregulatory Properties of Human Milk

The T-regulatory cytokines TGF-β1, TGF-β2 and IL-10 have been found in human milk in varying quantities. Variation between studies in the reported concentrations of cytokines in human milk may be due in part to measurement techniques, stage of lactation, and/or the characteristics of study mothers. TGF-β1 and TGF-β2 have been shown to be present in significant quantities in human milk and particularly in colostrum (Hawkes et al. 1999; Kalliomaki et al. 1999; Laiho et al. 2003). IL-10 has been found in fewer human milk samples and in much lower quantities than TGF-β1 and TGF-β2, at any stage of lactation (Böttcher et al. 2000b; Laiho et al. 2003; Srivastava et al. 1996). However, Garofalo et al. (1995) reported that IL-10 was detected in high concentrations in colostrum samples collected within 80 hours postpartum.

The cytokines in human milk appear to have immunoregulatory functions in the developing infant. Field and colleagues (2000) measured production of IL-10 by stimulated peripheral blood lymphocytes in breastfed infants, at ages 14 and 42 weeks, compared with infants fed standard formula and infants fed formula enriched in long-chain polyunsaturated fatty acids. They found that the IL-10 concentration in stimulated peripheral blood lymphocytes was significantly higher in breastfed infants compared with the formula groups. A longitudinal study of 15 breast- and 15 bottle-fed infants found that production of IFN-γ (a Th1 cytokine) by mononuclear leukocytes was lower in breastfed infants (Stephens et al. 1986), indicating that breastfeeding tends to maintain a Th2 phenotype in the young infant. However, among breastfed infants, there is variation in dose exposure to the immunoregulatory properties of human milk given varying degrees of breastfeeding and cytokine concentrations in milk from different mothers. Studies suggest that the variation in concentrations of human milk cytokines may be biologically relevant to infant health. For example, TGF-β1 has been found in lower concentration in colostrum from mothers whose infants had IgE-mediated cow's milk allergy than from mothers whose infants had non-IgE-mediated cow's milk allergy (Saarinen et al. 1999). Kalliomaki et al. (1999) reported TGF-β1 and TGF- β2 in significantly higher amounts in maternal colostrum, but not in mature milk and infants' serum, in infants with postweaning-onset atopic disease compared with infants who developed atopic disease while breastfeeding. Oddy et al. (2003b) conducted a study of 243 breastfeeding mother-infant pairs. Maternal milk samples collected at a mean of 11 days postpartum were assayed for TGF-β1, TNF-α, and IL-10 cytokines. They found that duration of breastfeeding and the concentration of TGF-β1 in maternal milk were associated inversely with risk of wheezing in infancy.

Given the potential significance of the immunoregulatory cytokines, it is important to understand factors that control their expression in human milk. Evidence suggests that milk concentrations reflect maternal immune status. In a double-blinded, placebo-controlled study, Rautava et al. (2002) administered probiotics to 62 pregnant and lactating mothers. The concentration of TGF-β2 was significantly higher in the milk of mothers receiving probiotics than in milk of mothers receiving placebo (2,885 vs. 1,340 pg/mL). Taken together, these studies suggest that maternal immune status and gastrointestinal tract health are relevant to the expression of immune factors in human milk, and specifically, that maternal ingestion of probiotics can increase the expression of TGF-β cytokines in her milk.

5.2. Composition of Human Milk in Relation to Risk of Asthma

In order for breastfeeding by atopic mothers to confer greater risk of asthma to the child, as suggested by Wright et al. (2001a, 2001b), one must postulate that milk constituents differ between atopic and non-atopic mothers. In fact, there is evidence of differences in cytokine composition by maternal atopic status. Böttcher et al. (2000c) analyzed the composition of milk from 24 allergic and 25 nonallergic mothers and found that concentrations of Th2 cytokines (IL-4, IL-13, and IL-5) were higher in the milk of allergic mothers. These cytokines are thought to play a major role in development of manifestations of allergic disease via the generation of IgE, and the regulation of the differentiation, recruitment and activation of eosinophils (Wills-Karp et al. 2001), suggesting the possibility that milk from allergic mothers might prime the child's immune system toward a Th2 phenotype. Conversely, Böttcher et al. (2003a) analyzed the effects of human milk on mitogen- and allergen-induced cytokine production from cord blood mononuclear cells. They found that colostrum from both nonallergic and allergic mothers enhanced allergen-specific Th2 cytokine production in infants. Further confirming its anti-inflammatory effects, they found that human milk inhibits IFN-γ production, with no difference in effect between the milk of allergic and nonallergic mothers. Böttcher and colleagues (2003b) further examined the levels of cytokines, chemokines, and IgA antibodies in human milk and found no association between the levels of these factors in human milk and infants' skin prick test positivity, development of allergic symptoms, or salivary secretory IgA levels during the first 2 years of life. This finding is consistent with previous studies showing breastfeeding protection against allergy or no increased risk of allergy associated with breastfeeding among children in the first five years of life. However, Wright et al. (2001a, 2001b) have suggested that breastfeeding does not increase the risk of allergy per se in the first few years of life, but rather, primes their development of allergic disease at later ages by prolonging the Th2 phenotype through early childhood.

Further, human milk may contain allergens and various chemical toxins (e.g. ozone, cotinine) that may enhance allergen sensitization in the infant; infants have been shown to develop antibody responses to antigens conveyed in human milk (Takahashi et al. 2002). Similarly, infants can be sensitized to food antigens consumed by the mother (Hirose et al. 2001; Vadas et al. 2001). However, the extent to which inhalant allergens are present in human milk and whether these antigens are present in different amounts in milk from allergic and nonallergic mothers is not known. It is, however, possible that as a result of recent changes in the environment in westernized countries, that mothers may transfer elevated levels of allergens, pollutants, and environmental chemicals to their infants during pregnancy or breastfeeding. However, analysis of the amount of chemical contaminants present in human milk to date have shown no direct effect on breastfed infants, except for severe cases of contamination such as in hexachlorobenzene-induced pemba yara, and polychlorinated biphenyl-induced growth retardation and abnormal skin pigmentation (Landrigan et al. 2002; Berlin et al. 2002). Thus, additional studies are needed to examine the relationship between asthma and the presence of toxic chemicals in human milk.

5.3. Effects of Human Milk on Diversity of Gastrointestinal Tract Flora

Another potential mechanism by which human milk may influence allergic status of the infant is via its well-established role in mucosal immunity of the gastrointestinal tract.

The high composition of nondigestible oligosaccharides in human milk promotes the colony formation of *Bifidobacteria* and *Lactobacilli*, also known as probiotics. Probiotics are suspected to have gut-barrier functions, give maturation signals for the gut-associated lymphoid tissues, and balance the generation of pro- and anti-inflammatory cytokines, thereby creating healthy interactions between the host and microbes in the gut that are needed to keep inflammatory responses regulated (Isolauri et al. 1999). However, breastfeeding may reduce diversity of flora in the gastrointestinal tract resulting in lack of Th1 conditioning; exclusively breastfed infants have lower levels of Gram-negative enterobacteria in their intestinal tracts (Yoshioka et al. 1983) and less diversity of colonization species (Wold 1998).

6. CONCLUSIONS

The prevalence, morbidity, and mortality of asthma have increased dramatically over the last few decades in industrialized countries. Because the genetic make-up of the population has not changed significantly over this time period, the increases must be due to changes in the environment. A plausible explanation for this phenomenon, referred to as the "hygiene hypothesis," suggests that changes have occurred in the western lifestyle that have resulted in reduced exposures to microbial infections and products. A myriad of changes in the westernized lifestyle may be responsible for the reduction in microbial exposures, such as smaller family size, antibiotic use, transition from farm to city dwelling, vaccination against infections, and general improvements in sanitation. Although the exact mechanisms underlying the expansion of pathogenic Th2 cells are unknown, early life influences are known to play a significant role.

The role of breastfeeding in relation to asthma is important to understand and is likely to be multidimensional. Breastfeeding is consistently associated with protection against infectious diseases, wheezing, and atopic eczema in the first few years of life. The immune factors in human milk responsible for this protection are becoming known. Yet, the clear maternal influence on development of asthma in the child suggests that the asthmatic mother conveys to the child either during gestation or through breastfeeding, or both, factors that increase the risk of developing later-onset asthma in the child. Studies suggest that the milk of atopic mothers may convey allergens and/or a cytokine balance that modulates the immune response of the child, predisposing towards an atopic response to later exposures. Further studies are required to elucidate the relationships between breastfeeding and asthma. The need for such information is critical in this era of increasing asthma prevalence and severity.

7. ACKNOWLEDGMENT

This work was supported by a program project grant from the National Institute of Child Health and Human Development (HD13021).

8. REFERENCES

Aaby P, Shaheen SO, Heyes CB, Goudiaby A, Hall AJ, Shiell AW, Jensen H, Marchant A. Early BCG vaccination and reduction in atopy in Guinea-Bissau. Clin Exp Allergy 2000;30:644-650.

Adlerberth I, Carlsson B, de Man P, Jalil F, Khan SR, Larsson P, Mellander L, Svanborg C, Wold AE, Hanson LA. Intestinal colonization with Enterobacteriaceae in Pakistani and Swedish hospital-delivered infants. Acta Paediatr Scand 1991;80:602-610.

Adlerberth I, Jalil F, Carlsson B, Mellander L, Hanson LA, Larsson P, Khalil K, Wold AE. High turnover rate of Escherichia coli strains in the intestinal flora of infants in Pakistan. Epidemiol Infect 1998;121:587-598.

Alm JS, Lilja G, Pershagen G, Scheynius A. Early BCG vaccination and development of atopy. Lancet 1997;350:400-403.

Atabani SF, Byrnes AA, Jaye A, Kidd IM, Magnusen AF, Whittle H, Karp CL. Natural measles causes prolonged suppression of interleukin-12 production. J Infect Dis 2001;184:1-9.

Azim T, Ahmad SM, Sefat EK, Sarker MS, Unicomb LE, De S, Hamadani JD, Salam MA, Wahed MA, Albert MJ. Immune response of children who develop persistent diarrhea following rotavirus infection. Clin Diagn Lab Immunol 1999;6:690-695.

Azzawi M, Bradley B, Jeffery PK, Frew AJ, Wardlaw AJ, Knowles G, Assoufi B, Collins JV, Durham S, Kay AB. Identification of activated T lymphocytes and eosinophils in bronchial biopsies in stable atopic asthma. Am Rev Respir Dis 1990;142:1407-1413.

Ball TM, Castro-Rodriguez JA, Griffith KA, Holberg CJ, Martinez FD, Wright AL. Siblings, day-care attendance, and the risk of asthma and wheezing during childhood. N Engl J Med 2000;343:538-543.

Barnes PF, Lu S, Abrams JS, Wang E, Yamamura M, Modlin RL. Cytokine production at the site of disease in human tuberculosis. Infect Immun 1993;61:3482-3489.

Barrios C, Brawand P, Berney M, Brandt C, Lambert PH, Siegrist CA. Neonatal and early life immune responses to various forms of vaccine antigens qualitatively differ from adult responses: predominance of a Th2-biased pattern which persists after adult boosting. Eur J Immunol 1996;26:1489-1496.

Beasley R. The burden of asthma with specific reference to the United States. J Allergy Clin Immunol 2002;109:S482-489.

Becquet R, Leroy V, Salmi LR. Breastfeeding, atopy, and asthma. Lancet 2003;361:174; author reply 175-176.

Berlin CM, Jr., Kacew S, Lawrence R, LaKind JS, Campbell R. Criteria for chemical selection for programs on human milk surveillance and research for environmental chemicals. J Toxicol Environ Health A 2002;65:1839-1851.

Bjorksten B. The environmental influence on childhood asthma. Allergy 1999;54 Suppl 49:17-23.

Bjorksten B, Naaber P, Sepp E, Mikelsaar M. The intestinal microflora in allergic Estonian and Swedish 2-year-old children. Clin Exp Allergy 1999;29:342-346.

Bjorksten F, Suoniemi I, Koski V. Neonatal birch-pollen contact and subsequent allergy to birch pollen. Clin Allergy 1980;10:585-591.

Bodner C, Godden D, Seaton A. Family size, childhood infections and atopic diseases. The Aberdeen WHEASE Group. Thorax 1998;53:28-32.

Borish L, Aarons A, Rumbyrt J, Cvietusa P, Negri J, Wenzel S. Interleukin-10 regulation in normal subjects and patients with asthma. J Allergy Clin Immunol 1996;97:1288-1296.

Böttcher MF, Nordin EK, Sandin A, Midtvedt T, Bjorksten B. Microflora-associated characteristics in faeces from allergic and nonallergic infants. Clin Exp Allergy 2000a;30:1590-1596.

Böttcher MF, Jenmalm MC, Bjorksten B, Garofalo RP. Chemoattractant factors in breast milk from allergic and nonallergic mothers. Pediatr Res 2000b;47:592-597.

Böttcher MF, Jenmalm MC, Garofalo RP, Bjorksten B. Cytokines in breast milk from allergic and nonallergic mothers. Pediatr Res 2000c;47:157-162.

Böttcher MF, Fredriksson J, Hellquist A, Jenmalm MC. Effects of breast milk from allergic and non-allergic mothers on mitogen- and allergen-induced cytokine production. Pediatr Allergy Immunol 2003a;14:27-34.

Böttcher MF, Jenmalm MC, Bjorksten B. Cytokine, chemokine and secretory IgA levels in human milk in relation to atopic disease and IgA production in infants. Pediatr Allergy Immunol 2003b;14:35-41.

Bottini N, Borgiani P, Otsu A, Saccucci P, Stefanini L, Greco E, Fontana L, Hopkin JM, Mao XQ, Shirakawa T. IL-4 receptor alpha chain genetic polymorphism and total IgE levels in the English population: two-locus haplotypes are more informative than individual SNPs. Clin Genet 2002;61:288-292.

Brandtzaeg PE. Current understanding of gastrointestinal immunoregulation and its relation to food allergy. Ann N Y Acad Sci 2002;964:13-45.

Buescher ES. Anti-inflammatory characteristics of human milk: how, where, why. Adv Exp Med Biol 2001;501:207-222.

Busse WW. The relationship between viral infections and onset of allergic diseases and asthma. Clin Exp Allergy 1989;19:1-9.

Carosso A, Ruffino C, Bugiani M. The effect of birth season on pollenosis. Ann Allergy 1986;56:300-303.

Chulada PC, Arbes SJ, Jr., Dunson D, Zeldin DC. Breast-feeding and the prevalence of asthma and wheeze in children: analyses from the Third National Health and Nutrition Examination Survey, 1988-1994. J Allergy Clin Immunol 2003;111:328-336.

Cookson WO, Sharp PA, Faux JA, Hopkin JM. Linkage between immunoglobulin E responses underlying asthma and rhinitis and chromosome 11q. Lancet 1989;1:1292-1295.

Coppa GV, Pierani P, Zampini L, Bruni S, Carloni I, Gabrielli O. Characterization of oligosaccharides in milk and feces of breast-fed infants by high-performance anion-exchange chromatography. Adv Exp Med Biol 2001;501:307-314.

Corrigan CJ, Kay AB. CD4 T-lymphocyte activation in acute severe asthma. Relationship to disease severity and atopic status. Am Rev Respir Dis 1990;141:970-977.

Crater SE, Platts-Mills TA. Searching for the cause of the increase in asthma. Curr Opin Pediatr 1998;10:594-599.

Dell S, To T. Breastfeeding and asthma in young children: findings from a population-based study. Arch Pediatr Adolesc Med 2001;155:1261-1265.

Diaz-Sanchez D, Garcia MP, Wang M, Jyrala M, Saxon A. Nasal challenge with diesel exhaust particles can induce sensitization to a neoallergen in the human mucosa. J Allergy Clin Immunol 1999;104:1183-1188.

Erb KJ, Kirman J, Delahunt B, Moll H, Le Gros G. Infection of mice with Mycobacterium bovis-BCG induces both Th1 and Th2 immune responses in the absence of interferon-gamma signalling. Eur Cytokine Netw 1999;10:147-154.

Falliers CJ, de Cardoso RR, Bane HN, Coffey R, Middleton E, Jr. Discordant allergic manifestations in monozygotic twins: genetic identity versus clinical, physiologic, and biochemical differences. J Allergy 1971;47:207-219.

Farooqi IS, Hopkin JM. Early childhood infection and atopic disorder. Thorax 1998;53:927-932.

Field CJ, Thomson CA, Van Aerde JE, Parrott A, Euler A, Lien E, Clandinin MT. Lower proportion of CD45R0+ cells and deficient interleukin-10 production by formula-fed infants, compared with human-fed, is corrected with supplementation of long-chain polyunsaturated fatty acids. J Pediatr Gastroenterol Nutr 2000;31:291-299.

Garofalo R, Chheda S, Mei F, Palkowetz KH, Rudloff HE, Schmalstieg FC, Rassin DK, Goldman AS. Interleukin-10 in human milk. Pediatr Res 1995;37:444-449.

Gruchalla RS, Gan V, Roy L, Bokovoy J, McDermott S, Lawrence G, Hynan L, Luckett P. Results of an inner-city school-based asthma and allergy screening pilot study: a combined approach using written questionnaires and step testing. Ann Allergy Asthma Immunol 2003;90:491-499.

Hamosh M. The milky way: from mammary gland to milk to newborn--Macy-Gyorgy Award presentation (1999). Adv Exp Med Biol 2002;503:17-25.

Hanson LA, Silfverdal SA, Korotkova M, Erling V, Strombeck L, Olcen P, Ulanova M, Hahn-Zoric M, Zaman S, Ashraf R, Telemo E. Immune system modulation by human milk. Adv Exp Med Biol 2002;503:99-106.

Hawkes JS, Bryan DL, James MJ, Gibson RA. Cytokines (IL-1beta, IL-6, TNF-alpha, TGF-beta1, and TGF-beta2) and prostaglandin E2 in human milk during the first three months postpartum. Pediatr Res 1999;46:194-199.

Heinzmann A, Mao XQ, Akaiwa M, Kreomer RT, Gao PS, Ohshima K, Umeshita R, Abe Y, Braun S, Yamashita T, Roberts MH, Sugimoto R, Arima K, Arinobu Y, Yu B, Kruse S, Enomoto T, Dake Y, Kawai M, Shimazu S, Sasaki S, Adra CN, Kitaichi M, Inoue H, Yamauchi K, Tomichi N, Kurimoto F, Hamasaki N, Hopkin JM, Izuhara K, Shirakawa T, Deichmann KA. Genetic variants of IL-13 signalling and human asthma and atopy. Hum Mol Genet 2000;9:549-559.

Hershey GK, Friedrich MF, Esswein LA, Thomas ML, Chatila TA. The association of atopy with a gain-of-function mutation in the alpha subunit of the interleukin-4 receptor. N Engl J Med 1997;337:1720-1725.

Hirose J, Ito S, Hirata N, Kido S, Kitabatake N, Narita H. Occurrence of the major food allergen, ovomucoid, in human breast milk as an immune complex. Biosci Biotechnol Biochem 2001;65:1438-1440.

Hsieh CS, Macatonia SE, Tripp CS, Wolf SF, O'Garra A, Murphy KM. Development of TH1 CD4+ T cells through IL-12 produced by Listeria-induced macrophages. Science 1993;260:547-549.

[ISAAC] The International Study of Asthma and Allergies in Childhood Steering Committee. Worldwide variation in prevalence of symptoms of asthma, allergic rhinoconjunctivitis, and atopic eczema. Lancet 1998;351:1225-1232.

Isolauri E, Tahvanainen A, Peltola T, Arvola T. Breast-feeding of allergic infants. J Pediatr 1999;134:27-32.

Johns DR. The other human genome: mitochondrial DNA and disease. Nat Med 1996;2:1065-1068.

Kalliomaki M, Ouwehand A, Arvilommi H, Kero P, Isolauri E. Transforming growth factor-beta in breast milk: a potential regulator of atopic disease at an early age. J Allergy Clin Immunol 1999;104:1251-1257.

Kalliomaki M, Kirjavainen P, Eerola E, Kero P, Salminen S, Isolauri E. Distinct patterns of neonatal gut microflora in infants in whom atopy was and was not developing. J Allergy Clin Immunol 2001;107:129-134.

Kaufmann SH, Ladel CH, Flesch IE. T cells and cytokines in intracellular bacterial infections: experiences with Mycobacterium bovis BCG. Ciba Found Symp 1995;195:123-132; discussion 132-126.

Kay AB. Allergy and allergic diseases. First of two parts. N Engl J Med 2001;344:30-37.

Kero J, Gissler M, Gronlund MM, Kero P, Koskinen P, Hemminki E, Isolauri E. Mode of delivery and asthma: is there a connection? Pediatr Res 2002;52:6-11.

Kilpelainen M, Terho EO, Helenius H, Koskenvuo M. Farm environment in childhood prevents the development of allergies. Clin Exp Allergy 2000;30:201-208.

Kim JH, Ohsawa M. Oral tolerance to ovalbumin in mice as a model for detecting modulators of the immunologic tolerance to a specific antigen. Biol Pharm Bull 1995;18:854-858.

Kline JN, Waldschmidt TJ, Businga TR, Lemish JE, Weinstock JV, Thorne PS, Krieg AM. Modulation of airway inflammation by CpG oligodeoxynucleotides in a murine model of asthma. J Immunol 1998;160:2555-2559.

Kramer MS, Chalmers B, Hodnett ED, Sevkovskaya Z, Dzikovich I, Shapiro S, Collet JP, Vanilovich I, Mezen I, Ducruet T, Shishko G, Zubovich V, Mknuik D, Gluchanina E, Dombrovskiy V, Ustinovitch A, Kot T, Bogdanovich N, Ovchinikova L, Helsing E. Promotion of Breastfeeding Intervention Trial (PROBIT): a randomized trial in the Republic of Belarus. JAMA 2001;285:413-420.

Kuhn R, Lohler J, Rennick D, Rajewsky K, Muller W. Interleukin-10-deficient mice develop chronic enterocolitis. Cell 1993;75:263-274.

Laiho K, Lampi AM, Hamalainen M, Moilanen E, Piironen V, Arvola T, Syrjanen S, Isolauri E. Breast milk fatty acids, eicosanoids, and cytokines in mothers with and without allergic disease. Pediatr Res 2003;53:642-647.

Landrigan PJ, Sonawane B, Mattison D, McCally M, Garg A. Chemical contaminants in breast milk and their impacts on children's health: an overview. Environ Health Perspect 2002;110:A313-315.

Loibichler C, Pichler J, Gerstmayr M, Bohle B, Kisst H, Urbanek R, Szepfalusi Z. Materno-fetal passage of nutritive and inhalant allergens across placentas of term and pre-term deliveries perfused in vitro. Clin Exp Allergy 2002;32:1546-1551.

Lynch NR, Hagel I, Perez M, Di Prisco MC, Lopez R, Alvarez N. Effect of anthelmintic treatment on the allergic reactivity of children in a tropical slum. J Allergy Clin Immunol 1993;92:404-411.

Mannino DM, Homa DM, Pertowski CA, Ashizawa A, Nixon LL, Johnson CA, Ball LB, Jack E, Kang DS. Surveillance for asthma--United States, 1960-1995. MMWR CDC Surveill Summ 1998;47:1-27.

Marsh DG, Neely JD, Breazeale DR, Ghosh B, Freidhoff LR, Ehrlich-Kautzky E, Schou C, Krishnaswamy G, Beaty TH. Linkage analysis of IL4 and other chromosome 5q31.1 markers and total serum immunoglobulin E concentrations. Science 1994;264:1152-1156.

Martinez FD. Viral infections and the development of asthma. Am J Respir Crit Care Med 1995;151:1644-1647; discussion 1647-1648.

Martinez FD, Stern DA, Wright AL, Holberg CJ, Taussig LM, Halonen M. Association of interleukin-2 and interferon-gamma production by blood mononuclear cells in infancy with parental allergy skin tests and with subsequent development of atopy. J Allergy Clin Immunol 1995a;96:652-660.

Martinez FD, Wright AL, Taussig LM, Holberg CJ, Halonen M, Morgan WJ. Asthma and wheezing in the first six years of life. The Group Health Medical Associates. N Engl J Med 1995b;332:133-138.

Martinez FD. Development of wheezing disorders and asthma in preschool children. Pediatrics 2002;109:362-367.

Matricardi PM, Franzinelli F, Franco A, Caprio G, Murru F, Cioffi D, Ferrigno L, Palermo A, Ciccarelli N, Rosmini F. Sibship size, birth order, and atopy in 11,371 Italian young men. J Allergy Clin Immunol 1998;101:439-444.

[MMWR] Asthma--United States, 1982-1992. MMWR Morb Mortal Wkly Rep 1995;43(51-52):952-955.

Morrow AL, Guerrero ML, Shults J, Calva JJ, Lutter C, Bravo J, Ruiz-Palacios G, Morrow RC, Butterfoss FD. Efficacy of home-based peer counselling to promote exclusive breastfeeding: a randomised controlled trial. Lancet 1999;353:1226-1231.

Mosmann TR, Cherwinski H, Bond MW, Giedlin MA, Coffman RL. Two types of murine helper T cell clone. I. Definition according to profiles of lymphokine activities and secreted proteins. J Immunol 1986;136:2348-2357.

[NHLBI/WHO] Global Strategy for Asthma Management and Prevention NHLBI/WHO Workshop Report, 1995.

Nicolai T, von Mutius E. Pollution and the development of allergy: the East and West Germany story. Arch Toxicol Suppl 1997;19:201-206.

Ober C. Susceptibility genes in asthma and allergy. Curr Allergy Asthma Rep 2001;1:174-179.

Oddy WH, Holt PG, Sly PD, Read AW, Landau LI, Stanley FJ, Kendall GE, Burton PR. Association between breast feeding and asthma in 6 year old children: findings of a prospective birth cohort study. BMJ 1999;319:815-819.

Oddy WH, Sly PD, de Klerk NH, Landau LI, Kendall GE, Holt PG, Stanley FJ. Breast feeding and respiratory morbidity in infancy: a birth cohort study. Arch Dis Child 2003a;88:224-228.

Oddy WH, Halonen M, Martinez FD, Lohman IC, Stern DA, Kurzius-Spencer M, Guerra S, Wright AL. TGF-beta in human milk is associated with wheeze in infancy. J Allergy Clin Immunol 2003b;112:723-728.

Pabst R. The anatomical basis for the immune function of the gut. Anat Embryol (Berl) 1987;176:135-144.

Pessi T, Sutas Y, Hurme M, Isolauri E. Interleukin-10 generation in atopic children following oral Lactobacillus rhamnosus GG. Clin Exp Allergy 2000;30:1804-1808.

Postma DS, Bleecker ER, Amelung PJ, Holroyd KJ, Xu J, Panhuysen CI, Meyers DA, Levitt RC. Genetic susceptibility to asthma--bronchial hyperresponsiveness coinherited with a major gene for atopy. N Engl J Med 1995;333:894-900.

Prescott SL, Macaubas C, Holt BJ, Smallacombe TB, Loh R, Sly PD, Holt PG. Transplacental priming of the human immune system to environmental allergens: universal skewing of initial T cell responses toward the Th2 cytokine profile. J Immunol 1998a;160:4730-4737.

Prescott SL, Macaubas C, Smallacombe T, Holt BJ, Sly PD, Loh R, Holt PG. Reciprocal age-related patterns of allergen-specific T-cell immunity in normal vs. atopic infants. Clin Exp Allergy 1998b;28 Suppl 5:39-44; discussion 50-31.

Prescott SL, Macaubas C, Smallacombe T, Holt BJ, Sly PD, Holt PG. Development of allergen-specific T-cell memory in atopic and normal children. Lancet 1999;353:196-200.

Raqib R, Lindberg AA, Wretlind B, Bardhan PK, Andersson U, Andersson J. Persistence of local cytokine production in shigellosis in acute and convalescent stages. Infect Immun 1995;63:289-296.

Rautava S, Kalliomaki M, Isolauri E. Probiotics during pregnancy and breast-feeding might confer immunomodulatory protection against atopic disease in the infant. J Allergy Clin Immunol 2002;109:119-121.

Reik W, Walter J. Imprinting mechanisms in mammals. Curr Opin Genet Dev 1998;8:154-164.

Remes ST, Castro-Rodriguez JA, Holberg CJ, Martinez FD, Wright AL. Dog exposure in infancy decreases the subsequent risk of frequent wheeze but not of atopy. J Allergy Clin Immunol 2001;108:509-515.

Saarinen KM, Vaarala O, Klemetti P, Savilahti E. Transforming growth factor-beta1 in mothers' colostrum and immune responses to cows' milk proteins in infants with cows' milk allergy. J Allergy Clin Immunol 1999;104:1093-1098.

Sandford A, Weir T, Pare P. The genetics of asthma. Am J Respir Crit Care Med 1996;153:1749-1765.

Sears MR, Greene JM, Willan AR, Taylor DR, Flannery EM, Cowan JO, Herbison GP, Poulton R. Long-term relation between breastfeeding and development of atopy and asthma in children and young adults: a longitudinal study. Lancet 2002;360:901-907.

Shevach EM, McHugh RS, Piccirillo CA, Thornton AM. Control of T-cell activation by CD4+ CD25+ suppressor T cells. Immunol Rev 2001;182:58-67.

Shirakawa T, Enomoto T, Shimazu S, Hopkin JM. The inverse association between tuberculin responses and atopic disorder. Science 1997;275:77-79.

Srivastava MD, Srivastava A, Brouhard B, Saneto R, Groh-Wargo S, Kubit J. Cytokines in human milk. Res Commun Mol Pathol Pharmacol 1996;93:263-287.

Stein RT, Holberg CJ, Morgan WJ, Wright AL, Lombardi E, Taussig L, Martinez FD. Peak flow variability, methacholine responsiveness and atopy as markers for detecting different wheezing phenotypes in childhood. Thorax 1997;52:946-952.

Stene LC, Nafstad P. Relation between occurrence of type 1 diabetes and asthma. Lancet 2001;357:607-608.

Stephens S, Duffy SW, Page C. A longitudinal study of gamma-interferon production by peripheral blood mononuclear cells from breast- and bottle-fed infants. Clin Exp Immunol 1986;65:396-400.

Strachan DP. Hay fever, hygiene, and household size. BMJ 1989;299:1259-1260.

Street NE, Mosmann TR. Functional diversity of T lymphocytes due to secretion of different cytokine patterns. FASEB J 1991;5:171-177.

Sudo N, Sawamura S, Tanaka K, Aiba Y, Kubo C, Koga Y. The requirement of intestinal bacterial flora for the development of an IgE production system fully susceptible to oral tolerance induction. J Immunol 1997;159:1739-1745.

Takahashi T, Yoshida Y, Hatano S, Sugita-Konishi Y, Igimi S, Yajima M, Kojima T, Kanno T, Yonekubo A, Yajima T, Kuwata T. Reactivity of secretory IgA antibodies in breast milk from 107 Japanese mothers to 20 environmental antigens. Biol Neonate 2002;82:238-242.

Taussig LM, Wright AL, Holberg CJ, Halonen M, Morgan WJ, Martinez FD. Tucson Children's Respiratory Study: 1980 to present. J Allergy Clin Immunol 2003;111:661-675; quiz 676.

Usha Kiran TS, Jayawickrama NS. Who is responsible for the rising caesarean section rate? J Obstet Gynaecol 2002;22:363-365.

Vadas P, Wai Y, Burks W, Perelman B. Detection of peanut allergens in breast milk of lactating women. JAMA 2001;285:1746-1748.

van den Biggelaar AH, van Ree R, Rodrigues LC, Lell B, Deelder AM, Kremsner PG, Yazdanbakhsh M. Decreased atopy in children infected with Schistosoma haematobium: a role for parasite-induced interleukin-10. Lancet 2000;356:1723-1727.

van Odijk J, Kull I, Borres MP, Brandtzaeg P, Edberg U, Hanson LA, Host A, Kuitunen M, Olsen SF, Skerfving S, Sundell J, Wille S. Breastfeeding and allergic disease: a multidisciplinary review of the literature (1966-2001) on the mode of early feeding in infancy and its impact on later atopic manifestations. Allergy 2003;58:833-843.

Wahn U, Lau S, Bergmann R, Kulig M, Forster J, Bergmann K, Bauer CP, Guggenmoos-Holzmann I. Indoor allergen exposure is a risk factor for sensitization during the first three years of life. J Allergy Clin Immunol 1997;99:763-769.

Wang CC, Nolan TJ, Schad GA, Abraham D. Infection of mice with the helminth Strongyloides stercoralis suppresses pulmonary allergic responses to ovalbumin. Clin Exp Allergy 2001;31:495-503.

Warner JA, Miles EA, Jones AC, Quint DJ, Colwell BM, Warner JO. Is deficiency of interferon gamma production by allergen triggered cord blood cells a predictor of atopic eczema? Clin Exp Allergy 1994;24:423-430.

Weiland SK, von Mutius E, Hirsch T, Duhme H, Fritzsch C, Werner B, Husing A, Stender M, Renz H, Leupold W, Keil U. Prevalence of respiratory and atopic disorders among children in the East and West of Germany five years after unification. Eur Respir J 1999;14:862-870.

Wickens K, Pearce N, Crane J, Beasley R. Antibiotic use in early childhood and the development of asthma. Clin Exp Allergy 1999;29:766-771.

Wilkinson JR, Lane SJ, Lee TH. Effects of corticosteroids on cytokine generation and expression of activation antigens by monocytes in bronchial asthma. Int Arch Allergy Appl Immunol 1991;94:220-221.

Wills-Karp M. Immunologic basis of antigen-induced airway hyperresponsiveness. Annu Rev Immunol 1999;17:255-281.

Wills-Karp M, Santeliz J, Karp CL. The germless theory of allergic disease: revisiting the hygiene hypothesis. Nat Rev Immunol 2001;1:69-75.

Wilson AF, Novey HS, Berke RA, Surprenant EL. Deposition of inhaled pollen and pollen extract in human airways. N Engl J Med 1973;288:1056-1058.

Wold AE. The hygiene hypothesis revised: is the rising frequency of allergy due to changes in the intestinal flora? Allergy 1998;53:20-25.

Wright AL, Holberg CJ, Martinez FD, Morgan WJ, Taussig LM. Breast feeding and lower respiratory tract illness in the first year of life. Group Health Medical Associates. BMJ 1989;299:946-949.

Wright AL, Holberg CJ, Taussig LM, Martinez FD. Factors influencing the relation of infant feeding to asthma and recurrent wheeze in childhood. Thorax 2001a;56:192-197.

Wright AL, Stern DA, Halonen M. The association of allergic sensitization in mother and child in breast-fed and formula-fed infants. Adv Exp Med Biol 2001b;501:249-255.

Xanthou M. Immune protection of human milk. Biol Neonate 1998;74:121-133.

Yoshioka H, Iseki K, Fujita K. Development and differences of intestinal flora in the neonatal period in breast-fed and bottle-fed infants. Pediatrics 1983;72:317-321.

SECTION V

RISK OF VIRAL TRANSMISSION BY BREASTFEEDING

HUMAN IMMUNODEFICIENCY VIRUS TRANSMISSION DURING BREASTFEEDING

Knowledge, Gaps, and Challenges for the Future

Ellen G. Piwoz[1], Jay Ross[2], and Jean Humphrey[3]

1. ABSTRACT

A number of risk factors for HIV transmission during breastfeeding have been identified. The experience counseling HIV-infected women on infant feeding options has expanded to consider these risk factors. Programmatic evidence is limited, but the review presented here strongly argues for an end to the polarized debate about whether HIV-infected women should breast or formula feed. In reality, neither alternative is risk-free for HIV-exposed infants, and the balance of risks varies in different settings and over time.

2. INTRODUCTION

Each year, approximately 600,000 infants and young children worldwide become infected with HIV, the virus causing AIDS, through vertical transmission, also known as mother-to-child or parent-to-child transmission of HIV (UNAIDS 2002). HIV transmission from mother to infant occurs during pregnancy, at the time of childbirth, and postnatally through breastfeeding. Breastfeeding is the cause of approximately 240,000 new HIV infections worldwide each year, or about 40 percent of total mother-to-child transmission (MTCT).

In the absence of interventions to prevent MTCT, 5 to 10 percent of HIV-infected pregnant women who give birth to live infants are estimated to transmit HIV during pregnancy; another 10 to 20 percent will pass the virus during labor and delivery; and another 10 to 20 percent will pass the virus during breastfeeding to at least 18 months of age (De Cock et al. 2000). HIV transmission during breastfeeding also occurs in

[1]SARA Project, Academy for Educational Development, 1825 Connecticut Avenue, NW, Washington, DC 20009
[2]LINKAGES Project, Academy for Educational Development, Washington, DC
[3]The Johns Hopkins Bloomberg School of Public Health, Baltimore, MD, USA, and the ZVITAMBO Project, Harare, Zimbabwe

approximately 30 percent of infants born to mothers who become infected while breastfeeding (Dunn et al. 1992). The majority of infants born to HIV-positive mothers, 50 to 75 percent, will remain uninfected even if breastfed.

The subject of HIV and breastfeeding has been a lightening rod for controversy, often unproductively pitting those whose primary mandate is slowing the devastating spread of HIV against breastfeeding and child survival advocates who have worked tirelessly to promote the well-being, growth, and development of all children living in resource-poor settings. In this chapter we will review current knowledge about HIV transmission during breastfeeding and discuss experience in programs that have counseled HIV-infected women on different feeding options. We also will make the case for reframing the public health dialogue about HIV and infant feeding in order to avoid unnecessary polarization of this issue in the future.

3. HIV TRANSMISSION DURING BREASTFEEDING: AN OVERVIEW

3.1. Mechanisms of Transmission

The exact mechanisms by which infants become infected through breastfeeding are not yet known. Cell-free and cell-associated HIV in maternal blood pass into human milk. Evidence suggests that HIV also may enter human milk directly from infected macrophages, lymphocytes, and epithelial cells in the mammary gland (Becquart et al. 2002). The breastfeeding infant consumes HIV, which then causes infection following entrance through permeable mucosal surfaces, lymphoid tissues, and/or lesions in the gastrointestinal tract.

A study in Kenya estimated that the breastfeeding infant may consume more than 60,000 HIV-infected cells and more than half a million cell-free virions every day (Lewis et al. 1998). With this level of exposure, it is remarkable that the majority of infants do not become HIV-infected. Immune factors in human milk, such as virus-specific CD8 T-lymphocytes (Sabbaj et al. 2002), HIV-specific immunoglobulins (Van de Perre et al. 1993, 1999), human milk erythropoeitin (Miller et al. 2002), and immune factors in infant saliva (Farquhar et al. 2002) are believed to play a role in preventing infection.

3.2. Risk Factors for Postnatal HIV Transmission

Several review papers have been published since 2000 that identify the risk factors for MTCT, including HIV transmission during breastfeeding (Fowler & Newell 2002; Bulterys et al. 2002; Coovadia & Coutsoudis 2001; Newell 2001). Risk factors for HIV transmission during breastfeeding can be divided into maternal, infant, and viral characteristics. In this chapter we will discuss maternal and infant characteristics only. Our discussion centers around transmission of HIV-1, the strain most often associated with vertical transmission.

Maternal risk factors for HIV transmission during breastfeeding include viral load in blood (John et al. 2001a; Fawzi et al. 2002) and human milk (Rousseau et al. 2003; Pillay et al. 2000); immune status (Leroy et al. 2002; Fawzi et al. 2002); breast health (Semba et al. 1999; Embree et al. 2000; Ekpini et al. 1997); and nutritional status, including hemoglobin and serum retinol levels (Fawzi et al. 2002; Semba et al. 1994). Infant risk factors include breastfeeding duration (Miotti et al. 1999; Embree et al. 2000); type of breastfeeding (Coutsoudis et al. 1999, 2001a); infant age (John et al. 2001b); and oral lesions (Embree et al. 2000; Ekpini et al. 1997). These risk factors should be addressed in MTCT counseling and prevention programs.

3.3. Maternal Viral Load, Immune Status, and Breast Health

The amount of virus in the mother's blood is an important risk factor for HIV transmission at all stages, including during breastfeeding (Leroy et al. 2001; John et al. 2001a; Fawzi et al. 2002). Viral load is high immediately following HIV infection before the immune system can mount a response, and later in HIV disease when the immune system is compromised and unable to control HIV replication.

The health of an HIV-affected immune system usually is measured by the number of CD4 T+ lymphocytes, one of the cells that HIV attacks and destroys. Antiretroviral therapy is initiated in the presence of clinical AIDS or in adults when CD4 lymphocyte counts drop below 200 cells/μL (WHO 2002). CD4 lymphocye counts indirectly may reflect the length of time a person has been infected, as well as the general health status of the individual.

Maternal CD4 lymphocyte counts are consistently strong predictors of HIV transmission at all stages, including during breastfeeding. Data from West Africa and Tanzania illustrate this relationship. In a placebo-controlled study to examine the efficacy of short-course zidovudine (ZDV) prophylaxis in West Africa, investigators reported that postnatal transmission (measured from 6 weeks through 24 months of age in breastfeeding infants) was 10 to 14 percent in mothers with baseline CD4 lymphocyte counts below 500 (measured in pregnancy). However, transmission was less than 3 percent during this same time period among women with baseline CD4 lymphocyte counts ≥500 (Leroy et al. 2002). Likewise, in Tanzania, investigators studying the efficacy of vitamin A and multivitamin supplementation on MTCT reported that postnatal transmission risks were 2.13 and 2.99 times greater in women with CD4 lymphocyte counts below 200 and between 200 and 499 cells/μL, respectively, when compared with women who had CD4 lymphocyte counts ≥500 in pregnancy (Fawzi et al. 2002). Thus, keeping HIV-infected mothers healthy may be one of the most important interventions for preventing infant HIV infection. As test costs decrease in the future, testing CD4 lymphocyte counts in HIV-infected women may be useful for counseling about infant feeding as well as for initiation of antiretroviral treatment.

Maternal breast health is another important risk factor for postnatal HIV transmission that also has relevance for our MTCT counseling and prevention programs. Breast problems such as cracked nipples, subclinical and clinical mastitis, and breast abscesses, which generally are more common in early lactation, are associated with increased human milk viral load (Willumsen et al. 2003; Semba et al. 1999), and a 2- to 4-fold increase in the risk of HIV transmission (Semba et al. 1999; Embree et al. 2000; John et al. 2001a; Fawzi et al. 2002). Although methods for recording these conditions varied across studies, reported prevalence rates for subclinical and clinical mastitis, and cracked and bleeding nipples in HIV-positive African mothers range from 7 to 21 percent (Table 1). These rates are similar to rates observed in non-HIV-affected populations (Semba et al. 1999; Filteau et al. 1999).

Breast health is of interest to counseling and prevention programs because the conditions associated with increased transmission risk can be prevented with lactation counseling, and easily treated when they occur. To date, no studies have been conducted to evaluate the impact of lactation counseling with appropriate management and

Table 1. Prevalence of subclinical and clinical mastitis, nipple lesions, and breast abscesses in HIV-infected mothers in African studies

Country (reference)	Mastitis	Nipple lesions	Breast abscesses
Kenya (Embree et al. 2000)	7% (clinical exam)	13% (clinical exam)	—
Kenya (John et al. 2001a)	11% (clinical exam)	13% (clinical exam)	12% (clinical exam)
South Africa (Willumsen et al. 2000)	21, 11, and 12% at 1, 6, and 14 weeks, respectively (Na+/K >1.0)	—	—
Malawi (Semba et al. 2001)	16% at 6 weeks (Na+ >12 mmol/L)	—	—
Côte d'lvoire (Ekpini et al. 1997)	—	10% (interview)	3% (interview)
Zimbabwe (Kambarami et al. 1997)	—	11% (clinical exam of mothers of hospitalized infants)	—

treatment of breast problems on postnatal HIV transmission. Additional research on this issue is needed.

However, to better understand the possible contribution of these conditions to total MTCT, we applied the following formula (Kleinbaum et al. 1982) for calculating population attributable risk (PAR) to the observed prevalence rates and adjusted risk estimates associated with subclinical (Semba et al. 1999) and clinical mastitis (John et al. 2001a) in studies in Malawi and Kenya, respectively.

Formula: $PAR = prevalence\ (RR\text{-}1)\ /\ 1{+}prevalence\ (RR\text{-}1)$

Malawi: $18\ percent = (0.164)\ (2.3\text{-}1)\ /\ 1{+}\ (0.164)\ (2.3\text{-}1)$

Kenya: $21\ percent = (0.11)\ (3.4\text{-}1)\ /\ 1 + (0.11)\ (3.4\text{-}1)$

Based on these calculations, although relatively uncommon, subclinical and clinical mastitis were responsible for 18 to 21 percent of total mother-to-child HIV transmission in these populations. Since breast conditions only affect postnatal transmission, which accounts for about 40 percent of total MTCT, we estimate that preventable and treatable breast conditions may be responsible for about half of breastfeeding transmission (e.g., 21/40 percent).

A study conducted in Bangladesh demonstrated that lactation management and support postdelivery significantly reduced the incidence of breast inflammation indicative of subclinical and clinical mastitis in HIV-negative mothers (Flores & Filteau 2002). These findings suggest that early breastfeeding counseling and support and prompt management and treatment of breast conditions should be an important component of infant feeding counseling for HIV-infected mothers who choose to breastfeed.

3.4. Breastfeeding Duration and Pattern

The risk of HIV transmission persists for as long as breastfeeding is practiced. Some studies indicate that the risk of HIV transmission may be higher in the first months of life (Nduati et al. 2000; John et al. 2001b). There are several possible explanations, including: the higher prevalence of mastitis and other breast conditions in the early months; the infant gut is more immature and thus also more vulnerable and permeable to HIV; and there is greater exposure to HIV because more milk is consumed in the early months of infancy.

A meta-analysis is underway to assess the timing of HIV transmission during breastfeeding (Read et al. 2002). This analysis, known as the Breastfeeding and HIV International Transmission Study (BHITS), uses data from 4,343 children born to HIV-infected mothers in studies throughout Africa (Kenya, Tanzania, South Africa, Uganda, Cote d'Ivoire, Burkina Faso). Nine hundred ninety-nine children were HIV-infected, but the timing of transmission during the postnatal period could be ascertained for only 55 percent. The BHITS meta-analysis defines HIV transmission as early (a positive test result before 4 weeks of age) and late (a negative test result at or after 4 weeks of age followed by a positive test result at some point during follow-up). Late transmission is attributed to breastfeeding; however, early infection (by 4 weeks of age) may have occurred during pregnancy, delivery, or early breastfeeding and the timing cannot be determined with tests that currently are available.

Findings from BHITS analysis suggest that the risk of HIV infection due to breastfeeding after 4 weeks of age is relatively constant over time. Preliminary reports of cumulative infection rates were 4 percent from 4 weeks to 6 months of age; 9 percent from 4 weeks to 12 months of age; and 16 percent up to 18 months of age. Breastfeeding (after 4 weeks) was responsible for about 42 percent of MTCT (Read et al. 2002).

One question that remains to be answered is "how much HIV transmission occurs during the first month of infant life?" This is difficult to answer because a positive HIV test result, using PCR technology, in the first 4 weeks may reflect seroconversion following late pregnancy, labor and delivery, or early postnatal HIV transmission. We attempted to estimate indirectly early breastfeeding transmission from available studies where cumulative HIV infection rates were reported for nonbreastfed and breastfed infants over time in the same population (Fig. 1).

Using this methodology, the difference in HIV seroconversion rates from birth to 4 weeks of age (absolute or pro-rated when measurements were taken at 6 to 8 weeks of age) between breastfed and nonbreastfed infants ranges from 1.8 percent to 4.5 percent, with a median value of 2.3 percent in the first month of life (Nduati et al. 2000; Coutsoudis et al. 2001a; Moodley et al. 2003; Petra Study Team 2002). This value is considerably greater than the 0.8 percent per month from the BHITS analysis for breastfeeding transmission after 1 month (Read et al. 2002), suggesting that total HIV transmission through breastfeeding is greater than previously estimated, and that breastfeeding during the first month of life may be a period of increased risk. Studies are

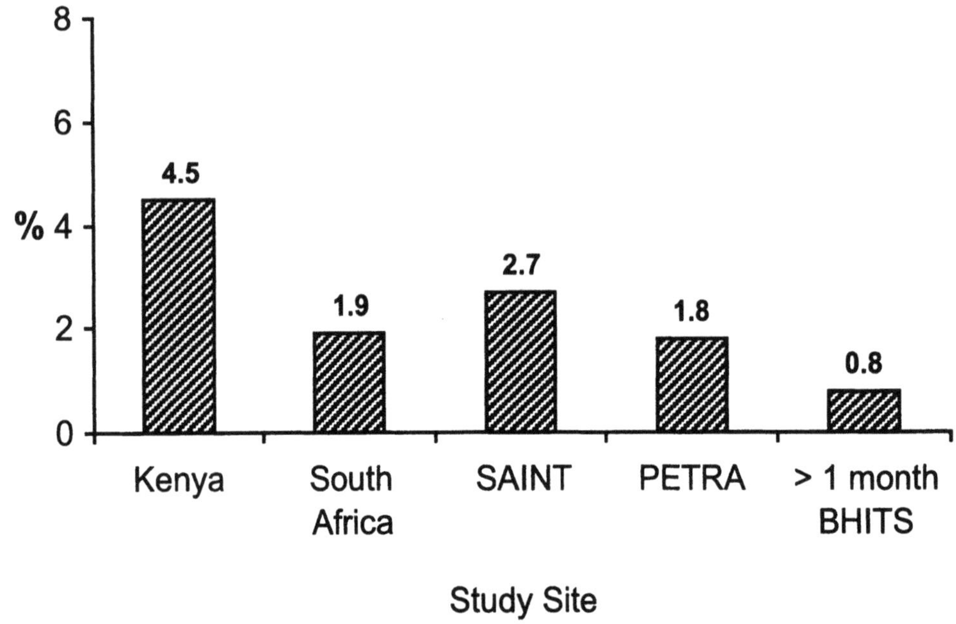

Figure 1. Estimated risk of postnatal HIV transmission during the first month (4 weeks) of life in Nairobi, Kenya (Nduati et al. 2000); Durban, South Africa (Coutsoudis et al. 2001a); the SAINT Trial, South Africa (Moodley et al. 2003); and the PETRA Study: Uganda, Tanzania, and South Africa (Petra Study Team 2002), compared with estimated monthly transmission risk after 4 weeks (Read et al. 2002).

now underway in Zimbabwe, South Africa, Ethiopia, and Malawi to assess the impact of extended infant antiretroviral prophylaxis to reduce the risk of breastfeeding HIV transmission in the first 4 to 6 weeks of infancy.

Although the risk of infant HIV infection through breastfeeding may be highest during the first month of life, the cumulative risk of HIV infection with continued breastfeeding beyond 6 months of age also is considerable. Figure 2 shows the estimated proportion of HIV infections occurring after 6 months of age in several studies in Africa. The proportions exclude the first 4 to 6 weeks of life because it is not possible to ascertain whether these infections are due to breastfeeding or other causes. These data suggest that continued breastfeeding (beyond 6 months of age) is responsible for one-half to three-quarters of all breastfeeding transmission (52–76 percent). If a 3 to 4 percent risk of breastfeeding transmission in the first 4 to 6 weeks is assumed, then the contribution of continued breastfeeding (beyond 6 months) is about 50 percent in all studies except Nduati et al. (2000). These findings suggest that early breastfeeding cessation (e.g., about 6 months) would prevent a significant proportion of breastfeeding-related HIV transmission and would promote HIV-free survival if cessation can be done safely with nutritionally adequate and appropriate replacement feeding. The challenges associated with early breastfeeding cessation and safe replacement feeding are discussed later in this chapter.

The type of breastfeeding practiced also may be an important determinant of postnatal HIV transmission. A study conducted in Durban, South Africa compared rates of HIV infection in infants who were never breastfed, breastfed exclusively for at least three months (no other liquids, solids, or milk given), and partially breastfed in the first

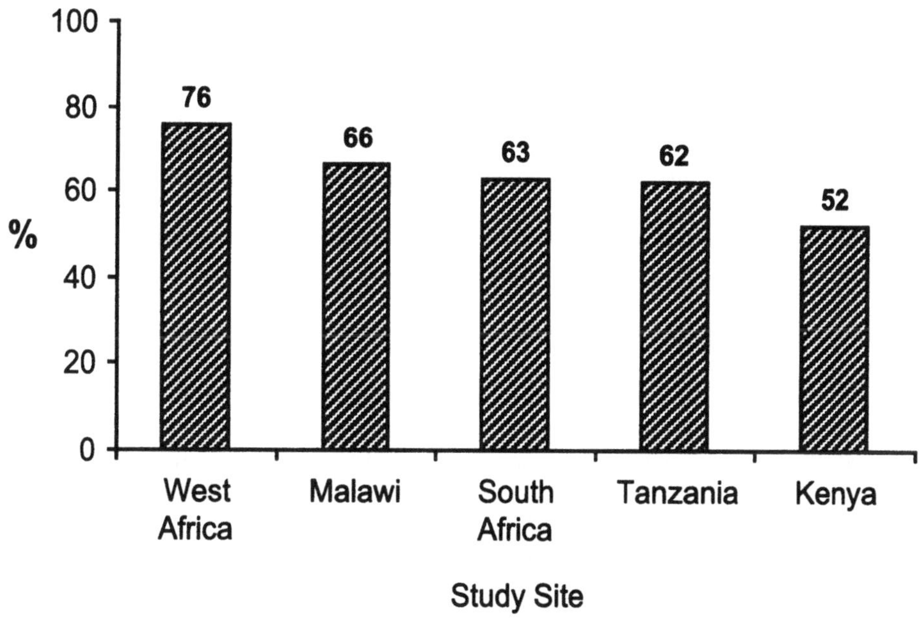

Figure 2. Estimated proportion of late postnatal transmission occurring after 6 months of age in West Africa (Leroy et al. 2002); Malawi (Miotti et al. 1999); South Africa (Coutsoudis et al. 2001); Tanzania (Fawzi et al. 2002); and Kenya (Nduati et al. 2000).

three months (other liquids, milks, or solids given before 3 months of age). Infection rates at birth were similar in the three groups; however, the partially breastfed infants had significantly higher rates of HIV infection at 3, 6, and 15 months of age (Coutsoudis et al. 1999, 2001a). This finding is extremely important because, until these results were reported, most policy and research organizations were promoting the avoidance of all breastfeeding as the best means for preventing postnatal HIV infection, rather than emphasizing ways to make breastfeeding safer for HIV-infected mothers and their infants. After the results were released, many organizations and scientists began promoting exclusive breastfeeding followed by abrupt cessation to prevent HIV transmission associated with mixed feeding.

Although the Durban study was first released in 1999, there are no additional data confirming these results. This is because such studies are complex and require extended follow-up. Early studies of HIV and breastfeeding did not collect detailed information on patterns of breastfeeding that would allow posthoc comparisons (Preble & Piwoz 1998). WHO has developed a tool to measure breastfeeding practices in MTCT research studies that will facilitate cross-study comparisons (Gaillard et al. 2002). Studies are being carried out in Zimbabwe, Zambia, Botswana, and South Africa that will compare HIV transmission among infants who are exclusively versus partially breastfed. The Zimbabwe study, known as ZVITAMBO, enrolled 4,500 HIV-positive mothers at delivery and followed them for at least 12 months. Detailed infant feeding data were collected prospectively to allow for comparisons between breastfeeding groups. The study was completed in 2001 and findings on HIV transmission, mortality, and HIV-free survival by infant feeding classification will be available in 2003.

3.5. Effects of Breastfeeding on Maternal Survival

The effects of pregnancy and breastfeeding on disease progression and survival of HIV-infected women, particularly women with compromised nutritional status, frequently has been discussed (French & Brocklehurst 1998). A meta-analysis to examine the effects of breastfeeding on the survival of HIV-infected women is now underway. A randomized trial of breastfeeding versus formula-feeding carried out in Nairobi reported that mothers who breastfed were three times more likely to die in the 24-month follow-up period (18 percent) compared with mothers who formula-fed (6 percent) (Nduati et al. 2001). This study raised considerable controversy, leading many to suggest that while exclusive breastfeeding may save infants' lives, it is not safe for HIV-infected mothers.

Careful review of the Nairobi report yields several important observations. Nearly half of the women in the study who died had advanced immune deficiency (CD4 <200 lymphocytes/μL) at enrollment, and 91 percent had baseline CD4 lymphocyte counts below 500. The relative risk of maternal death was 14.7 for women with CD4 lymphocyte counts <200, irrespective of infant feeding pattern, when compared with women who had no immune deficiency (CD4 >500 lymphocytes/μL). The findings were similar for maternal viral load (RR=8.0 if viral load was greater than 43,000 copies/mL) and postpartum weight loss (RR 3.4 per kg lost). Breastfeeding did convey an increased risk of maternal death (RR=2.9), which cannot be ignored, but most deaths in the study were among women who initially were immune compromised. Another report from the Durban, South Africa study found no difference in maternal morbidity or mortality in breastfeeding versus formula-feeding mothers, although total mortality in study women was <2 percent during 15 months of follow-up (Coutsoudis et al. 2001b). Based on the available information, we suggest that, where possible, breastfeeding should be avoided by HIV-infected women who have advanced immune deficiency because of increased risks of HIV transmission and possible adverse consequences to maternal health. However, findings from the meta-analysis will provide additional information related to this recommendation.

4. FEASIBILITY OF DIFFERENT INFANT FEEDING OPTIONS FOR HIV-INFECTED MOTHERS

The current WHO recommendations on infant feeding by HIV-infected mothers states the following (2001):

> When replacement feeding is acceptable, feasible, affordable, sustainable and safe, avoidance of all breastfeeding by HIV-infected mothers is recommended. Otherwise, exclusive breastfeeding is recommended during the first months of life. To minimize HIV transmission risk, breastfeeding should be discontinued as soon as feasible, taking into account local circumstances, the individual woman's situation and the risks of replacement feeding (including infections other than HIV and malnutrition).

Although this guidance sounds straightforward and sensible, making the decision to breastfeed or practice replacement feeding involves complex concepts that are difficult to assess and highly variable over time. Neither of the choices is risk-free. The guidance places the decision-making burden in the hands of the families to decide what practice is *acceptable*, given the social value of breastfeeding and concerns about revealing one's HIV status if replacement feeding is selected. *Feasibility* is also a personal issue that has economic as well as behavioral aspects, requiring skills and resources. *Sustainability* also may be difficult to determine and to achieve. If replacement feeding is chosen, it must be practiced (sustained) every day and every night, exclusively and without breastfeeding, for at least 6 months, when the challenge of providing nourishing complementary feeds must then be confronted.

Finally, there is the question of *safety*: infant feeding should be free from contamination, nutritious, as well as socially safe. The increased risks of infant mortality from replacement feeding in settings where infectious diseases are common and hygiene and sanitation are poor have been well documented (WHO Collaborative Study 2000; Humphrey & Iliff 2001). In addition to the health risks, several studies in Africa reveal social risks with replacement feeding. In these studies women who do not breastfeed were reported to arouse suspicion and were stigmatized by family and neighbors as being promiscuous or HIV-positive. This stigma, in turn, is passed on to the child who also is assumed to be HIV infected (Chopra et al. 2002; Piwoz et al. 1999; Gavin et al. 1999).

WHO-recommended feeding options for HIV-infected mothers include exclusive breastfeeding; feeding with heat-treated human milk or milk from a milk bank; wet-nursing by an HIV-negative woman; and early breastfeeding cessation or exclusive replacement feeding with commercial or home-prepared infant formula (UNAIDS/UNICEF/WHO 1998). Most experience to date has come from programs that support exclusive breastfeeding or the use of commercial infant formula. Data on the feasibility, sustainability, and safety of other feeding options are limited. Next we will review evidence concerning the feasibility, acceptability, sustainability, and safety of these feeding options using published and unpublished data.

4.1. Feasibility of Exclusive Breastfeeding

Experience from the Baby Friendly Hospital Initiative (BFHI), the Integrated Management of Childhood Illness (IMCI) program, and various research studies suggest that rates of exclusive breastfeeding in the general population can be increased through a comprehensive approach to promote, support, and protect breastfeeding, beginning with antenatal counseling, conducive hospital practices that facilitate immediate and unrestricted breastfeeding after delivery, and community or peer support in the postnatal period (WHO 1998a; Morrow et al. 1999; Haider et al. 2000; Kramer et al. 2001). However, rates of exclusive breastfeeding seldom exceed 70 percent, and timing and measurement methods vary between studies, which can influence prevalence estimates (Piwoz et al. 1995).

Experience in programs to promote exclusive breastfeeding among HIV-positive mothers have produced mixed and largely disappointing results, possibly because the interventions have not included all known elements for achieving successful breast-feeding described above. Preliminary estimates of exclusive breastfeeding in MTCT prevention programs reported at the Barcelona AIDS Conference ranged from 31 percent in Botswana (Mompati et al. 2002) to 87 percent in Zambia (Kuhn et al. 2002). Reports from Botswana (Shapiro et al. 2002), Uganda (Magoni et al. 2002), and Cote d'Ivoire (Malkin et al. 2002) suggest that adherence to exclusive breastfeeding is lower than adherence to exclusive replacement feeding.

4.2. Feasibility of Early and Rapid Breastfeeding Cessation

Many programs are promoting exclusive breastfeeding followed by rapid or abrupt breastfeeding cessation to minimize the additional risks of HIV transmission associated with early, partial breastfeeding. The possible risks of early and rapid breastfeeding cessation for infant, mother, and family have been summarized by Piwoz et al. (2002). Preliminary reports from Zambia (Thea et al. 2002), Uganda (Kisakye et al. 2002), and Botswana (Mompati et al. 2002) suggest that early and rapid cessation is possible to achieve with counseling support. The most common problems encountered with this practice were breast engorgement, mastitis, crying of infants, appetite loss, diarrhea, family objections, and importantly, financial constraints associated with replacement feeding. Problems were more common among infants less than 6 months of age (Mompati et al. 2002).

It is important to point out that the impact of early, rapid breastfeeding cessation on HIV transmission and HIV-free survival is not yet known, and studies are underway to determine this. Dietary intake data show that human milk provides more than half of the energy (55–67 percent); protein (44–59 percent); vitamin A (84–89 percent); calcium (65–79 percent); zinc (35–50 percent); riboflavin (59–71 percent); and folic acid (62–83 percent) consumed by infants from 6 to 11 months of age in developing countries (WHO 1998b). The contribution of human milk after one year is lower but still significant.

The recommendation for HIV-positive mothers to stop breastfeeding early to avoid HIV infection must take into account the increased risk of malnutrition after 6 months that occurs worldwide in resource-poor settings. Malnutrition is an underlying cause of 60 percent of all child deaths from 6 to 59 months of life, and in the year 2000, underweight was the cause of 1 out of 15 deaths globally (Ezzati et al. 2002). Most of the deaths due to underweight occurred in children less than 5 years of age, and suboptimal breastfeeding and complementary feeding practices are a major cause of underweight in children. Clearly, if HIV-positive mothers stop breastfeeding early, appropriate human milk substitutes must be made available and provided to prevent malnutrition and non-HIV-related mortality.

4.3. Feasibility of Other Breastfeeding Options

Data are limited on the feasibility of other breastfeeding options, including wet-nursing, heat-treated human milk, and milk banks for daily infant feeding by HIV-infected women. Some reports suggest that wet-nursing has become less common in rural and urban communities in Southern Africa because of HIV (Piwoz et al. 1999; Chopra et al. 2000). A study in South Africa found that indirect heating of human milk to 56 to 62.5°C for 12 to 15 minutes through a method known as Pretoria Pasteurization inactivates HIV, preventing viral replication (Jeffery et al. 2001). Although a promising approach for making breastfeeding safer, expressing and heat-treating milk involves two new practices that have to be sustained on a daily basis, possibly arousing suspicion among neighbors and family. Furthermore, milk must be handled and stored properly to avoid bacterial contamination. Because of the time, resources, and support required, this feeding option may be most useful for mothers with sick and low-birth-weight infants being fed in hospitals, for mothers with mastitis, and during the transition from exclusive breastfeeding to complete replacement (UNAIDS/UNICEF/WHO 2003, in preparation).

4.4. Feasibility of Commercial Infant Formula

Data presented at the Barcelona AIDS conference indicate high acceptance of free or subsidized commercial infant formula in PMTCT programs in countries such as Thailand (100 percent), Brazil (100 percent), and Botswana (89 percent), where infant mortality is relatively low, health care and safe water are available, and formula use is neither exceptional nor stigmatizing. In South Africa, a recent evaluation revealed large differences in the acceptance of commercial infant formula across provinces and between rural and urban areas, suggesting that replacement feeding can be done safely in many urban areas, but may still be unacceptable in poor rural areas within the same country (McCoy et al. 2002).

Data are limited on the growth, morbidity, and mortality of children born to HIV-infected mothers who breastfeed versus replacement feed. A study in India reported that nonbreastfed infants had significantly higher rates of hospitalization than breastfed infants born to HIV-infected mothers receiving ZDV prophylaxis (Phadke et al. 2002). A randomized trial in Kenya reported no significant differences in diarrhea and pneumonia, but slightly better nutritional status in breastfed versus formula-fed infants at 24 months of age (Mbori-Ngacha et al. 2001). Mortality at 24 months was similar in breastfed (24 percent) and formula-fed (20 percent) infants, although HIV-free survival was significantly greater in children who were formula-fed (Nduati et al. 2000). However, findings from clinical trials with strict screening and enrollment criteria, and frequent, free follow-up cannot be generalized automatically to larger populations that do not have access to the same services. It is likely that the risks of preventable deaths and disability are under-estimated in such trials because many of the barriers to quality health care common in these settings are removed.

4.5. Feasibility of Home-Prepared Infant Formula

For mothers who choose not to breastfeed and cannot provide commercial infant formula, WHO recommends home-prepared infant formula made from boiled animal milk (cow, goat, sheep, buffalo) mixed with water and sugar (UNAIDS/UNICEF/WHO 1998). Home-prepared milk formulas are low in several essential nutrients and infants fed from birth with modified animal milk also require micronutrient supplements.

There are limited data on the feasibility, acceptability, and health outcomes of HIV-exposed children fed on home-prepared infant formula. A study conducted in rural South Africa found that home-prepared formula made from fresh and powdered full-cream milk required 20 to 30 minutes to prepare at a cost of U.S. $10 per month or roughly 20 percent of the average family monthly income. Even when locally available micronutrient supplements were provided, the diets of infants fed in this way were dangerously low in vitamins A, C, and E; folic acid; pantothenic acid; zinc; copper; selenium; and essential fatty acids (Papathakis & Rollins 2002). Thus, safe feeding with home-prepared infant formula is complex (requiring adequate hygiene and proper dilution and mixing), and special micronutrient formulations will be required for use in areas where this feeding option is practiced.

5. CONCLUSIONS AND RECOMMENDATIONS

We propose that the issue of HIV and infant feeding shift its focus away from debate about which option is best, and instead place emphasis on feeding strategies that will promote HIV-free survival in different contexts. Furthermore, programs to prevent MTCT should focus more on maternal health and nutrition. Keeping HIV-infected mothers healthy may be one of the most important things that can be done to prevent postnatal HIV transmission. As noted earlier, the risk of breastfeeding transmission was two to three times greater in women with CD4 lymphocyte counts <500 (Fawzi et al. 2002; Leroy et al. 2002). Postpartum weight loss was associated with an increased risk of maternal death in breastfeeding and nonbreastfeeding mothers in a setting where maternal death also was associated with a higher risk of child death, irrespective of child HIV status (Nduati et al. 2001). How to improve the health and nutrition of HIV-infected mothers through ARV treatment, improved maternal care, and through other health and nutrition interventions is being studied.

For mothers who choose to breastfeed, greater attention should be given to minimizing risks of HIV transmission, while promoting good nutrition and preventing other childhood illnesses. Exclusive breastfeeding is recommended for all uninfected mothers and mothers of unknown HIV status, as well as for HIV-infected women who choose to breastfeed (WHO 2001). Good breastfeeding techniques and prompt treatment of breast and systemic infections will have benefits for all mothers and infants and also may prevent postnatal HIV transmission. Safe sex practices should also be encouraged to prevent new infections in women, particularly during the breastfeeding period.

In addition to making early breastfeeding safer for HIV-infected mothers, we also have to assist families to make appropriate decisions about early breastfeeding cessation. This decision about when to stop breastfeeding should be based on an assessment of the health status of the mother and the infant. Parents need to prepare for early cessation to ensure that the transition is safe. This includes teaching infants to feed from a cup, teaching parents how to safely and hygienically prepare replacement milks and foods, and helping parents to address any pressure or stigma in the community (Piwoz et al. 2002). Heat-treating human milk may help in the transition process, and where culturally acceptable, heat-treating should be taught.

Early breastfeeding cessation will prevent a sizeable fraction of postnatal transmission—50 percent or more if cessation is around 6 months. However, in order to prevent malnutrition and ensure adequate child growth and development, early cessation must be accompanied by adequate nutrition for the infant. Since human milk is an essential part of the infant diet throughout the first year and beyond, programs that encourage early cessation should insure that nutritious human milk substitutes and/or multinutrient supplements are available. Low-cost, locally produced, fortified foods, such as the nutrient-dense spreads currently used for community-based therapeutic feeding (Briend 2001) should be developed and tested for this purpose.

Safe replacement feeding from birth requires, at a minimum, access to replacement milks, clean water, preparation and feeding skills, and family support. In Africa, only 55 percent of the total population has access to safe water (Humphrey & Iliff 2001). In settings where HIV-infected women are provided with replacement milks, interventions must be put into place to make it safer, as well as to prevent spillover in the general population (Botswana MOH/UNICEF 2002).

For individual counseling about infant feeding, it may make the greatest sense to screen HIV-infected mothers, and focus counseling on replacement feeding to women most at risk of passing HIV during breastfeeding, such as among mothers with low CD4 lymphocyte counts or a clinical diagnosis of AIDS. Future research should identify easy-to-measure, sensitive indicators of maternal immune deficiency to help make this type of individually tailored information a reality.

Based on the data and analysis presented here, because of the HIV pandemic we must strengthen our efforts to promote and support optimal infant feeding. Abandoning support for infant feeding will increase HIV transmission and reduce child survival.

6. ACKNOWLEDGMENTS

Funding for this paper was provided by the Bureau for Africa, Office of Sustainable Development of the United States Agency for International Development (USAID) under the terms of Contract AOT-C-00-99-00237-00, and by the Bureau for Global Health, GH/HIDN Cooperative Agreement No. HRN-A-00-97-000007-00. The opinions expressed herein are those of the authors and do not necessarily reflect the views of USAID, AED, or the Johns Hopkins University Bloomberg School of Public Health.

7. REFERENCES

Becquart P, Chomont N, Roques P, Ayouba A, Kazatchkine M, Belec L, Hocini H. Compartmentalization of HIV-1 between breast milk and blood of HIV-infected mothers. Virology 2002;300:109-117.

Botswana Ministry of Health, UNICEF, Program Review Team, PMTCT Advisory Group, and Infant Feeding Study Group. Prevention of mother-to-child transmission: evaluation of a pilot programme and a follow-up study of infant feeding practices during the scaled-up progamme in Botswana. Evaluation and Program Planning 2002;25(4):421-431.

Briend A. Highly nutrient-dense spreads: a new approach to delivering multiple micronutrients to high-risk groups. Br J Nutr 2001;85(Suppl 2):S175-S179.

Bulterys M, Nolan ML, Jamieson DJ, Dominguez K, Fowler MG. Advances in the prevention of mother-to-child transmission: current issues, future challenges. AIDScience 2002;2(4):February 28.

Chopra M, Schaay N, Sanders D, Sengwana J, Puoane T, Piwoz EG, Dunnett L. Summary of the findings and recommendations from a formative research study with the Khayelitsha MTCT Programme, South Africa. Cape Town: University of the Western Cape Public Health Programme; May 2000.

Chopra M, Piwoz E, Sengwana J, Schaay N, Dunnett L, Sanders D. Effect of a mother-to-child HIV prevention programme on infant feeding and caring practices in South Africa. S Afr Med J 2002;92:298-302.

Coovadia HM, Coutsoudis A. Problems and advances in reducing transmission of HIV-1 through breastfeeding in developing countries. AIDScience 2001;1(4):July.

Coutsoudis A, Pillay K, Spooner E, Kuhn L, Coovadia HM. Influence of infant-feeding patterns on early mother-to-child transmission of HIV-1 in Durban, South Africa: a prospective cohort study. South African Vitamin A Study Group. Lancet 1999;354:471-476.

Coutsoudis A, Pillay K, Kuhn L, Spooner E, Tsai W-Y, Coovadia HM. Method of feeding and transmission of HIV-1 from mothers to children by 15 months of age: prospective cohort study from Durban, South Africa. AIDS 2001a;15:379-387.

Coutsoudis A, Coovadia H, Pillay K, Kuhn L. Are HIV-infected women who breastfeed at increased risk of mortality? AIDS 2001b;15:653-655.

De Cock KM, Fowler MG, Mercier E, de Vincenzi I, Saba J, Hoff E, Alnwick DJ, Rogers M, Shaffer N. Prevention of mother-to-child HIV transmission in resource-poor countries: translating research into policy and practice. JAMA 2000;283:1175-1182.

Dunn DT, Newell ML, Ades AE, Peckham CS. Risk of human immunodeficiency virus type 1 transmission through breastfeeding. Lancet 1992;340:585-588.

Ekpini ER, Wiktor SZ, Satten GA, Adjorlolo-Johnson GT, Sibailly TS, Ou CY, Karon JM, Brattegaard K, Whitaker JP, Gnaore E, De Cock KM, Greenberg, AE. Late postnatal mother-to-child transmission of HIV-1 in Abidjan, Cote d'Ivoire. Lancet 1997;349:1054-1059.

Embree JE, Njenga S, Datta P, Nagelkerke NJ, Ndinya-Achola JO, Mohammed Z, Ramdahin S, Bwayo JJ, Plummer FA. Risk factors for postnatal mother-child transmission of HIV-1. AIDS 2000;14:2535-2541.

Ezzati M, Lopez AD, Rodgers A, Vander Horn S, Murray CJ, and the Comparative Risk Assessment Collaborating Group. Selected major risk factors and global and regional burden of disease. Lancet 2002;360:1347-1360.

Farquhar C, VanCott TC, Mbori-Ngacha DA, Horani L, Bosire RK, Kreiss JK, Richardson BA, John-Stewart GC. Salivary secretory leukocyte protease inhibitor is associated with reduced transmission of human immunodeficiency virus type 1 through breast milk. J Infect Dis 2002;186:1173-1176.

Fawzi W, Msamanga G, Spiegelman D, Renjifo B, Bang H, Kapiga S, Coley J, Hertzmark E, Essex M, Hunter D. Transmission of HIV-1 through breastfeeding among women in Dar es Salaam, Tanzania. J Acquir Immune Defic Syndr 2002;31:331-338.

Filteau SM, Rice AL, Ball JL, Chakraborty J, Stoltzfus R, A.de Francisco J, Willumsen. Breast milk immune factors in Bangladeshi women in supplemented postpartum with retinol or beta-carotene. Am J Clin Nutr 1999;69:953-958.

Flores M, Filteau S. Effect of lactation counselling on subclinical mastitis among Bangladeshi women. Ann Trop Paediatr 2002;22:85-88.

Fowler MG, Newell ML. Breastfeeding and HIV-1 transmission in resource-limited settings. J Acquir Immune Defic Syndr 2002;30:230-239.

French R, Brocklehurst P. The effect of pregnancy on survival in women infected with HIV: a systematic review of the literature and meta-analysis. Br J Obstet Gynaecol 1998;105:827-835.

Gaillard P, Piwoz EG, Farley T. Collection of standardized information on infant feeding in the context of mother-to-child transmission of HIV. Stat Med 2001;20(23):3525-3537.

Gavin L, Tavengwa N, Iliff P, Nathoo K, Humphrey J. The development of an intervention to inform women about infant feeding in the context of HIV. Second Conference on Global Strategies for the Prevention of HIV Transmission from Mothers to Infants. Montreal; September 1999. Abstract Number 269.

Haider R, Ashworth A, Kabir I, Huttly SR. Effect of community-based peer counsellors on exclusive breastfeeding practices in Dhaka, Bangladesh: a randomised controlled trial. Lancet 2000;356:1643-1647.

Humphrey J, Iliff P. Is breast not best? Feeding babies born to HIV-positive mothers: Bringing balance to a complex issue. Nutr Rev 2001;59(4):119-127.

Jeffery BS, Webber L, Mokhondo KR, Erasmus D. Determination of the effectiveness of inactivation of human immunodeficiency virus by Pretoria pasteurization. J Trop Pediatr 2001;47:345-349

John GC, Nduati RW, Mbori-Ngacha DA, Richardson BA, Panteleeff D, Mwatha A, Overbaugh J, Bwayo J, Ndinya-Achola JO, Kreiss JK. Correlates of mother-to-child human immunodeficiency virus type 1 (HIV-1) transmission: association with maternal plasma HIV-1 RNA load, genital HIV-1 DNA shedding, and breast infections. J Infect Dis 2001a;183:206-212.

John GC, Richardson BA, Nduati RW, Mbori-Ngacha D, Kreiss JK. Timing of breast milk HIV-1 transmission: a meta-analysis. East Afr Med J 2001b;78:75-79.

Kambarambi RA, Kowo H. The prevalence of nipple disease among breastfeeding mothers of HIV seropositive infants. Cent Afr J Med 1997;43(1):20-22.

Kisakye H, Kukandwa KJ, Ndagire L, Nakyanzi T, Mugula RK, Bakaki PM. Experiences with early abrupt cessation of breastfeeding among HIV infected women in Kampala, Uganda. XIV International AIDS Conference. Barcelona; July 2002. Abstract MoPeE3739.

Kleinbaum DG, Kupper LL, Morgenstern H. Epidemiologic Research: Principles and Quantitative Methods. New York: Van Nostrand Reinhold; 1982.

Kramer MS, Chalmers B, Hodnett ED, Sevkovskaya Z, Dzikovich I, Shapiro S, Collet JP, Vanilovich I, Mezen I, Ducruet T, Shishko G, Zubovich V, Mknuik D, Gluchanina E, Dombrovskiy V, Ustinovitch A, Kot T, Bogdanovich N, Ovchinikova L, Helsing E; PROBIT Study Group. Promotion of Breastfeeding Intervention Trial (PROBIT): a randomized trial in the Republic of Belarus. JAMA 2001;285:413-420.

Kuhn L, Kasonde P, Vwalika C, Shutes E, Sinkala M, Kankasa C, Aldrovandi G, Thea D. Uptake of interventions to reduce mother-to-child HIV transmission: nevirapine and exclusive breastfeeding in the Zambia Exclusive Breastfeeding Study (ZEBS). XIV International AIDS Conference. Barcelona; July 2002. Abstract TuOrB1176.

Leroy V, Montcho C, Manigart O, Van de Perre P, Dabis F, Msellati P, Meda N, You B, Simonon A, Rouzioux C. Maternal plasma viral load, zidovudine and mother-to-child transmission of HIV-1 in Africa: DITRAME ANRS 049a trial. AIDS 2001;15:517-522.

Leroy V, Karon JM, Alioum A, Ekpini ER, Meda N, Greenberg AE, Msellati P, Hudgens M, Dabis F, Wiktor SZ. Twenty-four month efficacy of a maternal short-course zidovudine regimen to prevent mother-to-child transmission of HIV-1 in West Africa. West Africa PMTCT Study Group. AIDS 2002;16:631-641.

Lewis P, Nduati R, Kreiss JK, John GC, Richardson BA, Mbori-Ngacha D, Ndinya-Achola J, Overbaugh J. Cell-free human immunodeficiency virus type 1 in breast milk. J Infect Dis 1998;177:34-39.

Magoni M, Kituuka P, Okong P, Bassani L, Merminario E, Massella M, Guiliano M. Effectiveness of the prevention of mother to child transmission program and the influence of feeding options in an urban hospital in Kampala, Uganda. XIV Int. AIDS Conference. Barcelona; July 2002. Abstract TuOrB1178.

Malkin JE, Noba V, Coulibaly M, Ekpeni A, Chambon JF. Follow up of newborn after prevention of mother-to-child transmission (PMTCT) intervention regarding the method of feeding in Abidjan (Cote d'Ivoire). XIV International AIDS Conference. Barcelona; July 2002. Abstract MoPeD3679.

Mbori-Ngacha D, Nduati R, John G, Reilly M, Richardson B, Mwatha A, Ndinya-Achola J, Bwayo J, Kreiss J. Morbidity and mortality in breastfed and formula-fed infants of HIV-1-infected women: A randomized clinical trial. JAMA 2001;286:2413-2420.

McCoy D, Besser M, Visser R, Doherty T. Interim findings on the National PMTCT Pilot Sites: Lessons and Recommendations. Cape Town, South Africa: Health Systems Trust; 2002.

Miller M, Iliff P, Stoltzfus RJ, Humphrey J. Breastmilk erythropoietin and mother-to-child HIV transmission through breastmilk. Lancet 2002;360:1246-1248.

Miotti P, Taha TET, Kumwenda NI, Broadhead R, Mtimavalye LAR, Van der Hoeven L, Chiphangwi JD, Liomba G, Biggar RJ. HIV transmission through breastfeeding: A study in Malawi. JAMA 1999;282:744-749.

Mompati K, Luo C, Rollins N, Willumsen J, Kleitjes S, Phegelo M. Evaluation of infant feeding practices in PMTCT and non-PMTCT sites in Botswana. XIV International AIDS Conference. Barcelona; July 2002. Abstract TuPeF5408.

Moodley D, Moodley J, Coovadia H, Gray G, McIntyre J, Hofmyer J, Nikodem C, Hall D, Gigliotti M, Robinson P, Boshoff L, Sullivan JL, South African Intrapartum Nevirapine Trial (SAINT) Investigators. A multicenter randomized controlled clincial trial of nevirapine versus a combination of zidovudine and lamivudine to reduce intrapartum and early postpartum mother-to-child transmission of human immunodeficiency virus type1. J Infect Dis 2003;187(5):725-735.

Morrow AL, Guerrero ML, Shults J, Calva JJ, Lutter C, Bravo J, Ruiz-Palacios G, Morrow RC, Butterfoss FD. Efficacy of home-based peer counselling to promote exclusive breastfeeding: a randomised controlled trial. Lancet 1999;353:1226-1231.

Nduati R, John G, Mbori-Ngacha D, Richardson B, Overbaugh J, Mwatha A, Ndinya-Achola J, Bwayo J, Onyango FE, Hughes J, Kreiss J. Effect of breast feeding and formula feeding on transmission of HIV-1: A randomised clinical trial. JAMA 2000;283:1167-1174.

Nduati R, Richardson BA, John G, Mbori-Ngacha D, Mwatha A, Ndinya-Achola J, Bwayo J, Onyango FE, Kreiss J. Effect of breastfeeding on mortality among HIV-1 infected women: a randomised trial. Lancet 2001;357:1651-1655.

Newell ML. Prevention of mother-to-child transmission of HIV: Challenges for the current decade. Bull WHO 2001;79(12):1138-1144.

Papathakis PC, Rollins N. Adequacy of feeding recommendations for infants of HIV-infected mothers: assessment of nutrient content, cost and preparation time of breast milk replacements in the South African context. XIV International AIDS Conference. Barcelona; July 2002. Abstract MoOrF1030.

Petra Study Team. Efficacy of three short-course regimens of zidovudine and lamivudine in preventing early and late transmission of HIV-1 from mother to child in Tanzania, South Africa, and Uganda (Petra study): a randomised, double-blind, placebo-controlled trial. Lancet 2002;359:1178-1186.

Phadke MA, Bharucha KE, Shrotri AN, Sastry J, Gupte NA, Brookmeyer R, Joshi PL, Bollinger RC. High post-partum morbidity in replacement fed infants born to HIV-infected women in India, receiving short-course zidovudine. XIV International AIDS Conference. Barcelona; July 2002. Abstract WePeB5926.

Pillay K, Coutsoudis A, York D, Kuhn L, Coovadia HM Cell-free virus in breast milk of HIV-1-seropositive women. J Acquir Immune Defic Syndr 2000;24:330-336.

Piwoz EG, Creed de Kanashiro H, Lopez de Romaña G, Black RE, Brown KH. Potential misclassification of infants' usual feeding practices using 24-hour dietary assessment methods. J Nutr 1995;125(1):57-65.

Piwoz, EG, Chintu M, Ntombela N, Siyandi R, Kaliwile C, Nyirenda T, Banda A, Maambo L, Maambo R, van den Wyngaart A. Infant feeding options for HIV+ women: Findings and recommendations from a formative research study in Ndola, Zambia. Second Conference on Global Strategies for the Prevention of HIV Transmission from Mothers to Babies. Montreal; September 1999. Abstract Number 484.

Piwoz EG, Huffman SL, Lusk D, Zehner ER, O'Gara C. Issues, risks, and challenges of early breastfeeding cessation to reduce postnatal transmission of HIV in Africa. Washington, DC: Academy for Educational Development; 2002.

Preble EA, Piwoz EG. HIV and Infant Feeding: A chronology of research and policy advances and their implications for programs. Washington, DC: Academy for Educational Development; 1998.

Read JS, Newell ML, Dabis F, Leroy V. Breastfeeding and late postnatal transmission of HIV-1: An individual patient data meta-analysis (Breastfeeding and HIV International Transmission Study). XIV International AIDS Conference. Barcelona; July 2002. Abstract TuOrB1177.

Rousseau CM, Nduati RW, Richardson BA, Steele MS, John-Stewart GC, Mbori-Ngacha DA, Kreiss JK, Overbaugh J. Longitudinal analysis of human immunodeficiency virus type 1 RNA in breast milk and of its relationship to infant infection and maternal disease. J Infect Dis 2003;187(5):741-747.

Sabbaj S, Edwards BH, Ghosh MK, Semrau K, Cheelo S, Thea DM, Kuhn L, Ritter GD, Mulligan MJ, Goepfert PA, Aldrovandi GM. Human immunodeficiency virus-specific CD8(+) T cells in human breast milk. J Virol 2002;76:7365-7373.

Semba RD, Miotti PG, Chiphangwi JD, Saah AJ, Canner Jk, Dallabetta GA, Hoover JR. Maternal vitamin A deficiency and mother-to-child transmission of HIV-1. Lancet 1994;343:1593-1597.

Semba RD, Kumwenda N, Hoover DR, Taha TE, Quinn TC, Mtimavalye L, Biggar J, Broadhead R, Miotti PG, Sokoll LJ, van der Hoeven L, Chiphangwi JD. Human immunodeficiency virus load in breast milk, mastitis, and mother-to-child transmission of human immunodeficiency virus type 1. J Infect Dis 1999;180:93-98.

Shapiro RL, Lockman S, Thior I, Stocking L, Kebaabetswe P, Wester C, Peter T, Marlink R, Essex M, Heymann SJ. Low adherence to recommended infant feeding strategies in the pilot phase of a randomized trial to prevent mother-to-child HIV transmission in rural Botswana. XIV International AIDS Conference. Barcelona; July 2002. Abstract MoPeD3683.

Thea DM, Piwoz EG, Kasonde P, Vwalika C, Shutes E, Sinkala M, Kankasa C, Aldrovandi G, Kuhn L. The feasibility of early rapid breastfeeding cessation to reduce postnatal transmission of HIV in Lusaka, Zambia. XIV International AIDS Conference, Barcelona; July 2002. Abstract TuPeF5393.

UNAIDS. Report on the global HIV/AIDS epidemic. Geneva: UNAIDS/02.26E; 2002.

UNAIDS/UNICEF/WHO. HIV and Infant Feeding: Guidelines for decision-makers. WHO/FRH/NUT/CHD/ 98.1. WHO/UNAIDS; 1998.

UNAIDS/UNICEF/WHO. HIV and Infant Feeding: Guidelines for decision-makers. Update, 2003, in preparation.

Van de Perre P, Simonon A, Hitimana D, Dabis F, Msellati P, Mukamabano B, Butera JB, Van Goethem C, Karita E, Lepage P. Infective and anti-infective properties of breastmilk from HIV-infected women. Lancet 1993;341:914-918.

Van de Perre P. Transmission of human immunodeficiency virus type 1 through breastfeeding: How can it be prevented? J Infect Dis 1999;179(Suppl 3):S405-407.

[WHO] World Health Organization, Division of Child Health and Development. Evidence for the ten steps to successful breastfeeding. Geneva: World Health Organization; 1998a.

[WHO] World Health Organization. Complementary feeding of young children in developing countries: A review of current scientific knowledge. WHO/NUT/98.1. Geneva: World Health Organization; 1998b.

[WHO] World Health Organization. New data on the prevention of mother-to-child transmission of HIV and their policy implications: Conclusions and recommendations. Geneva: World Health Organization; 11-13 October 2000, approved January 15, 2001 [Cited 2001 Jan 19]. Available at: www.unaids.org/ publications/documents/mtct.

[WHO] World Health Organization, Collaborative Team on the Role of Breastfeeding in the Prevention of Infant Mortality. Effect of breastfeeding on infant and child mortality due to infectious diseases in less developed countries: a pooled analysis. Lancet 2000;355:451-455

[WHO] World Health Organization, Department of HIV/AIDS, Family and Community Health Cluster. Scaling up antiretroviral therapy in resource limited settings. Guidelines for a public health approach. Geneva: World Health Organization; 2002.

Willumsen JF, Filteau SM, Coutsoudis A, Uebel KE, Newell ML, Tomkins AM. Subclinical mastitis as a risk factor for mother-infant HIV transmission. Adv Exp Med Biol 2000;478;211-223.

Willumsen JF, Filteau SM, Coutsoudis A, Newell ML, Rollins NC, Coovadia HM, Tomkins AM. Breastmilk RNA viral load in HIV-infected South African women: Effects of sub-clinical mastitis and infant feeding. AIDS 2003;17 (3):407-414.

MOTHER-TO-INFANT HEPATITIS C VIRUS TRANSMISSION AND BREASTFEEDING

Eric E. Mast

1. ABSTRACT

Hepatitis C virus (HCV) is a blood-borne virus that is transmitted most efficiently by direct percutaneous exposures to blood. Infants are at risk of HCV infection primarily as a result of transmission from their infected mothers. However, there is no evidence of mother-to-infant transmission from breastfeeding. According to guidelines from the Centers for Disease Control and Prevention and the American Academy of Pediatrics, maternal HCV infection is not a contraindication to breastfeeding. It may be prudent for mothers who are HCV-infected and who choose to breastfeed to consider abstaining from breastfeeding if their nipples are cracked and bleeding.

2. INTRODUCTION

Hepatitis C virus (HCV) is transmitted most efficiently by direct percutaneous exposures to blood (Alter 2002). Approximately 1% of pregnant women in the United States have serologic evidence of HCV infection with detectable antibody to HCV (anti-HCV); about two-thirds of these women are infected chronically with detectable HCV RNA by polymerase chain reaction testing. Thus, approximately 30,000 to 40,000 infants born to HCV-infected pregnant women each year in the United States are at risk of infection. Maternal HCV infection generally has no effect on the course of pregnancy, and no clinical effects of maternal infection on the fetus or neonate have been reported. Infants are at risk of infection primarily as a result of perinatal transmission that usually occurs at or around the time of delivery.

HCV-infected infants typically have no clinical signs or symptoms of liver disease, and no cases of fulminant hepatitis have been reported among infected infants. However, the majority becomes chronically infected and most of these infants have evidence of chronic liver disease with elevated alanine aminotransfersase (ALT) levels (Resti et al. 1998). Limited data suggest that infants infected with HCV have few clinical signs or

Division of Viral Hepatitis, National Center for Infectious Diseases, Centers for Disease Control and Prevention, Mailstop G37, 1600 Clifton Road, Atlanta, GA 30333

symptoms of disease in the first several years of life. However, no follow-up data are available to assess the long-term consequences of perinatally acquired HCV infection. Among infected adults, the course of chronic liver disease is usually insidious, progressing at a slow rate without symptoms or physical signs in the majority of patients for the first two or more decades after infection. In long-term follow-up studies of adults with chronic HCV infection, cirrhosis developed in 10% to 20% of persons, and hepatocellular carcinoma in 1% to 5% of persons over a period of 20 to 30 years (Di Bisceglie et al. 1991; Seeff et al. 1992).

This chapter reviews available data on HCV transmission from mother to infant, focusing on studies that have evaluated the risk of HCV transmission from breastfeeding. In addition, existing recommendations for counseling pregnant and lactating women and for management of infants born to HCV-infected mothers are reviewed.

3. STUDIES OF HCV TRANSMISSION FROM MOTHER TO INFANT

In published studies of HCV transmission from mother to infant, the average rate of transmission from mothers who were anti-HCV positive was 5.8% (range, 0–25%) (Table 1). Factors that have been found to be consistently associated with an increased risk of transmission include the presence of HCV RNA in the mother at the time of delivery and maternal co-infection with HCV and human immunodeficiency virus (HIV). In addition, an association between higher transmission rates and increased serum HCV RNA titers has been reported in some studies.

In 11 studies in which maternal HCV RNA results were reported, HCV RNA has been detected in the mother at the time of delivery in virtually all cases of mother-to-infant transmission; only two cases of transmission to infants have been reported from

Table 1. Studies of hepatitis C virus transmission from mother to infant[a]

Maternal characteristic	No. of studies	Mother-infant pairs tested	Infants infected, (%)
Anti-HCV positive	66	7891	(5.8)
HCV RNA detected in serum	55		
Yes		4265	(8.5)
No		750	(0.3)
HIV-HCV co-infection	11		
Yes		627	(18.7)
No		2435	(5.4)
Mode of delivery	13		
Vaginal		2376	(8.0)
Caesarian section		825	(7.0)

[a]Adapted from Yeung et al. (2001); includes data from three additional references published after this review (Resti et al. 2002; Mast et al. 1999; Gibb et al. 2000).

more than 750 HCV RNA-negative mothers (Table 1). In studies that have included HCV-infected women with and without HIV co-infection, rates of HCV transmission were approximately three to four times higher from HCV-HIV co-infected women than from mothers with HCV infection alone (Table 1). However, one study found an association of transmission with injecting drug use, but not with HCV-HIV co-infection (Resti et al. 2002). Studies that have evaluated the effect of maternal HCV RNA titer on transmission to infants have yielded inconsistent results; some studies have found that increased HCV RNA titers were associated with increased transmission rates while others found no association. In addition, different methods have been used to quantitate HCV RNA titers in these studies and different titer levels have been related to transmission (Yeung et al. 2001).

Mode of delivery of an infant generally has not been found to be associated with transmission from mother to infant, with similar rates of transmission following vaginal delivery and caesarian section (C-section) (Table 1). However, increased transmission rates were associated with longer duration of membrane rupture in two studies (Spencer et al. 1997; Mast et al. 1999) and with use of internal fetal monitoring in one study (Mast et al. 1999). In addition, one study found a lower transmission rate from mothers who had elective C-sections compared with mothers who had emergency C-sections (Gibb et al. 2000). Thus, further investigation is needed to determine the possible role of using delivery techniques that decrease an infant's exposure to maternal blood (e.g., avoidance of scalp electrodes, elective C-section) to reduce transmission.

4. RISK OF HCV TRANSMISSION THROUGH BREASTFEEDING

The findings of studies that have tested human milk and/or colostrum samples for HCV RNA by PCR are difficult to interpret because PCR tests for HCV RNA only recently have been validated and licensed. In addition, different methods of processing human milk/colostrum specimens have been used. In 12 published studies, HCV RNA has been detected in 0% to 100% (median, 14.5%) of human milk and/or colostrum specimens from HCV RNA-positive mothers (Table 2). No association has been found between detection of HCV RNA in human milk and HCV titers in maternal serum (Mast et al. 1999; Lin et al. 1995).

Although HCV RNA has been detected in human milk, transmission of HCV through breastfeeding has not been documented. In 12 published studies that have evaluated breastfeeding as a risk factor for transmission from HCV-infected mothers, rates of transmission were similar in breastfed and formula-fed infants (Table 3). In addition, the timing of detection of HCV RNA in infants who acquire infection during the first several months of life is consistent with transmission occurring at or around the time of delivery (Mast et al. 1999; Ohto et al. 1994; Zuccotti et al. 1995). Late infections occurring after the first several months have not been documented in breastfed infants.

Table 2. Detection of HCV RNA in human milk specimens from HCV RNA-positive mothers

Study	No. of mothers tested	HCV RNA detected in human milk, No. (%)
Lin et al. 1995	15	15 (100)
Mast et al. 1999	37	19 (51)
Ruiz-Extremera et al. 2000	20	4 (20)
Zimmerman et al. 1995	10	2 (20)
Aizaki et al. 1996	5	1 (20)
Croxson et al. 1997	30	5 (17)
Koseki 1994	25	3 (12)
Dal Molin et al. 2002	13	1 (8)
Kurauchi et al. 1993	17	0 (0)
Polywka et al. 1999	37	0 (0)
Spencer et al. 1997	38	0 (0)
Ogasawara et al. 1993	10	0 (0)

Table 3. HCV transmission from mother to infant among breastfed and formula-fed infants

		Formula-fed		Breastfed	
Study	Maternal testing method	No. tested	Infected, No. (%)	No. tested	Infected No. (%)
Resti et al. 2002	HCV RNA	626	72 (11.5)	217	22 (10.1)
Dal Molin et al. 2002	HCV RNA	37	3 (8.1)	39	2 (5.1)
Mast et al. 1999	HCV RNA	121	5 (4.1)	63	2 (3.2)
Moriya et al. 1995	HCV RNA	15	1 (6.7)	55	1 (1.8)
Total		799	81 (10.1)	374	27 (7.2)
Tajiri et al. 2001	anti-HCV	16	0 (0)	98	9 (9.2)
Gibb et al. 2000	anti-HCV	355	24 (6.7)	59	5 (7.7)
Ruiz-Extremera et al. 2000	anti-HCV	30	1 (3.3)	43	7 (16.3)
Conte et al. 2000	anti-HCV	280	6 (2.1)	90	2 (2.2)
Mazza et al. 1998	anti-HCV	40	5 (12.5)	27	1 (3.7)
Tovo et al. 1997	anti-HCV	43	2 (4.6)	33	1 (3.0)
Zanetti et al. 1995	anti-HCV	23	0 (0)	71	0 (0)
Paccagnini et al. 1995	anti-HCV	57	12 (21.1)	13	2 (15.4)
Total		844	50 (16.8)	434	27 (6.2)

5. COUNSELING AND MANAGEMENT GUIDELINES

Guidelines for counseling HCV-infected pregnant women and for management of infants born to HCV-infected mothers have been developed by the Centers for Disease Control and Prevention (1998) and by the American Academy of Pediatrics (2003). Routine serologic testing of pregnant women for HCV infection is not recommended because no measures are available to prevent perinatal transmission, and there is no licensed therapy or guidelines for treatment of HCV-infected infants or children. However, health-care professionals in settings where pregnant women are evaluated or receive routine care should take risk histories from their patients to determine the need for testing (CDC 1998). Maternal HCV infection is not considered to be a contra-indication to breastfeeding. However, it may be prudent for mothers who are HCV-infected who choose to breastfeed to consider abstaining from breastfeeding if their nipples are cracked and bleeding. In addition, no evidence exists that mode of delivery is related to transmission; therefore, determining the need for cesarean delivery versus vaginal delivery should not be made solely on the basis of HCV infection status.

Because of their recognized exposure, children born to HCV-infected women should be tested for HCV infection. Testing of infants for anti-HCV should be performed no sooner than 15 to 18 months of age, when passively-transferred maternal anti-HCV declines below detectable levels. For earlier diagnosis of HCV infection, testing infant serum for HCV RNA may be performed on or after the infant's first well-child visit at 1 to 2 months of age and should be repeated at a subsequent visit. Umbilical cord blood should not be used for diagnosis of perinatal HCV infection because cord blood can be contaminated with maternal blood. If positive for either anti-HCV or HCV RNA, children should be evaluated with serial liver function tests for the presence or development of liver disease. Children with persistently abnormal serum ALT levels should be referred to a pediatric gastroenterologist for management.

6. REFERENCES

Aizaki H, Saito A, Kusakawa I, Ashiwara Y, Nagamori S, Toda G, Suzuki T, Ishii K, Matsuura Y, Miyamura T. Mother-to-child transmission of a hepatitis C virus variant with an insertional mutation in its hypervariable region. J Hepatol 1996;25:608-613.

Alter MJ. Prevention of spread of hepatitis C. Hepatology 2002;36 (Suppl 1):S93-S98.

American Academy of Pediatrics. Hepatitis C. In: Pickering LK, editor. 2003 Redbook: Report of the Committee on Infectious Diseases. 26th Edition. Elk Grove Village, IL: American Academy of Pediatrics, 2003; pp 336-340.

[CDC] Centers for Disease Control and Prevention. Recommendations for prevention and control of hepatitis C virus (HCV) infection and HCV-related chronic liver disease. MMWR 1998;47(No. RR-19):1-38.

Conte D, Fraquelli M, Prati D, Colucci A, Minola E. Prevalence and clinical course of chronic hepatitis C virus (HCV) infection and rate of HCV vertical transmission in a cohort of 15,250 pregnant women. Hepatology 2000;31:751-755.

Croxon M, Couper A, Voss L, Groves D, Gunn T. Vertical transmission of hepatitis C virus in New Zealand. NZ Med J 1997;110:165-167.

Dal Molin G, D'Agaro P, Ansaldi F, Ciana G, Fertz C, Alberico S, Campello C. Mother-to-infant transmission of hepatitis C virus: rate of infection and assessment of viral load and IgM anti-HCV as risk factors. J Med Virl 2002;67:137-142.

Di Bisceglie AM, Goodman ZD, Ishak KG, Hoofnagle JH, Melpolder JJ, Alter HJ. Long-term clinical and histopathological follow-up of chronic posttransfusion hepatitis. Hepatology 1991;14:969-974.

Gibb DM, Goodall RL, Dunn DT, Healy M, Neave P, Cafferkey M, Butler K. Mother to child transmission of hepatitis C virus: evidence for preventable peripartum transmission. Lancet 2000;356:904-907.

Koseki S. Mother-to-infant transmission of hepatitis C virus. Acta Obstet Gynaecol Jpn 1994;46:1322-1328.

Kurauchi O, Furui T, Itakura A, Ishiko H, Sugiyama M, Ohno Y, Ando H, Tanamura A, Ishida T, Nawa A, et al. Studies on transmission of hepatitis C virus from mother to child in the perinatal period. Arch Gynecol Obstet 1993;253:121-126.

Lin HH, Kao JH, Hsu HY, Ni YH, Chang MH, Huang SC, Hwang LH, Chen PJ, Chen DS Absence of infection in breast-fed infants born to hepatitis C virus-infected mothers. J Pediatr 1995;126:589-591.

Mast EE, Hwang LY, Seto D, Nolte FS, Kelly MG, Alter MJ. Perinatal hepatitis C virus transmission: maternal risk factors and optimal timing of diagnosis. Hepatology 1999;30:499A.

Mazza C, Ravaggi A, Rodella A, Padula D, Duse M, Lomini M, Puoti M, Rossini A, Cariani. Prospective study of mother-to-infant transmission of hepatitis C virus infection. Study Group for Vertical Transmission. J Med Virol 1998;54:12-19.

Moriya T, Sasaki F, Mizui M, Ohno N, Mohri H, Mishiro S, Yoshizawa H. Transmission of hepatitis C virus from mothers to infants: its frequency and risk factors revisited. Biomed Pharmacother 1995;49:59-64.

Ogasawara S, Kage M, Kosai K-I, Shimamatsu K, Kojiro M. Hepatitis C virus RNA in saliva and breastmilk of hepatitis C virus carrier mothers. Lancet 1993;341:561.

Hitoshi Ohto, Sousuke Terazawa, Nobuhiko Sasaki, Nobutaka Sasaki, Kunihiko Hino, Chieko Ishiwata, Makoto Kako, Niro Ujiie, Chikara Endo, Akira Matsui, Hiroaki Okamoto, Shunji Mishiro, for The Vertical Transmission of Hepatitis C Virus Collaborative Study Group. Transmission of hepatitis C virus from mothers to infants. N Engl J Med 1994;330:744-750.

Paccagnini S, Principi N, Massironi E, Tanzi E, Romano L, Muggiasca ML, Ragni MC, Salvaggio L. Perinatal transmission and manifestation of hepatitis C virus infection in a high risk population. Pediatr Infect Dis J 1995; 14:195-199.

Polywka S, Schroter M, Feucht HH, Zollner B, Laufs R. Low risk of vertical transmission of hepatitis C virus by breast milk. Clin Infect Dis 1999; 29:1327-1329.

Resti M, Azzari C, Mannelli F, Moriondo M, Novembre E, de Martino M, Vierucci A. Mother to child transmission of hepatitis C virus: prospective study of risk factors and timing of infection in children born to women seronegative for HIV-1. Tuscany Study Group on Hepatitis C Virus Infection. Br Med J 1998;17:437-441.

Resti M, Azzari C, Galli L, Zuin G, Giacchino R, Bortolotti F, Marcellini M, Moriondo M, de Martino M, Vierucci A; Italian Study Group on Mother-to-Infant Hepatitis C Virus Transmission. Maternal drug use is a preeminent risk factor for mother-to-child hepatitis C virus transmission: results of a multicenter study of 1372 mother-infant pairs. J Infect Dis 2002;18:567-572.

Ruiz-Extremera A, Salmeron J, Torres C, De Rueda PM, Gimenez F, Robles C, Miranda MT. Follow-up of transmission of hepatitis C to babies of human immunodeficiency virus (HHIV)-negative women: the role of breastfeeding in transmission. Pediatr Infect Dis J 2000;19:511-516.

Seeff LB, Buskell-Bales Z, Wright EC, Durako SJ, Alter HJ, Iber FL, Hollinger FB, Gitnick G, Knodell RG, Perrillo RP, Stevens CE, Hollingsworth CG, and the National Heart, Lung, and Blood Institute Study Group. Long-term mortality after transfusion-associated non-A, non-B hepatitis. N Engl J Med 1992;327:1906-1911.

Spencer JD, Latt N, Beeby PJ, Collins E, Saunders JB, McCaughan GW, Cossart YE. Transmission of hepatitis C virus to infants of human immunodeficiency virus-negative intravenous drug-using mothers: rate of infection and assessment of risk factors for transmission. J Viral Hepat 1997;4:395-409.

Tajiri H, Miyoshi Y, Funada S, Etani Y, Abe J, Onodera T, Goto M, Funato M, Ida S, Noda C, Nakayama M, Okada S. Prospective study of mother-to-infant transmission of hepatitis C virus. Pediar Infect Dis J 2001;20:10-14.

Tovo PA, Palomba E, Ferraris G, Principi N, Ruga E, Dallacasa P, Maccabruni A. Increased risk of maternal-infant hepatitis C virus transmission for women coinfected with human immunodeficiency virus type 1. Clin Infect Dis 1997;25:1121-1124.

Yeung LTF, King SM, Roberts EA. Mother-to-infant transmission of hepatitis C virus. Hepatology 2001;34:223-229.

Zanetti AR, Tanzi E, Paccagnini S, Principi N, Pizzocolo G, Caccamo ML, D'Amico E, Cambie G, Vecchi L: Lombardy Study Group Mother-to-infant transmission of hepatitis C virus. Lombardy Study Group on Vertical HCV Transmission. Lancet 1995;345:289-291.

Zimmerman R, Perucchin D, Fauchére J-C, Joller-Jemelka H, Geyer M, Huch R, Huch A. Hepatitis C virus in breast milk. Lancet 1995;345:928.

Zuccotti GV, Ribero ML, Giovannini M, Fasola M, Riva E, Portera G, Biasucci G, Decarlis S, Profeta ML, Tagger A. Effect of hepatitis C genotype on mother-to-infant transmission of virus. J Pediatr 1995;127:278-280.

SECTION VI

CELLULAR AND MOLECULAR BIOLOGY OF MAMMARY GLAND DEVELOPMENT AND LACTATION

MORPHOGENESIS OF MAMMARY GLAND DEVELOPMENT

Russell C. Hovey and Josephine F. Trott

1. ABSTRACT

Development of the mammary gland in females is a dynamic, orchestrated process that occurs throughout postnatal development. Initiated during embryogenesis, epithelial cells advance into the underlying stromal matrix to form a primitive rudimentary structure. With the onset of puberty this anlage then responds to hormonal and local cues to rapidly establish a ductal network. Whereas in mice this network is relatively simple, in humans there is significantly more branching morphogenesis to develop terminal duct lobular unit structures. With the onset of pregnancy and associated changes in the hormonal and local environment, alveolar development progresses to establish a gland that is densely filled with alveolar structures by the end of pregnancy. Concomitantly, mammary epithelial cells within the gland begin to attain their unique ability to synthesize various milk constituents, such that by parturition, functional lactogenesis can be realized.

2. INTRODUCTION

The functional state of the mammary gland is realized when it attains the ability to synthesize and secrete milk following the onset of lactogenesis. However, the mammary gland must develop through distinct postnatal stages before it can reach this state. Several levels of regulation are in place to carefully engineer this process during embryonic and postnatal life. This course of mammary gland development involves marked changes in the proliferation of mammary epithelial cells (MEC) leading to the concomitant formation of parenchymal structures that ultimately are required for milk production. At the same time, these dynamic changes occur within an extracellular stromal matrix that can impart both positive and negative local signals onto proximate MEC. Ultimately these processes are coordinated at the systemic level by key hormones whose levels alternate with reproductive stage.

Lactation and Mammary Gland Biology Group, Department of Animal Science, University of Vermont, 570 Main Street, Burlington, VT 05405

Protecting Infants through Human Milk, edited by Pickering *et al.*
Kluwer Academic/Plenum Publishers, 2004

3. THE STAGES OF MAMMARY GLAND DEVELOPMENT

Mammary gland growth is initiated in the embryo as the result of ectodermal thickening and cell migration to form mammary 'buds' that correspond to the areolus and nipple in the mature female. In the widely studied mouse model this process initiates around embryonic day 11 whereas in humans the process is first evident during the fourth week of embryonic life. Associated with this remodeling are changes in the underlying mesenchyme. In mice this leads to the invagination of mammary buds that become enveloped in several layers of dense connective tissue, while more distally there is a parallel accumulation of a loose, adipose-precursor mesenchyme (Kimata et al. 1985). By the time of birth the epithelial anlage has extended into the adipose tissue of the mammary fat pad (MFP) to become a simply branched ductal rudiment. In humans, the branching of this anlage in utero gives rise to 15 to 25 solid cords that ultimately exit as multiple openings (galactophores) in each nipple (Tobon & Salazar 1974).

In newborn females the mammary rudiment is composed of relatively simple ducts positioned within the subtending mammary stroma. Prior to puberty these structures are relatively dormant, growing at a rate that is isometric with body weight gain (Flux 1954). Following the onset of ovarian function in mice at puberty, MEC undergo extensive proliferation that leads to ductal extension and allometric growth of the mammary parenchyma in association with pronounced morphological changes (see below). Ramification of ductal structures into the MFP continues during recurrent estrous cycles until they reach its bounds, thereby establishing a network of ducts ultimately capable of draining milk to the nipple (Hovey et al. 2002).

The final stage of mammary development involves the formation of sac-like alveolar structures that arise from ducts and function as the principal milk-secreting structures of the mammary gland. During the estrous cycle in nulliparous mice there is a minor degree of alveolar budding within the mammary gland that is strain- and stage of cycle-dependent (Hovey et al. 2002). By contrast, alveolar development in the human breast is variable both within the breast and between individuals (see below). With the onset of pregnancy the mammary gland then enters a period of rapid alveolar proliferation whereby the interductal spaces of the mammary fat pad are displaced by alveoli arranged into discrete lobules, where lobules are arranged into lobes. During the later stages of pregnancy MEC also undergo terminal differentiation (lactogenesis I) whereby they acquire the ability to express milk-specific genes (Robinson et al. 1995). As parturition nears, MEC within the gland continue to proliferate while also being readied for secretory activation and responsiveness to the milk ejection stimulus (Neville et al. 2002).

4. MAMMARY GLAND MORPHOGENESIS

Significant morphologic changes occur in the gland during the process of mammary development. At birth, the epithelial anlage within the MFP of mice is a simple structure that has several branches arising from a single primary sprout, where each duct consists of multiple epithelial layers. With the onset of puberty, MEC in the ducts of mice respond to ovarian secretory activity by initiating rapid proliferation, primarily at their distal tips, in order to facilitate ductal extension (Daniel & Silberstein 1987). This terminal zone of proliferation consequently becomes enlarged and bulbous, and is widely referred to as the 'terminal end bud' (TEB). Several cell type subpopulations can be identified in this structure. The outermost, most distal layer of cells is referred to as the 'cap cell' layer and is a pale-staining, pluripotent population that gives rise to MEC within the body of the end bud as well as contractile myoepithelial cells that surround the subtending duct (Daniel & Silberstein 1987). Within the end bud, considerable tissue remodeling facilitates lumen formation within the subtending duct through a balance of extensive MEC proliferation that occurs concomitant with appreciable apoptosis (Humphreys 1999).

As the mammary ducts in mice extend they also branch into secondary, and then tertiary, ducts in order to fill the interductal spaces of the MFP, but never grow closer than 0.25 mm to each other. Alveolar development represents a separate morphogenetic process that builds upon the ductal framework. Alveoli bud from primary, secondary, and tertiary ducts to a limited extent during the estrous cycle, and then continue this process extensively during pregnancy (Brisken 2002). As each alveolus develops it concomitantly becomes encapsulated in a basketweave of myoepithelial cells. Alveolar development continues during pregnancy to form lobular clusters that, by parturition, almost entirely occupy the gland. Once the suckling stimulus is removed at weaning, alveoli undergo rapid postlactational involution by apoptosis so that within several days the gland's parenchymal morphology in many ways resembles that present in the mature, nulliparous female (Vonderhaar 1984).

The human breast undergoes an appreciably more complex morphogenesis compared with the mouse. At birth, the multiple ductal sprouts in the human breast are characterized by the presence of significantly more lobulation, a distinction that is sustained throughout development (Tobon & Salazar 1974). Around puberty, each of approximately 8 to 15 ductal sprouts undergoes primary extension through the formation of an end bud that likely is analogous to that in the mouse (Russo et al. 2001). However, at the same time the parenchyma displays both branching and alveolar morphogenesis in the form of terminal duct lobular units (TDLUs) that have been described and classified in detail by Russo et al. (Russo & Russo 1987). Developing TDLUs in nulliparous women are composed of clustered, short ductal sprouts (ductules) that continually develop during the progression from lobules type 1 to type 3, showing corresponding increases in their complexity (types 1, 2, and 3 have approximately 11, 47, and 81 ductules, respectively) (Russo et al. 2001). With pregnancy, these TDLU structures become even more dense and complex, generally progressing to TDLUs of types 3 and then 4. This is associated with an increase in MEC volume while terminally differentiated alveoli form and acquire the ability to synthesize and secrete milk constituents. Following involution, type 3 TDLUs predominate within the human breast whereas after menopause there is considerable regression to the TDLU type 1 (Russo et al. 2001).

5. HORMONAL REGULATION OF MAMMARY DEVELOPMENT

As evident from Section 4, mammary development is precisely defined by a female's reproductive stage, and hence is largely under hormonal regulation. While this regulation is complex, the following section outlines the major hormonal effects that occur during different stages of development.

5.1. Sexual Dimorphism and Embryonic Development

One of the earliest hormone-regulated events is sexually-dimorphic ablation of mammary gland development in the male embryo. In mice this involves the action of testosterone on androgen receptor-positive mesenchymal cells that encapsulate the ectodermal bud, causing them to condense around the mammary bud leading either to its destruction or pinching off from the developing nipple (Sakakura 1991). In humans, however, sexual dimorphism does not occur until puberty. Development of the mammary rudiment in female mice and humans is unlikely to depend directly on positive hormonal influences given that females of gene knockout models for the major hormones or their receptors undergo successful development of their mammary glands to the anlage stage (Hovey et al. 2002).

5.2. Ductal Extension

The first major phase of hormonal regulation commences with the onset of ovarian function around puberty, leading to end bud formation and ductal extension in response to increased serum estrogen levels. The importance of estrogen is indicated by the fact that ovariectomy of mice ablates ductal elongation that can be restored by exogenous estrogen (Flux 1954). In addition, estrogen receptor-α knockout mice do not develop a ductal network (Couse & Korach 1999), whereas in pubertal girls, exogenous estrogen clearly stimulates mammary development (Hovey et al. 2002).

The action of estrogen occurs through the transcription-regulating estrogen receptor (ER). In mammary glands of mice, ER are present in body cells but not cap cells of the end bud, in ductal MEC, and in the stroma (Woodward et al. 1998). In fact, the effect of estrogen on stromal cells is critical for ductal extension in mice. By contrast, in the human breast, ER are only expressed by MEC suggesting a direct effect of estrogen on these cells (Anderson et al. 1998). However, in both mice and humans, ER are expressed in a subpopulation of MEC that are nonproliferating (Grimm et al. 2002; Russo et al. 2001).

In addition to estrogen, growth hormone (GH) also serves a critical role in ductal extension. In fact, estrogen-induced ductal extension in mice cannot proceed in the absence of GH, where the combination of estrogen and GH is most efficacious in stimulating ductal growth (Lyons et al. 1958). GH most likely acts upon stromal GH receptors, consistent with its ability to interact with estrogen that also acts on the stroma via stromal ER. Unfortunately, limited information exists concerning the role for GH in human breast development, although a good correlation exists between serum GH and mammary growth during puberty in girls (Rose et al. 1991).

Although it is unclear whether other hormones participate in ductal extension per se, they are probably not critical. For example, we identified that mRNA for both the prolactin receptor (PRLR) and progesterone receptor (PR) is expressed in the ductal end bud (Hovey et al. 2001b). Furthermore, exogenous progesterone administered to ovary-intact female mice induces end bud formation as well as ductal elongation and branching (Atwood et al. 2000), and PR and PRLR are expressed homogeneously in the mammary ducts early in puberty (Hovey et al. 2001b). However, neither the PRLR nor the PR knockout mouse models have impaired ductal extension (Horseman et al. 1997; Ormandy et al. 1997), leaving the precise roles of these hormones unclear. Similarly, follicle-stimulating hormone and luteinizing hormone have been implicated in human breast development during puberty but, again, their exact roles are unclear.

5.3. Branching Morphogenesis

The period of ductal extension is both accompanied by, and then added to, by ductal branching, and both processes are primarily under hormonal regulation during puberty and pregnancy. In mice, one major effector of branching morphogenesis is progesterone. When administered to intact pubertal mice, progesterone induces an increase in ductal branching (Atwood et al. 2000) whereas conversely, female PR knockout mice have impaired ductal branching (Lydon et al. 1995). These findings coincide with the demonstration that PR are homogeneously expressed by MEC prior to puberty, but are then heterogeneously expressed within the ducts beyond 6 yo 7 seeks of age (Hovey et al. 2001b). Interestingly, this timing coincides with the age when exogenous estrogen is able to induce PR in ductal MEC (Woodward et al. 1998). Combined, these data have led to proposals that a subset of MEC are pluripotent in their ability to respond to progesterone through their expression of PR, and respond to progesterone by giving rise to subsequent ductal branching and alveolar development.

Ductal branching also is influenced by estrogen, particularly through its ability to interact with progesterone. Estrogen induces PR expression, where in both mice and humans ER and PR frequently are expressed in the same nonproliferating MEC, leading to suggestions that their ligands evoke their effects via paracrine stimulation. More recent evidence utilizing the α-ER knockout mouse model also indicates that both MEC and stromal ER participate in the regulation of estrogen plus progesterone-induced branching morphogenesis, alveolar development, and induction of PR in MEC (Mueller et al. 2002). Certainly it is clear that estrogen and progesterone cooperatively stimulate this development. While estrogen administered to mice promotes end bud formation, progesterone is without effect on MEC proliferaiton, whereas their combination induces significant MEC proliferation, tertiary branching, and alveolar development (Hovey et al. 2002). Similarly, combined treatment of postmenopausal women with estrogen plus progesterone induces significant lobular development compared with the lesser effects of estrogen, and nonapparent effects of progesterone (Haslam et al. 2002).

Another primary determinant of mammary morphogenesis is prolactin (PRL). Presently it appears unlikely that PRl alone regulates ductal branching per se given results from PRL- and PRLR-knockout models, although exogenous PRL does induce proliferation by MEC in sexually immature and mature female mice (Hovey et al. 2001b). Furthermore, we identified that as for PR, mRNA for PRLR is homogeneously expressed in MEC of the mammary gland prior to puberty, and thereafter becomes heterogeneously distributed in the same pattern as PR. Based on these observations we subsequently demonstrated a cooperative, synergistic effect of progesterone and PRL on ductal branch growth and MEC proliferation (Hovey et al. 2001b). These results therefore suggest that, as for estrogen and progesterone above, progesterone acting in concert with PRL also can facilitate ductal branching morphogenesis in mice.

Currently there is only limited information concerning the precise hormonal regulation of branching morphogenesis in humans. MEC within TDLU type 1 have a higher proliferation rate than those in types 2 or 3, and more of their MEC are ER and PR positive (Russo et al. 2001). While human MEC show maximal DNA synthesis during the luteal phase when levels of progesterone are high, breast tissue heterografted to mice is unresponsive to progesterone either alone or with supplemental estrogen (Laidlaw et al. 1995). There is also the potential for PRL regulation of lobule development given the effects of PRL on the mammary glands of mice and in human breast cancer. Along these lines, we have recently identified several new forms of the hPRLR that arise from splicing to a novel exon 11 (Trott et al. 2003). Two of these isoforms (PRLRSF1a and 1b) function as dominant-negatives to the long form of the PRLR, thereby inhibiting its signaling for milk protein gene transcription. These isoforms are distinct in both their ability to bind ligand and to function as a dominant negative receptor. A third isoform, Δ 7/11, is unique in that it contains the PRLR extracellular domain but no transmembrane domain that results in its secretion as a PRL binding protein (Trott et al. 2003). While the full biological significance of these new isoforms remains to be established, they are expressed in both normal and cancerous breast tissue and, hence, may regulate effects of PRL on the breast during normal development.

5.4. Alveolar Development

Once mammary ducts and branches are established, alveolar development can occur in response to hormonal influences during the estrous cycle, then proceeds extensively during pregnancy (Brisken 2002). This development continues to respond to estrogen and progesterone, where their combination stimulates significant alveologenesis in mice. Data from knockout studies indicate that the actions of PR are indispensable for alveolar development (Lydon et al. 1999), whereas ER-α appears not to be essential (Mueller et al. 2002).

There is also an essential role for PRL during alveologenesis, as demonstrated by both PRLR and PRL knockout mouse models (Horseman et al. 1997; Ormandy et al. 1997). Likewise, when PRL is provided to the mammary gland through pituitary isografts in vivo or in whole organ culture in vitro, extensive alveolar development results. This response is first initiated in pregnant mice by postcoital surges of PRL secretion during the first 8 to 10 days of pregnancy.

Alveolar development ultimately is coordinated by the actions of multiple hormones. This most clearly is indicated by demonstration that in hormone-ablated mice, the minimum requirement for lobulo-alveolar development is a combination of estrogen, progesterone, adrenal corticoid, and prolactin or growth hormone, where the presence of both these pituitary hormones facilitates greater alveolar development than either alone (Lyons et al. 1958). In an in vitro whole organ culture environment, greatest hormonal stimulation of lobulo-alveolar development is achieved using a combination of insulin, aldosterone, and PRL either with or without GH (Ichinose & Nandi 1966).

It is not precisely clear which hormones regulate alveolar development in humans, although it is likely that a similar combination to those detailed above is involved. Further work is essential in this area if human lactation is to be more precisely understood.

6. THE MAMMARY STROMA

Up to this point this review has focused on the MEC population and its proliferation and morphogenesis. In reviewing this, however, the role of nonepithelial elements must also be considered. In mice, MEC commence development during embryogenesis in a bed of mesenchymal cells. These ultimately give rise to a depot of white adipose tissue, the MFP, in which ductal and alveolar development subsequently occurs (Hovey et al. 1999). At the same time the MFP supports extensive lymphatic and vascular networks (Hovey et al. 1999).

It has become clear that the stroma is a major determinant of mammary development. For example, mouse MEC will only develop to their full potential in the MFP. The MFP is a major target of hormones including estrogen, GH, and PRL that exert effects on various constituents of the MFP (Hovey et al. 1999, 2001b). At the same time the MFP is also a major source of extracellular matrix and growth factors (see below) that impart significant effects on MEC proliferation and morphogenesis.

By comparison, the stromal matrix in humans contains considerably more connective tissue that separates MEC from directly interacting with adipocytes. Indeed, in addition to adipose tissue, two stromal connective tissues can be identified; a less-dense interlobular stroma and a denser intralobular stroma that have significantly different collagen content. This distinction between the stroma of mice and humans also parallels differences in parenchymal histomorphology and appears to indicate specific functions of the stroma across species (Hovey et al. 2001b). When human MEC were transplanted into the mouse MFP, they were unable to develop normally, whereas the parallel introduction of human mammary fibroblasts supported normal growth of human MEC in mice (Parmar et al. 2002).

In both mice and humans the mammary stroma undergoes significant changes during development. As TEB advance into the MFP, stromal cells proliferate and respond by reorganizing, a phenomenon similarly recorded in breast cancer (Hovey et al. 1999). During the menstrual cycle in humans the stroma also shows marked changes in its density. Ultimately, however, in both mice and humans the MFP becomes largely occupied by alveoli during pregnancy, reflecting the depletion of lipid from adipocytes and the remodeling of connective tissues.

7. LOCALLY DERIVED FACTORS

As discussed above, several notable hormones evoke marked changes within the mammary glands. However, these hormones do not necessarily act on the target MEC population to directly elicit a response, but rather achieve diverse responses through their ability to induce locally derived autocrine/paracrine growth factors.

One of the first of such molecules to receive considerable attention was insulin-like growth factor (IGF)-I. A known mitogen and effector of GH action in various tissues, IGF-I subsequently was identified as being induced by GH in the rodent mammary gland, and later, more specifically in stromal cells of the MFP (Kleinberg et al. 2000). This induction of IGF-I by GH is also enhanced by estrogen treatment (Kleinberg et al. 2000). Parallel studies showed that exogenous IGF-I could induce TEB formation, raising the likelihood that IGF-I was a primary mediator of GH- and estrgoen-induced ductal extension. Indeed, the stimulation of ductal extension by GH-induced, stroma-derived IGF-I has been confirmed recently using various genetic models (see Hadsell 2004; this volume).

Other stroma-derived factors have been implicated as mediators of hormone action on the mammary gland. The actions of estrogen can be linked to the local synthesis of potent mitogens such as transforming growth factor-α and hepatocyte growth factor (HGF). While the link between the action of estrogen on ductal growth and the local production of HGF is still tenuous, HGF has pronounced effects on ductal branching morphogenesis and extension that are consistent with this proposal (Zhang et al. 2002).

Most recently, we along with others have examined whether similar locally derived factors facilitate the effects of PRL in the mammary gland. Indeed it appears that IGF-II, a molecule similar to, yet distinct from, IGF-I functions as a local effector of PRL action during alveolar development (Hovey et al. 2003). Combined with findings for IGF-I, evolutionarily similar GH and PRL appear to have achieved the ability to signal distinct effects (ductal extension and alveolar development, respectively) through the differential induction of specific IGF family members in the mammary gland.

In addition to the parenchymal and stromal changes that occur in the mammary gland as outlined above, there is considerable parallel development of the vascular network. During ductal development, vessels grow and branch and then form a dense and intricate capillary bed during pregnancy and lactation (Djonov et al. 2001). Recently we have been investigating aspects of angiogenesis in the mammary gland by examining the expression of a potent regulator of endothelial cell function—vascular endothelial growth factor (VEGF). During development, specific isoforms of VEGF are expressed in the mammary stroma while during later stages the expression of one isoform, VEGF188, is down-regulated due to epithelial occupation of the MFP (Hovey et al. 2001a). Following parturition there is a notable up-regulation of VEGF expression in the mammary gland that corresponds to expression of VEGF by MEC, likely inducing the recruitment and permeability of capillaries in response to nutrient needs of MEC for milk synthesis.

Regulation of angiogenesis in the developing human breast is less well characterized, although it clearly shows developmental changes. Surrounding type 1 lobules is appreciable vascularization that decreases with stage of lobule development, indicating that the active growth sites and increased steroid receptivity in lobules type 1 is matched by increased blood supply (Russo et al. 2001). Given the clear role for blood flow in both lactation and human breast cancer, further information is necessary to provide a better understanding in this area.

8. ACKNOWLEDGMENTS

We would like to sincerely thank Dr. Barbara K. Vonderhaar, Anita Goldhar, and Erika Ginsburg of the National Institutes of Health for ongoing assistance and stimulating discussion.

9. REFERENCES

Anderson E, Clarke RB, Howell A. Estrogen responsiveness and control of normal human breast proliferation. J Mammary Gland Biol Neoplasia 1998;3:23-35.

Atwood CS, Hovey RC, Glover JP, Chepko G, Ginsburg E, Robison WG, Vonderhaar BK. Progesterone induces side-branching of the ductal epithelium in the mammary glands of peripubertal mice. J Endocrinol 2000;167:39-52.

Brisken C. Hormonal control of alveolar development and its implications for breast carcinogenesis. J Mammary Gland Biol Neoplasia 2002;7:39-48.

Couse JF, Korach KS. Estrogen receptor null mice: what have we learned and where will they lead us? Endocr Rev 1999;20:358-417.

Daniel CW, Silberstein G. Postnatal development of the rodent mammary gland. In: Neville MC, Daniel CW, editors. The Mammary Gland: Development, Regulation, and Function. New York: Plenum Press, 1987; pp 3-36.

Djonov V, Andres AC, Ziemiecki A. Vascular remodelling during the normal and malignant life cycle of the mammary gland. Microsc Res Tech 2001;52:182-189.

Flux DS. Growth of the mammary duct system in intact and ovariectomized mice of the chi strain. J Endocrinol 1954;11:223-237.

Grimm SL, Seagroves TN, Kabotyanski EB, Hovey RC, Vonderhaar BK, Lydon JP, Miyoshi K, Hennighausen L, Ormandy CJ, Lee AV, Stull MA, Wood TL, Rosen JM. Disruption of steroid and prolactin receptor patterning in the mammary gland correlates with a block in lobuloalveolar development. Mol Endocrinol 2002;16:2675-2691.

Hadsell DL. Genetic manipulation of mammary gland development and lacation. In: Pickering LK, Morrow AL, Ruiz-Palacios GM, Schanler RJ. Protecting Infants through Human Milk: Advancing the Scientific Evidence. Advances in Experimental Medicine and Biology Series. New York: Kluwer Academic/Plenum Publishers, 2004; this volume.

Haslam SZ, Osuch JR, Raafat AM, Hofseth LJ. Postmenopausal hormone replacement therapy: effects on normal mammary gland in humans and in a mouse postmenopausal model. J Mammary Gland Biol Neoplasia 2002;7:93-105.

Horseman ND, Zhao W, Montecino-Rodriquez E, Tanaka M, Nakashima K, Engle SJ, Smith F, Markoff E, Dorskind K. Defective mammopoiesis, but normal hematopoiesis, in mice with a targeted disruption of the prolactin gene. EMBO J 1997;16:6926-6935.

Hovey RC, McFadden TB, Akers RM. Regulation of mammary gland growth and morphogenesis by the mammary fat pad: a species comparison. J Mammary Gland Biol Neoplasia 1999;4:53-68.

Hovey RC, Goldhar AS, Baffi J, Vonderhaar BK. Transcriptional regulation of vascular endothelial growth factor expression in epithelial and stromal cells during mouse mammary gland development. Mol Endocrinol 2001a;15:819-831.

Hovey RC, Trott JF, Ginsburg E, Goldhar A, Sasaki MM, Fountain SJ, Sundararajan K, Vonderhaar BK. Transcriptional and spatiotemporal regulation of prolactin receptor mRNA and cooperativity with progesterone receptor function during ductal branch growth in the mammary gland. Dev Dyn 2001b;222:192-205.

Hovey RC, Trott JF, Vonderhaar BK. Establishing a framework for the functional mammary gland: from endocrinology to morphology. J Mammary Gland Biol Neoplasia 2002;7:17-38.

Hovey RC, Harris J, Hadsell DL, Lee AV, Ormandy CJ, Vonderhaar BK. Local insulin-like growth factor-II mediates prolactin-induced mammary gland development. Mol Endocrinol 2003;17:460-471.

Humphreys RC. Programmed cell death in the terminal end bud. J Mammary Gland Biol Neoplasia 1999;4:213-220.

Ichinose RR, Nandi S. Influence of hormones on lobulo-alveolar differentiation of mouse mammary glands in vitro. J Endocrinol 1966;35:331-340.

Kimata K, Sakakura T, Inaguma Y, Kato M, Nishizuka Y. Participation of two different mesenchymes in the developing mouse mammary gland: synthesis of basement membrane components by fat pad precursor cells. J Embryol Exp Morphol 1985;89:243-257.

Kleinberg DL, Feldman M, Ruan W. IGF-I: an essential factor in terminal end bud formation and ductal morphogenesis. J Mammary Gland Biol Neoplasia 2000;5:7-17.

Laidlaw IJ, Clarke RB, Howell A, Owen WMC, Potten CS, Anderson E. Proliferation of normal human breast tissue implanted in athymic nude mice is stimulated by estrogen and not progesterone. Endocrinology 1995;136:164-171.

Lydon JP, DeMayo FJ, Funk CR, Mani SK, Hughes AR, Montgomery CA Jr, Shyamala G, Conneely OM, O'Malley BW. Mice lacking progesterone receptor exhibit pleiotropic reproductive abnormalities. Genes Dev 1995;9:2266-2278.

Lydon JP, Ge G, Kittrell FS, Medina O, O'Malley BW. Murine mammary gland carcinogenesis is critically dependent on progesterone receptor function. Cancer Res 1999;59:4276-4284.

Lyons WR, Li CH, Johnson RE. The hormonal control of mammary growth and lactation. Recent Prog Horm Res 1958;14:219-254.

Mueller SO, Clark JA, Myers PH, Korach KS. Mammary gland development in adult mice requires epithelial and stromal estrogen receptor alpha. Endocrinology 2002;143:2357-2365.

Neville MC, McFadden TB, Forsyth I. Hormonal regulation of mammary differentiation and milk secretion. J Mammary Gland Biol Neoplasia 2002;7;49-66.

Ormandy CJ, Camus A, Barra J, Damotte D, Lucas B, Buteau H, Edery M, Brousse N, Babinet C, Binart N, Kelly PA. Null mutation of the prolactin receptor gene produces multiple reproductive defects in the mouse. Genes Dev 1997;11:167-178.

Parmar H, Young P, Emerman JT, Neve RM, Dairkee S, Cunha GR. A novel method for growing human breast epithelium in vivo using mouse and human mammary fibroblasts. Endocrinology 2002;143:4886-4896.

Robinson GW, McKnight RA, Smith GH, Hennighausen L. Mammary epithelial cells undergo secretory differentiation in cycling virgins but require pregnancy for the establishment of terminal differentiation. Development 1995;121:2079-2090.

Rose SR, Municchi G, Barnes KM, Kamp GA, Uriarte MM, Ross JL, Cassorla F, Cutler GB Jr. Spontaneous growth hormone secretion increases during puberty in normal girls and boys. J Clin Endocrinol Metab 1991;73:428-435.

Russo J, Russo IH. Development of the human mammary gland. In: Neville MC, Daniel CW, editors. The Mammary Gland: Development, Regulation, and Function. New York: Plenum Press, 1987; pp 67-93.

Russo J, Hu YF, Silva IDCG, Russo IH. Cancer risk related to mammary gland structure and development. Microsc Res Tech 2001;52:204-223.

Sakakura T. New aspects of stroma-parenchyma relations in mammary gland differentiation. Int Rev Cytol 1991;125:165-202.

Tobon H, Salazar H. Ultrastructure of the human mammary gland. I. Development of the fetal gland throughout gestation. J Clin Endocrinol Metab 1974;39:443-456.

Trott JF, Hovey RC, Koduri S, Vonderhaar BK. Alternative splicing to exon 11 of human prolactin receptor gene results in multiple isoforms including a secreted prolactin binding protein. J Mol Endocrinol 2003;30:31-47.

Vonderhaar BK. Hormones and growth factors in mammary gland development. In: Veneziale CM, editor. Control of Cell Growth and Proliferation. New York: Van Noostrand, Reinhold, 1984; pp 11-33.

Woodward TL, Xie JW, Haslam SZ. The role of mammary stroma in modulating the proliferative response to ovarian hormones in the normal mammary gland. J Mammary Gland Biol Neoplasia 1998;3:117-131.

Zhang HZ, Bennett JM, Smith KT, Sunil N, Haslam SZ. Estrogen mediates mammary epithelial cell proliferation in serum-free culture indirectly via mammary stroma-derived hepatocyte growth factor. Endocrinology 2002;143:3427-3434.

GENETIC MANIPULATION OF MAMMARY GLAND DEVELOPMENT AND LACTATION

Darryl L. Hadsell

1. ABSTRACT

The mammalian genome is believed to contain some 30,000 to 40,000 different genes. Of these an estimated 42% have no known function. Genetically engineered mouse models (GEMM) have been a powerful tool available for determining gene function in vivo. In the mammary gland, a variety of genetic engineering approaches have been applied successfully to understanding the importance of specific gene products to mammary gland development and lactation. Our own laboratory has applied genetically engineered mice to facilitate understanding of the regulation of mammary gland development and lactation by insulin-like growth factors (IGF) and by the transcription factor, upstream stimulatory factor (USF-2). Our studies on transgenic mice that overexpress IGF-I have demonstrated the importance of IGF-dependent signaling pathways to maintenance of mammary epithelial cells during the declining phase of lactation. Our analysis of early developmental processes in mammary tissue from mice that carry a targeted mutation in the IGF-I receptor gene suggests that IGF-dependent stimulation of cell cycle progression is more important to early mammary gland development than potential antiapoptotic effects. Lastly, our studies on mice that carry a targeted mutation of the *Usf2* gene have demonstrated that this gene is necessary for normal lactation and have highlighted the importance of this gene to the maintenance of protein synthesis. These studies, as well as studies of others, have highlighted both the strengths and limitations inherent in the use of GEMM. Limitations serve as the driving force behind development of new experimental strategies and genetic engineering schemes that will allow for a full understanding of gene function within the mammary gland.

The USDA/ARS Children's Nutrition Research Center, Department of Pediatrics, Baylor College of Medicine, 1100 Bates Street, Suite 10072, Houston TX 77030

Protecting Infants through Human Milk, edited by Pickering *et al.*
Kluwer Academic/Plenum Publishers, 2004

2. INTRODUCTION

One of the most important goals for lactation biology has been to understand the factors that determine milk yield. This goal has been a longstanding one in the arena of dairy production, and also has had increased support in the area of human lactation. Increasing the rates of breastfeeding initiation and duration is a national health objective and one of the goals of Healthy People 2000 (Working Group on Breastfeeding 1997) and 2010. The target is to "increase to at least 75% the proportion of mothers who breastfeed their babies in the early postpartum period and to at least 50% the proportion who continue breastfeeding until their babies are 5 to 6 months old." As of 2001, these proportions were at 69.5% and 32.5%, respectively (Ryan et al. 2002). This is well below the above goal and suggests that a large percentage of women in the United States is incapable of establishing a normal lactation. However, even during a "normal" lactation tremendous variations have been observed in both milk volume and milk composition and while these variations are of course most dramatic across species (Oftedal 1984), they also are quite spectacular within species.

Within the mouse, even in the same strain, milk volume varies by as much as 5-fold (Johnson MS et al. 2001). In humans, milk volume has been reported to vary by 1.5- to 2.9-fold (Cox et al. 1996; Butte et al. 1984). In Holstein dairy cows during the year 2001, milk volume was found to vary by as much as 10-fold (http://aipl.arsusda.gov). There are many reasons for such variation, but genetics is one important reason. The importance of genetic components to this variation is quite clear from the demonstration that genetic selection strategies have been successful at influencing milk volume or overall lactational performance (Hansen 2000; Nagai & Sarkar 1978). In addition, a number of groups have identified potential quantitative trait loci (QTL) important to milk yield, milk composition, or lactational performance in both dairy animals and mice (Peripato et al. 2002; Grisart et al. 2002; Arranz et al. 1998). On the basis of these types of studies, genetic contribution to the variation in milk yield and composition has been suggested to range from 27% to 55% and continued efforts are in progress to refine the QTL mapping to the point where specific genes can be identified.

In the year 2000 the human genome sequence was first published in draft form (Venter et al. 2001). Following this initial report, a completed genome sequence has now been reported for the mouse, and preliminary data have been obtained on the genome sequence of the cow (Waterston et al. 2002; Adam 2002). The analysis of the data resulting from this Herculean effort produced a number of novel findings about the biology of humans, but also produced a number of new tools, not the least of which is the sequence and location of some 30,000 to 40,000 genes. Of these genes, an estimated 42% have not yet been assigned a function. Some of this information will come from development and application of haplotype maps (Wiltshire et al. 2003; Johnson GC et al. 2001; Daly et al. 2001). However, the use of reverse genetic models also will be necessary to establish a full understanding of newly identified genes. This review will summarize the current state of knowledge concerning the application of genetically engineered mouse models (GEMM) to the analysis of normal mammary gland development and lactation. I will highlight examples of work from our own laboratory on the IGF system and on a bHLH/zip transcription factor, upstream stimulatory factor 2.

3. GENETICALLY ENGINEERED MOUSE MODELS (GEMM): A BRIEF HISTORY

The GEMM has been a part of the biologist's tool kit for almost a quarter of a century. The first reported creation of a transgenic mouse occurred in 1980 (Gordon et al. 1980). Shortly after this, in 1982, the power of transgenesis was illustrated by the dramatically increased growth observed in mice overexpressing human growth hormone (Palmiter et al. 1982). Within the few short years that followed this initial report, a number of groups began to apply this technology to problems of biomedical interest such as thalasemia, diabetes, and cancer (Lacy et al. 1983; Lacy & Costantini 1983; van der Putten et al. 1984; Brinster et al. 1984). In 1984 the first transgenic model of breast cancer was described based on the use of the MMTV-LTR (Stewart et al. 1984). Shortly after this, reports also appeared using mammary-specific milk protein gene promoters for genes such as the whey acidic protein (WAP) and the β-casein (Andres et al. 1987; Lee et al. 1988). At about this same time in the late 1980s techniques were being developed to mutate or ablate specific gene targets in mice through the use of homologous recombination (Thomas & Capecchi 1987). The first heterozygous mutant mouse strains produced through these techniques were reported in 1989 (Thompson et al. 1989; Schwartzberg et al. 1989; Zijlstra et al. 1989). Within a year, it became clear that with some genes, germline targeting would result in early lethality that could limit application of this approach to postnatal developmental processes (Sawai et al. 1991; Lufkin et al. 1991). In addition, lethality as well as infertility also were recognized as limitations to transgenic approaches (Stacey et al. 1988; Covarrubias et al. 1986; Soriano et al. 1987; Ornitz et al. 1991). These observations served as the driving force behind development of binary transgenic systems (Byrne & Ruddle 1989; Ornitz et al. 1991). Several systems, based on the use of transcriptional activators from bacteria, viruses, or insects have been developed that allow for both tissue-specific and temporal regulation of transgene expression in mice (Epstein-Baak et al. 1992; No et al. 1996; Furth et al. 1994; Wang et al. 1997). The most widely used of these is the tetracycline-transactivator system (Gossen & Bujard 2002). Along with these transgenic systems, the knowledge on site-specific recombinases from yeast and bacteriophage was being applied to develop systems that would allow for tissue-specific gene deletions (Lakso et al. 1992; Dymecki 2003). The Cre/LOX system has found wide use in study of the mammary gland (Wagner et al. 2001). Based on these developments, there are about six different types of genetic approaches that are being used to manipulate gene expression in the mouse mammary gland. These include: 1) targeted germline mutations; 2) mammary specific transgenes; 3) tissue specific, condition, gene deletion; 4) inducible transgenes; 5) transgenic expression of dominant negative gene products; and 6) mammary epithelial transplants established from transgenic or mutant mice. In addition, advances with a phenomenon known as RNAi have added to this repertoire a seventh technique that may revolutionize the creation of targeted deficiencies in gene expression. The application of these techniques to mammary gland development and lactation is discussed below.

4. APPLICATIONS OF GEMM MAMMARY GLAND DEVELOPMENT

The application of GEMM to early mammary gland development began with studies in the breast cancer field. In these studies the mouse mammary tumor virus long terminal repeat (MMTV) was used to target the expression of oncogenes to the mammary glands of virgin mice (Stewart et al. 1984; Sinn et al. 1987; Muller et al. 1988). In addition to the noted abilities of the overexpressed oncogenes to cause mammary tumors, several of these early studies also reported profound effects on early mammary gland development (Guy et al. 1992; Lin et al. 1992; Tsukamoto et al. 1988). The application of knockout mice to studies in early mammary gland development started with three reports. The first focused on estrogen action and described the effects of targeted deletion of the estrogen receptor on a variety of organ systems in mice (Korach 1994). The second demonstrated loss of cyclin D1 impaired pregnancy-dependent mammary gland development (Sicinski et al. 1995). The third demonstrated the importance of the src proto-oncogene to mammary tumorigenesis by crossing src-null mice to transgenic mice that overexpressed polyomavirus middle t under the control of MMTV (Guy et al. 1996). Following these reports a number of studies were published analyzing the impact of various germline mutations on mammary gland development in mice. Among these were the genes for progesterone receptor, estrogen receptor, prolactin receptor, p-cadherin, inhibin βB and the receptor tyrosine phosphatase, LAR (Ormandy et al. 1997; Humphreys et al. 1997; Radice et al. 1997; Robinson & Hennighausen 1997; Schaapveld et al. 1997; Cunha et al. 1997). A number of these studies also illustrated the importance of mammary tissue transplantation as a way to study mutant mammary epithelium within the context of a wild type host (Cunha et al. 1997; Humphreys et al. 1997; Robinson & Hennighausen 1997). Mammary tissue transplantation has been a useful technique in the cancer biology field for over 40 years (DeOme et al. 1959). By applying this approach to germline mutants, scientists have not only been able to rescue epithelium from null animals that exhibited infertility or early lethality, but also more clearly define the roles of mammary stroma and epithelium in ductal development through the use of tissue recombination (Cunha et al. 1997). Our own work on mammary development has combined the use of tissue transplantation to understand the actions of IGF-I during mammary ductal development.

5. IGF-I ACTIONS ON EARLY MAMMARY GLAND DEVELOPMENT

IGF-I belongs to a class of peptides known as the insulin (Insl) family. This family consisted of at least ten members: insulin, IGF-I, IGF-II, relaxin H1, relaxin H2, relaxin 3, relaxin-like factor, Placentin, INSL5, and INSL6 (Lok et al. 2000; Ivell & Bathgate 2002). This family is characterized by a three-domain structure possessing conserved cysteine motifs (Lok et al. 2000). Of these, insulin, IGF-I, and IGF-II are the most closely related at the amino acid level and constitute a subgroup of the family that interacts with two well-characterized tetrameric receptor tyrosine kinases, the insulin and IGF-I receptors. The remainder of the family members appear to more closely resemble relaxin, which is now known to interact with a G-protein coupled receptor (Hsu et al. 2002). IGF-I has been thought to play a role in normal mammary gland development and lactation for a number of years. Several reviews have been published on the actions of this growth factor system in the mammary gland (Hadsell et al. 2002; Hadsell & Bonnette 2000; Wood et al. 2000; Kleinberg et al. 2000; Flint et al. 2000).

Much of the work on IGF-I action in the mammary gland was stimulated by a handful of early observations on the actions of growth hormone. The importance of growth hormone to normal mammary gland development in pubertal mice was first established by the work of Lyons and coworkers (1958) and Nandi (1958). The work of Salmon and Daughaday (1957) on growth hormone (GH) action in cartilage led to the formulation of the somatomedin hypothesis and the ultimate identification of IGF-I and -II (VanWyk et al. 1971; Rinderknecht & Humbel 1978a, 1978b; Dulak & Temin 1972; Marquardt et al. 1981). In the mammary gland, the first indication that IGF-I could mediate GH action came with the observation that expression of the mRNA for this growth factor was elevated following treatment with estrogen and GH (Kleinberg et al. 1990). This observation was then followed by the finding that localized administration of exogenous IGF-I to the mammary gland stimulated ductal development and increased the number and size of mammary terminal end buds (TEB) (Ruan et al. 1992). These effects of IGF-I subsequently were shown to depend on the presence of estradiol (Ruan et al. 1995). Most importantly, analysis of IGF-I null mice demonstrated that loss of IGF-I dramatically diminished mammary ductal development (Ruan & Kleinberg 1999). In addition, ductal development in these mice could be effectively restored by administration of both estradiol and IGF-I, but not with estradiol alone, suggesting that the effect of the IGF-I null allele was mediated by direct effects of IGF-I on the mammary epithelium. The results demonstrated the importance of IGF-I to mammary ductal development but stopped short of defining the mechanism through which IGF-I acts.

Because IGFs and insulin possess a high degree of sequence similarity and because these ligands interact both with their own and each other's receptors, it was important to determine the importance of IGF-IR and IR to mammary gland development. Reports of mice homozygous for germline deletions in the IGF-IR (*Igf1r*$^{-/-}$) and IR (*IR*$^{-/-}$) failed to survive for very long after birth (Baker et al. 1997; Accili et al. 1996). At birth, *Igf1r*$^{-/-}$ mice were shown to weigh only 30% of their wild type siblings and die within minutes. In contrast *Ir*$^{-/-}$ mice had normal birth weights, but died within days of birth due to metabolic abnormalities. To study the impact of these gene deletions on mammary gland development transplantation studies had to be conducted (Bonnette & Hadsell 2001; Hadsell et al. 2000; Robinson et al. 2000). In both cases mammary tissue was taken from mid- to late-gestation fetuses and transplanted into the cleared inguinal fat pads of 3-week-old recipient female mice. For IR, the work of Robinson and coworkers (2000) demonstrated that loss of this receptor had only a mildly negative effect on mammary gland development and little effect on expression of the milk protein genes at day 1 of lactation. In contrast, work in our laboratory demonstrated that complete loss of IGF-IR causes a profound decrease in the extent of mammary ductal development (Bonnette & Hadsell 2001). In grafts harvested from virgin recipients, this diminished development was associated with decreases in branching and decreases in both the number and size of TEB. In addition, complete loss of IGF-IR in these grafts results in decreased cell proliferation within the TEB, with no effect on epithelial cell death. We also observed that pregnancy was capable of dramatically increasing the extent of ductal development to *Igf1r*$^{-/-}$ grafts (Fig. 1A, B). This increased development was associated with a 2-fold increase in TEB cell proliferation (Fig. 1C). Despite this, mammary development was never fully restored to normal, and cell proliferation rates in ductal and alveolar epithelium were still below that observed in *Igfr1*$^{+/+}$ grafts. Interestingly, grafts prepared from *Igf1r*$^{+/-}$ mammary tissue had no defect in the overall extent of development but did display decreased branching and increased cell death when harvested from virgin recipients. These observations support the conclusion that IGF-IR is an important component in the regulation of mammary ductal development. The observations also suggest that the IGF-IR may act in qualitatively different ways on ductal epithelium and TEBs. The important questions that remain, however, are: 1) what signaling mechanism does the IGF-IR use to regulate mammary ductal development? and 2) can differences in

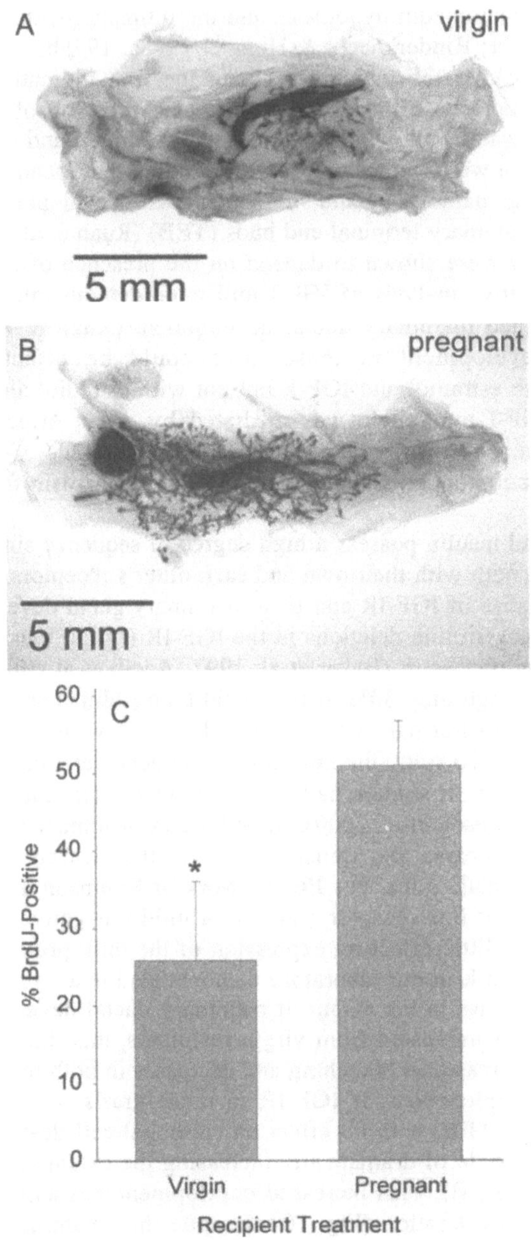

Figure 1. Pregnancy enhances ductal development and mammary cell proliferations in grafts of IGF-IR null epithelium. Grafts were established from mammary anlagen or day-16 female mouse fetuses as described previously (Bonnette & Hadsell 2001). The grafts were allowed to develop for four weeks in either a virgin recipient (A) or a recipient that was mated and allowed to go through 10 days of pregnancy (B). Each recipient was injected with bromodeoxyuridine (BrdU) 2 h prior to the collection of the grafts. TEB cell proliferation as measured by immunohistochemistry for BrdU was then compared among grafts harvested from virgin or pregnant recipients (C). The asterisk indicates a statistically significant difference ($P<0.05$). Each bar represents the mean±SEM for 4 to 6 grafts.

the responses of the epithelium to IGF-IR activation be accounted for by differential use of these signaling pathways? To address these questions, we have taken two approaches. The first relies on the use of IHC to analyze the expression of signaling proteins that are thought to mediate actions of IGF-IR. The second has relied again on the use of GEMM that display altered expression of specific IGF-IR signaling proteins.

Insulin receptor substrates (IRS) belong to the class of scaffolding proteins and have been demonstrated to serve as substrates for both the insulin and IGF-I receptors. Of the family members that have been demonstrated to date, two of these, IRS-1 and -2, are necessary for insulin and IGF action (Araki et al. 1994; Withers et al. 1998; Kubota et al. 2000). This is illustrated by the observation that IRS-1 knockout mice display reduced growth and mild insulin resistance, while IRS-2 knockout mice display more severe insulin resistance, but no growth defect. The third and fourth members of the IRS family (IRS-3 and -4) do not appear to be essential in and of themselves (Fantin et al. 2001; Liu et al. 1999), but may provide for redundancy in some organs (Laustsen et al. 2002).

Only a handful of observations have been made on the functions of IRS proteins in normal mammary cells. Studies on primary cultures of mouse mammary cells have demonstrated that the ability of insulin or IGF-I to inhibit apoptosis is associated with increased phosphorylation of IRS-1 (Farrelly et al. 1999). Our studies on the expression of IRS-1 and -2 in the mammary gland have shown that these proteins are dramatically increased with the onset of lactation, can be induced by exogenous prolactin, and are lost during forced mammary involution (Lee et al. 2003; Hadsell et al. 2001; Hovey et al. 2002). In addition, through both immunohistochemistry and immunofluorescence, we have demonstrated that IRS-1 and -2 have a unique pattern of expression within the TEB (Lee et al. 2003). For IRS-1, expression was observed in a punctate pattern within body cells but not cap cells. For IRS-2, the expression was uniform across both body and cap cells. At present, the significance of these differences in expression pattern are unclear. We also have analyzed mammary gland development in virgin IRS-1 null mice and find that ductal morphogenesis is normal (Lee et al. 2003). These observations support the conclusion that IRS-1 is likely not an important mediator of IGF-IR action in the TEB. However, much remains to be done on the subject of IGF-IR signaling in the TEB. Specifically, the actions of IRS-2, as well as a number of other candidate signaling proteins such as Akt and Erk, remain to be tested. In addition, the role of these signaling proteins in other stages of mammary gland development is just beginning to be described.

6. APPLICATION OF GEMM TO LACTATION

The use of GEMM as tools to understand the regulation of lactation developed out of the biotechnology field. This development was motivated by three ideas. The first idea was that pharmaceutical grade proteins might be produced in large amounts by harnessing the biosynthetic capacity of the mammary gland and using it as a bioreactor. The first example of this was published in 1987 with the reported overexpression of β-lactoglobulin in milk of transgenic mice (Simons et al. 1987). Shortly following were reports describing the overexpresion of tissue plasminogen activator and a soluble form of an human immunodeficiency virus receptor, CD4 (Pittius et al. 1988; Yu et al. 1989). To date, a wide array of proteins have now been produced in milk of transgenic animals and a number of review articles have been published describing the state of this technology (Clark 1998; Vilotte 2002; Houdebine 2000). The second idea underlying the use of GEMM during lactation was that the nutritional quality of milk could be altered or enhanced (Bremel et al. 1989). Much of the work in this area has involved the alteration of α-lactalbumin to reduce milk water content (L'Huillier et al. 1996; Soulier et al. 1999; Stinnakre et al. 1994; Stacey et al. 1995). However, work also has been done on modifying the milk proteins themselves and, more recently, success also has been demonstrated in the manipulation of milk fat content (Schwertfeger et al. 2003; Gutierrez et al. 1996; Gutierrez-Adan et al. 1996). The last idea motivating the application of transgenic approaches to lactation was that overall milk yield might be improved through such approaches. In this area, there have also been some successes both in mice and animals of agricultural importance (Noble et al. 2002; Iavnilovitch et al. 2002). Unfortunately, a survey of the literature on this subject demonstrates that there are many more examples of genetic manipulations that impair lactation than there are of those that enhance lactation. Although the reason for this discrepancy is unclear, it suggests that either more work is needed on the application of GEMM to the enhancement of lactation, or that it is much easier to impair normal lactation than it is to improve it. Our own work on genetic manipulation of lactation has focused on two areas: 1) IGF-I action, and 2) the bHLH-zip protein USF-2.

7. IGF-I ACTIONS DURING LACTATION

Our work on IGF-I action during lactation was motivated primarily by the connection between GH and lactation and between GH and IGF-I. The ability of GH to increase milk yield is well documented in dairy animals (Peel et al. 1981). In addition, GH is required for normal lactation, and under certain circumstances exogenous GH can enhance lactation in rodents (Madon et al. 1986; Capuco et al. 1999). Because IGF-I was believed to mediate many of the actions of GH, it was reasonable to hypothesize that transgenic overexpression of IGF-I within the mammary gland during lactation would enhance milk synthesis. To target the expression of IGF-I to the mammary gland we constructed a minigene construct using a PCR-based approach, termed splicing by overlap extension (Horton et al. 1989). The construction of this minigene allowed us to effectively reduce the coding information contained within the 80-Kb IGF-I gene to a gene only 3 Kb in size (Hadsell et al. 1996). In our original work we produced transgenic mice that overexpressed both IGF-I (WAP-IGF-I) and an N-terminal truncated IGF-I, termed des(1-3)IGF-I (WAP-DES). The truncated IGF-I that was produced is well known to be more potent because of reduced affinity for IGF binding proteins (Clemmons et al. 1992; Gillespie et al. 1990). Most of the work done with these mice has been with the WAP-DES construct. This work has produced a number of interesting findings. Firstly, overexpression of des(1-3)IGF-I does not enhance milk yield or alter milk composition during early lactation (Hadsell et al. 2002). This finding is not unique to des(1-3)IGF-I, as other transgenic models of IGF-I overexpression also fail to demonstrate significant increases in milk synthesis (Wolf et al. 1997). In addition, the high concentrations of des(1-3)IGF-I in the milk of these transgenic mice had minimal effect on the growth and development of the suckling pups, supporting the suggestion that oral IGF-I has minimal activity (Burrin et al. 1999). The most interesting initial finding from the WAP-DES mice was that overexpression of des(1-3)IGF-I can inhibit mammary gland involution (Hadsell et al. 1996). In agreement with this finding, Neunschwander and coworkers (1996) demonstrated that overexpressed IGF-I or IGFBP-3 also could inhibit mammary involution. Later studies found that overexpressed IGF-II also was capable of inhibiting mammary involution (Moorehead et al. 2001). From these studies it was clear that although IGFs when overexpressed may not have been able to enhance milk yield, they were capable of delaying mammary gland involution. This delay in mammary involution was shown to be associated with decreased epithelial cell apoptosis. In addition, overexpression of both des(1-3)IGF-I and IGF-II also resulted in increased frequency of mammary gland tumors (Hadsell et al. 2000; Bates et al. 1996; Pravtcheva & Wise 1999). However, despite the similarities among these models, there was one major difference: both IGF-I and -II could inhibit forced mammary involution while des(1-3)IGF-I could not.

During normal lactation in the mouse, peak milk synthesis occurs about 10 days postpartum. About 18 days postpartum the mammary gland begins to involute as a result of the gradual weaning of the pups (Quarrie et al. 1996). This involution also can be induced by either forced weaning of the pups or by sealing the teats to prevent milk removal (Li et al. 1997). Mammary involution also can be delayed by crossfostering of younger suckling pups onto the dam to maintain suckling stimulus and milk removal (Shipman et al. 1987; Li et al. 1997). Our initial observation suggesting that mammary involution was inhibited in the WAP-DES mice was based on the comparison of mammary whole mounts collected at 7 days following the end of a 21-day lactation (Hadsell et al. 1996). Following this we observed in two independent studies that overexpression of des(1-3)IGF-I inhibited apoptosis during natural mammary gland involution (Hadsell et al. 2000; Hadsell et al. 2001). However, when forced mammary involution was induced at day 16 postpartum, the overexpressed des(1-3)IGF-I had little ability to inhibit mammary cell apoptosis (Hadsell et al. 2001).

To determine the basis for this differential effect we examined both the expression profile of the WAP-DES transgene, and the expression and activation of several intracellular signaling proteins that are known to mediate IGF-IR action. This analysis revealed that the inability of des(1-3)IGF-I to inhibit mammary gland involution coincided with a dramatic decrease in the abundance of IRS-1 and -2 (Hadsell et al. 2001). This decrease also was associated with a significant decrease in the phosphorylation of the serine/threonine kinase Akt. Activation of this kinase is largely dependent on IRS proteins (Murata et al. 2003). Transgenic overexpression of Akt in the mammary gland is known to inhibit mammary involution (Schwertfeger et al. 2001; Hutchinson et al. 2001; Ackler et al. 2002). Taken together, these results suggest that action of des(1-3)IGF-I, unlike that of IGF-I or -II, requires the expression of signaling proteins necessary for the activation of Akt. The basis for this differential requirement, however, is still unclear. One possibility is that des(1-3)IGF-I, because of its inability to interact with IGFBP, is targeted through different intracellular trafficking mechanisms than wild type IGF-I or -II. In this respect, it is still unclear how transgenic proteins, which predominantly are secreted into the milk from the apical side of the epithelium, would be capable of stimulating receptors that are present on the basolateral side. One possibility that has been suggested is through a paracellular route during times when the tight junctions might be open, such as during lactogenesis (Tonner et al. 2002; Nguyen et al. 2001).

Regardless of the mechanistic differences between the IGF analogs, the fact that IRS-1 and -2 expression in the mammary gland increases with lactation and is lost during forced mammary involution supports the hypothesis that IGF signaling is important to maintenance of lactation and that expression of IRS proteins is a point of regulation (Lee et al. 2003). This hypothesis is being tested on transgenic mice that overexpress IRS-1 or -2 in the mammary gland. In addition, studies also are being conducted on mice that carry germline mutations in the IRS-1 and -2 genes to determine the importance of these proteins to normal lactation.

The original description of IRS-1 knockout mice suggested that knockout females were both fertile and capable of lactation (Araki et al. 1994). However, it was unclear from this paper if the mice referred to in those original studies were heterozygous or homozygous for the deletion. Furthermore, homozygous IRS-I null mice are growth deficient and display mild glucose intolerance (Araki et al. 1994). The actual capacity of homozygous IRS-I null mice to lactate appears to have not been measured. Data from our own observations on the IRS-1 knockout mice suggest that while heterozygotes are both fertile and capable of lactation, homozygous females are subfertile and give birth to small litters. Heterozygous IRS-2 knockout mice are both fertile and apparently capable of lactation (Burks et al. 2000). Homozygous IRS-2 knockout mice, however, are subfertile, obese, and insulin-resistant displaying many of the symptoms associated with polycystic ovary syndrome (PCOS) in women (Burks et al. 2000). These observations support the conclusion that if a lactation defect is observed in these mice it will be complex, possibly involving both systemic effects as well as mammary cell autonomous effects.

The analysis of IRS knockout mice also has taken a more physiologically relevant approach focusing on studies of compound heterozygotes. The basis for these experiments has been that type II diabetes is thought to often be a polygenic phenomenon resulting from multiple gene deficiencies rather than the complete loss of a single gene product (Kido et al. 2000). These types of studies have demonstrated that compound haploinsufficiency for insulin receptor in combination IRS-1 and/or IRS-2 results in more severe insulin resistance than that observed with the loss of just a single allele (Kido et al. 2000; Withers et al. 1999). Yet the severity of the phenotype is less severe than complete loss of IRS-2. Compound haploinsufficiency for *Igf1r* and IRS-2 has produced similar results (Withers et al. 1999). Insulin resistance and PCOS in humans have been associated with polymorphisms in IRS-1 and -2 (Le Fur et al. 2002; El Mkadem et al. 2001). In addition, lactational insufficiency has been reported in women with PCOS (Marasco et al. 2000). Therefore, although the phenotypes in these mice may be pleotropic in nature, the analysis should be useful to understanding physiologic processes underlying the impact of insulin resistance and PCOS on lactation.

8. UPSTREAM STIMULATORY FACTOR-2 IS IMPORTANT FOR LACTATION

Upstream stimulatory factor (USF) is a myc-related transcription factor that consists of the helix-loop-helix/zipper (bHLH/zip) proteins USF-1 and -2 (Gregor et al. 1990). Binding (Sirito et al. 1994; Sawadogo 1988) and in vitro transcription studies (Sawadogo 1988) have demonstrated that these proteins function as heterodimers to activate transcription through binding to E-box elements (Sawadogo & Roeder 1985) identical in sequence to those to which myc binds (Blackwell et al. 1990; Bendall & Molloy 1994). In addition, both USF and myc interact with TFII-I to form complexes at promoter initiator elements that activate or repress transcription, respectively (Roy et al. 1993; Roy et al. 1997). Binding of myc has been shown to activate transcription of genes required for cell cycle progression and/or cell growth (Grandori et al. 2001). The ability of USF to compete with myc for the same DNA-binding site supports the idea that USF cooperates with the myc/max/mad network to regulate cellular function.

In mammary epithelial cells, myc is an important regulator of cell cycle progression. Transgenic- or retroviral-mediated overexpression of myc in the mouse mammary gland causes abnormal increases in mammary cell proliferation (Edwards et al. 1988; Stewart et al. 1984). This proliferative phenotype has been observed in conjunction with a lactational defect. Despite these observations little work has been reported on the functional significance of the myc/max/mad network to the processes governing normal mammary gland development and lactation. In addition, the mechanism by which myc regulates mammary cell function and the importance of myc-related proteins such as USF-1 and -2 to normal mammary gland development and lactation are poorly understood.

Mice that carry targeted germline mutations in the genes for USF-1 or -2 have been characterized. Targeted deletion of the *Usf1* gene has little apparent effect on overall development (Vallet et al. 1998; Sirito et al. 1998). In contrast, USF-2 null mice have been reported to exhibit decreased viability, growth retardation, and decreased lifespan (Sirito et al. 1998; Vallet et al. 1997). During the course of initial studies on the *Usf2* null mice, the offspring of female homozygous USF-2 null mice were observed to be non-viable. Our own work on these mice has demonstrated that this lack of viability is due to reduced lactational capacity.

To obtain a relative estimate of lactational performance in the USF-2 null mice, the growth of crossfostered pups was measured over the first eight days of lactation. This analysis revealed that USF-2 null dams had about half the capacity to support the growth of suckling pups as their wild type or heterozygous littermates (Fig. 2). This diminished capacity was associated with reduced mammary gland wet weight as well as reductions in milk lactose and total milk nitrogen and in the volume of milk that could be obtained following administration of exogenous oxytocin. Surprisingly, however, there were no obvious differences in the extent of mammary gland development or in the expression of the major milk protein genes (Fig. 3). The USF-2 null mice had no obvious defects in maternal behavior and when pup retrieval latency was measured they displayed only a mild deficiency on day 1 postpartum. The USF-2 null mice also had normal levels of blood prolactin, but a 45% reduction in blood oxytocin. The most striking finding in the USF-2 null mice in terms of a potential mechanism was that the protein-to-DNA ratio in the mammary tissue of these mice was reduced. We also have observed that the abundance of eIF4E and eIF4G is significantly reduced in mammary glands from USF-2 null mice. These translation initiation factors are known to function at a key regulatory point in protein synthesis (McKendrick et al. 1999; Keiper et al. 1999). These observations support the conclusion that the decreased lactational performance USF-2 of null mice occurs through a defect in mammary cell protein synthesis. However, at this point there is no indication as to whether this defect is due to systemic effects or to a mammary cell autonomous effect. These results illustrate the utility of analyzing lactation defects in GEMM, but also illustrate an important limitation of studies in germline mutants, a lack of tissue specificity.

9. GEMM: LIMITATIONS AND PROMISES

The utility of the various GEMM for studies at the four key stages of mammary gland development is outlined in Figure 4. The germline mutation models can be of some use to the analysis of mammary gland development and lactation, but this use may be

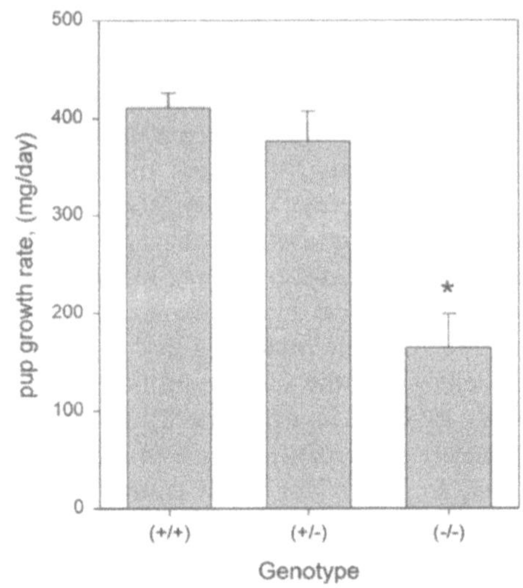

Figure 2. Lactation performance is decreased in Usf2-/- dams. Growth rates of the suckling pups over the first 8 days postpartum were used as an indicator of lactational performance. Average rates of pup growth were determined by linear regression from average daily body weight estimates obtained by measuring litter weight in litters (12 pups/litter) suckled on Usf2+/+, Usf2+/- or Usf2-/- dams. The asterisk indicates a significant decrease in the growth rate of pups suckled on Usf2-/- dams.

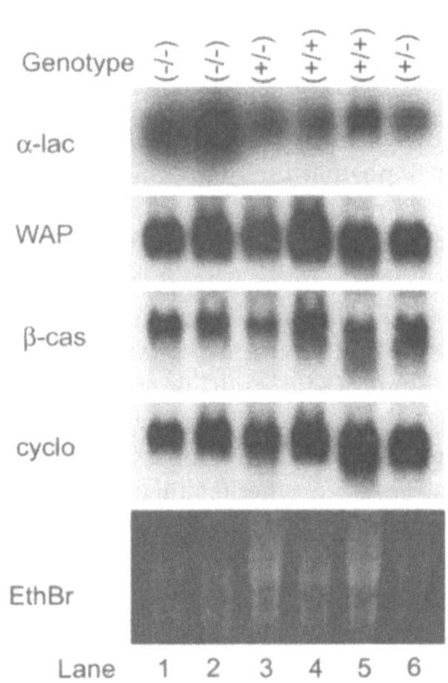

Figure 3. Decreased lactation performance is not associated with decreased milk protein mRNA abundance. Total RNA was prepared from mammary tissue of Usf2+/+, Usf2+/- or Usf2-/- mice at day 1 postpartum. Total RNA (10 μg) was then electrophoresed on a denaturing agarose gel and then blotted to a nylon membrane. The resulting blot was then probed with 32P-labeled cDNA probes for α-lactalbumin (α-lac), whey acidic protein (WAP), β-casein (β-cas), and cyclophilin (cyclo). The gel was stained with ethidium bromide (ethBr) to confirm the loading of each lane.

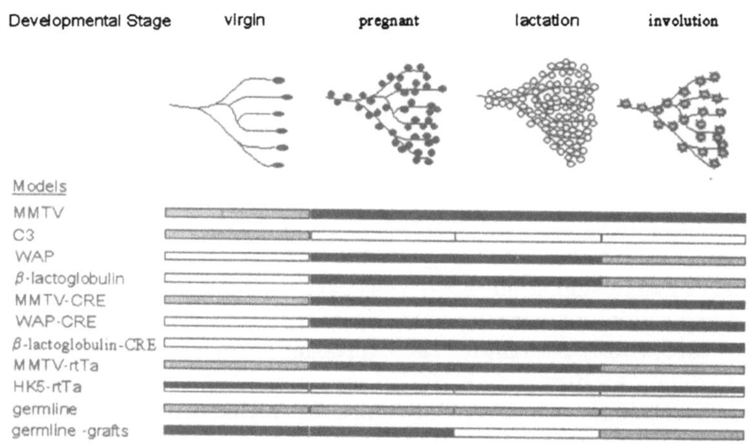

Figure 4. The utility of different GEMM varies with stage of mammary gland development. The applicability of different transgenic promoters or gene targeting schemes is indicated as a function of the four main stages of postnatal mammary gland development. The utility of the models is illustrated by differentially shaded bars: ■, highly applicable; ■, some possible limitations due to tissue specificity or expression levels; □, applicability untested or clearly limited by tissue specificity or developmental stage; ■, cell-type restrictions or tissue specificity restrictions.

limited by difficulties in pinpointing mechanisms of action. In this respect, if a lactation phenotype is found to be due to prepartum developmental effects, then transplantation (grafts) studies are an obvious solution for addressing questions pertaining to mechanisms. If the phenotype is not associated with prepartum developmental defects, the only currently available option is the use a tissue-specific targeting approach.

As described above, the tissue-specific gene targeting approaches have been developed through transgenic models using any of a number of mammary-specific promoters (Fig. 4). Several of these have been used successfully in conjunction with the CRE-LOX system (Wintermantel et al. 2002; Chapman et al. 2000; Selbert et al. 1998; Walton et al. 2001; Le Provost et al. 2002; Seagroves et al. 2003). With these, however, limitations have often been observed in the timing, cell-type specificity, or absolute levels of transgene expression depending on the model. For example MMTV-based transgenes have had much success in studies aimed at late-stage ductal development, alveologenesis, and lactation. Yet the utility of this promoter to drive the expression of transgenes to the mammary epithelium during early ductal development can be limited by lack of tissue specificity, site of integration-dependent variability in expression levels, and mosaic expression (Wagner et al. 1997, 2001; Hennighausen et al. 1995). The C3 promoter also has been described as expressed in the virgin gland (Maroulakou et al. 1994). However, the utility of this promoter to studies in mammary development and lactation is presently unclear. Cell-type-specific promoters, such as those for keratins, also have had some success (Dunbar et al. 2001). The K14 promoter has been used successfully to drive transgene expression to myoepithelial cells (Wysolmerski et al. 1995). These, however, may be limited by a lack of tissue specificity and by their restricted expression within the mammary epithelium. As discussed earlier in this review, the milk protein genes such as WAP and α-lactoglobulin have been applied successfully to studies of pregnancy and lactation. Yet with these systems, mechanisms relating specifically to lactation cannot be separated from those related to pregnancy-dependent mammary gland development. In this respect, it is clear that the use of tissue-specific, inducible transgenes needs to be expanded so that milk synthesis phenotypes can be separated effectively from developmental phenotypes. The same is necessary for currently available inducible gene ablation models based on CRE-LOX. In addition, gene ablation through CRE-LOX is irreversible. This could be viewed as a limitation depending on the circumstances of the intended studies. Recently, a gene targeting approach has emerged based on the use of small inhibitory RNAs and the phenomenon of RNA inhibition. This approach has the promise of revolutionizing the way in which genes are ablated and may accelerate the rate at which genes can be evaluated using GEMM.

The process of RNA inhibition (RNAi) has been used effectively for several years to suppress gene expression in a variety of organisms (Zamore 2002). More recently, RNAi has been used successfully to inhibit gene expression in mammalian cells and in mice (Carmell et al. 2003; McCaffrey et al. 2002; Lewis et al. 2002; Paddison et al. 2002; Yu et al. 2002). The technique, also referred to as post-transcriptional gene silencing (PTGS), exploits a biologic system that is believed to have evolved as a type of genomic immune system to protect against viruses and transposons (Plasterk 2002). Double stranded RNA (dsRNA) containing sequences identical to endogenous genes normally is not found at high concentrations within cells. When artificially introduced into cells, this dsRNA is cleaved into small inhibitory (si) RNAs of about 20 nt in length. These siRNAs are incorporated into an active siRNA complex, which can then recognize and anneal to specific mRNAs based on sequence complementarity. This siRNA complex then recruits a nucleolytic activity that cleaves and initiates the degradation of the mRNA.

In simpler organisms such as *C. elegans* and *Drosophila*, effective PTGS can be accomplished with dsRNAs of a variety of sizes and structural configurations. In mammalian cells, however, there exists an upper limit on the size of the dsRNA. When large dsRNAs are introduced into mammalian cells, they respond with both an inflammatory response that involves induction of interferons and a nonspecific RNA degradation response mediated by activation of the protein kinase, PKR (Manche et al. 1992; Minks et al. 1979; Stark et al. 1998). In contrast, siRNAs of 21 nt will inhibit gene expression effectively in a variety of formats without induction of interferon production (Elbashir et al. 2001). Most importantly, siRNAs are effective in cultured cells and animals when expressed as transgenes (Carmell et al. 2003; McCaffrey et al. 2002; Kunath et al. 2003). Until recently, however, this approach was limited by two main drawbacks. The first is that identification of a target site, or sites, within the mRNA of interest was based on time-consuming screens that have not always been successful (Bohula et al. 2003; Sohail et al. 2003). The second was the requirement that any transgenes used to target the siRNAs had to be driven by polymerase III-type promoters making the possibility of tissue specificity unlikely (Paddison et al. 2002).

Recently there have been two independently published reports of successful targeting of siRNAs based on polymerase II type promoters. The first demonstrated that CMV promoter could be used to target siRNA effectively provided that the space between the transcriptional start site and the siRNA was minimized to 6 bp and that the construct contained only the minimal poly-adenylation sequence (Xia et al. 2002). The second and more exciting finding was that the CMV promoter could actually be used to target large (~500 bp) inverted repeats to generate siRNAs, provided that the 5′ and 3′ ends of the transcript are engineered to prevent export from the nucleus (Shinagawa & Ishii 2003). This later finding means that screening for effective target sequences will no longer be a necessary part of producing effective siNA transgenes. Lastly, the fact that this approach is based on standard transgenic approaches rather than the use of embryonic stem cells and blastocyst injections suggests that a multigenic approach may be possible through the use of coinjection. This will greatly facilitate the generation and analysis of poly-transgenic animals to allow for the analysis of families of gene products. Work is on-going in our laboratory to apply this technology to the IRS proteins.

10. CONCLUSIONS

The use of GEMM in the study of mammary gland development and lactation continues to provide valuable models that contribute to our understanding of mammary cell biology. The contribution that these models have made to our understanding biology of IGFs and HLH proteins in the mammary gland is just one of several examples. The main challenge now is for us to improve both the speed and precision with which genetic manipulations can be accomplished. This too will happen.

11. ACKNOWLEDGMENTS

Thanks to Dr. Sharon Bonnette, Ms. Jessy George, and Mr. Daniel Torres for technical assistance. Thanks also to Dr. Adrian Lee for insightful discussions relating to this work. The work described in this review was funded by the grants from the NIDDK (DK52197) and the USDA (58-62550-6-001).

12. REFERENCES

Accili D, Drago J, Lee EJ, Johnson MD, Cool MH, Salvatore P, Asico LD, Jose PA, Taylor SI, Westphal H. Early neonatal death in mice homozygous for a null allele of the insulin receptor gene. Nat Genet 1996;12:106-109.

Ackler S, Ahmad S, Tobias C, Johnson MD, Glazer RI. Delayed mammary gland involution in mmtv-akt1 transgenic mice. Oncogene 2002;21:198-206.

Adam D. Draft cow genome heads the field. Nature 2002;417:778.

Andres AC, Schonenberger CA, Groner B, Hennighausen L, LeMeur M, Gerlinger P. Ha-ras oncogene expression directed by a milk protein gene promoter: tissue specificity, hormonal regulation, and tumor induction in transgenic mice. Proc Natl Acad Sci USA 1987;84:1299-1303.

Araki E, Lipes MA, Patti ME, Bruning JC, Haag B, Johnson RS, Kahn CR. Alternative pathway of insulin signalling in mice with targeted disruption of the IRS-1 gene. Nature 1994;372:186-190.

Arranz JJ, Coppieters W, Berzi P, Cambisano N, Grisart B, Karim L, Marcq F, Moreau L, Mezer C, Riquet J, Simon P, Vanmanshoven P, Wagenaar D, Georges M. A QTL affecting milk yield and composition maps to bovine chromosome 20: a confirmation. Anim Genet 1998;29:107-115.

Baker J, Liu J-P, Robertson E, Efstratiadis A. Role of insulin-like growth factors in embryonic and postnatal growth. Cell 1997;75:73-82.

Bates P, Fisher R, Ward A, Richardson L, Hill DJ, Graham CF. Mammary cancer in transgenic mice expressing insulin-like growth factor II (IGF-II). Br J Cancer 1996;72:1189-1193.

Bendall AJ, Molloy PL. Base preferences for DNA binding by the bHLH-Zip protein USF: effects of MgCl2 on specificity and comparison with binding of Myc family members. Nucleic Acids Res 1994;22:2801-2810.

Blackwell TK, Kretzner L, Blackwood EM, Eisenman RN, Weintraub H. Sequence-specific DNA binding by the c-myc protein. Science 1990;250:1149-1151.

Bohula EA, Salisbury AJ, Sohail M, Playford MP, Riedemann J, Southern EM, Macaulay VM. The efficacy of small interfering RNAs targeted to the type 1 insulin-like growth factor receptor (IGF1R) is influenced by secondary structure in the IGF1R transcript. J Biol Chem 2003;278:15991-15997.

Bonnette SG, Hadsell DL. Targeted disruption of the insulin-like growth factor I receptor gene inhibits cellular proliferation in mammary terminal endbuds (TEB). Endocrinology 2001;142:4937-4945.

Bremel RD, Yom HC, Bleck GT. Alteration of milk composition using molecular genetics. J Dairy Sci 1989;72:2826-2833.

Brinster RL, Chen HY, Messing A, Van Dyke T, Levine AJ, Palmiter RD. Transgenic mice harboring SV40 T-antigen genes develop characteristic brain tumors. Cell 1984;37:367-379.

Burks DJ, Font de Mora J, Schubert M, Withers DJ, Myers MG, Towery HH, Altamuro SL, Flint CL, White MF. IRS-2 pathways integrate female reproduction and energy homeostasis. Nature 2000;407:377-382.

Burrin DG, Fiorotto ML, Hadsell DL. Transgenic hypersecretion of des(1-3)human insulin-like growth factor I in mouse milk has limited effects on the gastrointestinal tract in suckling pups. J Nutr 1999;129;51-56.

Butte NF, Garza C, Smith EO, Nichols BL. Human milk intake and growth in exclusively breast-fed infants. J Pediatr 1984;104:187-195.

Byrne GW, Ruddle FH Multiplex gene regulation: a two-tiered approach to transgene regulation in transgenic mice. Proc Natl Acad Sci USA 1989;86:5473-5477.

Capuco AV, Kahl S, Jack LJ, Bishop JO, Wallace H. Prolactin and growth hormone stimulation of lactation in mice requires thyroid hormones. Proc Soc Exp Biol Med 1999;221:345-351.

Carmell MA, Zhang L, Conklin D, Hannon GJ, Rosenquist TA. Germline transmission of RNAi in mice. Nat Struct Biol 2003;10:91-92.

Chapman RS, Lourenco P, Tonner E, Flint D, Selbert S, Takeda K, Akira S, Clarke AR, Watson CJ. The role of Stat3 in apoptosis and mammary gland involution. Conditional deletion of Stat3. Adv Exp Med Biol 2000;480:129-138.

Clark AJ. The mammary gland as a bioreactor: expression processing, and production of recombinant proteins. J Mammary Gland Biol Neoplasia 1998;3:337-350.

Clemmons DR, Dehoff MH, Busby WH, Bayne ML, Cascieri MA. Competition for binding to insulin-like growth factor (IGF) binding protein-2, 3, 4, and 5 by IGFs and IGF analogs. Endocrinology 1992;131:890-895.

Covarrubias L, Nishida Y, Mintz B. Early postimplantation embryo lethality due to DNA rearrangements in a transgenic mouse strain. Proc Natl Acad Sci USA 1986;83:6020-6024.

Cox DB, Owens RA, Hartmann PE. Blood and milk prolactin and the rate of milk synthesis in women. Exp Physiol 1996;81:1007-1020.

Cunha GR, Young P, Hom YK, Cooke PS, Taylor JA, Lubahn DB. Elucidation of a role for stromal steroid hormone receptors in mammary gland growth and development using tissue recombinants. J Mammary Gland Biol Neoplasia **1997**;2:393-402.

Daly MJ, Rioux JD, Schaffner SF, Hudson TJ, Lander ES. High-resolution haplotype structure in the human genome. Nat Genet 2001;29:229-232.

DeOme KB, Faulkin LJ Jr, Bern HA, Blair PE. Development of mammary tumors from hyperplastic alveolar nodules transplanted into gland-free mammary fat pads of female C3H mice. Cancer Res 1959;19:515-520.

Dulak N, Temin HM. A partially purified polypeptide fraction from rat liver cell conditioned medium with multiplication stimulating activity for embryo fibroblasts. J Cell Physiol 1972;81:153-160.

Dunbar ME, Dann P, Brown CW, Van Houton J, Dreyer B, Philbrick WP, Wysolmerski JJ. Temporally regulated overexpression of parathyroid hormone-related protein in the mammary gland reveals distinct fetal and pubertal phenotypes. J Endocrinol 2001;171:403-416.

Dymecki SM. Flp recombinase promotes site-specific DNA recombination in embryonic stem cells and transgenic mice. Proc Natl Acad Sci USA 2003;93:6191-6196.

Edwards PAW, Ward JL, Bradbury JM. Alteration of morphogenesis by the v-myc oncogene in transplants of mammary gland. Oncogene 1988;2:407-412.

El Mkadem SA, Lautier C, Macari F, Molinari N, Lefèbvre P, Renard E, Gris JC, Cros G, Daurès JP, Bringer J, White MF, Grigorescu F. Role of allelic variants Gly972Arg of IRS-1 and Gly1057Asp of IRS-2 in moderate-to-severe insulin resistance of women with polycystic ovary syndrome. Diabetes 2001;50:2164-2168.

Elbashir SM, Harborth J, Lendeckel W, Yalcin A, Weber K, Tuschl T. Duplexes of 21-nucleotide RNAs mediate RNA interference in cultured mammalian cells. Nature 2001;411:494-498.

Epstein-Baak R, Lin Y, Bradshaw V, Cohn M. Inducible transformation of cells from transgenic mice expressing SV40 under lac operon control. Cell Growth Differ 1992;3:127-134.

Fantin VR, Wang Q, Lienhard GE, Keller SR. Mice lacking insulin receptor substrate 4 exhibit mild defects in growth reproduction and glucose homeostasis. Am J Physiol Endocrinol Metab 2001;278:E127-E133.

Farrelly N, Lee YJ, Oliver J, Dive C, Streuli CH. Extracellular matrix regulates apoptosis in mammary epithelium through a control on insulin signaling. J Cell Biol 1999;144:1337-1348.

Flint DJ, Tonner E, Allan GJ. Insulin-like growth factor binding proteins:IGF-dependent and -independent effects in the mammary gland. J Mammary Gland Biol Neoplasia 2000;5:65-73.

Furth PA, St Onge L, Boger H, Gruss P, Gossen M, Kistner A, Bujard H, Hennighausen L. Temporal control of gene expression in transgenic mice by a tetracycline-responsive promoter. Proc Natl Acad Sci USA 1994;91:9302-9306.

Gillespie C, Read LC, Bagley CJ, Ballard FJ. Enhanced potency of truncated insulin-like growth factor-I (des(1-3)IGF-I) relative to IGF-I in lit/lit mice. J Endocrinol 1990;127:401-405.

Gordon JW, Scangos GA, Plotkin DJ, Barbosa JA, Ruddle FH. Genetic transformation of mouse embryos by microinjection of purified DNA. Proc Natl Acad Sci USA 1980;77:7380-7384.

Gossen M, Bujard H. Studying gene function in eukaryotes by conditional gene inactivation. Annu Rev Genet 2002;36:153-173.

Grandori C, Cowley SM, James LP, Eisenman RN. The myc/max/mad network and the transcriptional control of cell behavior. Annu Rev Cell Dev Biol 2001;16 653-699.

Gregor PD, Sawadogo M, Roeder RG. The adenovirus major late transcription factor USF is a member of the helix-loop-helix group of regulatory proteins and binds to DNA as a dimer. Genes Dev 1990;4:1730-1740.

Grisart B, Coppieters W, Farnir F, Karim L, Ford C, Berzi P, Cambisano N, Mni M, Reid S, Simon P, Spelman R, Georges M, Snell R. Positional candidate cloning of a QTL in dairy cattle: identification of a missense mutation in the bovine DGAT1 gene with major effect on milk yield and composition. Genome Res 2002;12:222-231.

Gutierrez A, Meade HM, Ditullio P, Pollock D, Harvey M, Jimenez-Flores R, Anderson GB, Murray JD, Medrano JF. Expression of a bovine kappa-CN cDNA in the mammary gland of transgenic mice utilizing a genomic milk protein gene as an expression cassette. Transgenic Res 1996;5:271-279.

Gutierrez-Adan A, Maga EA, Meade HM, Shoemaker CF, Medrano JF, Anderson GB, Murray JD. Alterations of the physical characteristics of milk from transgenic mice producing bovine k-casein. J Dairy Sci 1996;79:791-799.

Guy CT, Cardiff RD, Muller WJ. Induction of mammary tumors by expression of polyomavirus middle T oncogene: a transgenic mouse model for metastatic disease. Mol Cell Biol 1992;12:954-961.

Guy CT, Muthuswamy SK, Cardiff RD, Soriano P, Muller WJ. Activation of the c-src tyrosine kinase is required for the induction of mammary tumors in transgenic mice. Genes Dev 1996;8:23-32.

Hadsell D, Greenberg NM, Fligger JM, Baumrucker CM, Rosen JM. Targeted expression of des (1-3) human insulin-like growth factor I in transgenic mice influences mammary gland development and IGF-binding protein expression. Endocrinology 1996;137:321-330.

Hadsell DL, Bonnette SG. IGF and insulin action in the mammary gland: lessons from transgenic and knockout models. J Mammary Gland Biol Neoplasia 2000;5:19-30.

Hadsell DL, Murphy KL, Reece N, Alexeenko T, Lascerica R, Rosen JM. Cooperation between des(1-3)IGF-I and mutant p53 accelerates mammary gland carcinogenesis in bigenic mice. Oncogene 2000;19:889-898.

Hadsell DL, Alexeenko T, Klemintidis Y, Torres D, Lee AV. Inability of overexpressed des(1-3)human insulin-like growth factor I (IGF-I) to inhibit forced mammary gland involution is associated with decreased expression of IGF signaling molecules. Endocrinology 2001;142:1479-1488.

Hadsell DL, Bonnette SG, Lee AV. Genetic manipulation of the IGF-I axis to regulate mammary gland development and function. J Dairy Sci 2002;85:365-377.

Hansen LB. Consequences of selection for milk yield from a geneticist's viewpoint. J Dairy Sci 2000;83:1145-1150.

Hennighausen L, Wall RJ, Tillmann U, Li M, Furth PA. Conditional gene expression in secretory tissues and skin of transgenic mice using the MMTV-LTR and the tetracycline responsive system. J Cell Biochem 1995;59:463-472.

Horton RM, Hunt HD, Ho SN, Pullen JK, Pease LR. Engineering hybrid genes without the use of restriction enzymes: gene splicing by overlap extension. Gene 1989;77:61-68.

Houdebine LM. Transgenic animals as bioreactors. Transgenic Res 2000;9:305-320.

Hovey RC, Harris J, Hadsell DL, Lee AV, Ormandy CJ, Vonderhaar BK. Local insulin-like growth factor-II mediates PRL-induced mammary gland development. Mol Endocrinol 2002;17:460-471.

Hsu SY, Nakabayashi K, Nishi S, Kumagi J, Kudo M, Sherwood OD, Hsueh AJW. Activation of orphan receptors by the hormone relaxin. Science 2002;295:671-674.

Humphreys RC, Lydon J, O'Malley BW, Rosen JM. Mammary gland development is mediated by both stromal and epithelial progesterone receptors. Mol Endocrinol 1997;11:801-811.

Hutchinson J, Jin J, Cardiff RD, Woodgett JR, Muller WJ. Activation of Akt (protein kinase B) in mammary epithelium provides a critical cell survival signal required for tumor progression. Mol Cell Biol 2001;21;2203-2212.

Iavnilovitch E, Groner B, Barash I. Overexpression and forced activation of stat5 in mammary gland of transgenic mice promotes cellular proliferation, enhances differentiation, and delays postlactational apoptosis. Mol Cancer Res 2002;1;32-47.

Ivell R, Bathgate RAD. Reproductive biology of the relaxin-like growth factor (RFL/INSL3). Biology Reprod 2002;67:699-705.

Johnson GC, Esposito L, Barratt BJ, Smith AN, Heward J, Di Genova G, Ueda H, Cordell HJ, Eaves IA, Dudbridge F, Twells RC, Payne F, Hughes W, Nutland S, Stevens H, Carr P, Tuomilehto-Wolf E, Tuomilehto J, Gough SC, Clayton DG, Todd JA. Haplotype tagging for the identification of common disease genes. Nat Genet 2001;29:233-237.

Johnson MS, Thomson SC, Speakman JR. Limits to sustained energy intake. I. lactation in the laboratory mouse Mus musculus. J Exp Biol 2001;204:1925-1935.

Keiper BD, Gan W, Rhoads RE. Protein synthesis initiation factor 4G. Int J Biochem Cell Biol 1999;31:37-41.

Kido Y, Burks DJ, Withers D, Bruning JC, Kahn CR, White MF, Accili D. Tissue-specific insulin resistance in mice with mutations in the insulin receptor, IRS-1 and IRS-2. J Clin Invest 2000;105:199-205.

Kleinberg DL, Ruan W, Catanese V, Newman CB, Feldman M. Non-lactogenic effects of growth hormone on growth and insulin-like growth factor-I messenger ribonucleic acid of rat mammary gland [published erratum appears in Endocrinology 1990 Oct;127(4):1977]. Endocrinology 1990;126:3274-3276.

Kleinberg DL, Feldman M, Ruan W. IGF-I:An essential factor in terminal end bud formation and ductal morphogenesis. J Mammary Gland Biol Neoplasia 2000;5:7-18.

Korach KS. Insights from the study of animal lacking functional estrogen receptor. Science 1994;266:1524-1527.

Kubota N, Tobe K, Terauchi Y, Kazuhiro E, Yamauchi T, Suzuki R, Tsubamoto Y, Komeda K, Nakano R, Miki H, Satoh S, Sekihara H, Sciacchitano S, Lesniak M, Aizawa S, Nagai R, Kimura S, Akanuma Y, Taylor SI, Kadowaki T. Disruption of insulin receptor substrate 2 causes type 2 diabetes because of liver insulin resistance and lack of compensatory β-cell hyperplasia. Diabetes 2000;49:1880-1889.

Kunath T, Gish G, Lickert H, Jones N, Pawson T, Rossant J. Transgenic RNA interference in ES cell-derived embryos recapitulates a genetic null phenotype. Nature Biotechnol 2003;21:559-561.

L'Huillier PJ, Soulier S, Stinnakre MG, Lepourry L, Davis SR, Mercier JC, Vilotte JL. Efficient and specific ribozyme-mediated reduction of bovine alpha-lactalbumin expression in double transgenic mice. Proc Natl Acad Sci USA 1996;93:6698-6703.

Lacy E, Costantini FD. Structure and expression of foreign globin genes in transgenic mice. Prog Clin Biol Res 1983;134:13-25.

Lacy E, Roberts S, Evans EP, Burtenshaw MD, Costantini FD. A foreign beta-globin gene in transgenic mice: integration at abnormal chromosomal positions and expression in inappropriate tissues. Cell 1983;34:343-358.

Lakso M, Sauer B, Mosinger B Jr, Lee EJ, Manning RW, Yu S-H, Mulder KL, Westphal H. Targeted oncogene activation by site-specific recombination in transgenic mice. Proc Natl Acad Sci USA 1992;89:6232-6236.

Laustsen PG, Michael MD, Crute BE, Cohen SE, Ueki K, Kulkarni RN, Keller SR, Lienhard GE, Kahn CR. Lipoatrophic diabetes in $Irs1^{-/-}Irs3^{-/-}$ double knockout mice. Genes Dev 2002;16:3213-3222.

Le Fur S, Le Stunff C, Bougnères P. Increased insulin resistance in obese children who have both 972 IRS-1 and 1057 IRS-2 polymorphisms. Diabetes 2002;51:S304-S307.

Le Provost F, Riedlinger G, Hee YS, Benedict J, Gonzalez FJ, Flaws J, Hennighausen L. The aryl hydrocarbon receptor (AhR) and its nuclear translocator (Arnt) are dispensable for normal mammary gland development but are required for fertility. Genesis 2002;32;231-239.

Lee KF, DeMayo FJ, Atiee SH, Rosen JM. Tissue-specific expression of the rat β-casein gene in transgenic mice. Nucleic Acids Res 1988;16:1027-1041.

Lee AV, Zhang P, Ivanova M, Bonnette S, Oesterreich S, Rosen JM, Grimm S, Hovey RC, Vonderhaar BK, Kahn CR, Torres D, George J, Mohsin S, Allred DC, Hadsell DL. Developmental and hormonal signals dramatically alter the localization and abundance of insulin receptor substrate proteins in the mammary gland. Endocrinology 2003;144:2683-2694.

Lewis DL, Hagstrom JE, Loomis AG, Wolff JA, Herweijer H. Efficient delivery of siRNA for inhibition of gene expression in postnatal mice. Nat Genet 2002;32:107-108.

Li M, Liu X, Robinson G, Bar-Peled U, Wagner K, Young WS, Hennighausen L, Furth PA. Mammary-derived signals activate programmed cell dath during the first stage of mammary gland involution. Proc Natl Acad Sci USA 1997;94:3425-3430.

Lin TP, Guzman RC, Osborn RC, Thordarson G, Nandi S. Role of endocrine, autocrine and paracrine interactions in the development of mammary hyperplasia in wnt-1 transgenic mice. Cancer Res 1992;56:4413-4419.

Liu SC, Wang Q, Lienhard GE, Keller SR. Insulin receptor substrate 3 is not essential for growth or glucose homeostasis. J Biol Chem 1999;274:18093-18099.

Lok S, Johnston DS, Conklin D, Lofton-Day CE, Adams RL, Jelmberg AC, Whitmore TE, Schrader S, Griswold MD, Jaspers SR. Identification of INSL6, a new member of the insulin family that is expressed in the testis of the human and rat. Biol Reprod 2000;62:1593-1599.

Lufkin T, Dierich A, LeMeur M, Mark M, Chambon P. Disruption of the Hox-1.6 homeobox gene results in defects in a region corresponding to its rostral domain of expression. Cell 1991;66:1105-1119.

Lyons WR, Li CH, Johnson RE. The hormonal control of mammary growth and lactation. Recent Prog Horm Res 1958;4:219-248.
Madon RJ, Ensor DM, Knight CH, Flint DJ. Effects of an antiserum to rat growth hormone on lactation in the rat. J Endocrinol 1986;111:117-123.
Manche L, Green SR, Schmedt C, Mathews MB. Interactions between double-stranded RNA regulators and the proteins kinase DAI. Mol Cell Biol 1992;12:5238-5248.
Marasco L, Marmet C, Shell E. Polycystic ovary syndrome: a connection to insufficient milk supply? J Hum Lact 2000;16:143-148.
Maroulakou IG, Anver M, Garrett L, Green JE. Prostate and mammary adenocarcinoma in transgenic mice carrying a rat C3(1) simian virus 40 large tumor antigen fusion gene. Proc Natl Acad Sci USA 1994;91:11236-11240.
Marquardt H, Todaro GJ, Henderson LE, Oroszlan S. Purification and primary structure of a polypeptide with multiplication-stimulating activity from rat liver cell cultures. J Biol Chem 1981;256:6859-6865.
McCaffrey AP, Meuse L, Pham TT, Conklin DS, Hannon GJ, Kay MA. RNA interference in adult mice. Nature 2002;418:38-39.
McKendrick L, Pain VM, Morley SJ. Translation initiation factor 4E. Int J Biol Chem 1999;31:31-35.
Minks MA, West DK, Envin S, Aglioni C. Structural requirements of double-stranded RNA for the activations of 2', 5' -oligo(A) polymerase and protein kinase of interferon-treated HeLa cells. J Biol Chem 1979;254:10180-10183.
Moorehead RA, Fata JE, Johnson MB, Khokha R. Inhibition of mammary epithelial apoptosis and sustained phosphorylation of Akt/PKB in MMTV-IGF-II transgenic mice. Cell Death Differ 2001;8:16-29.
Muller WJ, Sinn E, Pattengale PK, Wallace R, Leder P. Single-step induction of mammary adenocarcinoma in transgenic mice bearing the activated c-neu oncogene. Cell 1988;1:105-115.
Murata H, Hresko RC, Mueckler M. Reconstitution of PI 3-kinasae-dependent insulin signaling in a cell-free system. J Biol Chem 2003;13:21607-21614.
Nagai J, Sarkar NK. Relationship between milk yield and mammary gland development in mice. J Dairy Sci 1978;61:733-739.
Nandi S. Endocrine control of mammary gland development and function in the C3 11/HE Crgl mouse. J Natl Cancer Inst 1958;21:1039-1062.
Neuenschwander S, Schwartz A, Wood TL, Roberts CTJ, Henninghausen L, LeRoith D. Involution of the lactating mammary gland is inhibited by the IGF system in a transgenic mouse model. J Clin Invest 1996;97:2225-2232.
Nguyen DA, Parlow AF, Neville MC. Hormonal regulation of tight junction closure in the mouse mammary epithelium during the transition from pregnancy to lactation. J Endocrinol 2001;170:347-356.
No D, Yao TP, Evans RM. Ecdysone-inducible gene expression in mammalian cells and transgenic mice. Proc Natl Acad Sci USA 1996;93:3346-3351.
Noble MS, Rodriguez-Zas S, Cook JB, Bleck GT, Hurley WL, Wheeler MB. Lactational performance of first-parity transgenic gilts expressing bovine alpha-lactalbumin in their milk. J Anim Sci 2002;80:1090-1096.
Oftedal OT. Milk composition, milk yield and energy output at peak lactation: a comparative review. Symp Zoolog Soc (London) 1984;51:33-85.
Ormandy CJ, Binart N, Kelly PA. Mammary gland development in prolactin receptor knockout mice. J Mammary Gland Biol Neoplasia 1997;2:355-364.
Ornitz DM, Moreadith RW, Leder P. Binary system for regulating transgene expression in mice: targeting int-2 gene expression with yeast GAL4/UAS control elements. Proc Natl Acad Sci USA 1991;88:698-702.
Paddison PJ, Caudy AA, Bernstein E, Hannon GJ. Short hairpin RNAs (shRNAs) induce sequence-specific silencing in mammalian cells. Genes Dev 2002;16:948-958.
Palmiter RD, Brinster RL, Hammer RE, Trumbauer ME, Rosenfeld MG, Birnberg NC, Evans RM. Dramatic growth of mice that develop from eggs microinjected with metallothione in growth hormone fusion genes. Nature 1982;300:611-615.
Peel CJ, Bauman DE, Gorewit RC, Sniffen CJ. Effect of exogenous growth hormone on lactational performance in high yielding dairy cows. J Nutr 1981;111:1662-1671.
Peripato AC, de Brito RA, Vaughn TT, Pletscher LS, Matioli SR, Cheverud JM. Quantitative trait loci for maternal performance for offspring survival in mice. Genetics 2002;162:1341-1353.
Pittius CW, Hennighausen L, Lee E, Westphal H, Nicols E, Vitale J, Gordon K. A milk protein gene promoter directs the expression of human tissue plasminogen activator cDNA to the mammary gland in transgenic mice. Proc Natl Acad Sci USA 1988;85:5874-5878.
Plasterk RHA. RNA silencing: the genome's immune system. Science 2002;296:1263-1265.
Pravtcheva DD, Wise TL. Metastasizing mammary carcinomas in H19 enhancers-Igf2 transgenic mice. J Exp Zool 1999;281:43-57.
Quarrie LH, Addey CV, Wilde CJ. Programmed cell death during mammary tissue involution induced by weaning, litter removal, and milk stasis. J Cell Physiol 1996;168:559-569.

Radice GL, Ferreira-Cornwell MC, Robinson SD, Rayburn H, Chodosh LA, Takeichi M, Hynes RO. Precocious mammary gland development in P-cadherin-deficient mice. J Cell Biol 1997;139:1025-1032.
Rinderknecht E, Humbel RE. Primary structure of human insulin-like growth factor II. FEBS Lett 1978a;89:283-286.
Rinderknecht E, Humbel RE. The amino acid sequence of human insulin-like growth factor I and its structural homology with proinsulin. J Biol Chem 1978b;253:2769-2776.
Robinson GW, Hennighausen L. Inhibins and activins regulate mammary epithelial cell differentiation through mesenchymal-epithelial interactions. Development 1997;124:2701-2708.
Robinson GW, Accili D, Hennighausen L. Rescue of mammary epithelium of early lethal phenotypes by embryonic mammary gland transplantation as exemplified with insulin receptor null mice. In: Ip MM, Asch BB, editors. Methods in Mammary Gland Biology and Breast Cancer Research. New York: Kluwer Academic/Plenum Publishers, 2000; pp 307-316.
Roy AL, Carruthers C, Gutjahr T, Roeder RG. Direct role for Myc in transcription initiation mediated by interactions with TFII-I. Nature 1993;365:359-361.
Roy AL, Du H, Gregor PD, Novina CD, Martinez E, Roeder RG. Cloning of an Inr- and E-box-binding protein, TFII-I, that interacts physically and functionally with USF-1. EMBO J 1997;16:7091-7104.
Ruan W, Kleinberg DL. Insulin-like growth factor I is essential for terminal end bud formation and ductal morphogenesis during mammary development. Endocrinology 1999;140:5075-5081.
Ruan W, Newman CB, Kleinberg DL. Intact and amino-terminally shortened forms of insulin-like growth factor I induce mammary gland differentiation and development. Proc Natl Acad Sci USA 1992;89:10872-10876.
Ruan W, Catanese V, Wieczorek R, Feldman M, Kleinberg DL. Estradiol enhances the stimulatory effect of insulin-like growth factor-I (IGF-I) on mammary development and growth hormone-induced IGF-I messenger ribonucleic acid. Endocrinology 1995;136:1296-1302.
Ryan AS, Wenjun Z, Acosta A. Breastfeeding continues into the new millennium. Pediatrics 2002;110:1103-1109.
Salmon WD Jr, Daughaday WH. A hormonal controlled serum factor which stimulates sulfate incorporation by cartilage in vitro. J Lab Clin Med 1957;49:825-826.
Sawadogo M. Multiple forms of the human gene-specific transcription factor USF. II. DNA binding properties and transcriptional activity of the purified HeLa USF. J Biol Chem 1988;263:11994-12001.
Sawadogo M, Roeder RG. Interaction of a gene-specific transcription factor with adenovirus major late promoter upstream of the TATA box region. Cell 1985;43:165-175.
Sawai S, Shimono A, Hanaoka K, Kondoh H. Embryonic lethality resulting from disruption of both N-myc alleles in mouse zygotes. New Biol 1991;3:861-869.
Schaapveld RQ, Schepens JT, Robinson GW, Attema J, Oerlemans FT, Fransen JA, Streuli M, Wieringa B, Hennighausen L, Hendriks WJ. Impaired mammary gland development and function in mice lacking LAR receptor-like tyrosine phosphatase activity. Dev Biol 1997;188:134-146.
Schwartzberg PL, Robertson EJ, Goff SP. Targeted gene disruption of the endogenous c-abl locus by homologous recombination with DNA encoding a selectable fusion protein. Proc Natl Acad Sci USA 1989;87:3210-3214.
Schwertfeger K, Richert MM, Anderson SM. Mammary gland involution is delayed by activated akt in transgenic mice. Mol Endocrinol 2001;15:867-881.
Schwertfeger KL, McManaman JL, Palmer CA, Neville MC, Anderson SM. Expression of constitutively activated Akt in the mammary gland leads to excess lipid synthesis during pregnancy and lactation. J Lipid Res 2003;44:1100-1112.
Seagroves TN, Hadsell D, McManaman J, Palmer C, Liao D, McNulty W, Welm B, Wagner KU, Neville M, Johnson RS. HIF1alpha is a critical regulator of secretory differentiation and activation, but not vascular expansion, in the mouse mammary gland. Development 2003;130:1713-1724.
Selbert S, Bentley DJ, Melton DW, Rannie D, Lourenco P, Watson CJ, Clarke AR. Efficient BLG-Cre mediated gene deletion in the mammary gland. Transgenic Res 1998;7:387-396.
Shinagawa T, Ishii S. Generation of Ski-knockdown mice by expressing a long double-strand RNA from an RNA polymerase II promoter. Genes Dev 2003;17:1340-1345.
Shipman LJ, Docherty AH, Knight CH, Wilde CJ. Metabolic adaptations in mouse mammary gland during a normal lactation cycle and in extended lactation. Q J Exp Physiol 1987;72:303-311.
Sicinski P, Donaher JL, Parker SB, Li T, Fazeli A, Gardner H, Haslma SZ, Bronson RT, Elledge SJ, Weinberg RA. Cyclin D1 provides a link between development and oncogenesis in the retina and breast. Cell 1995;82:621-630.
Simons JP, McClenaghan M, Clark AJ. Alteration of the quality of milk by expression of sheep beta-lactoglobulin in transgenic mice. Nature 1987;328:530-532.
Sinn E, Muller W, Pattengale P, Tepler I, Wallace R, Leder P. Coexpression of MMTV/v-Ha-ras and MMTV/c-myc genes in transgenic mice: synergistic action of oncogenes in vivo. Cell 1987;49:465-475.

Sirito M, Lin Q, Maity T, Sawadogo M. Ubiquitous expression of the 43- and 44-kDa forms of transcription factor USF in mammalian cells. Nucleic Acids Res1994;22:427-433.

Sirito M, Lin Q, Deng JM, Behringer RR, Sawadogo M. Overlapping roles and asymetrical cross-regulation of the USF proteins in mice. Proc Natl Acad Sci USA 1998;95:3758-3763.

Sohail M, Doran G, Riedemann J, Macaulay V, Southern EM. A simple and cost-effective method for producing small interfering RNAs with high efficacy. Nucleic Acids Res 2003;31:e38.

Soriano P, Gridley T, Jaenisch R. Retroviruses and insertional mutagenesis in mice: proviral integration at the Mov 34 locus leads to early embryonic death. Genes Dev1987;1:366-375.

Soulier S, Stinnakre MG, Lepourry L, Mercier JC, Vilotte JL. Use of doxycycline-controlled gene expression to reversibly alter milk-protein composition in transgenic mice. Eur J Biochem 1999;260:533-539.

Stacey A, Bateman J, Choi T, Mascara T, Cole W, Jaenisch R. Perinatal lethal osteogenesis imperfecta in transgenic mice bearing an engineered mutant pro-alpha 1(I) collagen gene. Nature 1988;332:131-136.

Stacey A, Schnieke A, Kerr M, Scott A, McKee C, Cottingham I, Binas B, Wilde C, Colman A. Lactation is disrupted by alpha-lactalbumin deficiency and can be restored by human alpha-lactalbumin gene replacement in mice. Proc Natl Acad Sci USA 1995;92:2835-2839.

Stark GR, Kerr IM, Williams BR, Silverman RH, Schreiber RD. How cells respond to interferons. Annu Rev Biochem 1998;67:227-264.

Stewart TA, Pattengale PK, Leder P. Spontaneous mammary adenocarcinomas in transgenic MTV/myc fusion genes. Cell 1984;38:627-637.

Stinnakre MG, Vilotte JL, Soulier S, Mercier JC. Creation and phenotypic analysis of alpha-lactalbumin-deficient mice. Proc Natl Acad Sci USA 1994;91:6544-6548.

Thomas KR, Capecchi MR. Site-directed mutagenesis by gene targeting in mouse embryo-derived stem cells. Cell 1987;51:503-512.

Thompson S, Clarke AR, Pow AM, Hooper ML, Melton DW. Germ line transmission and expression of a corrected HPRT gene produced by gene targeting in embryonic stem cells. Cell 1989;56:313-321.

Tonner E, Barber MC, Allan GJ, Beattie J, Webster J, Whitelaw CB, Flint DJ. Insulin-like growth factor binding protein-5 (IGFBP-5) induces premature cell death in the mammary glands of transgenic mice. Development 2002;129:4547-4557.

Tsukamoto AS, Grosshedl R, Guzman RC, Parslow T, Varmus HE. Expression of the int-1 gene in transgenic mice is associated with mammary gland hyperplasia and adenocarcinomas in male and female mice. Cell 1988;55:619-625.

Vallet VS, Henrion AA, Bucchini D, Casado M, Raymondjean M, Kahn A, Vaulont S. Glucose-dependent liver gene expression in upstream stimulatory factor 2 -/- mice. J Biol Chem 1997;272:21944-21949.

Vallet VS, Casado M, Henrion AA, Bucchini D, Raymondjean M, Kahn A, Vaulont S. Differential roles of upstream stimulatory factors 1 and 2 in the transcriptional response of liver genes to glucose. J Biol Chem 1998;273:20175-20179.

van der Putten H, Botteri F, Illmensee K. Developmental fate of a human insulin gene in a transgenic mouse. Mol Gen Genet 1984;198:128-138.

VanWyk JJ, Hall K, Van den Brande JL, Weaver RP. Further purification and characterization of sulfation factor and thymidine factor from acromegalic plasma. J Clin Endocrinol Metab 1971;32:389-403.

Venter JC, Adams MD, Myers EW, Li PW, Mural RJ, Sutton GG, Smith HO, Yandell M, Evans CA, Holt RA, Gocayne JD, Amanatides P, Ballew RM, Huson DH, Wortman JR, Zhang Q, Kodira CD, Zheng XH, Chen L, Skupski M, Subramanian G, Thomas PD, Zhang J, Gabor Miklos GL, Nelson C, Broder S, Clark AG, Nadeau J, McKusick VA, Zinder N, Levine AJ, Roberts RJ, Simon M, Slayman C, Hunkapiller M, Bolanos R, Delcher A, Dew I, Fasulo D, Flanigan M, Florea L, Halpern A, Hannenhalli S, Kravitz S, Levy S, Mobarry C, Reinert K, Remington K, Abu-Threideh J, Beasley E, Biddick K, Bonazzi V, Brandon R, Cargill M, Chandramouliswaran I, Charlab R, Chaturvedi K, Deng Z, Di F, V, Dunn P, Eilbeck K, Evangelista C, Gabrielian AE, Gan W, Ge W, Gong F, Gu Z, Guan P, Heiman TJ, Higgins ME, Ji RR, Ke Z, Ketchum KA, Lai Z, Lei Y, Li Z, Li J, Liang Y, Lin X, Lu F, Merkulov GV, Milshina N, Moore HM, Naik AK, Narayan VA, Neelam B, Nusskern D, Rusch DB, Salzberg S, Shao W, Shue B, Sun J, Wang Z, Wang A, Wang X, Wang J, Wei M, Wides R, Xiao C, Yan C, Yao A, Ye J, Zhan M, Zhang W, Zhang H, Zhao Q, Zheng L, Zhong F, Zhong W, Zhu S, Zhao S, Gilbert D, Baumhueter S, Spier G, Carter C, Cravchik A, Woodage T, Ali F, An H, Awe A, Baldwin D, Baden H, Barnstead M, Barrow I, Beeson K, Busam D, Carver A, Center A, Cheng ML, Curry L, Danaher S, Davenport L, Desilets R, Dietz S, Dodson K, Doup L, Ferriera S, Garg N, Gluecksmann A, Hart B, Haynes J, Haynes C, Heiner C, Hladun S, Hostin D, Houck J, Howland T, Ibegwam C, Johnson J, Kalush F, Kline L, Koduru S, Love A, Mann F, May D, McCawley S, McIntosh T, McMullen I, Moy M, Moy L, Murphy B, Nelson K, Pfannkoch C, Pratts E, Puri V, Qureshi H, Reardon M, Rodriguez R, Rogers YH, Romblad D, Ruhfel B, Scott R, Sitter C, Smallwood M, Stewart E, Strong R, Suh E, Thomas R, Tint NN, Tse S, Vech C, Wang G, Wetter J, Williams S, Williams M, Windsor S, Winn-Deen E, Wolfe K, Zaveri J, Zaveri K, Abril JF, Guigo R, Campbell MJ, Sjolander KV, Karlak B, Kejariwal A, Mi H, Lazareva B, Hatton T, Narechania A, Diemer

K, Muruganujan A, Guo N, Sato S, Bafna V, Istrail S, Lippert R, Schwartz R, Walenz B, Yooseph S, Allen D, Basu A, Baxendale J, Blick L, Caminha M, Carnes-Stine J, Caulk P, Chiang YH, Coyne M, Dahlke C, Mays A, Dombroski M, Donnelly M, Ely D, Esparham S, Fosler C, Gire H, Glanowski S, Glasser K, Glodek A, Gorokhov M, Graham K, Gropman B, Harris M, Heil J, Henderson S, Hoover J, Jennings D, Jordan C, Jordan J, Kasha J, Kagan L, Kraft C, Levitsky A, Lewis M, Liu X, Lopez J, Ma D, Majoros W, McDaniel J, Murphy S, Newman M, Nguyen T, Nguyen N, Nodell M. The sequence of the human genome. Science 2001;291:1304-1351.

Vilotte JL. Lowering the milk lactose in vivo: potential interests, strategies, and physiological consequences. Reprod Nutr Dev 2002;42:127-132.

Wagner KU, Wall RJ, St Onge L, Gruss P, Wynshaw-Boris A, Garrett L, Li M, Furth PA, Hennighausen L. Cre-mediated gene deletion in the mammary gland. Nucleic Acids Res 1997;25:4323-4330.

Wagner KU, McAllister K, Ward T, Davis B, Wiseman R, Hennighausen L. Spatial and temporal expression of the cre gene under the control of the MMTV-LTR in different lines of transgenic mice. Transgenic Res 2001;10:545-553.

Walton KD, Wagner KU, Rucker EB III, Shillingford JM, Miyoshi K, Hennighausen L. Conditional deletion of the bcl-x gene from mouse mammary epithelium results in accelerated apoptosis during involution but does not compromise cell function during lactation. Mech Dev 2001;109:281-293.

Wang Y, DeMayo FJ, Tsai SY, O'Malley BW. Ligand-inducible and liver-specific target gene expression in transgenic mice. Nat Biotechnol 1997;15:239-243.

Waterston RH, Lindblad-Toh K, Birney E, Rogers J, Abril JF, Agarwal P, Agarwala R, Ainscough R, Alexandersson M, An P, Antonarakis SE, Attwood J, Baertsch R, Bailey J, Barlow K, Beck S, Berry E, Birren B, Bloom T, Bork P, Botcherby M, Bray N, Brent MR, Brown DG, Brown SD, Bult C, Burton J, Butler J, Campbell RD, Carninci P, Cawley S, Chiaromonte F, Chinwalla AT, Church DM, Clamp M, Clee C, Collins FS, Cook LL, Copley RR, Coulson A, Couronne O, Cuff J, Curwen V, Cutts T, Daly M, David R, Davies J, Delehaunty KD, Deri J, Dermitzakis ET, Dewey C, Dickens NJ, Diekhans M, Dodge S, Dubchak I, Dunn DM, Eddy SR, Elnitski L, Emes RD, Eswara P, Eyras E, Felsenfeld A, Fewell GA, Flicek P, Foley K, Frankel WN, Fulton LA, Fulton RS, Furey TS, Gage D, Gibbs RA, Glusman G, Gnerre S, Goldman N, Goodstadt L, Grafham D, Graves TA, Green ED, Gregory S, Guigo R, Guyer M, Hardison RC, Haussler D, Hayashizaki Y, Hillier LW, Hinrichs A, Hlavina W, Holzer T, Hsu F, Hua A, Hubbard T, Hunt A, Jackson I, Jaffe DB, Johnson LS, Jones M, Jones TA, Joy A, Kamal M, Karlsson EK, Karolchik D, Kasprzyk A, Kawai J, Keibler E, Kells C, Kent WJ, Kirby A, Kolbe DL, Korf I, Kucherlapati RS, Kulbokas EJ, Kulp D, Landers T, Leger JP, Leonard S, Letunic I, Levine R, Li J, Li M, Lloyd C, Lucas S, Ma B, Maglott DR, Mardis ER, Matthews L, Mauceli E, Mayer JH, McCarthy M, McCombie WR, McLaren S, McLay K, McPherson JD, Meldrim J, Meredith B, Mesirov JP, Miller W, Miner TL, Mongin E, Montgomery KT, Morgan M, Mott R, Mullikin JC, Muzny DM, Nash WE, Nelson JO, Nhan MN, Nicol R, Ning Z, Nusbaum C, O'Connor MJ, Okazaki Y, Oliver K, Overton-Larty E, Pachter L, Parra G, Pepin KH, Peterson J, Pevzner P, Plumb R, Pohl CS, Poliakov A, Ponce TC, Ponting CP, Potter S, Quail M, Reymond A, Roe BA, Roskin KM, Rubin EM, Rust AG, Santos R, Sapojnikov V, Schultz B, Schultz J, Schwartz MS, Schwartz S, Scott C, Seaman S, Searle S, Sharpe T, Sheridan A, Shownkeen R, Sims S, Singer JB, Slater G, Smit A, Smith DR, Spencer B, Stabenau A, Stange-Thomann N, Sugnet C, Suyama M, Tesler G, Thompson J, Torrents D, Trevaskis E, Tromp J, Ucla C, Ureta-Vidal A, Vinson JP, Von Niederhausern AC, Wade CM, Wall M, Weber RJ, Weiss RB, Wendl MC, West AP, Wetterstrand K, Wheeler R, Whelan S, Wierzbowski J, Willey D, Williams S, Wilson RK, Winter E, Worley KC, Wyman D, Yang S, Yang SP, Zdobnov EM, Zody MC, Lander ES. Initial sequencing and comparative analysis of the mouse genome. Nature 2002;420:520-562.

Wiltshire T, Pletcher MT, Batalov S, Barnes SW, Tarantino LM, Cooke MP, Wu H, Smylie K, Santrosyan A, Copeland NG, Jenkins NA, Kalush F, Mural RJ, Glynne RJ, Kay SA, Adams MD, Fletcher CF. Genome-wide single-nucleotide polymorphism analysis defines haplotype patterns in mouse. Proc Natl Acad Sci USA 2003;100:3380-3385.

Wintermantel TM, Mayer AK, Schutz G, Greiner EF. Targeting mammary epithelial cells using a bacterial artificial chromosome. Genesis 2002;33:125-130.

Withers DJ, Gutierrez JS, Towery H, Burks DJ, Ren JM, Previs S, Zhang Y, Bernal D, Pons S, Shulman GI, Bonner-Wier S, White MF. Disruption of IRS-2 causes type 2 diabetes in mice. Nature 1998;391:900-904.

Withers DJ, Burks DJ, Towery HH, Altamuro SL, Flint CL, White MF. Irs-2 coordinates Igf-1 receptor-mediated β-cell development and perhipheral insulin signalling. Nat Genet 1999;23:32-40.

Wolf E, Jehle PM, Weber MM, Sauerwein H, Daxenberger A, Breier BH, Besenfelder U, Frenyo L, Brem G. Human insulin-like growth factor I (IGF-I) produced in the mammary glands of transgenic rabbits: yield, receptor binding, mitogenic activity, and effects on IGF-binding proteins. Endocrinology 1997;138:307-313.

Wood TL, Richert MM, Stull MA, Allar MA. The insulin-like growth factors (IGFs) and IGF binding proteins in postnatal development of murine mammary glands. J Mammary Gland Biol Neoplasia 2000;5:31-42.

Working Group on Breastfeeding. Breastfeeding and the use of human milk (RE9729). Pediatrics 1997;100:1035-1039.

Wysolmerski JJ, McCaughern-Carucci JF, Daifotis AG, Broadus AE, Philbrick WM. Overexpression of parathyroid hormone-related protein or parathyroid hormone in transgenic mice impairs branching morphogenesis during mammary gland development. Development 1995;121:3539-3547.

Xia H, Mao Q, Paulson HL, Davidson BL. siRNA-mediated gene silencing in vitro and in vivo. Nat Biotechnol 2002;20:1006-1010.

Yu SH, Deen KC, Lee E, Hennighausen L, Sweet RW, Rosenberg M, Westphal H. Functional human CD4 protein produced in milk of transgenic mice. Mol Biol Med 1989;6:255-261.

Yu J, DeRuiter SL, Turner DL. RNA interference by expression of short-interfering RNAs and hairpin RNAs in mammalian cells. Proc Natl Acad Sci USA 2002;99:6047-6052.

Zamore PD. Ancient pathways programmed by small RNAs. Science 2002;296:1265-1269.

Zijlstra M, Li E, Sajjadi F, Subramani S, Jaenisch R. Germ-line transmission of a disrupted beta 2-microglobulin gene produced by homologous recombination in embryonic stem cells. Nature 1989;342:435-438.

GLUCOSE TRANSPORT IN LACTATION

Peter M. Haney

1. ABSTRACT

Lactose is the major carbohydrate of human milk and is also the major osmotic constituent of human milk. Therefore, synthesis of lactose is the major determinant of the volume of milk produced by the lactating human mammary gland. Lactose is synthesized from free glucose and UDP-galactose. Thus, glucose transport is required not only across the plasma membrane but also across an intracellular membrane to the compartment of lactose synthesis. The latter requirement is unique to mammary epithelial cells. Historically, based primarily on subcellular fractionation studies, lactose synthesis was thought to occur in Golgi. Yet, the only known glucose transporter isoform expressed in mammary gland is GLUT1, a plasma membrane glucose transporter. We therefore comprehensively studied the possible role of GLUT1 as a glucose transporter. We tested the hypothesis that changes in the amount, activity, and subcellular targeting of GLUT1 during lactation are consistent with an important role for GLUT1 in the regulation of lactation. The experiments described here summarize our recent work in the lactating mouse mammary gland and in mouse mammary epithelial cells in culture. The results demonstrate that GLUT1 is targeted to an intracellular compartment. However, studies in mammary epithelial cells in culture demonstrate that this is not a Golgi compartment, but a low-density, exquisitely Brefeldin A-sensitive compartment of Golgi-related vesicles. This raises the possibility that lactose synthesis does not take place in the Golgi proper. The results strongly suggest that GLUT1 appears to be important in delivery of substrate to the site of lactose synthesis.

2. INTRODUCTION

Pediatricians and other health care professionals recommend that mothers breastfeed. This recommendation is supported by a wealth of evidence regarding the nutritional, neurodevelopmental, immunologic, and psychologic benefits of breastfeeding (AAP 1997). However, our understanding of the elaborate and elegant machinery of milk

---

Department of Pediatrics, Section of Neonatology, USDA/ARS, Children's Nutrition Research Center, Baylor College of Medicine, Houston, TX 77030

synthesis and secretion is primitive. This chapter will focus on exploring what is likely to be one of the simplest components of this process, the synthesis and secretion of lactose.

Lactose is the major carbohydrate of human milk and is also the major osmotic constituent of human milk. Therefore, synthesis of lactose is the major determinant of the volume of milk produced by the lactating human mammary gland. Lactose is synthesized from free glucose and UDP-galactose. Measurements of intracellular glucose concentration reveal that glucose transport is rate-limiting for lactose synthesis (Wilde & Kuhn 1981). Historically, based primarily on subcellular fractionation studies, lactose synthesis is thought to occur in Golgi. Thus, glucose transport is required not only across the plasma membrane but also across an intracellular membrane to the compartment of lactose synthesis. The latter requirement is unique to mammary epithelial cells. Yet, the only known glucose transporter isoform expressed in mammary gland is GLUT1, a plasma membrane glucose transporter.

Previous studies in the mammary gland provide conflicting evidence regarding whether GLUT1 is targeted to intracellular compartments. Subcellular fractionation and Western blotting studies of rat mammary glands at day 10 of lactation give results consistent with Golgi localization of GLUT1 (Madon et al. 1990), but studies relying on microscopy (Camps et al. 1994) identify GLUT1 as a plasma membrane protein, with no intracellular localization. We therefore comprehensively studied the possible role of GLUT1 as a glucose transporter. We tested the hypothesis that changes in the amount, activity, and subcellular targeting of GLUT1 during lactation are consistent with an important role for GLUT1 in the regulation of lactation. The experiments described here summarize our recent work in the lactating mouse mammary gland (Nemeth et al. 2000) and in mouse mammary epithelial cells in culture (Haney 2001). The results demonstrate that GLUT1 is targeted to an intracellular compartment. However, studies in mammary epithelial cells in culture demonstrate that this is not a Golgi compartment, but a low-density, exquisitely Brefeldin A-sensitive compartment of Golgi-related vesicles. The results strongly suggest that GLUT1 appears to be important in delivery of substrate to the site of lactose synthesis.

3. MATERIALS AND METHODS

3.1. Antisera

Rabbit antibody to human GLUT1 raised against a sysnthetic peptide including the 16 C-terminal amio acids was a gift from Dr. Mike Mueckler (Washington University, St. Louis, MO). This antibody was affinity purified using the same peptide bound to thio-propyl sepharose. Mouse monoclonal antibodies to rat GM130 were from Transduction Laboratories, Lexington, KY.

3.2. Cell Culture

CIT3 cells were supplied by Dr. Margaret Neville (University of Colorado, Denver, CO). Cells were maintained in growth medium, which included 10 μg/mL insulin and 5 ng/mL epidermal growth factor. To differentiate the cells, secretion medium, which lacked epidermal growth factor but did contain 10 μg/mL insulin, as well as 3 μg/mL prolactin and 3 μg/mL hydrocortisone, was used for 4 days. In certain experiments, cells were exposed to 500 nm or 5 μM Brefeldin A for 30 minutes at 37°C just prior to fixation.

3.3. Subcellular Fractionation and Density Gradient Centrifugation

Mammary glands were removed, rinsed, resuspended in a small amount of homogenization buffer (PBS, 1 mM EDTA), and homogenized. Centrifugations were 3,000×g for 10 minutes, 17,000×g for 10 minutes, and 100,000×g for 30 minutes. Density gradient centrifugation of the 17,000-g pellet was in a self-generating iodixanol density gradient (10–37%) at 180,000×g for 3 hours.

3.4. Western Blotting

SDS-PAGE and wet transfer of proteins to nitrocellulose were by standard methods. Primary antibody was the peptide affinity-purified GLUT1 antibody described above, at a concentration of 1 μg/mL. Differences were quantitated using laser densitometry and analyzed using ImageQuant software.

3.5. 2-Deoxyglucose Uptake

Uptake of [^{3}H]2-deoxyglucose was measured using standard methods (Tordjman et al. 1989). Noncarrier-mediated uptake was measured in the presence of 20 μM cytochalasin B. This was subtracted from total 2-deoxyglucose uptake and results therefore reflect specific carrier-mediated activity. Statistical significance was calculated using Student t-test for independent samples.

3.6. Confocal Microscopy

Primary antibodies described above were used at a concentration of 2.5 μg/mL for GLUT1 and 5 μg/mL for GM130. After rinsing, fluorescein-labeled goat anti-rabbit antibodies and Texas-red sheep anti-mouse antibodies were applied. Under these circumstances, yellow signal indicates colocalization. The inverted confocal laser scanning microscope used was a Molecular Dynamics Multiprobe 2010.

4. RESULTS AND DISCUSSION

GLUT1 expression in mouse mammary gland (Fig. 1) was studied throughout the lactation cycle. GLUT1 was present in low levels in virgins, gradually increased during pregnancy, rose abruptly about the time of delivery, peaked during midlactation, and abruptly fell to low levels upon weaning. This expression pattern reflects a protein whose role is tightly coupled to lactation.

Further evidence that GLUT1 is important to lactation via delivery of substrate to intracellular compartments was provided by evidence of a shift in GLUT1 targeting during the lactation cycle. Fractions enriched in Golgi (Fig. 2, lane 4) and plasma membrane (Fig. 2, lane 5) were prepared. Plasma membrane targeting was dominant in virgin mice, but by day 8 of lactation, targeting to the Golgi-enriched fraction was dominant. If this phenomenon was a key regulatory mechanism, we would expect to observe targeting to Golgi-enriched fractions regulated appropriately during forced

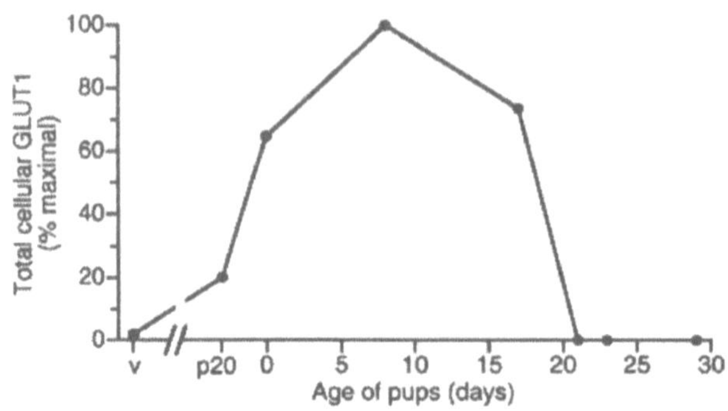

Figure 1. GLUT1 is expressed at low levels in virgin gland (v) and at low levels in late pregnancy (p), but at high levels during lactation, and then falls abruptly to low levels upon weaning. Levels of GLUT1 protein were determined by Western blotting and expressed as a percentage of the value on day 8.

weaning, when removal of pups curtails milk production and returning them causes a resumption of milk production. Indeed, we observed exactly this, as the preferential targeting of GLUT1 to Golgi-enriched fractions (Fig. 3, lane 4) during lactation held true after 90 minutes of forced weaning, but by 3 hours, GLUT1 was targeted preferentially to plasma membrane-enriched fractions (Fig. 3, lane 5). By 5 hours of forced weaning, GLUT1 was targeted almost exclusively to plasma membrane-enriched fractions. Furthermore, this effect was reversible. When pups were returned to the mother after 5 hours of forced weaning, just 5 hours later targeting of GLUT1 to Golgi-enriched fractions was substantially restored, and after 15 hours full restoration occurred (Fig. 4). The reversible character of the targeting of GLUT1 to Golgi-enriched fractions and the rapid manner in which this targeting is modulated indicate a dynamic process of glucose transporter targeting that requires frequent suckling to maintain optimal substrate delivery for lactose synthesis.

Immunocytochemical and immunofluorescence studies (data not shown) confirmed intracellular localization of GLUT1 during lactation and revealed partial colocalization with β-COP, a marker of Golgi as well as certain other related intracellular compartments. To further define the intracellular compartment, we turned to studies in culture of the CIT3 mammary epithelial cell. These cells were selected from Comma-1-D cells for their ability to form tight junctions, express β-casein, and exhibit polarized transport in response to prolactin and hydrocortisone (Toddywalla et al. 1997). Total cellular content of GLUT1 rose 15-fold in these cells in response to treatment with prolactin and hydrocortisone (Fig. 5). Despite the increased level of GLUT1 protein, 2-deoxyglucose uptake, which reflects glucose transport activity at the plasma membrane, declined 70% (Fig. 5), suggesting either decreased specific activity of the transporter or a lack of its availability at the plasma membrane. Consistent with results shown above in the lactating mammary gland, subcellular fractionation studies showed predominant GLUT1 targeting to plasma membrane-enriched fractions in the absence of prolactin and hydrocortisone, and predominant GLUT1 targeting to Golgi-enriched fractions in the presence of prolactin and hydrocortisone (Fig. 6). Iodoxanol density gradient centrifugation of the Golgi-enriched pellet demonstrated that GLUT1 was targeted to low density (1.05–1.08 g/cm^3) fractions, consistent with Golgi localization.

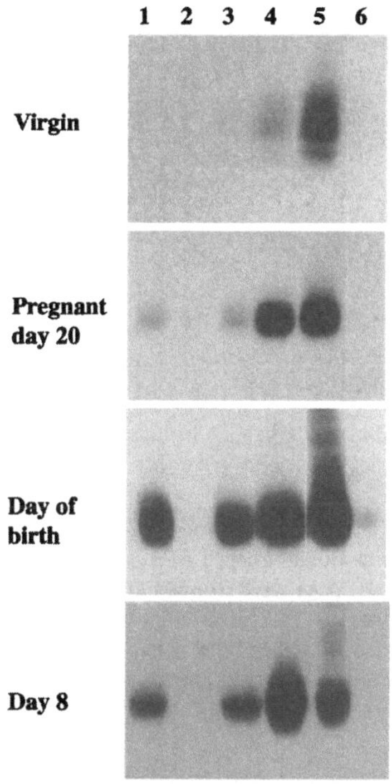

Figure 2. GLUT1 is targeted to Golgi-enriched fractions during lactation. Lane 1: homogenate; lane 2: 3,000-g (nuclear) pellet; lane 3: 3,000-g supernatant; lane 4: 17,000-g (Golgi-enriched) pellet; lane 5: 100,000-g (plasma membrane-enriched) pellet; lane 6: 100,000-g supernatant (cytosol). Samples contained 60 μg of protein except for virgin samples, which contained 25 μg. In virgin gland, GLUT1 is targeted predominantly to plasma membrane. There is approximately equivalent targeting to plasma membrane-enriched and Golgi-enriched fractions in late pregnancy and on the day of delivery. GLUT1 is predominantly targeted to the Golgi-enriched fraction on day 8.

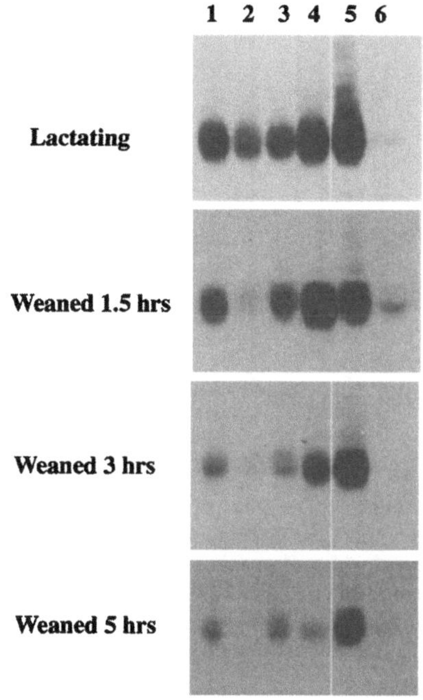

Figure 3. Forced weaning causes a decline in GLUT1 protein and in targeting of GLUT1 to Golgi-enriched fractions. Lane 1: homogenate; lane 2: 3,000-g (nuclear) pellet; lane 3: 3,000-g supernatant; lane 4: 17,000-g (Golgi-enriched) pellet; lane 5: 100,000-g (plasma membrane-enriched) pellet; lane 6: 100,000-g supernatant (cytosol). Samples contained 60 μg of protein. Declines in amount of GLUT1 and in its targeting to Golgi-enriched fractions are apparent after 3 hours and are pronounced after 5 hours.

Confocal immunofluorescent microscopy confirmed that GLUT1 targeting was primarily to plasma membrane in the absence of prolactin and hydrocortisone (Fig. 7A). In the presence of prolactin and hydrocortisone, GLUT1 showed an intracellular pattern with a perinuclear predominance, but also a punctate distribution throughout the cytoplasm (Fig. 7D). In neither case was there colocalization of GLUT1 with the trans-Golgi marker Brefeldin A (Figs. 7C and 7F). Since Brefeldin A sensitivity is a hallmark of Golgi, we tested the relative effect of low (500 nM) and high (5 μM) concentrations of Brefeldin A on the targeting of GLUT1 and GM130, a cis-Golgi marker, in cells exposed to prolactin and hydrocortisone. The results (Fig. 8) show that the perinuclear localization

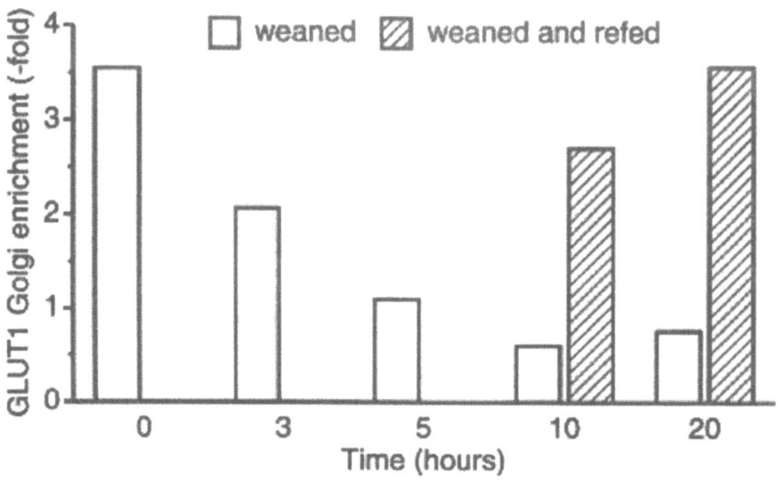

Figure 4. The effect of forced weaning on GLUT1 targeting to Golgi-enriched fractions is reversible. Values indicated in crosshatch are from mothers whose pups were returned after 5 hours of forced weaning. Targeting to Golgi-enriched fractions was lost by 5 hours and was not observed at 10 and 20 hours. However, when pups were returned to mothers after 5 hours of forced weaning, targeting of GLUT1 to Golgi-enriched fractions was observed 5 hours later, and was restored fully 15 hours later.

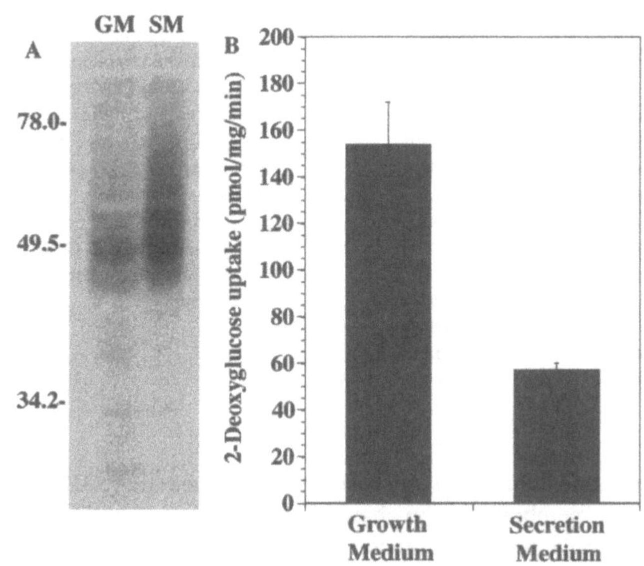

Figure 5. Lactogenic hormones increase the amount of GLUT1 but decrease the uptake of 2-deoxyglucose across the plasma membrane. CIT3 mouse mammary epithelial cells were grown in the absence (lane 1, 60 μg protein) and presence (lane 2, 20 μg protein) of prolactin and hydrocortisone. Difference in 2-deoxyglucose activity was significant ($P<0.003$). GM=growth medium; SM=secretion medium.

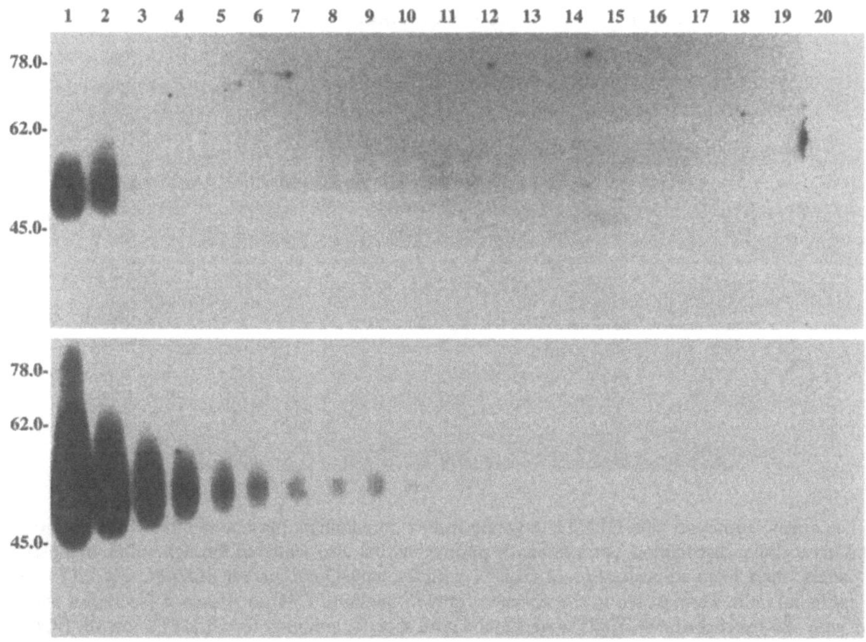

Figure 6. GLUT1 is targeted to low-density fractions. CIT3 mouse mammary epithelial cells were grown in the absence (upper panel) and presence (lower panel) of prolactin and hydrocortisone. Golgi-enriched fractions were subjected to iodixanol density gradient centrifugation, and 10 μg of protein from each fraction was subjected to SDS-PAGE and Western blotting. GLUT1 was concentrated in the least dense fractions (1.05–1.08 g/cm^3).

of GLUT1 is completely abolished at the low Brefeldin A concentration, while the high concentration is necessary to maximally disrupt GM130 targeting. In other words, GLUT1 is even more sensitive to Brefeldin A than the Golgi marker GM130. There is also no evidence of colocalization of GLUT1 with GM130. In other experiments not shown here, there was also no colocalization of GLUT1 with *i)* EYFP-Golgi, which contains the targeting domain of galactosyltransferase and is a medial-Golgi marker, *ii)* β-COP, which marks Golgi as well as certain other intermediate compartments, and *iii)* transferrin-Texas Red, a marker of early endosomes.

These results, as well as unpublished video microscopy in living cells we performed, indicate that although GLUT1 is targeted to a compartment that has both the low density and the Brefeldin A sensitivity characteristic of Golgi, this compartment does not represent classical Golgi proper. Rather, the intracellular GLUT1 compartment is an exquisitely Brefeldin A-sensitive, low-density, vesicular compartment that is presumably closely related to Golgi. These results have the potential to alter the current paradigm of lactose synthesis, which is thought to take place in the Golgi. Identifying the sorter that is responsible for the sequestration of GLUT1 in the lactose synthesis compartment is an important goal, as the activity of this sorter may well be an important regulator of substrate delivery for lactose synthesis, and therefore an important regulator of milk production.

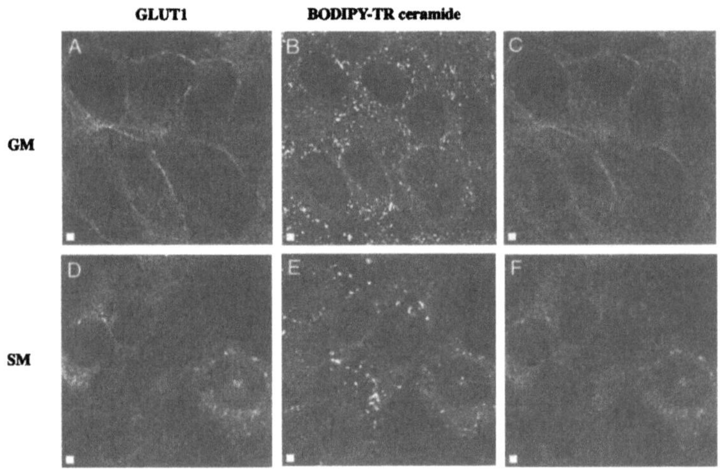

Figure 7. Lactogenic hormones alter GLUT1 targeting from a predominant plasma membrane distribution to a predominant intracellular distribution, predominantly perinuclear but also scattered throughout the cytoplasm in a punctate pattern; there is no colocalization of GLUT1 with the trans-Golgi marker BODIPY-TR. CIT3 mouse mammary epithelial cells were grown in the absence (growth medium, GM) or presence (secretion medium, SM) of prolactin and hydrocortisone. Cells were stained with specific antibody for GLUT1 and with BODIPY-TR ceramide, fixed, and studied by confocal microscopy.

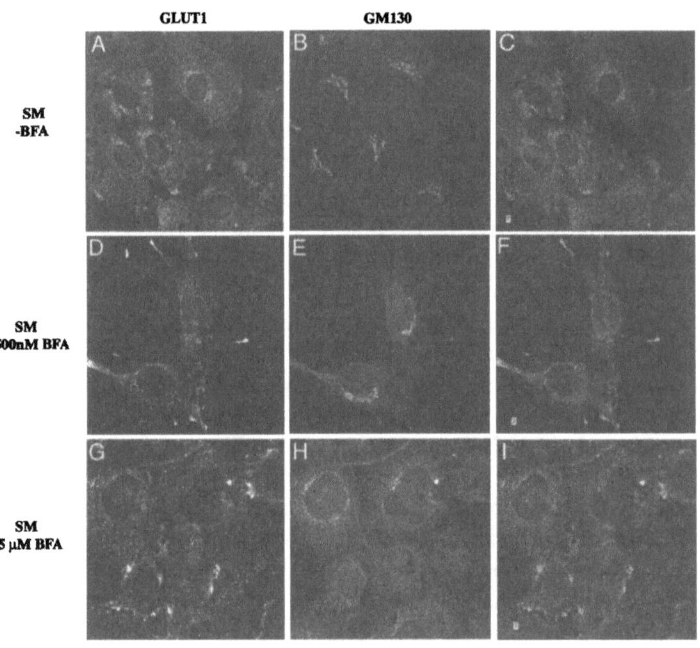

Figure 8. Perinuclear targeting of GLUT1 is exquisitely sensitive to Brefeldin A. CIT3 mouse mammary epithelial cells grown in no (upper panels), low concentration (500 nM), or high concentration (5 μM) Brefeldin A were stained with specific antibody for GLUT1 and the Golgi marker GM130, fixed, and studied by confocal microscopy. 500 nM Brefeldin A perturbed GM130 only slightly but completely abolished perinuclear localization of GLUT1. SM=secretory medium containing Brefeldin A (BFA).

5. ACKNOWLEDGMENTS

I wish to acknowledge the expert technical assistance of Ms. Stella Tsang and the dedicated work of Dr. Arieh Riskin. Support provided by U.S. Department of Defense grants DAMD17-94-J-4241 and DAMD17-96-1-6257 and by NIH grant 1R29HD/DK34701. This project of the USDA/ARS Children's Nutrition Research Center, Department of Pediatrics, Baylor College of Medicine, and Texas Children's Hospital has been funded in part with federal funds from the USDA/ARS under cooperative agreement number 58-6250-6-001. The contents of this publication do not necessarily reflect the views or policies of the U.S. Department of Agriculture, nor does mention of trade names, commercial products, or organizations imply endorsement by the U.S. government.

Figures 1 through 4 reprinted from Pediatric Research, Vol. 47, B.A. Nemeth et al., Golgi targeting of the GLUT1 glucose transporter in lactating mouse mammary gland, pp. 444-450, Copyright 2000, with permission from Pediatric Research. Figures 5 through 8 reprinted from Cell Biology International, Vol. 25, P.M. Haney, Localization of the GLUT1 glucose transporter to Brefeldin A-sensitive vesicles of differentiated CIT3 mouse mammary epithelial cells, pp. 277-288, Copyright (2001), with permission from Elsevier Science.

6. REFERENCES

[AAP] American Academy of Pediatrics. Work Group on Breastfeeding. Breastfeeding and the use of human milk. Pediatrics 1997;100;1035-1039.

Camps M, Vilaro S, Testar X, Palacin M, Zorzano Z. High and polarized expression of GLUT1 glucose transporters in epithelial cells from mammary gland: acute down-regulation of GLUT1 carriers by weaning. Endocrinology 1994;134:924-934.

Haney PM. Localization of the GLUT1 glucose transporter to brefeldin A-sensitive vesicles of differentiated CIT3 mouse mammary epithelial cells. Cell Biol Int 2001;25:277-288.

Madon RJ, Martin S, Davies A, Fawcett HA, Flint DJ, Baldwin SA. Identification and characterization of glucose transport proteins in plasma membrane- and Golgi vesicle-enriched fractions prepared from lactating rat mammary gland. Biochem J 1990;272:99-105.

Nemeth BA, Tsang SW, Geske RS, Haney PM. Golgi targeting of the GLUT1 glucose transporter in lactating mouse mammary gland. Pediatr Res 2000;47:444-450.

Toddywalla VS, Kari FW, Neville MC. Active transport of nitrofurantoin across a mouse mammary epithelial monolayer. J Pharmacol Exp Ther 1997;280:669-676.

Tordjman KM, Leingang KA, James DE, Mueckler MM. Differential regulation of two distinct glucose transporter species expressed in 3T3-L1 adipocytes: effect of chronic insulin and tolbutamide treatment. Proc Natl Acad Sci USA 1989;86:7761-7765.

Wilde CJ, Kuhn NJ. Lactose synthesis and the utilisation of glucose by rat mammary acini. Int J Biochem 1981;13:311-316.

REGULATION OF MILK LIPID FORMATION AND SECRETION IN THE MOUSE MAMMARY GLAND

James L. McManaman[1], Carol A. Palmer[2], Steven Anderson[3], Kaylee Schwertfeger[4], and Margaret C. Neville[1,4]

1. ABSTRACT

Cytosolic lipid droplets (CLDs), the immediate precursors of milk lipids in lactating animals, undergo cell-specific changes in their formation and intracellular distribution during mammary gland differentiation. Cell biological studies indicate that CLD formation in mammary epithelial cells is regulated in part by AKT-dependent increases in glucose uptake. Proteomic studies show that CLDs from lactating mammary epithelial cells possess a distinct protein composition enriched in molecules involved in their secretion and intracellular transport. CLD secretion is dependent on lactation and requires the purine catabolic enzyme xanthine oxidoreductase (XOR). Confocal immunofluorescence microscopy of XOR in lactating and nonlactating mammary glands and biochemical analysis of secreted CLDs link the secretion process to the formation of a stable tripartite complex between XOR, adipophilin (ADPH), and butyrophilin (Btn). Together these studies provide a molecular and cellular framework for understanding the process of milk lipid formation.

2. INTRODUCTION

Human milk is a complex fluid capable of sustaining the total nutrition of a human infant for six months or longer. In most mammalian species, including humans, lipids are a major constituent of milk; providing a large proportion of neonatal calories and essential fatty acids required for membrane synthesis. The composition of human milk reflects the activities of distinct secretion and transport processes of the mammary gland and mirrors the differing nutritional requirements of mammalian neonates. The various transport pathways involved in human milk production are depicted in Figure 1. Many of

[1]Division of Basic Reproductive Science, Department Obstetrics and Gynecology, University of Colorado Health Sciences Center (UCHSC), 4200 E. 9th Avenue, Denver, CO 80262
[2]Department of Physiology and Biophysics (UCHSC)
[3]Department of Pathology (UCHSC)
[4]Department of Cell Biology, Baylor College of Medicine, Houston, TX

Protecting Infants through Human Milk, edited by Pickering *et al.*
Kluwer Academic/Plenum Publishers, 2004

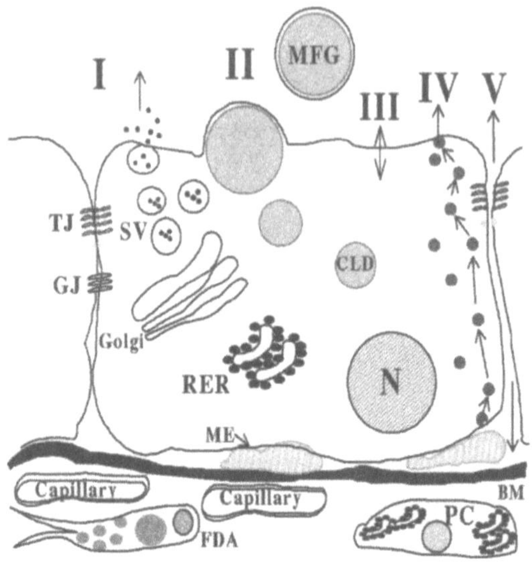

Figure 1. Pathways for milk secretion. I) Exocytotic pathway for secretion of lactose, milk protein, calcium, phosphate, and citrate. II) Synthesis and secretion of milk lipid. III) Apical membrane transporters for glucose, some amino acids, and monovalent ions. IV) Transcytotic pathway for immunoglobulins, other proteins. V) Paracellular pathway closed in lactation. TJ, tight junction; GJ, gap junction; D, desmosome; SV, secretory vesicle; RER, rough endoplasmic reticulum; ME, myoepithelial cell process; N, nucleus; CLD, cytoplasmic lipid droplet; MFG, milk fat globule. Adapted and used with permission from Kluwer Academic/Plenum Publishers (from Neville et al. In: Neville & Neifert, eds., 1983. Lactation: Physiology, Nutrition, and Breast-feeding).

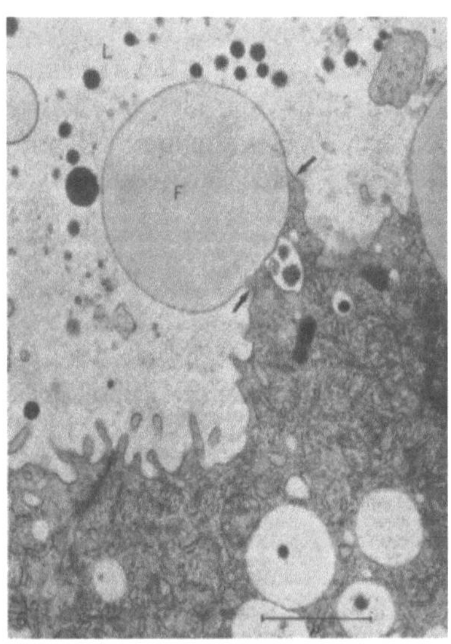

Figure 2. Electron micrograph showing a fat droplet (F) budding from an alveolar epithelial cell. Arrows indicate the continuity of the membrane surrounding the fat droplet and the apical plasma membrane of the cell. Reprinted with permission of the University of Pennsylvania Press (from Wellings SR. In: Monica Reynolds & SJ Foley, eds., 1969. Lactogenesis: The initiation of milk secretion at parturition).

these pathways, such as exocytosis of protein and lactose-containing vesicles (Pathway I) and transcytosis of immunoglobulins (Pathway IV), are similar to processes in the epithelia of many organs, although the nature of the compounds secreted is unique to the mammary gland. Lipids, however, are secreted by a novel pathway not duplicated in any other organ (Mather & Keenan 1998). Milk lipids originate from triglyceride and cholesterol ester containing cytoplasmic lipid droplets (CLDs), which are secreted by a novel membrane envelopment process (Pathway II). The details of this secretion process are understood poorly and still controversial (Mather & Keenan 1998). However, electron microscopic images showing CLDs contacting and being enveloped by the apical plasma membrane (Hollman 1974; Mather & Keenan 1998) in lactating mammary tissue imply the existence of specific CLD transport and docking mechanisms and have led to the hypothesis that CLD secretion occurs by a budding process (Fig. 2) that releases membrane bilayer-coated CLDs, commonly known as milk fat globules (MFG), into the alveolar lumen.

The lipid content of milk varies widely among species, ranging from <0.2% in rhinoceros milk to ~4% in humans and ruminants, to as much as 50% in seals and whales (Jenness 1979). Calculations of the amounts of milk lipid secreted by women and mice during a typical lactation period (Allen et al. 1991; Schwertfeger et al. 2003) indicate that for many species, including humans, the lactating mammary gland is among the most active of the lipogenic organs in the body. The substrate for lipid synthesis depends on diet. On a high fat diet such as the average American diet, about 90% of the fatty acids for triglyceride (TAG) synthesis are derived from dietary lipid or fat depots (Jensen et al. 1995; Hachey et al. 1987). TAG from VLDL and chylomicrons are broken down by lipoprotein lipase in the plasma compartment (Hamosh et al. 1970), and the resulting fatty acids, as well as those carried by albumin from fat stores, are transferred into the mammary alveolar cell to be re-esterified to TAG. In women on low-fat diets, as eaten in many economically developing areas, as well as by rodents on normal laboratory chow, the fatty acids for triglyceride synthesis are derived from glucose using well-described de novo lipogenic metabolic pathways (Dils 1983, 1986). Consequently milk lipid formation appears to be a highly regulated process requiring integration of biogenic, transport, and secretory functions. At present, we have only a limited understanding of both the molecular regulation of these functions and the cellular mechanisms that integrate their activities for efficient production of milk lipids during lactation.

Milk is secreted by a distinct population of epithelial cells that line the lumina of mammary alveoli. These alveolar epithelial cells undergo functional differentiation during the latter half of pregnancy in a complex process that is characterized by growth and proliferation of alveolar structures and expression of the necessary cellular elements for synthesis and secretion of milk components. This differentiation process, often referred to as lactogenesis, can be divided into initiation and secretory activation phases (Fleet et al. 1975; Hartmann 1973; Neville et al. 2002). The initiation phase, which begins around mid-pregnancy in most species, is associated with increase in alveolar size, lumenal expansion, and induction of milk protein gene expression. Although there is evidence that some epithelial cells become capable of secreting small quantities of milk specific components during this phase, overt secretion is held in check by high circulating levels of progesterone (Kuhn 1969). The decline in progesterone, which occurs around parturition in rodents, triggers the secretory activation phase that is characterized by concerted amplification of genes for milk proteins (Neville et al. 2002) and biosynthetic enzymes (Baldwin & Yang 1974), closure of tight junctions (Nguyen et al. 2001) and ultrastructural changes associated with copious milk secretion (Hollman 1974). Although many of the morphological and biochemical characteristics of this differentiation process are reasonably well established, less is known about the cellular and physiological changes required for alveolar epithelia cells to initiate milk secretion.

Genetic models have been helpful in defining critical processes and factors involved in regulating early stages of mammary gland development. However, at present only a limited number of models exist that possess specific defects in functional differentiation or milk secretion. Three distinct genetic models were described recently in which mammary epithelial cells undergo relatively normal alveologenesis but fail to lactate normally (Schwertfeger et al. 2003; Palmer et al. 2003; Vorbach et al. 2002). Interestingly, each model possessed defects in CLD formation and secretion that provide clues to mechanisms regulating lipogenesis and lipid secretion. Here we describe studies of the formation, trafficking, and secretion of CLDs in mouse mammary tissue utilizing developmental and genetic models.

3. CLD BIOGENESIS

CLDs are located in nearly all eukaryotic organisms, tissues, and cell types. Electron microscopy and biochemical analysis have shown that CLDs are complex assemblies composed of a TAG-enriched neutral lipid matrix surrounded by single phospholipid monolayer (Tauchi-Sato et al. 2002) and coated with specific populations of proteins (Murphy 2001). The TAGs in the matrix are formed primarily from cytosolic fatty acids and diacylglycerol by actions of acetyltransferases located in specific regions of the smooth endoplasmic reticulum (ER) membrane (Smith et al. 2000). Somehow TAG droplets are released from the ER membrane into the cytoplasm. The mechanisms of this release and CLD assembly are unknown. However, CLD surface associated proteins are thought to be important in the formation and/or stabilization of CLDs within the aqueous environment of the cytoplasm (Murphy & Vance 1999; Murphy 2001).

3.1. Mammary Gland CLDs Possess a Unique and Complex Protein Composition

Analyses of the composition and origins of CLD-associated proteins from different organisms, tissues, and cell types, indicate there may be multiple mechanisms for CLD assembly (Murphy & Vance 1999; Murphy 2001) and suggest that the composition of the surface-associated proteins may reflect cell-specific functions of these structures. Utilizing 2D gel electrophoresis and mass spectrometry to define the protein composition of CLDs in mammary and liver tissue of lactating mice (Wu et al. 2000), we found that the protein composition of CLDs isolated from mouse mammary glands is considerably more complex and qualitatively distinct from that of isolated liver CLDs. A partial list of CLD proteins that were identified by mass spectrometry are shown in Table 1. A key finding of these studies was that CLDs from the mammary gland, but not those from liver, possess components of microtubule motors and proteins that interact with the cytoskeleton. These observations suggest that protein composition of mammary CLDs may be specialized for transport and secretion of these structures and is consistent with earlier studies that implicated microtubules in milk lipid secretion (Patton et al. 1977).

A major protein component that was common to CLDs from both tissue types is adipophilin (Fig. 3). However, the isoform composition of ADPH isolated from mammary gland CLDs appeared to be different from that obtained from liver CLDs (Wu et al. 2000). The functional significance of these isoforms is uncertain. However, since

Table 1. Protein identification by mass spectrometry[a]

Map ID#	Identification (abbreviation)	MFGM	Mam. CLD	liver CLD	Mol. mass (kDa)	p*I* [b]
1	TER ATPase	+	+	–	89.3	5.13
2	Fibrinogen γ	+	–	–	99.2	5.57
3	Gephyrin	+	+	–	79.8	5.29
4	Pyruvate carboxylase	+	+	–	129.6	6.57
5	ERP99	+	+	–	91.2	4.91
6	Dynein intermediate chain	+	+	–	68.3	5.16
7	Hsp 70	+	+	–	70.0	6.37
8	Cholesterol esterase	+	–	–	65.8	6.30
9	Motor protein	+	+	–	79.7	6.71
10	TIF32/RPG1	+	+	–	40.1	6.10
11	ER carboxylesterase	+	+	–	30.9	6.31
12	Heterotrimeric G protein β	+	–	–	37.3	6.19
13	ERP29	+	+	–	28.9	6.37
14	Peroxiredoxin IV	+	+	–	28.3	6.50
15	FAS	+	–	–	272.0	5.96
16	Gelsolin	+	+	–	80.8	6.43

[a]A partial list of the proteins found on cytoplasmic lipid droplet (CLD) fractions from mouse mammary gland and liver and the membrane fraction from mouse milk fat globules (MFGM). Proteins were isolated by 2 dimensional gel electrophoresis and their identities were determined by mass spectrometry.
[b]p*I* = isoelectric point. Adapted and used with permission from Wiley-VCH Verlag GmbH, Weinheim, Germany (from Wu et al. Electrophoresis 2000;21:3470-3482).

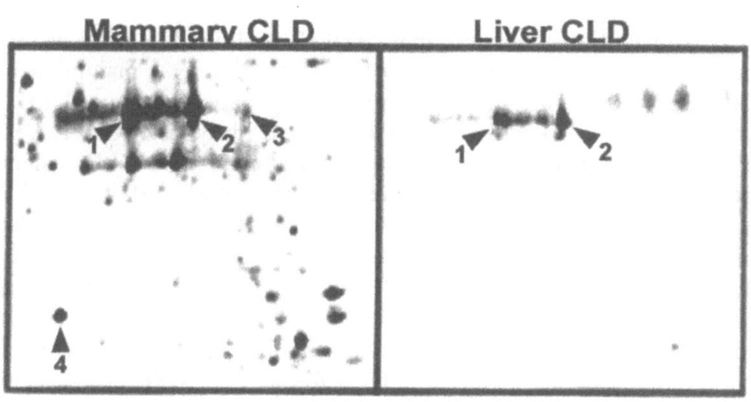

Figure 3. Differences in the protein complexity of mammary gland and liver cytoplasmic lipid droplets (CLDs). CLD proteins were analyzed by 2D gel electrophoresis. Spots 1, 2 and 3 are charge isoforms and spot 4 is a size isoform of ADPH. Note spots 3 and 4 are missing from 2D analysis of liver CLDs. Adapted and used with permission from Wiley-VCH Verlag GmbH, Weinheim, Germany (from Wu et al. Electrophoresis 2000;21:3470-3482).

ADPH appears to be a single gene product, the presence implies differences in post-translational processing of ADPH in mammary gland and liver.

3.2. ADPH Specifically Localizes to CLDs in Alveolar Epithelial Cells of the Mammary Gland

ADPH is a member of the genetic and structurally related perilipin family of lipid droplet binding proteins (Lu et al. 2001; Miura et al. 2002). In addition to ADPH and perilipin, other members of this family include the mannose-6 phosphate receptor targeting protein (TIP-47), and lipid droplet binding proteins of *drosophila* and *dictyostelium* (Miura et al. 2002). Immunohistochemical analysis demonstrated that ADPH localizes to CLDs in most mammalian cell types, either during their differentiation or at maturity (Heid et al. 1998; Brasaemle et al. 1997). Perilipin, on the other hand, is found selectively on lipid droplets in adipocytes and steroidogenic cells (Londos et al. 1995, 1999), where it has been shown to regulate lipid storage and mobilization by controlling access of lipases to the triglyceride matrix of CLDs (Souza et al. 1998, 2002; Londos et al. 1999).

Using immunofluorescence microscopy we (McManaman et al., in preparation), and others, found that ADPH localized specifically to CLDs in alveolar epithelial cells and was not detected in adipose tissue (Heid et al. 1998). Conversely, perilipin localized to mammary adipocytes and was not detected in epithelial cells. ADPH coated CLDs appeared about day 7 of pregnancy (P7) and gradually increased in number and size with some eventually reaching diameters of greater than 20 μm just before parturition. At parturition these lipid droplets move to the lumen and are replaced by small lipid droplets in the cytoplasm. These results demonstrate that alveolar epithelial cells develop the capacity to synthesize and store triglycerides early in the initial phase of functional development. However, since lipids are not secreted prior to parturition (Hollman 1974), the biogenesis of CLDs appears to be independent of their secretion.

3.3. ADPH Is An Essential Protein in Lipid Metabolism in Mammalian Cells

There is substantial evidence that ADPH is linked tightly to triglyceride accumulation and may be essential to CLD formation in diverse mammalian cell types, including mammary epithelial cells. Antisense oligonucleotides to ADPH have been shown to interfere with CLD accumulation in cultured fibroblasts (Gao & Serrero 1999) and ADPH expression also has been shown to correlate with CLD accumulation in macrophages (Vosper et al. 2001), monocytes (Buechler et al. 2001), liver (Steiner et al. 1996; Heid et al. 1998), colorectal tumor cells (Gupta et al. 2001), and fibroblasts (Gao et al. 2000) in response to pharmacological agents or conditions that induce lipogenesis. Consistent with the potential role of ADPH in CLD formation, we found that ADPH mRNA levels in the mouse mammary gland increased during differentiation and that this increase correlated with the observed increases in CLD accumulation (McManaman et al., in preparation). In addition to a role in CLD formation, ADPH has been suggested to be required for secretion of CLDs by mammary epithelial cells (Mather & Keenan 1998; McManaman et al. 2001; Wu et al. 2000). Therefore, ADPH may function in both the formation and secretion of milk lipids.

3.4. Role of ADPH in CLD Formation

To further evaluate the role of ADPH in CLD formation, we expressed full-length ADPH and truncation mutations of ADPH as a vesicular stomatitus virus (VSV) peptide tagged fusion protein in COS7 cells (McManaman et al. 2003). We found that both endogenous ADPH and the full-length ADPH-VSV fusion protein specifically target to CLDs. We used this technique to identify the regions of the ADPH molecule responsible for its targeting to lipid droplets (McManaman et al. 2003). Perilipin family members share significant sequence similarity in a ~100 AA region at their N-terminus. This region, termed the PAT (**P**erilipin, **A**dipophilin and **T**IP-47) domain (Lu et al. 2001; Miura et al. 2002), was postulated to control the association of these proteins with CLDs (Lu et al. 2001). However, when we expressed the PAT domain of mouse ADPH (amino acids 1-102) as a VSV tagged protein in COS cells, it did not target CLDs. However, the region C-terminal to the PAT domain (amino acids 98-425) did target CLDs. Thus, the PAT domain itself does not appear to be necessary or sufficient to target ADPH to CLDs. Although the structure of ADPH has not been determined, structural algorithms predict that it possesses significant amounts of alpha-helical structure in the region between amino acids 185 and 205. When an N-terminal sequence that contained this region (amino acids 1-220) was expressed as a VSV-tagged construct, it was found to target lipid droplets. However, a construct containing the region C-terminal to this helical region (amino acids 215-425) did not target to CLDs. Importantly, we found that the regions of APDH that target CLDs also increased CLD accumulation in COS cells. These results suggest that not only are limited regions of the ADPH sequence responsible for its interactions with CLDs but that these regions also may assist in regulating CLD formation. Interestingly, these results also raise the possibility that regions not involved in binding of ADPH to CLDs could participate in other cellular functions, such as CLD secretion.

3.5. AKT Activation Contributes to CLD Accumulation

Our preliminary in vivo evidence suggests that ADPH expression by itself may not be the only factor responsible for CLD accumulation. Lipid accumulation in 3T3 L1 adipocytes is induced by activation of the AKT (also known as PKB) signaling pathway. Activation of AKT in these cells appears to increase translocation of the GLUT4 glucose transporter to the plasma membrane, resulting in increased glucose uptake and de novo triglyceride synthesis (Delzenne et al. 2001; Magun et al. 1996). Our studies suggest that a similar pathway may contribute to CLD accumulation in mammary epithelial cells (Schwertfeger et al. 2003). Transgenic mice expressing a constitutively active (myristylated) form of AKT (myrAKT) under the control of the MMTV promoter were found to secrete milk that contained 2- to 3-times the amount of milk lipid found in wild-type mice (Schwertfeger et al. 2003). ADPH immunofluorescence microscopy also showed that there was premature CLD accumulation and increased CLD volume in the alveoli of these mice during lactogenesis (Schwertfeger et al. 2003). Quantitative RT-PCR, however, demonstrated that the steady-state levels of ADPH mRNA in the mammary glands of myrAKT mice were similar to those found in control animals (unpublished observations). These findings indicate that activation of AKT increases CLD formation without increasing ADPH expression. These results suggest both ADPH expression and induction of TAG biosynthesis contribute to CLD formation during lactogenesis.

3.6. Microarray Analysis Demonstrates Enhanced Expression of Lipogenic Pathways during Secretory Activation

Taken together these findings indicate that regulation of lipid biogenesis in the mammary gland may involve a number of distinct cellular pathways. To better define the cellular processes involved in lipogenesis in the mammary gland, we used microarray (Rudolph et al. 2003) analysis to identify global changes in gene expression induced during lactogenesis and the periparturient period of lactation. Specifically, gene expression profiles were analyzed in mammary glands from quadruplicate mice at days 12 (P12) and 17 (P17) of pregnancy, the day after overnight birth of the pups (defined as lactation day 1 or L1 here), lactation day 2 (L2) and lactation day 9 (L9) as morphological and biochemical data indicate that these time points are likely to represent critical boundary periods of initial functional differentiation (P12-P17), secretory activation (P17-L1), secretory maturation (L1-L2), and stable milk secretion (L2-L9). From this analysis we found that genes for the enzymes of fatty acid and cholesterol synthesis tended to remain flat between P12 and P17 but increased sharply (2- to 5-fold) from P17 to L1. Table 2 shows the relative changes of genes associated with triglyceride and cholesterol metabolism between P17 and L1. Genes for cholesterol and fatty acid synthesis have been found to be regulated in other tissues by either SREBP-2 (cholesterol synthesis) or SREBP-1c (fatty acid synthesis) (Mesenkamp et al. 2001; Kang & Davis 2000). We found levels of SREBP-1 mRNA also were increased between P17 and L1, raising the possibility that SREBP transcription factors play a significant role in regulating lipid synthesis and CLD accumulation during the secretory activation phase of functional differentiation.

Table 2. Lipogenic enzymes are upregulated during secretory activation[a]

Function	Gene name	Strain	Strain
		FVB	**CD-1**
Glucose transport	GLUT-1	↑↑	↑↑
Pentose phosphate shunt	G6PD	↑	↑
Glycerol-PO4 synthesis	Aldolase C	↑↑↑	↑↑↑
Oxaloacetate synthesis	Pyruvate carb	↑	↑↑↑
Pyruvate malate shuttle	Citrate transporter	↑↑↑	↑↑↑
Acetyl CoA synthesis	ATP Cit Lyase	↑↑↑	↑↑↑
Malonyl CoA synthesis	ACC		
Fatty Acid synthesis	FAS	↑	↑↑↑
Delta 9 desaturation	SCD2	↑	↑↑
Cholesterol synthesis	Lanosterol synthase	↑↑↑	↑↑↑
Cholesterol synthesis	FPPS	↑↑↑	↑↑↑
Regulator	SREBP-1	↑	↑↑

[a]Microarray analysis of mammary glands from FVB and CD-1 mouse strains showed significant increases in expression of several enzymes involved in fatty acid and cholesterol biosynthesis between day 17 of pregnancy and day 2 of lactation. The arrows indicate relative increases in mRNA levels for each enzyme in each strain. Ratio L1/P17: ↑↑↑, >3; ↑↑, >2<3; ↑, >1.4<2.

4. CLD SECRETION

The findings of marked decreases in CLD size and number and accumulation of CLDs at the apical plasma membrane shortly after parturition suggest that size and localization of CLDs are influenced by secretory activity. Two experimental models of impaired lactation were employed to test this hypothesis.

4.1. CLD Biogenesis and Secretion in Mice Over-Expressing Human Protein C

In the first model we investigated CLD size in transgenic mice that express the human form of the anti-coagulant factor, protein C (hPC), under control of the whey acid protein promoter (Palmer et al. 2003). Homozygous hPC animals appear to undergo normal pregnancy and delivery, possess histologically normal mammary alveoli during pregnancy and are capable of expressing some milk proteins (Palmer et al. 2003). However, these animals exhibit a profound lactational deficit and are unable to support their litters (Palmer et al. 2003). Histological analysis (Fig. 4) of these mice showed that their lipid droplets failed to decrease in size and move into the lumen at L1. Thus hPC animals appear to have the capacity to generate CLDs but lack the ability to secrete these structures. This possibility is supported by our preliminary analysis of the milk composition of hPC mice, which demonstrated that the lipid content of milk of hPC mice was only 1% to 2% of that found in the milk of control mice. These findings therefore suggest that lipid secretion may be impaired selectively in hPC mice and provide further evidence that the biosynthesis and secretion of CLDs are independently regulated processes.

4.2. Effects of Milk Stasis on CLD Formation and Secretion

The relationship between CLD biogenesis and secretion was further evaluated by determining the effects of milk stasis on CLD formation in control CD-1 mice. Milk stasis, induced by forced weaning at lactation day 10, interferes with secretion and results in decreased milk protein gene expression (McManaman et al. 2002). Figure 5 shows that CLDs were small and associated with the apical membrane in alveoli from normally suckled control animals. However, in mice in which milk secretion was impaired for 24 hours by forced weaning, there was a marked increase in CLD size and a loss of CLD polarization. These results indicate that milk stasis interferes with CLD secretion but not with CLD formation. Thus, there is evidence that CLD biogenesis and secretion are regulated independently in response to the loss of secretory function as well to its development.

5. MECHANISM OF CLD SECRETION

CLD secretion occurs only at the apical plasma membrane. Electron microscopic imaging and biochemical evidence support a process in which CLDs dock with, and are enveloped by, the apical plasma membrane of alveolar epithelial cells (see Fig. 2). The resulting membrane bilayer enveloped CLDs are then released into the lumen at which point they are referred to as milk fat globules (MFGs). The mechanism by which CLDs dock with, and are enveloped by, the apical plasma membrane is understood poorly but there is accumulating biochemical, microscopic, and genetic evidence that the secretion

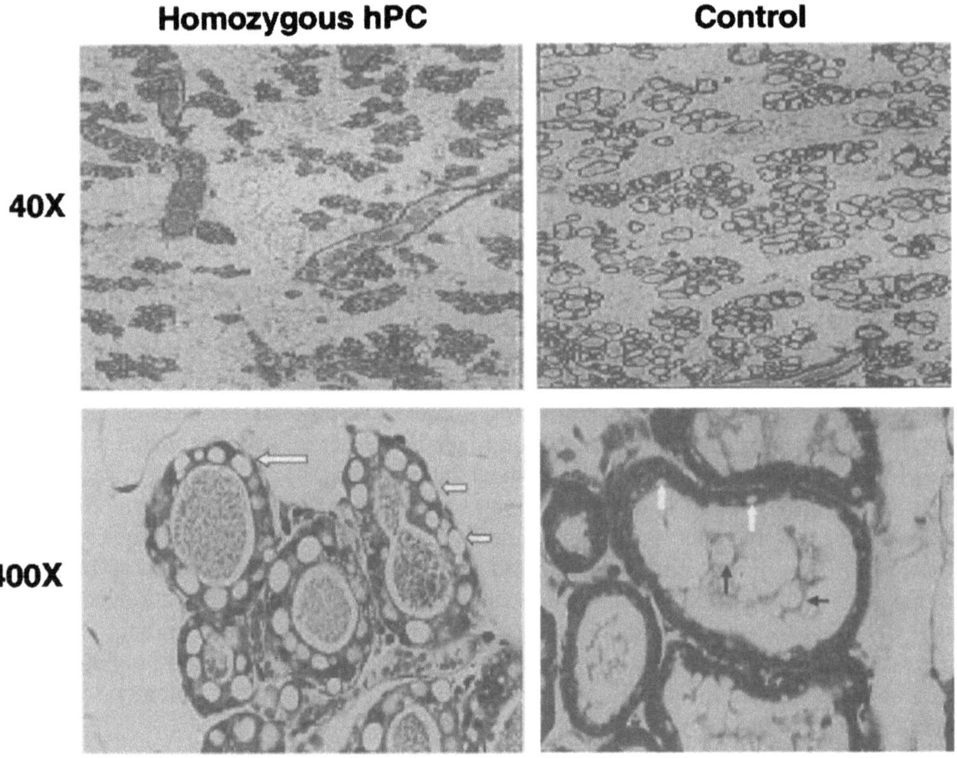

Figure 4. Alveolar morphology in hPC mice. Hematoxylin and eosin stained sections of lactation day one mammary glands at 40X and 400X magnification. In the lower magnification note the large areas of adipose tissue that remain in the transgenic sample. At the higher magnification note the larger cytoplasmic lipid droplets in the transgenic sample as compared to the control (white arrows). Also note presence of milk fat droplets in control (black arrows) but not transgenic lumen.

process involves formation of a tripartite complex between ADPH on the surface of CLDs, the peripheral membrane protein xanthine oxidoreductase (XOR), and a mammary gland specific transmembrane protein, butyrophilin (Btn) (Mather & Keenan 1998; McManaman et al. 2002).

5.1. Role of Xanthine Oxidoreductase (XOR)

Genetically induced XOR insufficiency results in a lactational defect characterized by CLD accumulation in alveolar epithelial cells (Vorbach et al. 2002). Our own studies indicate that the apical membrane association of XOR is key factor in CLD secretion (McManaman et al. 2002). The amount of XOR in mammary epithelial cells increases during the initial phase of functional differentiation, but immunofluorescence analysis shows that it localizes to the cytoplasm during this period (McManaman et al. 2002). However, within hours of parturition XOR was found at the apical plasma membrane (McManaman et al. 2002). These results indicate that the plasma membrane association of XOR is dependent on secretory activity of the mammary gland. This hypothesis was tested using the milk stasis model described above. We found that 24 hours after inducing milk stasis XOR had lost its apical membrane localization and was now found in the

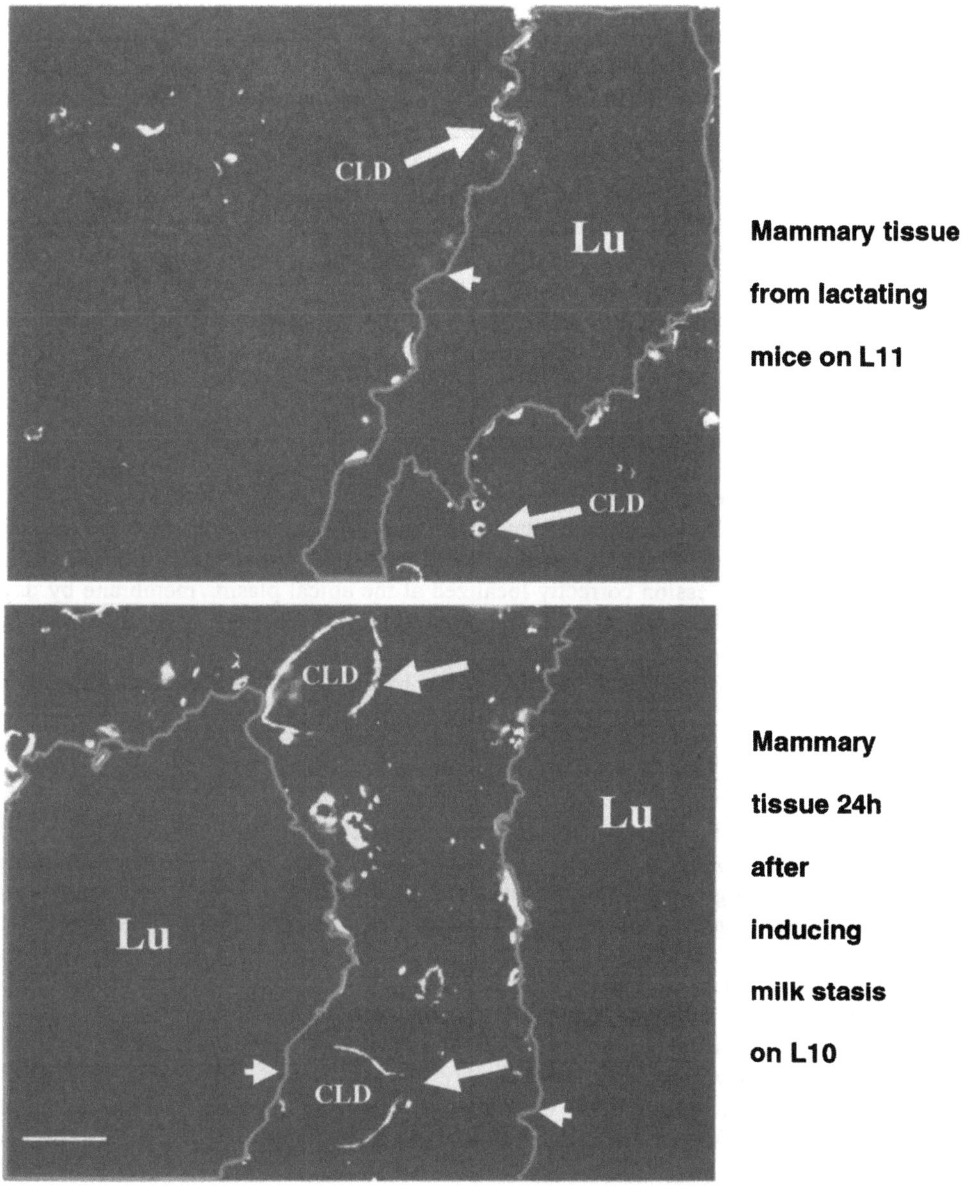

Figure 5. Effects of milk stasis on CLD size and localization. Milk stasis was induced on lactation day 10 in CD1 mice by forced weaning for 24 hours. Control animals were maintained with their litters for this same period. Mammary glands were then removed and processed for immunohistochemistry (McManaman et al. 2002). CLDs were identified by staining with anti-ADPH antibodies, luminal borders were identified by staining with FITC labeled wheat germ agglutinin, and nuclei were stained with DAPI. Representative APDH stained CLDs are indicated by the large arrows; Lu indicates luminal region; luminal borders are outlined by the gray lines (small arrows); nuclei are not shown. Bar=10 μm. Note the small size and apical membrane localization of CLDs found in control tissue compared with the large size (the arrows in the bottom panel indicate two CLDs with diameters in excess of 10 μm) and increased numbers of basally localized CLDs found in alveoli from animals subjected to forced weaning.

cytoplasm. In addition to altering its membrane association, milk stasis also resulted in a decrease in the steady-state mRNA levels of XOR (McManaman et al. 2002). By 24 hours after inducing milk stasis, the average XOR mRNA levels were 51±4% of control glands, and by 42 hours after inducing milk stasis they were only 13±4% of control glands. Although milk stasis is known to eventually lead to alveolar epithelial apoptosis and tissue remodeling as part of the involution process (Marti et al. 1997; Strange et al. 1992; Lund et al. 1996), the loss of XOR from the membrane and the decline in its mRNA levels occurred prior to disruption of alveolar morphology or the appearance of apoptotic nuclei (McManaman et al. 2002). Together these results demonstrate that the expression of XOR mRNA and the amount of this protein at the apical plasma membrane are regulated by secretory activity. Importantly, the dynamic nature of the association of XOR with the apical membrane is what would be predicted if this association regulated CLD secretion.

5.2. Effects of Secretory Activity on Btn Expression and Localization

Btn also is hypothesized to be required for CLD secretion (Mather & Keenan 1998). In agreement with this hypothesis, we found that Btn mRNA expression increased several fold during the later period of functional differentiation (McManaman et al., in preparation) and that this expression correctly localized at the apical plasma membrane by day 18 of pregnancy (McManaman et al. 2002). Although these findings are consistent with the proposed role of Btn in lipid secretion (Mather & Keenan 1998) they also suggest that the presence of Btn at the apical membrane is, by itself, not sufficient to drive the secretion process.

5.3. XOR, Btn, and ADPH Form a Complex during Lactation

If CLD secretion is dependent on formation of a complex between XOR, Btn and ADPH, then there should be evidence of this interaction on apical plasma membrane during lactation. Using confocal immunofluorescence microscopy we found significant co-localization between these proteins at the apical plasma membranes of lactating CD-1 mice (McManaman et al. 2002). Quantitation of the degree of staining overlap showed that the areas of overlap of XOR stain with Btn and ADPH stain corresponded to 76% and 73%, respectively, of the total apical membrane staining area of XOR (McManaman et al. 2002). Importantly, those areas of XOR staining not directly overlapping with Btn or ADPH staining were approximated closely to regions that did overlap and XOR staining at sites distant from regions of overlap were not observed. This high degree of co-localization of XOR with ADPH and Btn suggests that these interactions are highly specific and not simply adventitious events.

We also found that there was significant co-localization between these proteins on milk fat globules isolated from mouse milk and that membranes isolated from these droplets (milk fat globule membranes–MFGM) were enriched in these proteins (McManaman et al. 2002). To clarify interactions between these proteins, MFGMs were isolated, extracted with Triton X-100, and fractionated by size exclusion chromatography (McManaman et al. 2002). We found that 50% to 70% of the total XOR activity associated with isolated MFGM could be extracted by incubation in 1% Triton X-100, and that the extracted XOR enzymatic activity eluted as two peaks with distinct size properties (Fig. 6). The size of the earliest eluting peak (I) was greater than 600 kDa whereas the apparent size of the second peak (II) was similar to that of purified native

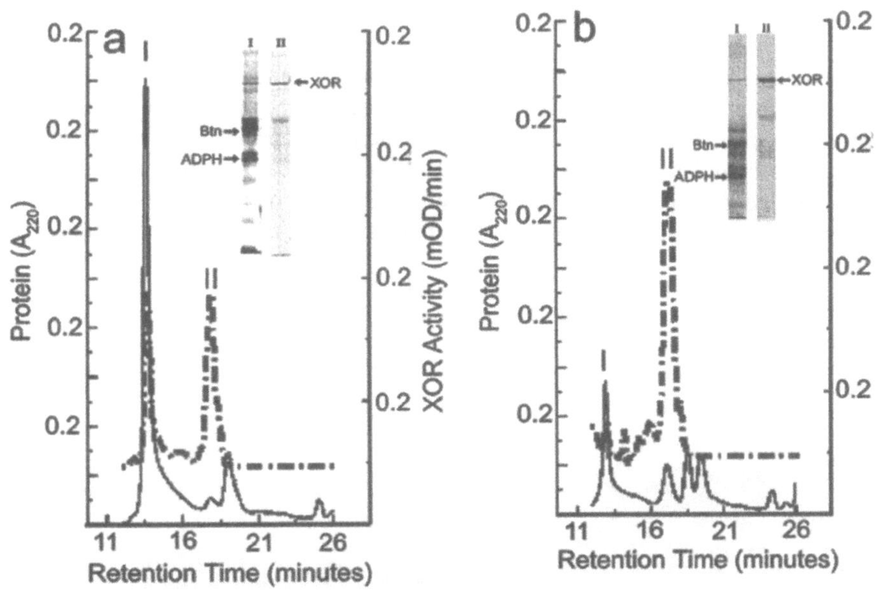

Figure 6. Size exclusion chromatography (SEC) analysis of interactions between XOR, Btn and ADPH isolated from milk lipid globule membranes. Panel a shows the elution properties of XOR enzymatic activity (dashed line) and 220 nm absorbing material (solid line) following SEC of Triton X-100 solubilized milk lipid globule membrane proteins. The inets shows a silver stained gel of proteins in peaks I and II separated SDS-PAGE. The identities of XOR, Btn and ADPH bands were confirmed by N-terminal microsequence analysis and are indicated. XOR bands in peaks I and II are indicated by the arrow at the right of the peak II lane. Panel b shows the elution properties of XOR, Btn and ADPH after incubating peak I with 5mM DTT. XOR activity and A220 nm absorbance are indicated by the dashed and solid lines respectively. Silver stained gels of proteins in peaks I and II are shown in the insets, and the positions of XOR, Btn, and ADPH are indicated as above. Adapted and used with permission from The Physiological Society, London, UK (from McManaman et al. J Physiol 2002;545.2:569-579).

mouse mammary gland XOR. The protein compositions of each peak, determined by SDS-PAGE in conjunction with silver staining, showed that peak I was enriched in bands that subsequently were identified as XOR, Btn and ADPH by microsequence analysis. Peak II however was composed primarily of XOR. These results indicate that significant amounts of MFGM-associated XOR exist as a Triton X-100 stable complex with Btn and ADPH. The nature of this complex was determined by reducing Peak I with dithiothreitol and reanalyzing the resulting solution by size exclusion chromatography (SEC). As shown in Figure 6 nearly all of the XOR activity now eluted in the peak II position. SDS-PAGE and silver stain analysis showed although some Btn and ADPH were still found in peak I but most of the XOR protein was now in peak II. In contrast SEC showed that if peak I was not reduced with DTT all of the XOR remained in peak I (McManaman et al. 2002). These results therefore indicate that the association of XOR with apical membranes is a dynamic process that involves at least in part, thiol-dependent interactions with Btn and/or ADPH.

5.4. Model of Milk Lipid Secretion

In summary, our studies provide evidence that the ability to secrete milk lipids develops in two stages (Fig. 7). CLD biogenesis occurs during the initiation phase of appears to correctly localize to the apical plasma membrane prior to CLD secretion, XOR is found in the cytoplasm (McManaman et al. 2002). Apical transport and secretion of CLDs is initiated during the secretory activation phase of differentiation. Although the mechanism of transport is unknown, our data suggest that it involves specific microtubule

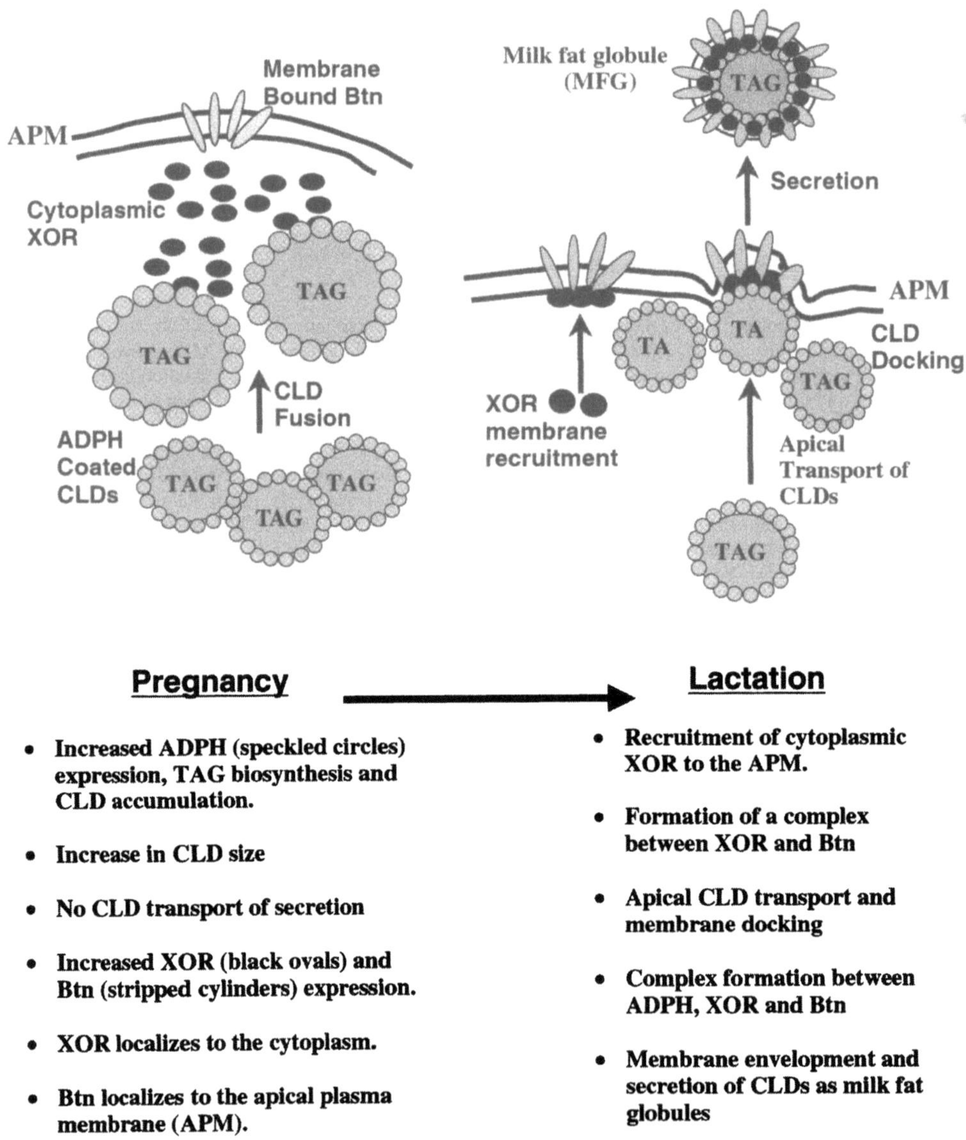

Figure 7. Model of milk lipid secretion

motors (Wu et al. 2000), and is closely linked to the secretion process, since it does not appear to occur in transgenic animals that fail to lactate or if secretion is inhibited in normal animals by milk stasis (McManaman et al., in preparation). The mechanism of CLD secretion also is unknown. The results of Vorbach and colleagues (2002), have demonstrated that it is dependent on XOR expression, and our studies suggest it involves thiol-dependent recruitment of XOR from the cytoplasm to the apical plasma membrane (McManaman et al. 2002) where it forms a complex with Btn (Mather & Keenan 1998). This complex is postulated to act as a site for CLD docking (Mather & Keenan 1998; Wu et al. 2000); the docking process in turn is hypothesized to involve specific interactions between APDH on the CLD surface and the XOR/ Btn complex. Because membrane recruitment of XOR is thus far the only process that correlates with CLD secretion, we hypothesize that this event is a primary regulator of the secretion process (McManaman et al. 2002). Our future studies will be directed at understanding how the membrane recruitment of XOR is regulated and defining the critical interactions between ADPH, XOR, and Btn that mediate CLD secretion.

6. ACKNOWLEDGMENTS

This work was supported by NIH grants HL 45582, R37 HD19547, PO1 HD 38129, and RO1 HD 15437.

7. REFERENCES

Allen JC, Keller RP, Archer P, Neville MC. Studies in human lactation: milk composition and daily secretion rates of macronutrients in the first year of lactation. Am J Clin Nutr 1991;54:69-80.

Baldwin RL, Yang YT. Enzymatic and metabolic changes in the development of lactation. In: Larson BL, Smith VR, editors. Lactation. New York: Academic Press, 1974; pp 349-407.

Buechler C, Ritter M, Duong CQ, Orso E, Kapinsky M, Schmitz G. Adipophilin is a sensitive marker for lipid loading in human blood monocytes. Biochim Biophys Acta 2001;1532:97-104.

Delzenne NM, Kok N. Effects of fructans-type prebiotics on lipid metabolism. Am J Clin Nutr 2001;73:456S-458S.

Dils RR. Comparative aspects of milk fat synthesis. J Dairy Sci 1986;69:904-910.

Dils RR. Milk fat synthesis. In: Mepham TB, editor. Biochemistry of Lactation. Amsterdam: Elsevier, 1983; pp 141-157.

Fleet IR, Goode JA, Hamon MH, Laurie MS, Linzell JL, Peaker M. Secretory activity of goat mammary glands during pregnancy and the onset of lactation. J Physiol 1975;251:763-773.

Gao J, Serrero G. Adipose differentiation related protein (ADRP) expressed in transfected COS-7 cells selectively stimulates long chain fatty acid uptake. J Biol Chem 1999;274:16825-16830.

Gao J, Ye H, Serrero G. Stimulation of adipose differentiation related protein (ADRP) expression in adipocyte precursors by long-chain fatty acids. J Cell Physiol 2000;182:297-302.

Gupta RA, Brockman JA, Sarraf P, Willson TM, DuBois RN. Target genes of peroxisome proliferator-activated receptor gamma in colorectal cancer cells. J Biol Chem 2001;276:29681-29687.

Hachey DL, Thomas MR, Emken EA, Garza C, Brown-Booth L, Adlof RO, Klein PD. Human lactation: maternal transfer of dietary triglycerides labeled with stable isotopes. J Lipid Res 1987;28:1185-1192.

Hamosh M, Clary TR, Chernick SS, Scow RO. Lipoprotein lipase activity of adipose and mammary tissue and plasma triglyceride in pregnant and lactating rats. Biochim Biophys Acta 1970;210:473-482.

Hartmann PE. Changes in the composition yield of the mammary secretion of cows during the initiation of lactation. Journal of Endocrinology 1973;59:231-247.

Heid HW, Moll R, Schwetlick I, Rackwitz HR, Keenan TW. Adipophilin is a specific marker of lipid accumulation in diverse cell types and diseases. Cell Tissue Res 1998;294;309-321.

Hollman KH. Cytology and fine structure of the mammary gland. In: Larson BL, Smith VR, editors. Lactation. New York: Academic Press, 1974; pp 3-95.

Jenness R. Comparative aspects of milk proteins. J Dairy Res 1979;46:197-210.

Jensen RG, Bitman J, Carlson SE, Couch SC, Hamosh M, Newburg DS. Milk lipids: A. Human milk lipids. In: Jensen RG, editor. Handbook of Milk Composition. San Diego: Academic Press, 1995; pp 495-542.

Kang S, Davis RA. Cholesterol and hepatic lipoprotein assembly and secretion. Biochim Biophys Acta 2000;1529:223-230.

Kuhn NJ. Progesterone withdrawal as the lactogenic trigger in the rat. J Endocrinol 1969;44:39-54.

Londos C, Brasaemle DL, Gruia-Gray J, Servetnick DA, Schultz CJ, Levin DM, Kimmel AR. Perilipin: unique proteins associated with intracellular neutral lipid droplets in adipocytes and steroidogenic cells. Biochem Soc Trans 1995;23:611-615.

Londos C, Brasaemle DL, Schultz CJ, Segrest JP, Kimmel AR. Perilipins, ADRP, and other proteins that associate with intracellular neutral lipid droplets in animal cells. Semin Cell Dev Biol 1999;10:51-58.

Lu X, Gruia-Gray J, Copeland NG, Gilbert DJ, Jenkins NA, Londos C, Kimmel AR. The murine perilipin gene: the lipid droplet-associated perilipins derive from tissue-specific, mRNA splice variants and define a gene family of ancient origin. Mamm Genome 2001;12:741-749.

Lund LR, Romer J, Thomasset N, Solberg H, Pyke C, Bissell MJ, Dano K, Werb Z. Two distinct phases of apoptosis in mammary gland involution: Proteinase-independent and -dependent pathways. Development 1999;122:181-193.

Magun R, Burgering BM, Coffer PJ, Pardasani D, Lin Y, Chabot J, Sorisky A. Expression of a constitutively activated form of protein kinase B (c-Akt) in 3T3-L1 preadipose cells causes spontaneous differentiation. Endocrinology 1996;137:3590-3593.

Marti A, Feng Z, Altermatt HJ, Jaggi R. Milk accumulation triggers apoptosis of mammary epithelial cells. Eur J Cell Biol 1997;73:158-165.

Mather IH, Keenan TW. Origin and secretion of milk lipids. J Mammary Gland Biol Neoplasia 1998;3:259-273.

McManaman JL, Palmer CA, Wright RM, Neville MC. Functional regulation of xanthine oxidoreductase expression and localization in the mouse mammary gland: evidence of a role in lipid secretion. J Physiol 2002;545:567-579.

McManaman JL, Zabaronick W, Schaack J, Orlicky D. Lipid targeting domains of adipophilin. J Lipid Res 2003;44:668-673.

Mensenkamp AR, Havekes LM, Romijn JA, Kuipers F. Hepatic steatosis and very low density lipoprotein secretion: the involvement of apolipoprotein E. J Hepatol 35;2001:816-822.

Miura S, Gan JW, Brzostowski J, Parisi MJ, Schultz CJ, Londos C, Oliver B, Kimmel AR. Functional conservation for lipid storage droplet association among Perilipin, ADRP, and TIP47 (PAT)-related proteins in mammals, Drosophila, and Dictyostelium. J Biol Chem 2002;277:32253-32257.

Murphy DJ, Vance J. Mechanisms of lipid-body formation. Trends Biochem Sci 1999;24:109-115.

Murphy DJ. The biogenesis and functions of lipid bodies in animals, plants and microorganisms. Prog Lipid Res 2001;40:325-438.

Neville MC, McFadden TB, Forsyth I. Hormonal regulation of mammary differentiation and milk secretion. J Mammary Gland Biol Neoplasia 2002;7:49-66.

Neville MC, Neifert MR, editors. Lactation: Physiology, Nutrition, and Breast-Feeding. New York: Plenum Press, 1983.

Nguyen D-AD, Parlow AF, Neville MC. Hormonal regulation of tight junction closure in the mouse mammary epithelium during the transition from pregnancy to lactation. J Endocrinol 2001;170:347-356.

Palmer CA, Lubon H, McManaman JL. Transgenic mice expressing recombinant human protein C exhibit defects in lactation and impaired mammary gland development. Transgenic Res 2003;12:283-292.

Patton, S., Stemberger, B. H., & Knudsen, C. M.. The suppression of milk fat globule secretion by colchicine: an effect coupled to inhibition of exocytosis. Biochim Biophys Acta 1977;499:404-410.

Rudolph M, McManaman JL, Hunter L, Phang T, Neville MC. Initiation of lactation in the mammary gland: Temporal analysis of a complex biological switch with expression profiling and trajectory clustering. J Mammary Gland Biol Neoplasia 2003;8:287-307.

Schwertfeger KL, McManaman JL, Palmer CA, Neville MC, Anderson SM. Expression of constitutively activated Akt in the mammary gland leads to excess lipid synthesis during pregnancy and lactation. J Lipid Res 2003;44:1100-1112.

Smith SJ, Cases S, Jensen DR, Chen HC, Sande E, Tow B, Sanan DA, Raber J, Eckel RH, Farese R V Jr. Obesity resistance and multiple mechanisms of triglyceride synthesis in mice lacking Dgat. Nat Genet 2000;25:87-90.

Souza SC, Muliro KV, Liscum L, Lien P, Yamamoto MT, Schaffer JE, Dallal GE, Wang X, Kraemer FB, Obin M, Greenberg AS. Modulation of hormone-sensitive lipase and protein kinase A-mediated lipolysis by perilipin A in an adenoviral reconstituted system. J Biol Chem 2002;277:8267-8272.

Souza SC, Yamamoto MT, Franciosa MD, Lien P, Greenberg AS. BRL 49653 blocks the lipolytic actions of tumor necrosis factor-alpha: a potential new insulin-sensitizing mechanism for thiazolidinediones. Diabetes 1998;47:691-695.

Steiner S, Wahl D, Mangold BL, Robison R, Raymackers J, Meheus L, Anderson NL, Cordier A. Induction of the adipose differentiation-related protein in liver of etomoxir-treated rats. Biochem Biophys Res Commun 1996;218:777-782.

Strange R, Li F, Saurer S, Burkhardt A, Friis RR. Apoptotic cell death and tissue remodelling during mouse mammary gland involution. Development 1992;115:49-58

Tauchi-Sato K, Ozeki S, Houjou T, Taguchi R, Fujimoto T. The surface of lipid droplets is a phospholipid monolayer with a unique Fatty Acid composition. J Biol Chem 2002;277:44507-44512.

Vorbach C, Scriven A, Capecchi MR. The housekeeping gene xanthine oxidoreductase is necessary for milk fat droplet enveloping and secretion: gene sharing in the lactating mammary gland. Genes Dev 2002;16:3223-3235.

Vosper H, Patel L, Graham TL, Khoudoli GA, Hill A, Macphee CH, Pinto I, Smith SA, Suckling KE, Wolf CR, Palmer CN. The peroxisome proliferator-activated receptor delta promotes lipid accumulation in human macrophages. J Biol Chem 2001;276:44258-44265.

Wellings SR. Ultrastructural basis of lactogenesis. In: Reynolds M, Folley SJ, editors. Lactogenesis. Philadelphia: University of Pennsylvania Press, 1969; pp 5-25.

Wu CC, Howell KE, Neville MC, Yates JR III, McManaman JL. Proteomics reveal a link between the endoplasmic reticulum and lipid secretory mechanisms in mammary epithelial cells. Electrophoresis 2000;21;3470-3482.

SECTION VII

EXTENDED ABSTRACTS

SOCIAL CAPITAL AND BREASTFEEDING INITIATION AMONG PUERTO RICAN WOMEN

Alex K. Anderson[1], David A. Himmelgreen[2], Yu-Kuei Peng[1], Sofia Segura-Pérez[3], and Rafael Pérez-Escamilla[1]

1. INTRODUCTION

Little is known about breastfeeding rates and factors that affect the likelihood for ever breastfeeding (BF) among Puerto Rican women residing in the continental United States. A cross-sectional study was designed to examine acculturation and food behaviors among low-income Latinos in Hartford, CT. We examined the association of social capital with the likelihood of BF among women 17 to 40 years of age with a child less than 6 years of age. Chi-square analyses were used to examine the bivariate association between BF and independent variables. Multivariate logistic regression was used to estimate the independent association between social capital and BF after controlling for confounders. Backward stepwise multivariate logistic regression results indicate that mothers who exchanged services with friends or relatives were more likely to have breastfed the previous child (OR=2.65; 95% CI=1.16–6.05) and also more likely to have ever breastfed the index child (OR=2.08; 95% CI=1.07–4.05) compared with their counterparts who did not exchange services. Mothers who listened to only Latino music (vs. those listening to non-Latino music) were less likely (OR=0.49; 95% CI=0.25–0.95) to have breastfed the index child. Findings suggest that social capital, as represented by exchange of services with friends or relatives, is associated with a higher likelihood of BF in this Puerto Rican community.

2. BACKGROUND

Latinos are the fastest growing minority population in the United States. However, research on BF has not paid adequate attention to the various ethnic/cultural groups within this subpopulation. Giachello (1994) reported that Mexican-American women were more likely to initiate breastfeeding than were their counterparts with Cuban and Puerto Rican ancestry based on data collected from 1982 to 1984 in the National Survey

[1]Department of Nutritional Sciences, University of Connecticut, Storrs, CT 06269
[2]Department of Anthropology, University of South Florida, Tampa, FL
[3]Hispanic Health Council, Inc., Hartford, CT

Protecting Infants through Human Milk, edited by Pickering *et al.*
Kluwer Academic/Plenum Publishers, 2004

of Family Growth and the Hispanic Health and Nutrition Examination Survey. Furthermore, among Latinos, Puerto Ricans experience the highest infant mortality rates (Carter-Porkas & Zambrana 2001). Pérez-Escamilla et al. (1998) previously have conducted studies to examine factors associated with breastfeeding initiation in the Puerto Rican community. However, these studies have not examined the link with social capital. Thus, the objective of this paper is to examine the independent association of social capital with ever breastfeeding among Puerto Rican women living in the continental United States.

3. STUDY DESIGN

This is a cross-sectional study conducted with 201 caretakers of children less than 6 years of age. Data on breastfeeding practices were determined retrospectively. The majority of respondents were recruited from the Hispanic Health Council (43%). The remainder of the respondents were recruited from WIC offices (30%), The Connecticut Children's Medical Center (9%), and other places (18%). Interviews were conducted by three trained bilingual/bicultural interviewers using a structured questionnaire. The great majority of the interviews (89%) were conducted at the respondent's home and 11% at the Hispanic Health Council. Most of the respondents (73%) preferred to be interviewed in Spanish. Each interview lasted between 60 and 90 minutes.

4. DATA ANALYSES

Social capital was divided into three dimensions: 1) exchange of services with friends, neighbors, or relatives (such as running errands, baby-sitting, and cooking), 2) lend or borrow money from friends, neighbors, or relatives, and 3) lend or borrow goods from friends, neighbors, or relatives. A total of 161 respondents who were the biological mothers of the study (index) child were included in these analyses. Chi-square analyses were used to examine the bivariate association between breastfeeding the previous child (yes/no) and ever breastfeeding the index child (yes/no), and each of the independent variables. Multivariate logistic regression was used to estimate the independent association between social capital and BF after controlling for confounders.

5. RESULTS

The mean age of respondents was 25 years, with 72% of them born in Puerto Rico and 49% being single mothers. While 60% had less than a high school education, 41% owned a car and 80% were receiving food stamps.

Backward stepwise multivariate logistic regression results indicate that mothers who exchanged services with friends or relatives were more likely to have BF the previous child (OR=2.65; 95% CI=1.16–6.05) and also more likely to have BF the index child (OR=2.08; 95% CI=1.07–4.05) compared with their counterparts who did not exchange services. Older respondents (≥30 years) were more likely than their younger counterparts to have breastfed the previous child (OR=3.50; 95% CI=1.19–10.30) and have breastfed the index child (OR=2.67; 95% CI=1.06–6.70). Mothers who listened to only Latino music (vs. those listening to non-Latino music) were less likely (OR=0.49; 95%

Table 1. Likelihood of ever breastfeeding (BF) the previous child and the index child

	BF previous child[a]			BF index child[b]		
	n	OR	95% CI	n	OR	95% CI
Exchange services with friends/relatives:						
Yes	46	2.65	1.16–6.05	76	2.08	1.07–4.05
ref: No	61	1.00		84	1.00	
Respondent's age:						
≥30 years	81	3.50	1.19–10.30	132	2.67	1.06–6.71
ref: <30 years	26	1.00		28	1.00	
Educational level:						
≥high school	43	2.11	0.90–5.00			
ref: <high school	64	1.00				
Kind of music to which respondent listens:						
Latino				77	0.49	0.25–0.95
ref: Non-Latino or mixed				83	1.00	
Respondent head of household:						
Yes				124	0.46	0.20–1.04
ref: No				36	1.00	

Backward stepwise logistic regression. Variables removed from model:
[a]Lend or borrow money from friends or relatives, lend or borrow goods from friends or relatives, respondent head of household and kind of music to which respondent listens
[b]Lend or borrow money from friends or relatives, lend or borrow goods from friends or relatives, parity of respondent and educational level of respondent

CI=0.25–0.95) to have breastfed the index child. The following variables were not associated (P>0.05) with BF in either the index (n=160) or the "previous child" (n=107) in multivariate models: exchange of goods, exchange of money, respondent's level of education, parity (only entered in index child model), and respondent's head of household status (Table 1).

6. CONCLUSIONS

Social capital by way of exchange of services and support is associated with a higher likelihood of breastfeeding in this Puerto Rican community. Social capital defined as either lending/borrowing money or exchanging goods was not associated with breastfeeding. This finding suggests that the construct of social capital is multidimensional and that it is important to capture its different dimensions in research studies. Older women are more likely to breastfeed their infants than their younger counterparts. Acculturation was associated positively with BF in this community. This contrasts with findings with Mexican Americans that have consistently found an inverse association between acculturation and BF. This suggests that the background BF culture in country or territory of origin (i.e., weak in Puerto Rico but strong in Mexico) modifies the association between acculturation and BF among Latinos in the continental United States.

7. REFERENCES

Carter-Porkas O, Zambrana RE. Latino health status. In: Aguirre-Molina M, Molina CW, Zambrana RE. Health Issues in the Latino Community. San Francisco: Jossey Bass, 2001; pp 23-54.

Giachello ALM. Maternal/perinatal health. In: Molina CW, Aguirre-Molina M, editors. Latino Health in the US: A Growing Challenge. Washington, DC: American Public Health Association, 1994; pp 135-187.

Pérez-Escamilla R, Himmelgreen D, Segura-Millán S, Ferris A, González A, Damio G, Bermúdez-Vega A. Breastfeeding initiation among inner-city Puerto Rican women from Hartford, Connecticut. J Am Diet Assoc 1998;98:657-663.

RACIAL/ETHNIC DISPARITIES IN PUBLIC OPINION ABOUT BREASTFEEDING: THE 1999-2000 HEALTHSTYLES SURVEYS IN THE UNITED STATES

Ruowei Li, Fred Fridinger, and Laurence Grummer-Strawn

1. INTRODUCTION

African American women in the United States have been reported to be less likely than whites to initiate and maintain breastfeeding (Li et al. 2002; Ryan 1997). Previous studies examining the basis of racial/ethnic disparities in breastfeeding behaviors mainly involved pregnant and lactating women (Scott 1999; Tan & Jeffery 1995). Because women's choices of feeding practice are influenced by attitudes of people with whom they have contact (Humphreys et al. 1998), understanding the racial/ethnic disparities in public opinions that shape women's breastfeeding behaviors is important. The purpose of this study was to examine racial/ethnic disparities in public knowledge about the health benefits of breastfeeding and public perceptions about barriers to breastfeeding.

2. METHODS

The Healthstyles Survey, conducted by Porter Novelli each summer, is a mail survey of men and women 18 years of age and older in the United States. Each year since 1999, several breastfeeding questions have been added to the survey. The 1999 Healthstyles Survey included two survey items related to the health benefits of breastfeeding; the 2000 survey included 10 items related to public perceptions of breastfeeding constraints. To each statement, respondents were asked to rate their agreement as Strongly Disagree (1), Moderately Disagree (2), Neither Disagree nor Agree (3), Moderately Agree (4), or Strongly Agree (5). In our analysis, we treated responses 1 and 2 jointly to indicate disagreement, responses 4 and 5 jointly to indicate agreement, and response 3 to indicate no opinion. The surveys for both years yield a sample of about 2,400 adults in the United States (response rate = 75%). There are many similarities in sociodemographic profile between the Healthstyles sample and the U.S. census data. To adjust for over- or

Division of Nutrition and Physical Activity, National Center for Chronic Disease Prevention and Health Promotion, Centers for Disease Control and Prevention, Mailstop K-25, 4770 Buford Highway NE, Atlanta, Georgia 30341-3717

Table 1. Percentage agreement with each statement about breastfeeding (%)

	Total	White	African American	Hispanic
Breastfeeding is healthier for babies than formula feeding	68	67	71	70
Feeding a baby formula instead of breastmilk increases the chances the baby will get sick	22	21	20	30
A mother who breastfeeds has to give up too many lifestyle habits	45	41	60	54
Breastfeeding will tie the mother down and interfere too much with her social life	9	8	13	13
A mother cannot breastfeed her baby and work or go to school	10	8	19	16
It is embarrassing for a mother to breastfeed in front of others	27	26	25	34
Women commonly have problems making enough milk for their babies	13	12	14	18
Breastfeeding is painful to mothers	8	7	9	9
Breastfeeding a baby correctly is hard to learn	9	9	10	8
Breastfed babies do not feel as close to their fathers and grandparents as bottle-fed babies	7	6	9	8
Breastfed babies cry a lot more than bottle-fed babies	5	4	6	8
Breastfeeding will spoil a baby	3	2	4	8

Table 2. Adjusted odds[a] of agreement with each breastfeeding statement using multiple logistic regression (OR, 95% CI)

	White	African American	Hispanic
Breastfeeding is healthier for babies than formula feeding	1.00	1.47 (0.76, 2.83)	1.36 (0.68, 2.73)
Feeding a baby formula instead of breastmilk increases the chances the baby will get sick	1.00	0.83 (0.54, 1.37)	1.25 (0.82, 1.92)
A mother who breastfeeds has to give up too many lifestyle habits	1.00	***2.57 (1.68, 3.93)***[b]	1.50 (0.96, 2.34)
Breastfeeding will tie the mother down and interfere too much with her social life	1.00	***2.32 (1.27, 4.42)***	1.54 (0.81, 2.93)
A mother cannot breastfeed her baby and work or go to school	1.00	***2.49 (1.51, 4.09)***	***2.28 (1.27, 4.12)***
It is embarrassing for a mother to breastfeed in front of others	1.00	0.85 (0.52, 1.39)	1.33 (0.83, 2.15)
Women commonly have problems making enough milk for their babies	1.00	1.29 (0.72, 2.32)	1.44 (0.76, 2.71)
Breastfeeding is painful to mothers	1.00	1.36 (0.66, 2.79)	1.06 (0.47, 2.38)
Breastfeeding a baby correctly is hard to learn	1.00	1.03 (0.48, 2.21)	0.83 (0.43, 1.60)
Breastfed babies do not feel as close to their fathers and grandparents as bottle-fed babies	1.00	1.70 (0.92, 3.16)	0.77 (0.31, 1.94)
Breastfed babies cry a lot more than bottle-fed babies	1.00	1.10 (0.50, 2.42)	1.33 (0.53, 3.34)
Breastfeeding will spoil a baby	1.00	1.99 (0.90, 4.40)	***4.42 (1.98, 9.90)***

[a]Adjusted for age, sex, household income, education, marital status, employment, population density, and region.
[b]Bold italics indicate a statistically significant odds ratio.

under-representation of a particular category according to the U.S. census, data were post-stratified and weighted on seven demographic variables, including age, sex, marital status, race/ethnicity, income, region, and household size. In this way, the Healthstyles sample distribution matches that of U.S. census data, and the survey sample reflects the general population.

SAS 6.12 (SAS, Cary, NC) was used to estimate the percentage agreement with breastfeeding items for each race/ethnicity. We applied multiple logistic regression analyses to examine the association of race/ethnicity with public opinions about breastfeeding after adjusting for age, sex, household income, education, marital status, employment, population density, and region.

3. RESULTS

The results show that almost 70% of adults in the United States believe that breastfeeding is healthier for infants than is formula feeding, and knowledge of the health benefits of breastfeeding is similar for whites and African Americans. Almost half of respondents agreed that a mother who breastfeeds has to give up too many lifestyle habits, and African Americans are more likely than whites to have this negative opinion (Table 1). The multiple logistic regression analyses indicate that African Americans are at least two times more likely than whites to believe that breastfeeding interferes with mothers' personal and social lives, and that a mother cannot breastfeed her baby and work or go to school (Table 2).

4. DISCUSSION

Because this study was a national survey involving a large and demographically diverse sample of people, survey results reflect current U.S. social and cultural norms regarding breastfeeding. Findings from this study indicate that African Americans tend to have positive attitudes toward the health benefits of breastfeeding, but negative perceptions about breastfeeding constraints. Survey results suggest that African Americans endorse breastfeeding as the best infant feeding method, but perceive that many barriers prohibit breastfeeding.

An ecological model of interventions involving individual and social environmental factors has been proposed for health promotion (McLeroy et al. 1988; Bentley et al. 1999). This model assumes that changes in the social environment will produce changes in individuals, and that the support of individuals in the population is essential for implementing environmental changes. This model focuses on the relational features of communities, and views behavior as being affected by multiple factors, including intra- and interpersonal, institutional, community, public policy, and media influences. Although this study does not provide direct evidence about how public perceptions influence a woman's breastfeeding behavior, it suggests the social and environmental causes of low breastfeeding practices among African Americans.

The *HHS Blueprint for Action on Breastfeeding* recommends that special attention be given to barriers to breastfeeding for all women, and especially African American women (USHHS 2000). Because social and cultural norms guide women's decisions about breastfeeding and influence support for this practice, strategies to increase breastfeeding rates should target individual and social environmental barriers. Promotional efforts addressing constraints to breastfeeding are needed, especially among African Americans.

5. REFERENCES

Bentley ME, Gavin L, Black MM, Teti L. Infant feeding practices of low-income, African American adolescent mothers: An ecological, multigenerational perspective. Soc Sci Med 1999;49:1085-1100.

Humphreys A, Thompson N, Miner K. Intention to breastfeed in low-income pregnant women: The role of social support and previous experience. Birth 1998;25:167-174.

Li R, Ogden C, Ballew C, Gillespie C, Grummer-Strawn L. The prevalence of exclusive breastfeeding among U.S. infants: The Third National Health and Nutrition Examination Survey. Am J Public Health 2002;92:1107-1110.

McLeroy KR, Bibeau D, Steckler A, Glanz K. An ecological perspective on health promotion programs. Health Edu Q 1988;15:251-377.

Ryan AS. The resurgence of breastfeeding in the United States. Pediatrics 1997;99:1-5.

Scott JA. Factors associated with the initiation and duration of breastfeeding: a review of the literature. Breastfeeding Rev 1999;7:5-16.

Tan JC, Jeffery HE. Factors that influence the choice of infant feeding. J Paediatr Child Health. 1995;31:375-378.

[USHHS] United States Department of Health and Human Services. HHS Blueprint for Action on Breastfeeding. Washington, DC: U.S. Government Printing Office, 2000.

A COMPARISON OF PATTERNS OF BREASTFEEDING AND COMPLEMENTARY FEEDING IN PERU AND GHANA

G.S. Marquis[1], M.E. Penny[2], E.K. Colecraft[1], and M.F. Lozada[2]

1. INTRODUCTION

During the second year of life, child growth is dependent in part on an adequately balanced intake of human milk and complementary foods. Results from Zeitlin and Ahmed (1995) suggested that the 12- to 18-month age period is challenging because toddlers may not sufficiently increase complementary food intake to compensate for decreasing intake of human milk. In Peru and Ghana, breastfeeding is widely practiced after 12 months of age with the mean duration being about 21 months (GSS 1998; INEI 2000). Food intake of children at this age is dependent on availability of food, beliefs about acceptability of foods for children, access of children to different eating events (such as snacking), and feeding styles. This study examined the patterns of child feeding in two countries that have similar breastfeeding practices but differences in these determinants of complementary feeding. These results may provide indications of practices that could be used to improve the nutritional status of all children after 12 months of life.

2. METHODS

2.1. Subjects

Women with healthy toddlers 12 to 18 months of age were recruited in Lima, Peru and Accra, Ghana. Peruvian children were enrolled through census of neighborhoods and referrals from other studies being conducted in a low- to lower-middle class community. Ten nonbreastfed toddlers were first identified and 10 breastfed toddlers were matched by age (±2 months) and surrounding neighborhood to ensure similar age and socioeconomic distribution of the two feeding groups. When more than one breastfed toddler was located as a match for the nonbreastfed toddler, the breastfed participant was chosen randomly.

---

[1]Department of Food Science & Human Nutrition, Iowa State University, Ames, IA 50011, USA
[2]Instituto de Investigación Nutricional, Lima, Peru

Protecting Infants through Human Milk, edited by Pickering *et al.*
Kluwer Academic/Plenum Publishers, 2004

These 20 children were observed for 12 daytime hours. Upon completion, an additional 10 breastfed children were observed for 24 hours. In Ghana, a field worker visited three times per week an outpatient clinic serving a low- to middle-income community where growth monitoring was conducted daily. Mothers of all 12- to 18-month-old healthy children sent to the weighing station were approached until fifteen studies (12 breastfed and 3 nonbreastfed) were completed. Although all mothers agreed to participate in the study at the time of enrollment at the clinic, two mothers were not at home when we went to commence the study and were replaced. Three of the breastfed children were selected randomly to be observed for 24 hours; all other children (breastfed and nonbreastfed) were observed for 12 daytime hours. Written informed consent was obtained from all mothers. This protocol was approved by the Human Subjects Office at Iowa State University, the Ethics Committee at the Instituto de Investigación Nutricional, and the Ghanaian Ministry of Health.

2.2. Data Collected

A similar questionnaire was used in both sites to collect information on family demographics and a variety of socioeconomic indicators, including housing quality, access to basic services (water, sewage, electricity), hygiene, and employment. Weight and height were measured with a precision of at least 20 g and 0.1 cm, respectively.

Human milk intake was measured by weighing the child before and after each feed using an electronic digital balance sensitive to 1 g (Neville 1995). Nighttime (12 hours) human milk intakes were estimated from 12-hour daytime human milk intake using country-specific equations based on data from the children who were studied for 24 hours (R^2=0.350 [Peru]; R^2=0.527 [Ghana]).

All liquids and foods were weighed before being offered to the child and any liquid and foods served but not consumed were weighed to determine total intake. When a food item was prepared at home, all raw ingredients were weighed; a list of ingredients for purchased foods was obtained from packages when available, recipes provided by vendors, or common recipes from the community. Macronutrient estimations of the diet were made using local and regional food composition tables and the USDA food composition tables when items were not available in the local tables.

2.3. Statistical Analysis

Mean group differences for continuous variables were tested with the Student t-test and analysis of variance (ANOVA); Kruskal-Wallis one-way ANOVA was used for variables with non-normal distribution. Frequency differences were tested with the Pearson and Mantel-Hantzel chi-square tests. Results are presented as mean ± standard error of the mean. All tests were two-tailed and statistical significance was set at $P<0.05$ unless otherwise indicated.

3. RESULTS

Demographic and socioeconomic characteristics of the participants are shown in Table 1. Children from the two sites were comparable by age; however, Peruvian children had significantly lower anthropometric measurements than Ghanaian children.

Table 1. Demographic and socioeconomic characteristics of Peruvian and Ghanaian participants[a]

	Peru		Ghana		
	Breastfed n=20	Weaned n=10	Breastfed n=12	Weaned n=3	P value[b]
Child characteristics					
Age (months)	14.4±0.4	16.2±0.5	15.1±0.6	14.7±1.7	
Anthropometry					
weight-for-age (z-score)	–0.4±0.2	–1.0±0.3	0.2±0.5	0.5±0.3	0.022
height-for-age (z-score)	–0.7±0.2	–1.6±0.3	–0.0±0.4	0.1±0.1	0.006
weight-for-height (z-score)	0.1±0.2	0.0±0.2	0.2±0.4	0.7±0.3	
Maternal characteristics					
Age (years)	20.4±1.2	22.5±2.7	27.9±1.7	33.3±1.8	<0.001
Employed outside home	0.0	10.0	41.3	100.0	<0.001
Municipal services					
In-house piped water	60.0	20.0	33.4	66.7	
In-house connected toilet	65.0	30.0	41.7	0.0	
Electricity	100.0	100.0	100.0	100.0	

[a]Mean±SEM or %

[b]Analysis of variance was used for continuous variables; only the main effect of the variable "country" was significant. Mantel-Hantzel chi-square was used for categorical variables.

Ghanaian mothers were older and working outside the home was the norm; only one Peruvian mother worked outside the home. Municipal services were similar.

The energy density of Peruvian complementary foods was significantly higher than Ghanaian foods (1.6±0.1 vs. 1.3±0.1 kcal/g, respectively; P=0.03). Peruvian toddlers consumed smaller quantities of food at one time but had access to food over more of the 24-hour period than Ghanaian children. Figure 1 demonstrates the intake distribution of complementary foods and human milk over 24 hours in breastfed children. Almost all of the energy from complementary foods was consumed during the day (7 AM to 7 PM) in Ghana (94.9±9.7%). In contrast, Peruvian children ate over a longer time; only 71.9±15.1% was consumed during the daytime (P<0.001). The percent of total 24-hour energy from human milk that was consumed during the day was similar for Ghanaians and Peruvians. Total 24-hour estimated human milk intakes (504.0±193.2 vs. 488.7±194.8 g), energy intake from complementary foods (544.6±269.1 vs. 522.1±214.3 kcal), and total energy per kilogram body weight (89.1±29.6 vs. 85.6±23.2 kcal/kg) were similar in Ghana and Peru, respectively.

The type of foods consumed by toddlers differed by country as well as breastfeeding status (Fig. 2). For Peruvian breastfed toddlers, daytime intake consisted of more energy from snacks and less energy from main dishes (e.g., rice and stew) than Ghanaians and nonbreastfed Peruvian toddlers (P<0.01). Almost half of Peruvian breastfed toddlers' energy was from savory snacks and sweets. Both breastfed and nonbreastfed Peruvian children consumed more energy from liquids (e.g., bovine milk) than Ghanaian children. Energy intake among Ghanaian toddlers was primarily in the form of meals and paps.

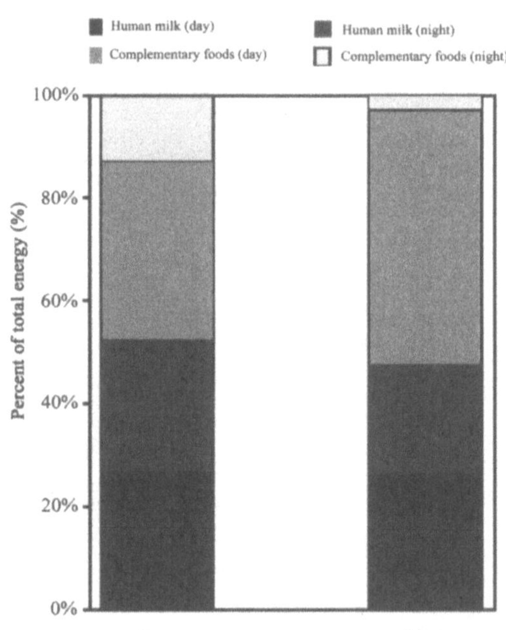

Figure 1. Intake of human milk and complementary foods by breastfed Ghanian and Peruvian toddlers, by time of day

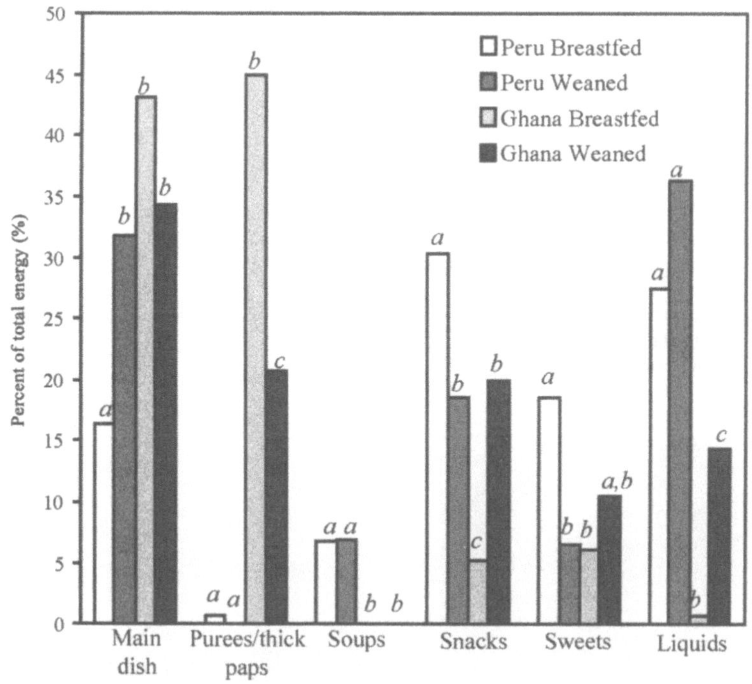

Figure 2. Sources of energy from complementary foods consumed during the day for Peruvian and Ghanian toddlers, by breastfeeding status. Different superscript letters denote significant differences among country/feeding groups.

4. DISCUSSION

Energy intake from human milk and complementary foods was similar for Peruvian and Ghanaian toddlers, but the children achieved their intakes differently. Peruvian children were more likely to eat small amounts during the day whereas Ghanaian children ate less often, with little food intake at night. Nonbreastfed toddlers did not simply eat more of the same foods than breastfed toddlers ate; dietary patterns were different. This was noted in the dramatic increase in the energy contribution of main dishes for Peruvian weaned toddlers and the decreased use of paps for Ghanaian weaned children. Different feeding patterns may be due to maternal perceptions of breastfed children as "still young" and, therefore, still fed as an infant. An important educational message in both countries may be related to providing regular family foods to breastfed toddlers. Whereas Ghanaian health educators may wish to help mothers introduce appropriate snacks and offer more food in the evening, this message would not be appropriate for Peruvians. In contrast, Peruvian messages may focus on reducing snacks and sweets to encourage eating the family meal. These results demonstrate the importance of making educational messages appropriate for the local community reality in which they are going to be used.

5. ACKNOWLEDGMENT

Funding was obtained from the Center for Designing Foods to Improve Nutrition (ISU).

6. REFERENCES

[GSS] Ghana Statistical Services. Demographic and Health Survey. Ghana, 1998.

[INEI] Instituto Nacional de Estadística e Informática. Encuesta Demográfica y de Salud Familiar 2000. Peru, 2000.

Neville MC. Volume and caloric density of human milk. In: Jensen RG, editor. Handbook of Milk Composition. San Diego: Academic Press, 1995; pp 99-113.

Zeitlin MF, Ahmed NU. Early Hum Dev 1995;41:97-110.

EARLY DETERMINANTS OF NON-EXCLUSIVE BREASTFEEDING AMONG GUATEMALAN INFANTS

Daniel W. Sellen[1,2], Amanda L. Thompson[1], Daniel J. Hruschka[1], Aryeh D. Stein[2], and Reynaldo Martorell[2]

1. INTRODUCTION

Ethnographic and observational studies suggest that during the perinatal period, physiological, psychosocial, and cultural factors influence initiation and maintenance of breastfeeding and patterns of feeding nonhuman milk substances (Pérez-Escamilla et al. 1996, 1998; Scott & Binns 1999; Chapman & Pérez-Escamilla 1999). Public health nutritionists need to understand the etiology of non-exclusive breastfeeding in the first 6 months of life because of the mismatch between actual and recommended breastfeeding practices (Lutter 2000; Sellen 2001). Studies have found that delayed lactogenesis stage II (LS-II) can be assessed by milk volume, human milk biomarkers, and maternal perception and recall of onset of lactation and if not resolved is a cause of actual and perceived difficulties with breastfeeding in the first days postpartum, persistent insufficient milk volume, early introduction of infant formula or other nonhuman milk substances, and reduced breastfeeding duration (Chapman & Pérez-Escamilla 1999, 2000a; Dewey 2001). To date, few studies have examined the causes or effects of delayed LS-II in rural populations in developing countries.

2. OBJECTIVES

We examined risk factors for later onset of lactation in a rural Guatemalan birth cohort born between June 1996 and July 1998 (n=341) and tested the hypothesis that delay undermines establishment of exclusive breastfeeding during the first week of life.

3. MATERIAL AND METHODS

Maternal and infant anthropometrics, survey data on maternal and household characteristics, and information about delivery were collected as part of a continuing

[1]Department of Anthropology, Emory University, 1557 Pierce Drive NE, Atlanta, GA 30322
[2]Department of International Health, Emory University, Atlanta, GA

Protecting Infants through Human Milk, edited by Pickering *et al.*
Kluwer Academic/Plenum Publishers, 2004

study of the intergenerational effects of undernutrition in four villages (Martorell et al. 1995). Data on daily feeding during the first week were elicited by maternal recall of frequency, quantities, and times of feeding of human milk and all other substances at day 8 during home interview, and by 24-hour recall at 1 and 3 months postpartum.

Onset of lactation was coded as the day (ordinal values 1, 2, 3, or 4–7 days postpartum) on which women reported perceiving that their milk had "come in" (Chapman & Pérez-Escamilla 2000b). Delayed onset of lactation was defined when onset of lactation was greater than 3 days postpartum. The method of feeding each infant was categorized daily during the first week of life and at 1 and 3 months following recent convention (WHO 1991). Infants were categorized as exclusively breastfed (EBF) on days when only water, medicinal supplements, or other non-nutritive liquids were given in addition to human milk; and as non-exclusively breastfed when any other substances were given in addition to human milk. Infants were coded as having established a pattern of EBF by the end of the first week if they were classified as EBF on all of days 5, 6, and 7 postpartum.

4. RESULTS

Most infants were term singletons (98%) born normally (89%) to multiparas (60%). A proportion was of low birth weight (<2500 g, 11%) and/or showed intrauterine growth retardation (<10th percentile BW, 8%). Initiation of breastfeeding was untimely for almost half of all infants (>1 hour postpartum, 47%), EBF continued throughout the first week of life in 30% of infants, and only 47% of infants established EBF by 5 to 7 days.

Adjusting for covariates, maternal obesity, short preceding birth interval (PBI), and above average maternal age were found to independently increased the odds of delayed onset of lactation (Table 1). Maternal obesity significantly increased the risk of failure to establish exclusive breastfeeding by 7 days (adjusted OR=8.03, 95% CI=1.7, 38.9). Infants EBF by 1 week showed greater odds of EBF at 1 and 3 months, and infants EBF at 1 month showed greater odds of EBF at 3 months (Table 2).

Table 1. Factors affecting the delayed onset of lactation (>3 days)

Main effect	Adjusted OR (95% CI)[a]
Maternal obesity (BMI>30)	2.7 (1.1, 6.5)
Maternal age (>median, 26 years)	1.8 (1.04, 3.0)
Short PBI[b] (<2 years)	2.1 (1.2, 3.7)

[a]Univariate odds ratios (OR) adjusted for primiparity, low BW, long labor (>10 hours), and abnormal delivery (Caesarian or forceps) using logistic regression
[b]PBI=preceding birth interval

Table 2. Association between early and later exclusive breastfeeding (EBF)

	OR (95% CI)	
	EBF at 1 month	EBF at 3 months
EBF by 7 days	5.7 (3.5, 9.5)	5.5 (3.3, 9.1)
EBF at 1 month	---	8.5 (5.1, 14.0)

5. CONCLUSIONS

Delayed onset of lactation undermines maternal capacity to establish EBF in the first week and at later ages in this population. Risk factors for delayed onset of lactation include maternal obesity, short preceding birth interval, and greater maternal age. Strategies to support the initiation and maintenance of exclusive breastfeeding should focus on risks for delayed onset of lactation.

6. ACKNOWLEDGMENTS

Supported by NIH grant HD-299-2706 and Emory College. Morgen Hickey assisted with data management.

7. REFERENCES

Chapman DJ, Perez-Escamilla R. Does delayed perception of the onset of lactation shorten breastfeeding duration? J Hum Lact 1999;15:107-111; quiz 137-109.

Chapman DJ, Pérez-Escamilla R. Lactogenesis stage II: Hormonal regulation, determinants and public health consequences. Recent Res Dev Nutr 2000a;3:43-63.

Chapman DJ, Perez-Escamilla R. Maternal perception of the onset of lactation is a valid, public health indicator of lactogenesis stage II. J Nutr 2000b;130:2972-2980.

Dewey KG. Maternal and fetal stress are associated with impaired lactogenesis in humans. J Nutr 2001;131:3012S-3015S.

Lutter C. Length of exclusive breastfeeding: linking biology and scientific evidence to a public health recommendation. J Nutr 2000;130:1335-1338.

Martorell R, Habicht JP, Rivera JA. History and design of the INCAP longitudinal study (1969-77) and its follow-up (1988-89). J Nutr 1995;125:1027S-1041S.

Perez-Escamilla R, Himmelgreen D, Segura-Millan S, Gonzalez A, Ferris AM, Damio G, Bermudez-Vega A. Prenatal and perinatal factors associated with breast-feeding initiation among inner-city Puerto Rican women. J Am Diet Assoc 1998;98:657-663.

Perez-Escamilla R, Segura-Millan S, Canahuati J, Allen H. Prelacteal feeds are negatively associated with breast-feeding outcomes in Honduras. J Nutr 1996;126:2765-2773.

Scott JA, Binns CW. Factors associated with the initiation and duration of breastfeeding: a review of the literature. Breastfeed Rev 1999;7:5-16.

Sellen DW. Comparison of infant feeding patterns reported for nonindustrial populations with current recommendations. J Nutr 2001;131:2707-2715.

[WHO] World Health Organization. Geneva, 1991.

ASSOCIATION OF DEGREE AND TIMING OF EXPOSURE TO BREASTFEEDING PEER COUNSELING SERVICES WITH BREASTFEEDING DURATION

Donna Chapman[1], Grace Damio[2], Sara Young[3], and
Rafael Pérez-Escamilla[1]

1. INTRODUCTION

Randomized trials conducted in developing countries have demonstrated that breastfeeding peer counseling increases rates of breastfeeding initiation and improves the duration of breastfeeding (Morrow et al. 1999; Haider et al. 2000). We are conducting a randomized community trial, designed to evaluate the effectiveness of an existing community-based breastfeeding peer counseling program serving mostly low income Latinas (i.e., women from Spanish-speaking countries in Latin America or the Caribbean) in Hartford, CT. Preliminary data from this on-going study previously have shown that subjects randomized to receive breastfeeding peer counseling have a median breastfeeding duration one month greater than their counterparts who did not receive breastfeeding peer counseling (1.75 mo vs. 0.8 mo, $P<0.05$) (Chapman et al. 2002). The objectives of this analysis are to: a) report on a process evaluation of the program, focusing on actual coverage of pre-, peri-, and postnatal services; and b) determine if differences in the degree and timing of the exposure to breastfeeding peer counseling services are associated with breastfeeding duration.

The program under evaluation, Breastfeeding: Heritage and Pride, is administered jointly by Hartford Hospital and the Hispanic Health Council. This program is comprised of 3.25 full-time equivalents (FTEs), including one bilingual internationally board certified lactation consultant, who serves as a working supervisor, and 2.25 FTE staff peer counselors. Entry-level peer counselors earn U.S. $12.00 per hour, and receive medical benefits if they are working full-time. The program is funded on a year-to-year basis from grant sources, including the University of Connecticut Family Nutrition Program and Reduce Infant Morbidity and Mortality Program funds. Peer counselors serve approximately 800 predominantly Latina clients annually.

[1]University of Connecticut, Department of Nutritional Sciences, Storrs, CT 06269-4017
[2]Hispanic Health Council, Hartford, CT
[3]Hartford Hospital, Hartford, CT

Protecting Infants through Human Milk, edited by Pickering *et al.*
Kluwer Academic/Plenum Publishers, 2004

2. METHODS

In this study, 157 pregnant women who were considering breastfeeding were recruited at <26 weeks gestation and randomized to receive: a) routine prenatal and perinatal breastfeeding education provided by Hartford Hospital (NO PC); or b) breastfeeding peer counseling services in addition to the routine breastfeeding education offered at Hartford Hospital (PC). The PC protocol specified that PCs meet with clients once prenatally, daily during the maternity stay, and at least twice during the early postpartum period. Subjects were interviewed in person within 48 hours of delivery and monthly through 6 months postpartum via telephone to assess infant feeding practices and peer counselor contact. Documentation of PC contact in the program files was reviewed. These analyses focus on the 60 subjects in the PC group who were eligible for the study at the time of delivery. Cox regression analyses were used to assess differences in breastfeeding duration for subjects with or without PC contact at specified time periods. Contact was determined to have occurred if either the subject reported PC contact or if the PC file documented a visit.

3. RESULTS

3.1. Process Evaluation

A summary of coverage provided by the PC program is shown in Table 1. Prenatal contact with a breastfeeding PC was reported by 50% of the subjects. On average, subjects receiving prenatal contact reported that the visit was approximately 65 minutes long. Specific content areas for the prenatal visits, along with the percentage of subjects reporting that the content areas were reviewed are as follows: breastfeeding positions (96%), breastfeeding brochures reviewed (92%), breastfeeding myths (92%), breast pump use (85%), breastfeeding video observed (54%). One-half of the subjects reported that they did not receive a prenatal home visit from a PC. The PC program files were reviewed to determine the reasons for the lack of a prenatal visit for these subjects. Frequently an appointment had been made, but there was not further documentation in the PC file (29%). Alternatively, subjects failed to return PC phone calls (13%), thus an appointment was never scheduled. Scheduled visits were rescheduled but did not occur in 13% of women without a prenatal visit. Two subjects refused the prenatal visit (8%), and in two cases there was no documentation of attempted contact by the PC (8%).

Table 1. Summary of peer counseling program coverage

	% Subjects recalling visit	% PC[a] files confirming visit	% Cases with confirmation by either subject or PC file	% Agreement between subject recall and PC file
Prenatal	50	39	55	90
Perinatal	93	96	98	95
Postnatal	45	47	62	78

[a]PC=peer counselor

Perinatal contact with a breastfeeding PC was reported by 94% of subjects. During their one-month postpartum interviews, subjects reported receiving 2.5±4.1 perinatal visits. On average the total amount of time subjects reported spending with PCs during their hospitalization was 58.9±135.5 minutes.

Among those subjects initiating breastfeeding, maternal report of PC contact by home visits and telephone calls during the first month postpartum was 45% and 51%, respectively. Of the subjects receiving PC home visits, the frequency of home visits during the first month postpartum was as follows: 1 visit (30%), 2 visits (26%), 3 visits (30%) and 4 or more home visits (13%). Among subjects reporting phone contact with PCs during the first month postpartum, 1, 2, 3, and 4 or more phone calls were received by 35%, 12%, 23%, and 31%, respectively. Maternal report of contact with PCs decreased dramatically during the second month postpartum with home visits and phone contact reported by 8% and 12% of subjects, respectively.

3.2. Association of Degree and Timing of Peer Counseling with Breastfeeding Duration

Among subjects initiating breastfeeding, the 25th percentile of breastfeeding duration for women with prenatal contact tended to be greater than that of women without prenatal contact (1.1 mo vs. 0.6 mo, respectively) (Fig. 1). Due to the high level of perinatal coverage, comparisons of breastfeeding duration are not presented. The first quartile of breastfeeding duration among women with PC home visits in the first month postpartum was significantly greater than that of their counterparts who did not receive home visits (1.8 mo vs. 0.5 mo, respectively; $P<0.05$). For subjects who received both perinatal and postpartum contact, the 25th percentile for breastfeeding duration was significantly greater (1.8 mo vs. 0.5 mo, respectively; $P<0.05$) than that of women who did not receive PC services at both of these times. Subjects receiving all three services (pre-, peri-, and postpartum) tended to have a greater first quartile of breastfeeding duration than subjects who did not (2.1 mo vs. 0.9 mo, respectively; $P=0.08$).

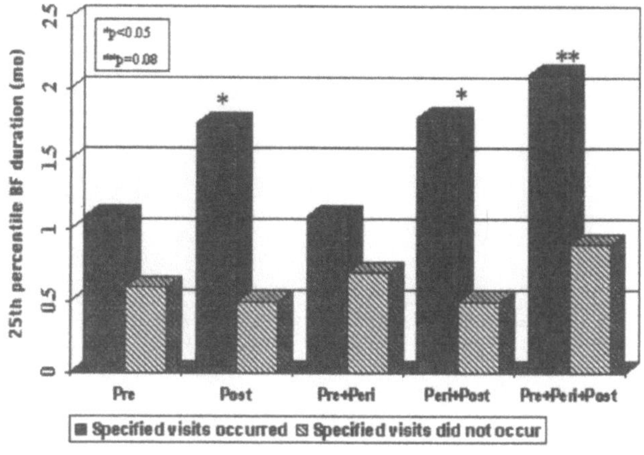

Figure 1. Association of degree and timing of peer counselor exposure with breastfeeding duration

4. CONCLUSIONS

These data reflect coverage levels for pre, peri, and postpartum services provided by an existing peer counseling program operating under "real world" conditions. While service levels do not meet the program's stated coverage goals, the overall levels of coverage are reasonable and sufficient to expect the differences in breastfeeding duration previously shown (Chapman et al. 2002).

These preliminary results suggest that postpartum peer counseling services effectively increase breastfeeding duration. This effect appears to be magnified when pre-, peri-, and postnatal services are combined. Further research is needed to confirm these preliminary findings and to further determine the impact of prenatal and perinatal peer counseling visits on breastfeeding duration. Because self selection and recall bias cannot be ruled out in this study, future randomized clinical trials evaluating the impact of the degree and timing of breastfeeding peer counseling are essential.

5. REFERENCES

Chapman DJ, Damio G, Young S, Pérez-Escamilla R. Impact of breastfeeding peer counseling services on breastfeeding initiation and duration among a low-income, Hispanic population: A randomized community trial. FASEB J 2002;16:A978.

Haider R, Ashworth A, Kabir I, Huttly SRA. Effect of community-based peer counselors on exclusive breastfeeding practices in Dhaka, Bangladesh: a randomized controlled trial. Lancet 2000;356:1643-1647.

Morrow AL, Guerrero ML, Shults J, Calva JJ, Lutter C, Bravo J, Ruiz-Palacios G, Morrow RC, Butterfoss FD. Efficacy of home-based peer counselling to promote exclusive breastfeeding: a randomised controlled trial. Lancet 1999;353:1226-1231.

EFFECT OF EDUCATION AND LACTATION SUPPORT ON MATERNAL DECISION TO PROVIDE HUMAN MILK FOR VERY-LOW-BIRTH-WEIGHT INFANTS

Paula M. Sisk, Cheryl A. Lovelady, and Robert G. Dillard

1. INTRODUCTION

Premature infants are at increased risk for infection, necrotizing enterocolitis, feeding intolerance, and developmental delay compared with term infants. When infants are fed human milk, the incidence of these problems is diminished (Schanler et al. 1999; Atkinson 2000). In the United States, the national breastfeeding initiation rate of mothers who deliver prematurely is 48%, compared with 60% for mothers of term infants. Incidence of breastfeeding is correlated negatively with infant gestational age and socioeconomic status of the mother (Ryan 1997). Family and hospital staff support has been found to increase lactation success in mothers of premature infants (Peitschnig et al. 2000). However, health care professionals may be reluctant to ask mothers to provide human milk for a number of reasons: 1) stress has been shown to interfere with milk production (Lau 1999) and preterm delivery has been shown to be stressful to parents, 2) the effort and time required might be considered burdensome and stressful when breastfeeding was not the mothers' feeding plan, and 3) the time and expertise required for adequate counseling of mothers could be costly when mothers' willingness and ability to express milk is uncertain. These concerns are countered by the view that mothers should be presented with all the evidence supporting human milk feeding in preterm infants in order for a well-informed decision to be made.

The aims of this study were to: 1) determine if counseling mothers on the benefits of human milk for their very-low-birth-weight (VLBW) infants would increase their stress and anxiety levels, 2) ascertain if mothers of VLBW infants who had not planned to breastfeed would express milk during the infants' hospital stay, and 3) compare the infant intake of human milk provided by the mothers who initially planned to breastfeed with that of mothers who initially planned to feed their infants formula during the first four weeks of their hospital stay.

Department of Nutrition, University of North Carolina at Greensboro, PO Box 25170, Greensboro, NC 27402

Protecting Infants through Human Milk, edited by Pickering *et al.*
Kluwer Academic/Plenum Publishers, 2004

2. METHODS

Mothers 18 years of age or older who delivered a VLBW infant between 700 and 1500 grams were enrolled within three days of delivery. Women were ineligible for the study if they had a medical condition that contraindicated providing human milk, reported substance abuse during the pregnancy, or were unable to speak English. The State Trait Anxiety Inventory measures a person's trait of anxiety and their present state of anxiety (Speilberger 1983). These self-evaluation questionnaires were administered before counseling. A board certified lactation consultant counseled all mothers on the benefits of human milk for premature infants and the procedure for collection and storage of milk. Mothers who decided to initiate lactation were given assistance with milk expression and procurement of an electric breast pump. The State Trait Anxiety Inventory and the Parental Stressor Scale: Neonatal Intensive Care Unit Questionnaire (Miles & Funk 2000) were administered after counseling. Infant intake of maternal milk was measured during the first four weeks of hospital stay. Group assignment [Breast (BR), n=64 or Formula (FO), n=31] was based on feeding preference stated at hospital admission prior to counseling. Women who initially decided to formula feed were divided into two subgroups. The first subgroup included women who initially decided to formula feed and then switched to breastfeeding after counseling (Formula-Breast). The other subgroup consisted of women who chose not to express milk after counseling (Formula-Formula). Means between groups were compared with ANOVA, Student t-test, and chi-square analysis.

3. RESULTS

Baseline characteristics of the mothers were similar except the BR mothers had a higher rate of marriage than the FO mothers (Table 1). When analyzing data with the three groups (BR, Formula to Breast, and Formula to Formula), the Formula to Formula infants had a significantly greater mean gestational age and birth weight. After counseling, 100% of the women who planned to breastfeed initiated milk expression and 84% of the women who planned to formula feed initiated milk expression. The State Anxiety scores at each time point were within the normal range (mean 36.17, standard deviation 10.96) for all women age 18 to 39 years (Table 2). There were no significant differences in State Anxiety scores between the BR and FO groups. There were no differences in anxiety scores before and after counseling between the two groups when controlling for trait score and initial anxiety score. This suggests that counseling did not increase stress and anxiety. There was no difference between the BR and FO groups in overall stress measured by the Parental Stressor Scale: NICU instrument. The scores were within the observed range (mean 2.61, standard deviation 0.75) for parents of newborns requiring intensive care. Infants of BR mothers received significantly more milk than the Formula to Breast mothers from week 1 to week 4 (Table 3.) A significantly higher percentage of infants of BR mothers compared with Formula to Breast mothers consumed human milk for over 50% of their enteral feedings at each time period (Fig. 1). However, over 50% of the Formula to Breast group received human milk for at least half of their enteral intake for the first month of life.

Table 1. Subject characteristics

	Breast-Breast n=64	Formula-Breast n=26	Formula-Formula n=5
Maternal Age (y)[a]	26.5 (0.8)	24.4 (0.9)	29.8 (2.8)
Maternal Education (y)[a]	11.8 (0.6)	9.5 (1.1)	13.0 (1.0)
Marital Status[b]			
Married (%)	40 (63)	6 (23)	4 (80)
Race (%)			
White	37 (58)	11 (42)	3 (60)
African-American	24 (38)	15 (58)	2 (40)
Hispanic	2 (3)	0	0
Asian	1 (2)	0	0
Medicaid (%)	35 (55)	18 (69)	3 (60)
Parity[a]	0.7 (0.1)	0.9 (0.2)	1.2 (0.6)
Previously Breastfed (%)	7 (11)	3 (12)	0 (0)
Birth weight (gm)[b]	1,169 (26)	1,058 (40)	1,382 (33)
Gestational Age (wk)[b]	28.7 (0.3)	28.3 (0.5)	31.6 (0.6)
Infant Gender (%)			
Female	50	54	60
Male	50	46	40

[a]Mean±SEM
[b]Significantly different, ANOVA, P<0.05

Table 2. Anxiety and stress of mothers of very-low-birth weight infants did not increase after counseling

	Breast-Breast n=64	Formula-Breast n=26	Formula-Formula n=5
Parental Stressor Scale–NICU[a]	2.4 (9.1)	2.1 (0.2)	2.8 (0.3)
Trait Anxiety Score[a]	36.7 (1.2)	40.1 (2.3)	43.6 (3.4)
State Anxiety 1[a] (before counseling)	45.2 (1.7)	42.5 (2.4)	43.4 (3.5)
State Anxiety 2[a] (after counseling)	42.4 (1.7)	39.3 (2.5)	43.2 (5.7)

[a]Mean±SEM

Table 3. Infant intake of human milk during weeks 1 to 4 of the hospital stay

Hospital time interval	Breast-Breast (mL)[a]	Formula-Breast (mL)[a]
Week 1	n=54 166 (28)	n=23 98 (42)
Week 2	n=55 631 (63)[b]	n=22 391 (117)
Week 3	n=49 942 (82)[b]	n=18 231 (90)
Week 4	n=44 1,042 (92)[b]	n=12 361 (184)

[a]Mean±SEM
[b]Significantly different, ANOVA, P≤0.001
Infants who were NPO (receiving nothing by mouth) for the entire week were excluded.

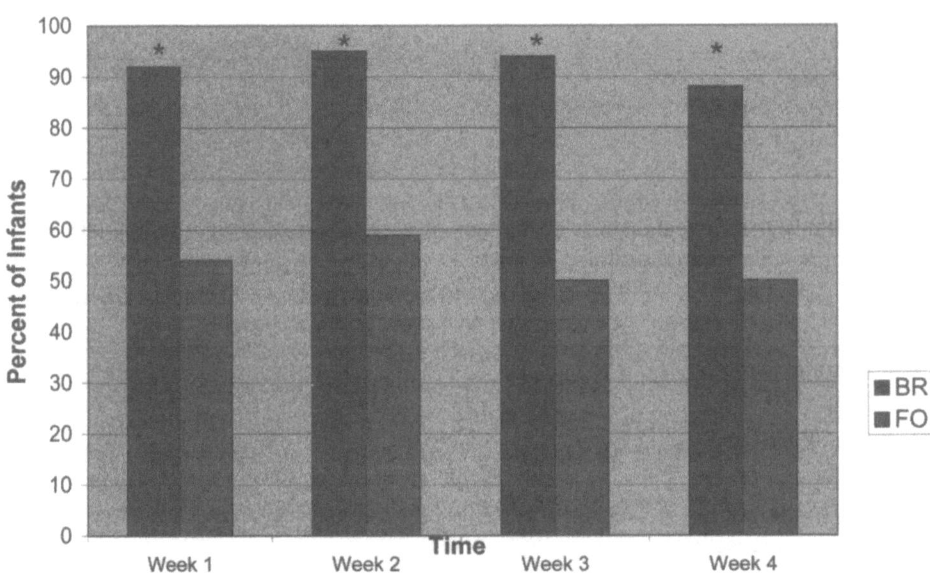

Figure 1. Percent of infants receiving greater than 50% of enteral feedings from human milk; *P<0.001

4. CONCLUSION

Counseling mothers of very-low-birth-weight infants about the benefits of human milk, when followed by assistance with milk expression, does not increase their anxiety and stress. The counseling was effective in that over 50% of mothers who had not planned to breastfeed and were able to provide human milk for at least half of their infants' enteral feedings during the first month of life.

5. REFERENCES

Atkinson S. Human milk feeding of the micropremie. Clin Perinatol 2000;27:235-246.

Lau C. Stress and lactation. In: Atkinson SA, Lemons JA, editors. Human Milk for Very-Low-Birth-Weight Infants. Report of 108th Ross Conference on Pediatric Research, Phoenix, AZ. Columbus, OH: Ross Products Division Abbot Laboratories, 1999; pp 109-119.

Miles MS, Funk SG. Parental Stressor Scale: Neonatal Intensive Care Unit. University of North Carolina at Chapel Hill, 2000.

Peitschnig B, Sklossy H, Gottling A, Posch M, Kafer A, Lischka A. Breastfeeding rates of VLBW-influence of professional breastfeeding support. Adv Exp Med Biol 2000;478:429-430.

Ryan A. The resurgence of breastfeeding in the United States. Pediatrics 1997;99:1-5.

Schanler R, Shulman F, Lau C. Feeding strategies for premature infants: beneficial outcomes of feeding fortified human milk versus preterm formula. Pediatrics 1999;103:1150-1157.

Speilberger C. Manual for the State-Trait Anxiety Inventory for Adults. Redwood City CA: Mind Garden, 1983.

INTERACTION OF STRESS AND LACTATION DIFFERS BETWEEN MOTHERS OF PREMATURE SINGLETONS AND MULTIPLES

C. Lau, N. Hurst, P. Burns, and R.J. Schanler

1. INTRODUCTION

Preterm mothers commonly have difficulty providing sufficient milk to meet the needs of their infants (Lau 2001). For many infants, lactation is halted prior to their hospital discharge. This early termination of lactation is often blamed on the stress mothers encounter as a result of the medical condition of their infants. Indeed, inhibition of lactation by stress routinely is acknowledged and a number of studies have reported significant psychological distress in preterm mothers (Lau 2001; Meyer et al. 1995; Miles et al. 1999; Singer et al. 1999). However, no study to our knowledge has investigated the relationship between stress and lactation in the same mothers. In 2002, we examined such interaction in mothers of infants born <30 weeks gestation. Lactation performance was measured as 24-hour milk collection. Maternal psychological distress was assessed as a function of anxiety, depression, and a parental stress score scale specifically designed for neonatal intensive care units [PSS:NICU] (Miles et al. 1993). Total duration of skin-to-skin holding during hospitalization and pumping frequency also were recorded. We reported that the lactation performance of these mothers was correlated negatively with depression, but not anxiety, and positively with skin-to-skin holding and pumping frequency (Lau et al. 2002). Given that multiple births account for a large proportion of premature deliveries (Blondel et al. 2002), determination of whether the interaction of stress and lactation differed between mothers of premature singletons and multiples is important. We hypothesized that mothers of multiples would have greater anxiety and depression, be less motivated to maintain pumping/breastfeeding schedules, and have more difficulty meeting the needs of their infants when compared with mothers of premature singletons.

Department of Pediatrics/Newborn, Baylor College of Medicine, One Baylor Plaza, Houston, TX 77004
(Dr. Schanler is currently located at Schneider Children's Hospital at North Shore, Manhasset, NY.)

Protecting Infants through Human Milk, edited by Pickering *et al.*
Kluwer Academic/Plenum Publishers, 2004

2. METHODS

This study was approved by the Baylor College of Medicine Institutional Review Board for Human Research. One hundred twenty-five mothers of infants, born <30 weeks gestation, were recruited. The study design consisted of five visits to the General Clinical Research Center (GCRC) at Texas Children's Hospital every other week beginning two weeks postpartum. At each visit, mothers were asked to answer a series of psychological questionnaires and to provide an accurate measure of their 24-hour milk collection.

2.1. Data Collection

At the time of their first visit, the socioeconomic status of the mothers was collected. Psychological assessment was monitored by the following tests: the Spielberger Trait and State Anxiety Inventory (Consulting Psychologists Press, Palo Alto, CA), the Beck Depression Inventory [BDI] (Psychological Corp., San Antonio, TX), and the Parental Stressor Scale: Neonatal Intensive Care Unit [PSS:NICU] (Miles et al. 1993). The Spielberger Trait Anxiety was given at the time of the subjects' first visit to the GCRC. The Spielberger State Anxiety Inventory, BDI, and PSS:NICU were given at every visit. The PSS:NICU comprised one general stress question and four categories of potential NICU-specific stressors: the sight and sound of the NICU, the appearance and behavior of the infant, parental role alteration, and staff behaviors and communication. To measure lactation performance, pumping frequency and volume per pumping during the 24 hours following each visit was used to calculate a 24-hour milk collection. Total duration of skin-to-skin holding during the infant's hospitalization was obtained from a record of all sessions.

2.2. Data Analyses

The independent t-test was used for comparisons of measures between mothers of singletons and multiples. Differences in socioeconomic status were assessed by the chi-square method. Binary logistic regression was used to examine factors correlated with mothers who maintained pumping/breastfeeding and mothers who did not within each group of mothers. Similarly, multiple regression was used to identify factors correlated with lactation performance within groups. These factors were first identified individually using the Pearson correlation method. Variables demonstrating P values ≤0.05 were entered into the regression analyses.

3. RESULTS

The socioeconomic status was similar between the two groups of mothers. Table 1 shows the respective maternal characteristics of the two groups. Only a between-group difference in the 24-hour milk volume was observed. There was no significant difference in any of the psychological measures (Table 2) nor in the percent of mothers who maintained pumping/breastfeeding during hospitalization (60%). However, the latter measure was correlated with different factors depending upon the groups. For mothers of singletons, this was correlated negatively with the Parental Role Alteration subset of the PSS:NICU (P=0.037, OR=0.44, 95% CI=0.20–0.95) and positively with the duration of skin-to-skin holding (P=0.018, OR=1.10, 95% CI=1.02–1.18). For mothers of multiples,

Table 1. Maternal characteristics

	Singletons	Multiples
Number	85	40
Maternal Age (years)	28.9±6.5	28.9±7.2
Gestational Age (weeks)	27.1±1.6	27.3±1.8
Birth Weight (g)	939±228 (n=85)	1001±272 (n=88)
Sets of twins/triplets	---	32/8
24-hour milk volume (mL)[a]	430±320	599±441
Pumping frequency (number/day)	5.2±1.4	5.3±1.1
Skin-to-skin holding (total hours)	14.8±23.5	17.4±21.5

[a]P=0.039

Table 2. Psychological scores

Spielberger Trait-State Anxiety Inventory

Anxiety (Mean±SD)	Trait (standard T score: 50 percentile)	State (standard T score: 50 percentile)
Singletons	36.5±9.1 (36)	37.7±11.2 (36)
Multiples	35.4±10.5	34.5±10.1

Beck Depression Inventory

	Score (Mean±SD)	Minimal (0–9)	Mild (10–16)	Moderate (17–29)	Severe (>30)
Singletons	8.6±6.1	68%	21%	11%	--
Multiples	9.1±7.1	61%	28%	8%	3%

PSS:NICU[a]

	Singletons (Mean±SD)	Multiples (Mean±SD)
Sight and sound	2±1	2±1
Baby's looks	3±1	3±1
Parental role	4±1	4±4
Staff behavior	2±1	2±1
General stress	4±1	4±1

[a]Stress Occurrence Level (Metric 1)

0 = not applicable
1 = not at all stressful
2 = a little stressful
3 = moderately stressful
4 = very stressful
5 = extremely stressful

it was correlated positively with maternal age only (P=0.03, OR=1.17, 95% CI=1.02–1.35). In a similar manner, 24-hour milk collection was correlated positively with pumping frequency for mothers of singletons ($P<0.01$, R^2 = 24.4%) and correlated negatively with depression and positively with duration of skin-to-skin for mothers of multiples (P=0.032 and P=0.005, respectively; R^2 = 40.1%). The percent of mothers of multiples able to meet 100% of *at least* one of their infant's need was similar to that of mothers who met the needs of their singleton (45% vs. 32%, respectively).

4. DISCUSSION AND CONCLUSION

Mothers of singletons and multiples exhibited similar characteristics, socioeconomic status, psychological distress scores, and motivation to maintain lactation. However, the 24-hour milk volume was reduced in mothers of singletons compared with mothers of multiples. Despite all similarities, their motivation to pump/breastfeed and their lactation performance were correlated with different factors. Motivation to maintain lactation was correlated with parental role alteration and skin-to-skin holding for mothers of singletons, but only to maternal age for mothers of multiples. Lactation performance was in turn correlated to pumping frequency for mothers of singletons and to the level of depression and skin-to-skin holding for mothers of multiples.

To our knowledge, this is the first study showing how the birth of singletons or multiples can differentially affect the lactation performance of mothers with very-low-birth-weight infants. This observation suggests that maternal affect and/or coping attributes likely differ depending upon whether singletons or multiples are involved. A better understanding of these differences would help in developing appropriate interventions to promote pumping/breastfeeding in mothers of premature infants.

5. REFERENCES

Blondel B, Kogan MD, Alexander GR, Dattani N, Kramer MS, Macfarlane A, Wen SW. The impact of the increasing number of multiple births on the rates of preterm birth and low birthweight: an international study. Am J Public Health 2002;92:1323-1330.

Lau C. Effects of stress on lactation. Pediatr Clin North Am 2001;48:221-234.

Lau C. The effect of stress on lactation--its significance for the preterm infant. Adv Exp Med Biol 2002;503:91-97.

Meyer EC, Garcia Coll CT, Seifer R, Ramos A, Kilis E, Oh W. Psychological distress in mothers of preterm infants. J Dev Behav Pediatr 1995;16:412-417.

Miles MS, Funk SG, Carlson J. Parental Stressor Scale: neonatal intensive care unit. Nurs Res 1993;42:148-152.

Miles MS, Holditch-Davis D, Burchinal P, Nelson D. Distress and growth outcomes in mothers of medically fragile infants. Nurs Res 1999;48:129-140.

Singer LT, Salvator A, Guo S, Collin M, Lilien L, Baley J. Maternal psychological distress and parenting stress after the birth of a very low-birth-weight infant. JAMA 1999;281:799-805.

MAKING MY BABY HEALTHY

Changing the Decision from Formula to Human Milk Feedings for Very-Low-Birth-Weight Infants

Donna J. Miracle[1], Paula P. Meier[2], and Patricia A. Bennett [3]

1. INTRODUCTION

The scientific literature is replete with health, growth, and developmental benefits when very-low-birth-weight (VLBW; ≤1,500 g) infants are provided their own mothers' milk (Lucas et al. 1992; 1994). These benefits are provided through a combination of nutritional, enzymatic, anti-inflammatory and anti-infective properties within human milk (Meier 2001; Schanler 2001; Mathur et al. 1990). Despite these documented benefits, fewer than half of women who give birth to VLBW infants in the United States initiate and maintain lactation (Ross/Abbott 2000). In the Rush Mothers' Milk Club program of breastfeeding interventions, all mothers of VLBW infants are targeted by NICU care providers and encouraged to provide human milk for their infants, regardless of initial feeding intent. The purpose of this study was to examine maternal decisions and responses to providing milk for a VLBW infant when the mother's initial intent had been to formula-feed.

2. METHODS

Using prospective, purposive sampling, semi-structured interviews were conducted with 21 of 23 eligible mothers over a consecutive nine-month period. All women indicated that they initially planned to formula-feed VLBW infants, but changed this decision when a physician or nurse told them about the importance of human milk for their infant. These mothers initiated lactation with a breast pump. Women who were still expressing milk at one-month post-birth became candidates for the semi-structured interview, which was audio-recorded and transcribed verbatim. Data were coded, categorized, and subjected to dimensional analysis (Schatzman 1991).

[1]Rush University, Chicago, IL
[2]Rush-Presbyterian St. Luke's Medical Center, Chicago, IL
[3]Anderson University, Anderson, IN

2.1. Characteristics of the Sample

Of the 21 women, 71% were African-American, 20% were Caucasian, and 9% were Latina; 62% were low-income (SSI, WIC-eligible). Further characteristics are depicted in Table 1.

Table 1. Additional characteristics of the study sample

Characteristic	Mean	Range
Maternal age (years)	26.5	18–38
Infant birth weight (g)	705.4	504–1310
Gestational age (weeks)	25.8	23–33

3. RESULTS

Of the 21 mothers, all expressed milk for >30 days, 19 went on to feed at breast, and 2 elected to complete certification through LaLeche League to become Breastfeeding Peer Counselors for the Rush Mothers' Milk Club. The women reported that the main reasons for initial plans to formula-feed were: "not knowing anyone who had breastfed" (n=13) and "pain associated with feeding or pumping" (n=10). All 21 women reported that they decided to "use the breast pump" when the nurse or physician talked with them about the health benefits of mothers' milk for their infant. All mothers reported being "thankful" that they were encouraged to provide milk, and all denied feeling "forced" into this decision. The analysis produced 12 themes organized into a dimensional matrix (Schatzman 1991), with the core concepts as: "I have to do this to make my baby healthy and to grow" and "this is the only thing I can do for my baby." Strategic process themes included: not listening to distracters, scheduling time to express milk, and "bonding" with the pump. Mothers perceived the outcome of providing milk as enhanced empowerment and confidence, as exemplified by: "I *can* do this for my baby" and "I can see a difference in my baby because of my milk".

4. CONCLUSION

These findings underscore the role of nurses and physicians in providing information about human milk to women who initially indicate they plan to formula-feed their VLBW infants. These data do not support concerns of NICU care providers that sharing the health benefits of human milk with these women will lead to feelings of coercion or guilt. Instead, the findings indicate that mothers can use this information to make informed choices about method of feeding for their VLBW infants.

5. REFERENCES

Lucas A, Morley R, Cole TJ, Lister G, Leeson-Payne C. Breast milk and subsequent intelligence quotient in children born preterm. Lancet 1992;339:261-264.

Lucas A, Morley R, Cole TJ, Gore SM. A randomised multicentre study of human milk versus formula and later development in preterm infants. Arch Dis Child Fetal Neonatal Ed 1994;70:F141-146.

Mathur NB, Dwarkadas AM, Sharma VK, Saha K, Jain N. Anti-infective factors in preterm human colostrum. Acta Paediatr Scand 1990;79:1039-1044.

Meier PP. Breastfeeding in the special care nursery. Prematures and infants with medical problems. Pediatr Clin North Am 2001;48:425-442.

[Ross/Abbott] Breastfeeding Trends. Mothers Survey. Columbus, OH: Ross Products Division, Abbott Laboratories, Inc., 2000.

Schanler R. The use of human milk for premature infants. Pediatr Clin North Am 2001;48:207-219.

Schatzman, L. Dimensional analysis: Notes on an alternative approach to the grounding of theory in qualitative research. In: Maines DR, editor. Social Organization and Social Process: Essays in Honor of Anselm Strauss. New York: D.E. Gruyter, 1991; pp 303-313.

COMFORT AND EFFECTIVENESS OF THE SYMPHONY BREAST PUMP FOR MOTHERS OF PRETERM INFANTS

Comparison of Three Suction Patterns

P. Meier[1], N. Hurst[2], N. Rodriguez[1], B. Ackerman[3], K. Howard[4], M. Allen[4], and J. Engstrom[5]

1. INTRODUCTION

Sustaining an adequate milk volume is difficult for mothers of very-low-birth-weight (≤1,500 g) infants who must use a breast pump long term. A comfortable, effective, and efficient pump facilitates efforts of mothers, and may result in a greater volume of milk.

2. PURPOSE

This is a report of an ongoing study designed to evaluate the comfort, effectiveness, and efficiency of a new breast pump (Symphony TM; Medela, Inc., McHenry, IL) among mothers of preterm infants. The Symphony pump is driven with a programmable card that cycles the pump in different suction patterns, mimicking the rhythm of a term infant. This study compares three suction patterns generated by the Symphony pump, which are evaluated by comparing the following outcomes: (1) mean daily milk volume; (2) mean milk volume per pumping; (3) mean seconds until milk ejection; (4) percent of milk volume expressed at 5 and 10 minutes; (5) degree of breast emptying; and (6) maternal perceptions of comfort and effectiveness.

[1]Rush University Medical Center (RUMC), 1653 West Congress Parkway Chicago, IL 60612
[2]Texas Children's Hospital, Houston, TX
[3]Yale-New Haven Medical Center, New Haven, CT
[4]Brigham and Women's Hospital, Boston, MA
[5]University of Illinois at Chicago, Chicago, IL

Protecting Infants through Human Milk, edited by Pickering *et al.*
Kluwer Academic/Plenum Publishers, 2004

3. METHODOLOGY

A total of 120 mothers of preterm infants (birth weight ≤1,250 g) will be enrolled in this multisite study. Mothers who are enrolled initiate lactation using the Classic TM (Medela) pump, and are instructed to pump 8 times daily. Care practices that influence milk volume are standardized among the four research sites, including: milk expression techniques, skin-to-skin holding of infants, and suckling at the emptied breast. All women record milk volume for each breast separately from the time of birth through completion of the study.

When milk volume is greater than 350 mL per day for 5 consecutive days, mothers are assigned randomly to test the Symphony pump. At Rush University Medical Center, 30 mothers are testing each of three patterns twice, for a total of 6 pumpings over 9 days. The order of patterns will be assigned randomly, and mothers will be blinded to which pattern they are using. At the other 3 sites, mothers will use 1 of the 3 patterns for all pumpings for 7 days, then return to using the Classic pump for 5 days. Mothers from all sites complete questionnaires that measure their perceptions of comfort and effectiveness for each pattern, and will allow them to compare these measures to the Classic pump, which all mothers use initially. Data collection is scheduled to be completed by early 2004.

4. RESULTS

In pilot studies (4 sites; n=39), mothers tested the 3 different patterns and were asked to rate their perceptions of comfort (on a scale from 1 to 10, with 10 being the most comfortable) using the Comfort and Effectiveness Questionnaire designed to be used in the larger study. The mean comfort score for the two-phase Symphony pattern was 9.6 (6–10). All mothers "agreed" or "strongly agreed" that "this pump is more comfortable than the one I'm using at home" (Classic or Lactina).

5. CONCLUSIONS

While the larger study will compare more variables, the findings from the pilot study show that mothers perceived the two-phase Symphony pattern as "more comfortable" than the Classic or Lactina. We speculate that maternal comfort is linked to greater milk volume, and a greater "dose" of milk for these infants.

6. ACKNOWLEDGMENT

Supported by Medela, Inc., McHenry; and NIH #F31NR07584

7. REFERENCES

Cregan MD, deMello TR, Hartmann P. Pre-term delivery and breast expression: Consequences for initiating lactation. Adv Exp Med Biol 2000;478:427-428.

Cregan MD, deMello TR, Kershaw D, McDougall K, Hartmann PE. Initiation of lactation in women after preterm delivery. Acta Obstet Gynecol Scand 2002;81;870-877.

Daly SEJ, Kent JC, Owens RA, Hartmann PE. Frequency and degree of milk removal and the short-term control of human milk synthesis. Exp Physiol 1996;81:861-875.

Meier PP. Breastfeeding in the special care nursery: Prematures and infants with medical problems. In: Schanler RJ, editor. Breastfeeding 2001: The Management. Pediatr Clin North Am 2001;48:425-442.

Mitoulas LR, Lai CT, Gurrin LC, Larsson M, Hartmann PE. Effect of vacuum profile on breast milk expression using an electric breast pump. J Hum Lact 2002;18:353-366.

Mitoulas LR, Lai CT, Gurrin LC, Larsson M, Hartmann PE. Efficacy of breast milk expression using an electric breast pump. J Hum Lact 2002;18:344-352.

Mitoulas LR, Sherriff JL, Hartmann PE. Short- and long-term variation in the production, content, and composition of human milk fat. Adv Exp Med Biol 2000;478:401-402.

Raisler J. Against the odds: breastfeeding experiences of low income. J Midwifery Womens Health 2000;45:253-263.

Schanler RJ. The use of human milk for premature infants. In: Schanler RJ, editor. Breastfeeding 2001: The evidence. Pediatr Clin North Am 2001;48:207-219.

IDENTIFICATION OF FACTORS AFFECTING BREAST PUMP EFFICACY

L.R. Mitoulas[1], D.T. Ramsay[1], J.C. Kent[1], M. Larsson[2], and P.E. Hartmann[1]

1. INTRODUCTION

Many studies have investigated the physical characteristics of sucking by breast- and bottle-fed infants (Woolridge 1986; Weber et al. 1986; Mathew & Bhatia 1989; Bamford et al. 1992). However, none have applied the same approach to human milk expression using an electric breast pump. In this regard there is a paucity of information regarding factors that can affect breast pump function. We have developed a method suitable for the objective determination of breast pump efficacy (Mitoulas et al. 2002a) and have used this method to compare a standard pumping pattern to an experimental pumping pattern in an effort to identify factors that may be responsible for breast pump efficacy.

2. METHODS

Mothers (n=12) of healthy, term-delivered infants (1–6 months of age) were recruited through either the Australian Breastfeeding Association, Western Australia Branch or private health care centers. All mothers supplied written, informed consent to participate in the studies, which were approved by the Human Research Ethics Committee, The University of Western Australia. All infants were exclusively breastfed on demand. Mothers expressed milk from one breast on two occasions using one of two randomly allocated pumping patterns; the Medela Classic pumping pattern (47 cycles/minute) and a 3-Phase experimental pumping pattern consisting of a stimulation phase (pre-milk ejection, 120 cycles/minute) and expression phases A (0–2 minutes post-milk ejection, 20 cycles/minute) and B (2–10 minutes post-milk ejection, range 55–78 cycles/minute). For both patterns, vacuum was variable (–50 to –250 mm Hg) and set to the comfort of the mother. The volume of milk expressed was recorded for each 30-second period, and milk ejection was determined by an acute increase in the diameter of a milk duct in the contra-lateral breast as monitored by ultrasound (Acuson XP-10).

[1]Biochemistry and Molecular Biology, School of Biomedical and Chemical Sciences, Faculty of Life and Physical Sciences, University of Western Australia, 35 Stirling Highway, Crawley, WA 6009, Australia
[2]Medela AG, Lattichstrasse 4b, 6341 Baar, Switzerland

Protecting Infants through Human Milk, edited by Pickering *et al.*
Kluwer Academic/Plenum Publishers, 2004

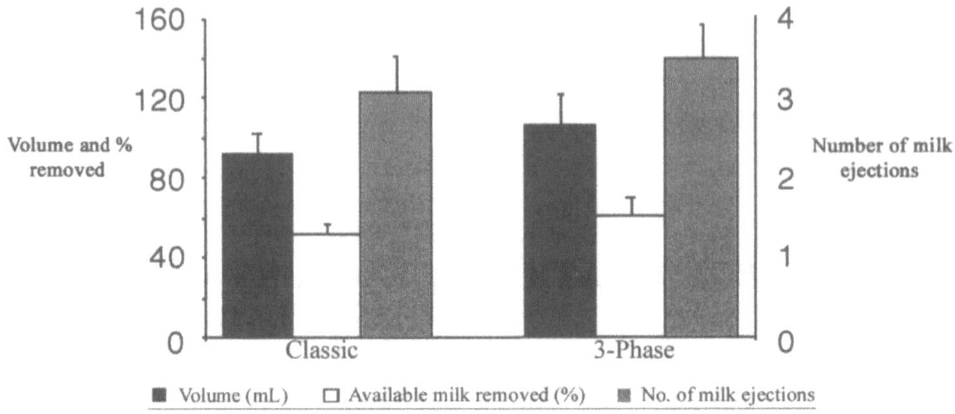

Figure 1. The mean (±SEM) total volume of milk, percentage of available milk expressed, and the number of milk ejections for the 10-minute expression period for the Classic and 3-Phase patterns.

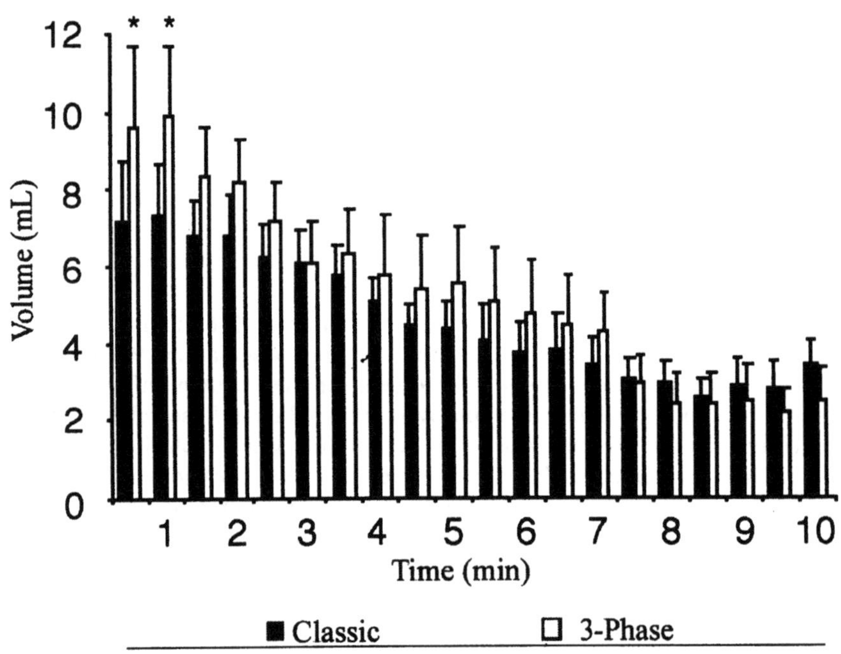

Figure 2. Volume (±SEM) of milk removed in each 30-second period by the Classic and 3-Phase patterns; (*P<0.05, Classic vs. 3-Phase).

3. RESULTS

The total volume of milk expressed (92.6±9.4 mL; 105.6±16.3 mL), the percentage of available milk removed (51.50±5.86%; 60.51±9.64%) and the total number of observed milk ejections (3.17±0.58; 3.58±0.28) did not differ between the Classic and 3-Phase patterns, respectively (Fig. 1). However, the rate of milk removal was greater for the 3-Phase pattern when compared with the Classic pattern for the first and second 30-second periods post-milk ejection [$P<0.05$] (Fig. 2).

4. CONCLUSIONS

Multiple milk ejections were observed during the 10-minute expression period with mothers experiencing approximately three milk ejections for both the Classic and 3-Phase patterns, respectively. In this regard, mothers usually sensed the first but not subsequent milk ejections. The consistency in the percentage of available milk removed in the immediate post-milk ejection periods (30 seconds) together with the lack of a relationship between total volume expressed and the number of milk ejections suggests that both patterns may need to be further optimized to take advantage of milk availability after a milk ejection. However, even though there was no difference in the total volume of milk removed over the entire 10-minute expression period, the 3-Phase pattern was more efficient than the Classic pattern in the first minute after the initial milk ejection. These data agree with previous results from this laboratory (Mitoulas et al. 2002b), and suggest a possible benefit of the vacuum curve dynamics of expression phase A of the 3-Phase pattern in the immediate post-milk ejection period.

5. ACKNOWLEDGMENTS

The authors thank the mothers and infants who participated in this study and the Australian Breastfeeding Association. Financial support for this study was provided by Medela AG (Switzerland), The Lotteries Commission of Western Australia, and the Women and Infants Research Foundation.

6. REFERENCES

Bamford O, Taciak V, Gewolb IH. The relationship between rhythmic swallowing and breathing during suckle feeding in term neonates. Pediatr Res 1992;31:619-624.

Mathew OP, Bhatia J. Sucking and breathing patterns during breast- and bottle-feeding in term neonates. Effects of nutrient delivery and composition. Am J Dis Child 1989;143:588-592.

Mitoulas LR, Lai CT, Gurrin LC, Larsson M, Hartmann PE. Efficacy of breast milk expression using an electric breast pump. J Hum Lact 2002a;18:344-352.

Mitoulas LR, Lai CT, Gurrin LC, Larsson M, Hartmann PE. Effect of vacuum profile on breast milk expression using an electric breast pump. J Hum Lact 2002b;18:353-360.

Weber F, Woolridge MW, Baum JD. An ultrasonographic study of the organisation of sucking and swallowing by newborn infants. Dev Med Child Neurol 1986;28:19-24.

Woolridge, M.W. The "anatomy" of infant sucking. Midwifery 1986;2:164-171.

PROTECTION OF BREASTFEEDING, MARKETING OF HUMAN MILK SUBSTITUTES AND ETHICS

M.F. Rea, F.F. Marcolino, A.J. Colameo, and L.A.Trevellin

1. INTRODUCTION

Although human milk provides adequate nutrition, many children are weaned early and fed human milk substitutes. Breastfeeding replacement by commercial infant formula represents an important source of profit generation for formula manufacturers. Therefore, selling and marketing these products are planned carefully as mothers stop breastfeeding. The World Health Organization (WHO) established an International Code of Marketing of Breast Milk Substitutes in 1981 (WHO-UNICEF 1981) [Fig. 1]. These WHO standards have been in effect in Brazil since 1988, and were revised twice: in 1992 (NBCAL 1992) and in 2002. The Code provides one special article dealing with Health Workers (Article 7), in which rules for ethical procedures of infant formula companies are defined. The Brazilian Code was disseminated to pediatricians by professional associations and the Minister of Health. Copies of the Code also were distributed to pediatricians by the largest infant food company in Brazil, indicating how the company interprets the national Code.

Pediatricians are important sources of information and influence decisions by mothers about infant feeding. In the early 20th century parents obtained most of their information about infant feeding from their child's physician because promotion of commercial human milk substitutes had not been fully implemented. After production of the first infant formula, companies realized the importance of having pediatricians as allies to sell their products and, therefore, the link between physicians and infant formula industry has been important (Sokol 1997). This link has never been documented scientifically, however, except by members of International Baby Food Action Network (IBFAN), as part of their advocacy activities (IBFAN 2001).

In May 2002, a revised Brazilian Code was adopted with clearer rules for commercial promotion through the health sector, not only for infant formula, but also for milks in general, baby foods, feeding bottles, and pacifiers. The purpose of this study was to document the influence of infant food representatives and infant formula manufacturers on pediatricians, to determine how physicians decide about feeding recommendations, and to assess the role of the Code in regard to the behavior of pediatricians in Brazil.

Instituto de Saude, Coordination of Institutes of Research, Secretaria de Estado da Saude de São Paulo, Brazil

Protecting Infants through Human Milk, edited by Pickering *et al.*
Kluwer Academic/Plenum Publishers, 2004

The "International Code of Marketing of Breast Milk Substitutes":

Key provisions relevant to health professionals

- There is a "legitimate market for infant formula," but "...in view of the vulnerability of infants in the early months of life and the risks involved in inappropriate feeding practices, including the unnecessary and improper use of breastmilk substitutes, the marketing of breastmilk substitutes requires special treatment, which makes usual marketing practices unsuitable for these products."
- "There should be no advertising or other form of promotion to the general public of products within the scope of this Code." Article 5.1
- No facility of a health care system should be used for the purpose of promoting infant formula or other products within the scope of this Code...." Article 6.2
- "those who are concerned...with maternal and infant nutrition should make themselves familiar with...the Code" (Article 7.1)
- "No financial or material inducements to promote products...should be offered...to health workers or members of their families, nor should these be accepted..." (Article 7.3)
- "Samples...of products within the scope of this Code...should not be provided...unless for professional evaluation or research at the institutional level..." (Article 7.4).

Related World Health Assembly Resolutions:

- "...no donations of free or subsidised supplies of breastmilk substitutes and other products...in any part of the health care system." Resolution WHA 47.5
- World Health Assembly Resolution 49.15 calls for measures to ensure that, "the financial support for professionals working in infant and young child health does not create conflicts of interest."

Figure 1. Codes of marketing of human milk substitutes

2. METHODS

In this cross-sectional study, a random sample of 360 pediatricians in São Paulo City were interviewed in their offices using an open-ended questionnaire containing questions related to infant food companies and pharmaceutical companies. A trained interviewer was responsible for the interviews. The results were coded and EPI-INFO was used for data management and analysis.

3. RESULTS

Pediatricians in all regions of São Paulo City were interviewed from October 2001 through September 2002.

The 360 pediatricians surveyed provided health care in private, public, or semi-public offices, and sometimes in ambulatory care facilities in hospitals. All pediatricians were visited routinely by representatives of infant formula and food companies, and dummy and pacifier companies. Approximately 31% of pediatricians surveyed declared a pediatric subspecialization and 22% indicated that they teach pediatrics. 72% of the pediatricians had been invited by companies for lunches or other meals; 16% declared that they had received funds from companies for paying registration fees, 10% for tickets, and 9% for hotels to attend events. Among those who had received sponsorship from companies, 40% were teachers of pediatrics.

Eighty-two percent of scientific events attended by the pediatricians surveyed were sponsored by infant formula companies. In events or in everyday practice, the pediatricians received gifts such pens, papers, paper-bags, and many other items.

Ninety-one percent were visited during the previous week by infant formula or food company representatives (43% Nestlé; 32% Gerber; 24% Support; 3% Mead-Johnson, and 2% Abbott) and 8% by feeding bottle and pacifier company representatives. During these office visits, 79% of pediatricians received samples of infant formula, baby foods, dummies or pacifiers, and 42% distributed them to mothers; the others kept it for personal use or distribution in institutions, such as crèches and hospitals.

When asked about the role of representatives in their clinical practices, many of the pediatricians responded that they are necessary for providing information about new products, and that they are influential and well prepared to convince them to use one product. However, the majority of pediatricians insisted that they prescribe only what is best for infants. Very few pediatricians indicated any criticism about the role of representatives or suggested new ways of learning about baby food products.

Questioned if they knew about the Brazilian Code of Marketing of Breast Milk Substitutes, Feeding Bottles, Dummies and Pacifiers, less than 10% responded yes.

The majority of pediatricians said they believe breastfeeding is the best way to feed infants but, in general, they felt in the Brazilian situation that it is necessary to enhance breastfeeding promotion.

4. CONCLUSIONS AND COMMENTS

Our findings indicate the influence of infant formula companies on daily activities of pediatricians in São Paulo. The different ways of promoting their products were documented, such as distribution of gifts, samples, written material, and support for participation in events. Samples of infant formula or other substitutes are received and many times distributed to patients, showing that pediatricians do not understand that this practice can be harmful for breastfeeding and is not allowed by the Code.

There is a trend of having more influential pediatricians, like teachers, funded to attend events, compared with others who do not teach. This practice indicates that companies are clear as to whom they consider to be more influential to disseminate their products. There is also a trend for more prescriptions of a product when the product representative visits a physician.

Conflict of interest exists each time professional attitude is influenced or even if influence is attempted. Both the Code (International and National) and the World Health Assembly Resolutions, using several ethical rules, called attention to this conflict in different ways. However, these documents apparently are not sufficient to avoid the possible conflict of interest and to impose ethical limits in the relationship between pediatricians and infant formula company representatives. Policies to protect breast-feeding practices from commercial interest must be reviewed, disseminated, understood, and practiced.

5. REFERENCES

[IBFAN] International Baby Food Action Network. Breaking the Rules, 2001. Penang, Malaysia.

[NBCAL] Norma Brasileira de Comercialização de Alimentos para Lactentes. Resolution 31/92 of October 1992, Minister of Health, Brazil (Code second version; revised).

Sokol E. The Code Handbook. International Code Documentation Centre, IBFAN Penang, Malaysia, 1997.

[WHO/UNICEF] International Code of Marketing of Breast Milk Substitutes. Geneva: World Health Organization, 1981.

MICRONUTRIENT STATUS OF BRAZILIAN LACTATING ADOLESCENTS

V.B. Azeredo, F.F. Bezerra, R. Figueiredo, C.M. Donangelo, and N.M.F. Trugo

1. INTRODUCTION

Pregnancy in Brazilian adolescents has increased in recent years. In 2000, 26% of children born in the Public Health System in Brazil were from adolescent mothers (Ribeiro et al. 2000). Brazilian women of reproductive age appear to have a high frequency of inadequate dietary intake for several micronutrients, especially during pregnancy and lactation (Borghi et al. 1997; Trugo 1997).

The high nutritional needs of pregnant and lactating adolescents associated with possible inadequate intakes may increase the risk of micronutrient deficiencies in this group with adverse consequences for maternal and child health. This information could be of value for implementing public policies and interventions specifically designed for this group. The purpose of this study was to evaluate the micronutrient status (iron, zinc, copper, folate, and vitamins B_{12}, A, and E) of Brazilian lactating adolescents.

2. METHODS

2.1. Study Group and Sample Collection

Nursing adolescents (n=35) participated in this study after informed consent. They were of low socioeconomic status and attended a Municipal Health Center in Rio de Janeiro. The adolescents were 16.6±1.1 years of age, at 9.1±6.0 weeks postpartum, and exclusively or predominantly breastfeeding (8.3±2.8 feedings/day). Fasting blood samples (20 mL) were obtained by venous puncture. Plasma was separated and divided in aliquots and stored at –20°C. Dietary intake was evaluated by three nonconsecutive 24 h-recall questionnaires. Nutrient intake was analyzed by use of the Food Processor software (Esha Research), adapted for Brazilian foods (database from IBGE 1996).

Laboratório de Bioquímica Nutricional e de Alimentos, Instituto de Química, Universidade Federal do Rio de Janeiro, Brazil

Protecting Infants through Human Milk, edited by Pickering *et al.*
Kluwer Academic/Plenum Publishers, 2004

Table 1. Micronutrient intake and frequency of inadequate intake in Brazilian lactating adolescents (n=35)

Nutrient	DRI[a]	Mean±SD	Median	Range	Frequency of inadequate intake
Iron (mg/day)	10[b]	11.2±5.2	9.3	3.5–23.1	56%
Zinc (mg/day)	14[b]	10.6±5.0	8.8	4.8–23.8	78%
Copper (mg/day)	1.3[b]	1.03±0.76	0.94	0.32–4.4	85%
Folate (μg/day)	500[c]	308±162	294	95.6–796	96%
Vitamin B_{12} (μg/day)	2.8[c]	6.0±14.5	3.0	0.75–77.9	48%
Vitamin E (mgTE/day)[a]	19[d]	6.7±6.4	5.3	1.55–29.9	94%
Vitamin A (μgRE/day)[a]	1200[b]	321±182	306	68–676	100%

[a]Definitions: DRI=Dietary Recommended Intake; TE=α-tocopherol equivalents; RE=Retinol equivalents
References: [b]Institute of Medicine 2001; [c]Institute of Medicine 1998a; [d]Institute of Medicine 2000

Table 2. Biochemical indices and frequency of inadequate intake of micronutrient status in Brazilian lactating adolescents (n=35)

	Cut-off values for marginal status	Mean±SD	Median	Range	Frequency of inadequate intake
Haematocrit (%)	<36[a]	38±3.4	38.4	31–44.2	20%
Hemoglobin (g/L)	<120[a]	122±15	120	83–150	34.3%
Plasma iron (μmol/L)	<7.2[b]	9.8±5.2	9.7	2.5–27.0	28.6%
Plasma transferrrin saturation (%)	<15[b]	19.3±12.0	19.0	3.8–56.3	40%
Plasma zinc (μmol/L)	<10.7[c]	11.8±2.8	11.4	7.6–17.8	32%
Plasma copper (μmol/L)	<10[c]	19.7±5.2	18.4	12.3–32.0	0
Plasma folate (nmol/L)	<13.6[b]	9.5±5.0	7.8	1.5–20.4	43.5%
Plasma vitamin B_{12} (pmol/L)	<150[b]	298±113	271	110–587	4.3%
Plasma α-tocopherol (μmol/L)	<11.6[d]	9.0±4.0	8.3	1.2–20.3	80%
Plasma retinol (μmol/L)	<1.05[c]	1.3±0.4	1.2	0.8–2.1	30%

References: [a]Institute of Medicine 1998b; [b]Sauberlich et al. 1984; [c]Institute of Medicine 2001; [d]Sokol 1996

2.2. Analytical Determinations

Hematocrit was determined by capillary centrifugation. Hemoglobin was measured by the cyanomethaemoglobin reaction (Bioclin kit, Brazil). Plasma iron, copper, and zinc were determined by inductively coupled plasma–atomic emission spectrometry (ICP-AES). Plasma transferrin saturation was obtained by the ratio between plasma iron and plasma total iron binding capacity (Analisa kit, Brazil). Erythrocyte folate and plasma folate and vitamin B_{12} were determined by radioisotope dilution assay (RIDA; Folate and DualCount kits, respectively; Diagnostic Products, USA). Plasma retinol and α-tocopherol were determined by reversed-phase HPLC (Hess et al. 1991).

2.3. Statistical Analysis

The software Statgraphics 4.0 (STSC, USA) was used for data description and statistical analysis. The effect of iron and folate supplementation during pregnancy on maternal status and the association between dietary intake and maternal status were determined by ANOVA and correlation analysis, respectively. Differences were considered statistically significant at $P<0.05$.

3. RESULTS

The dietary intake of the micronutrients studied and the frequency of inadequate intake are shown in Table 1. The mean intakes for zinc, copper, folate, vitamin E, and vitamin A were lower than the recommended intakes (IOM 1998, 2000, 2001), but mean intakes of iron and vitamin B_{12} were adequate. There was a high frequency of inadequate intake for all micronutrients studied, especially for vitamin A, folate, and vitamin E.

Results for the biochemical indices of nutritional status are shown in Table 2. The mean values of plasma folate and α-tocopherol were lower than the cut-off values used for characterization of marginal status. Moreover, there was a high frequency of inadequate intake for most of the indices evaluated, particularly for plasma α-tocopherol. These results indicate that lactating adolescents might be at nutritional risk of multiple micronutrient deficiencies.

There was no correlation between biochemical indices and dietary intakes, except for plasma and dietary folate ($r = 0.48$; $P<0.05$). The use of iron and folate supplementation during pregnancy did not affect their respective biochemical indices during lactation, but plasma copper was 22% lower ($P<0.05$) in lactating adolescents who used iron supplements. Hemoglobin increased ($r = 0.41$; $P<0.05$) and plasma copper and α-tocopherol decreased ($r = -0.36$ and $r = -0.42$, respectively; $P<0.05$) with advancing weeks postpartum.

4. CONCLUSION

In conclusion, Brazilian lactating adolescents present multiple micronutrient deficiencies, which may increase the risk of impaired maternal and infant development.

5. ACKNOWLEDGMENTS

This work was supported by CNPq, CAPES, FAPERJ, and FUJB (Brazil). FFB, RF, CMD, and NMFT acknowledge CNPq for fellowships.

6. REFERENCES

Borghi R, Baxter YC, Galletta MA, Maculevicius J, Zugaib M. Mudanças no comportamento alimentar em gestantes adolescentes. Rev Ginecol Obstet 1997;8:20-22.

Hess D, Keller HE, Oberlin B, Bonfanti R, Schuep W. Simultaneous determination of retinol, tocopherol, carotenes and lycopene in plasma by means of HPLC reversed phase. Int J Vitam Nutr Res 1991;61:232-238.

[IBGE] Instituto Brasileiro de Geografia e Estatística. Estudo Nacional da Despesa Familiar: Tabela de Composição de Alimentos. 5th Edition, 1999.

[IOM] Insitute of Medicine. Dietary Reference Intakes for Thiamin, Riboflavin, Niacin, Vitamin B_6, Folate, Vitamin B_{12}, Pantothenic Acid, Biotin and Choline. Washington, DC: National Academy Press, 1998a.

[IOM] Insitute of Medicine. Prevention of Micronutrient Deficiencies—Tools for Policymakers and Public Health Workers. Washington, DC: National Academy Press, 1998b.

[IOM] Insitute of Medicine. Dietary Reference Intakes for Vitamin C, Vitamin E, Selenium and Carotenoids. Washington, DC: National Academies Press, 2000.

[IOM] Insitute of Medicine. Dietary Reference Intakes for Vitamin A, K, Arsenic, Boron, Chromium, Cooper, Iodine, Iron, Manganese, Molybdenum, Nickel, Silicon, Vanadium and Zinc. Washington, DC: National Academies Press, 2001.

Ribeiro ER, Barbieri MA, Bettiol H, Silva AM. Comparação entre duas coortes de mães adolescentes em município do sudeste do Brasil. Rev Saúde Pública 2000;34:136-142.

Sauberlich HE, Dowdy RP, Skala JH. Laboratory Tests for Assessment of Nutritional Status. 7th Edition. Boca Raton, FL: CRC Press, 1984.

Sokol RJ. Vitamin E. In: Ziegler EE, Filler LJ, editors. Present Knowledge in Nutrition. 7th Edition. Washington, DC: ILSI Press, 1996; pp 130-136.

Trugo NMF. Micronutrient regulation in pregnant and lactating women from Rio de Janeiro. Arch Latinoam Nutr 1997;47:n° 2 (suppl 1).

NUTRITIONAL STATUS OF EXCLUSIVELY BREASTFEEDING ADOLESCENTS FROM NORTHWEST AND CENTRAL MEXICO

G. Caire[1], E. Casanueva[2], L.M. De Regil[1], A. Bolaños[1], and A.M. Calderón de la Barca[1]

1. INTRODUCTION

Breastfeeding may impair nutritional status of adolescent mothers, a vulnerable group due to their additional nutrient requirements. Data from countries with emerging economies (Geervani & Jayashree 1988; Casanueva et al. 1991) have found more weight and fat losses at three months postpartum in adolescent compared with adult lactating mothers. Mexico, a country in economic transition, presents contrasting social-cultural characteristics between northwest (NW) and central regions. There are no studies about the effect of breastfeeding on maternal nutritional status in the NW region, while this nutritional information from the central region is well known. This study evaluated the effect of breastfeeding at one and three months postpartum on the nutritional status of adolescent mothers from northwest and central Mexico.

2. METHODS

A longitudinal design was used to evaluate anthropometry and body composition of adolescent lactating women. Subjects were healthy, primiparous, and were exclusively breastfeeding their infants. Twenty-one women were enrolled: 11 from NW and 10 from the central regions. All of the women signed an informed consent. Sociodemographic indicators were collected at the first interview in the households. Maternal body weight (BW), height (H), dietary intake (DI), physical activity level (PAL), and total body water (TBW) were measured at one and three months postpartum. TBW was estimated by deuterium dilution and infrared spectroscopy (Caire et al. 2002). Body mass index ($BMI=BW/H^2$), fat free mass (FFM=TBW/0.73), and body fat (BF=BW–FFM) were calculated. Anthropometric comparisons by region and period and relationships between

[1]Centro de Investigación en Alimentación y Desarrollo, AC, Hermosillo, Sonora, México
[2]Instituto Nacional de Perinatologia, México, DF, México

Protecting Infants through Human Milk, edited by Pickering *et al.*
Kluwer Academic/Plenum Publishers, 2004

variables were evaluated using paired t-test, covariance analysis (DI and PAL as covariates), and multiple regression.

3. RESULTS

The mean age of adolescents from NW and central regions was 16.7±0.8 and 16.2±1 years, respectively. At one month postpartum, weight, BMI, and body fat were significantly ($P<0.01$) greater in adolescents from NW region (Table 1). In the central region group, weight loss was 1.75±1.26 kg/mo, representing 18.8 g/day. Adjusting by dietary energy and PAL, decline in body weight was not significant. Percentage of body fat decreased ($P<0.05$) in the central region group over time and at three months was lower ($P<0.001$) in adolescent mothers from the central region. From a public health perspective, weight and fat loss during lactation could contribute to maternal depletion in undernourished populations.

Although all women were from a low socioeconomic level, there were various categories, 80% of the adolescents from the central region and only 20% from the NW region were from the low income category. The inclusion of an interaction term between socioeconomic level and region in the regression model showed that determinants of BMI at one month were: weight gain during pregnancy, body fat, region, socioeconomic level, and the interaction term (R^2=0.630, P=0.0001). At three months, predictor variables were the same as those at one month, except for weight gain during pregnancy (R^2=0.501, $P<0.001$).

Table 1. Maternal anthropometry and body fat of adolescent mothers at time of lactation[a]

	1 month		3 months	
	Northwest (n=11)	Central (n=10)	Northwest (n=11)	Central (n=10)
Body weight (kg)	60.0±10.2[b]	48.9±3.2[c]	60.2±11.7[b]	47.2±3.2[d]
Height (m)	1.56±0.07[b]	1.53±0.05[b]	1.56 ±0.07[b]	1.53±0.05[b]
BMI (kg/m^2)	24.6±3.8[b]	20.9±1.4[c]	24.7±4.3[b]	20.5±1.6[c]
Body fat (%)	36.7±4.8[b]	29.3±6.2[c]	34.9±4.9[b]	24.4±6.4[d]

[a]Mean±SD
[b,c,d]Different letter superscripts across columns are significantly different from each other, P<0.05.

4. DISCUSSION

To explain differences in the nutritional status of the adolescent mothers from the two Mexican regions, the environmental factor may have had a greater influence than the physiological or ethnicity factors. Detriment of nutritional status of lactating adolescent mothers from the central area was associated with socioeconomic status. The increase in body fat during pregnancy was not enough to support breastfeeding for three months.

5. ACKNOWLEDGMENT

The study was partially supported by the International Atomic Energy Agency (9381).

6. REFERENCES

Caire JG, Calderón de la Barca AM, Bolaños AV, Valencia ME, Coward AW, Salazar G, Casanueva E. Measurement of deuterium oxide by infrared spectroscopy and isotope ratio mass spectrometry for quantifying daily milk intake in breast-fed infants and maternal body fat. Food Nutr Bull 2002;23(Suppl 3):38-41.

Casanueva E, Soberanis Y, Ortiz T, Bobadilla M. Cambios en la composición corporal en el período perinatal en un grupo de adolescentes. Perinatol Reprod Hum 1991;5:28-32.

Geervani P, Jayashree G. A study on nutritional status of adolescent and adult pregnant and lactating women and growth of their infants. J Trop Pediatr 1988;34:234-237.

BONE MINERAL DENSITY AND BONE TURNOVER IN ADOLESCENT MOTHERS AFTER LACTATION

E. Casanueva, M.E. Flores-Quijano, E. Frike, R. Samano, and S. De Santiago

1. INTRODUCTION

A woman gains 37% of her bone mass during adolescence. When an adolescent experiences pregnancy and lactation, her metabolism is challenged to support her own growth while providing the energy and nutrient requirements of fetal growth and milk synthesis.

Lactation represents a temporary catabolic state that promotes a significantly larger postpartum weight loss (lean and fat body mass) for breastfeeding teenagers than for adult mothers (Casanueva et al. 1991), illustrating young women's inability to compensate for the additional demand. In general terms there are few studies about bone health in breastfeeding teenagers. Therefore it is important to determine the effect of lactation on bone mineral density and bone turnover to establish if adolescents need calcium supplementation during breastfeeding (De Santiago 2002).

The objective of this study was to evaluate bone mineral density and bone turnover at nine months postpartum to identify if pregnancy and lactation affect the bone health of adolescent women.

2. METHODS

We studied three groups of adolescent and adult primigravidas [10 women per group]: a) nonpregnant, nonlactating; b) pregnant, nonlactating; and c) pregnant women who breastfed for three months. Women were seen on one occasion at nine months postpartum. Calcium intake was estimated by a food frequency questionnaire; bone mineral content of the lumbar spine (L2-L4) and femoral neck were measured by dual energy X-ray absorptiometry (DXA, Norland XR-26); serum osteocalcin was analyzed by commercial RIA; and urine N-telopeptide was measured using a commercial enzyme immunoassay.

Instituto Nacional de Perinatología, Instituto Nacional de Ciencias Médicas y Nutrición Salvador Zubirán and Universidad Iberoamericana, México D.F., México

Protecting Infants through Human Milk, edited by Pickering *et al.*
Kluwer Academic/Plenum Publishers, 2004

Table 1. Spearman rank correlations among the different variables (r values)[a]

	BMD[b] (L2–L4)	BMD[b] Trocanter	Osteocalcin	N-telopeptides
Age	0.321*	–0.007	–0.360**	–0.233
Full lactation time[c]	–0.088	0.043	0.421**	0.357**
Weight	0.369**	0.408**	0.021	–0.088
Height	0.251	0.343**	–0.084	–0.156
BMI[d]	0.278*	0.343**	0.053	0.045
BMD L2–L4	---	0.534**	–0.375**	–0.305*
BMD femoral neck	---	---	–0.230	–0.143
Osteocalcin	---	---	---	0.717***

[a]n=60 cases
[b]BMD=bone mineral density
[c]Full lactation time is defined as the number of weeks of exclusively breastfeeding.
[d]BMI=body mass index
*P<0.05; **P<0.01; ***P<0.001

Table 2. Bone mineral density by risk factors

Risk factor	Cases with BMD[a] <0.90 cm^2 (%)	Odds ratio	(CI 95%)
Femoral neck			
Pregnancy			
No	14/20 (70)		
Yes	16/40 (40)	3.50	1.11–11.07
BMI			
<21	16/23 (69)		
≥21	14/37 (38)	3.75	1.24–11.38
Height cm			
<160	24/28 (63)		
≥160	6/22 (27)	4.57	1.45–14.39
Body fat %			
<31	25/39 (64)		
≥31	5/21 (24)	5.71	1.72–18.9
Lumbar (L2–L4)			
BMI			
<21	15/23 (65)		
≥21	13/37 (35)	3.46	1.16–10.31
Body fat %			
<31	22/39 (56)		
≥31	6/21 (29)	3.23	1.03–10.10

[a]BMD=bone mineral density

3. RESULTS

The mean age of women was 16.3 and 25.6 years for adolescents and adults, respectively. There was no significant difference in weight, height, and body mass index (BMI) among the subjects. The mean BMI in adolescents was 21.3 and 22.1 in adults. Calcium intake (690±104 mg/day) was not different between the groups. No significant differences were observed between adolescents and adults in bone mineral density; however, lower values were observed in nulliparous adolescents. Lactating adolescents had higher concentrations of osteocalcin and N-telopeptides than the other two groups ($P<0.05$).

Bone mineral density (BMD) was correlated positively with age, weight, height, and BMI. Osteocalcin and N-telopeptides were correlated positively with full lactation time and negatively with age [$P<0.05$] (Table1).

The relative risk for low BMD (lumbar and trocanter) was associated with pregnancy, BMI, height (<160 cm), and body fat (<31%). Breastfeeding practice and duration, however, did not represent risk factors for low BMD (Table 2).

4. CONCLUSIONS

We observed that at nine months postpartum, lactating adolescents had almost total recovery of bone mineral density lost during lactation. However, pregnancy at an early age and high parity during adolescence represent a risk for bone demineralization.

5. REFERENCES

Casanueva E, Soberani Y, Ortiz T, Bobadilla M. Cambios en la composición corporal en el período perinatal en un grupo de adolescentes. [Changes in body composition during perinatal period in adolescents.] Perinatol Reprod Hum 1991;5:28-32.

De Santiago S, Alonso L, Halhali A, Larrea F, Isoard F, Bourges H. Negative calcium balance during lactation in rural Mexican women. Am J Clin Nutr 2002;76:845-51.

BREASTFEEDING AND FOOD TABOOS IN NURSING MOTHERS FROM MEXICO

Maria Irene Santos-Torres[1] and Edgar M. Vásquez-Garibay[2]

1. INTRODUCTION

The importance of human milk as the best and only food for infants under 6 months of age has a worldwide consensus, as has the value of promoting breastfeeding as a basic food beyond six months of age when infants also should receive adequate complementary feedings (WHO 1986). The purpose of this study was to identify food taboos of nursing women who participate in a breastfeeding support program.

2. METHODS

A cross-sectional study design included 493 nursing women interviewed 10 to 45 days after delivery. All of the women participated in the Baby Friendly Hospital program. A questionnaire was completed at birth and during their first postnatal clinic visit. From information provided, the following data were obtained: general characteristics of the nursing mother, obstetric and gynecologic background, postpartum conditions, characteristics of the newborn infant and the family, infant feeding practices, and foods avoided by the mother during lactation. A chi-square test was used to identify associations between food taboos, maternal characteristics, and demographic variables.

3. RESULTS

Seventy-two percent (72%) of the infants received full breastfeeding (31% exclusive and 41% almost exclusive), 17% partial breastfeeding (Labbock & Krasovec 1990), and 11% of infants received formula as initial feeding after hospital discharge. Fifty percent (50%) of the women avoided at least one food in their diet since childbirth due to belief that it was harmful while breastfeeding. Forty-seven percent (47%) avoided three or more foods. The majority of foods avoided were fruits and vegetables (62%) and legumes (20%). Fifty different foods were considered harmful by mothers during the first stages of

[1]Hospital General de Occidente, Secretaría de Salud, Zapopan, Jalisco, México
[2]Instituto de Nutrición Humana, Universidad de Guadalajara, Guadalajara, México

Protecting Infants through Human Milk, edited by Pickering *et al.*
Kluwer Academic/Plenum Publishers, 2004

nursing (<45 days). Mothers avoided such foods because they believed the foods may cause undesirable effects in the milk supply, or adversely affect the infant, or both (i.e., decreasing milk supply, causing infantile colic or diarrhea). Rejection of foods was associated with living more than 10 years in Guadalajara city (OR 1.95 [1.25–3.09], P=0.002), breastfeeding experience (OR 1.91 [1.18–3.12], P=0.005), no prenatal information about breastfeeding (OR 1.59 [1.08–2.34], P=0.01), and another person's decision (OR 1.61 [1.09–2.38], P=0.01).

4. DISCUSSION

Food taboos in specific stages of life such as pregnancy and nursing periods have been described as traditional in Asia, Africa, and Latin America, as well as in immigrant populations in the United States, Canada, and Australia (Manderson & Matthews 1981; Fishman et al. 1988). The underlying explanation is that birth is a moment of extreme vulnerability by excessive loss of heat during delivery. The mother should follow certain "precautions," which prohibit consumption of foods considered cold, such as many fruits and vegetables, and encourage the consumption of foods perceived as hot. These taboos form part of complex belief systems derived from medical humoral theory. In Mexico they probably can be traced from the Nahuatl perspective of the cold/hot theory (Castro 1995). There is almost no information about food taboos in nursing mothers in Mexico. It is therefore important that health professionals become more knowledgeable about the influence that culture has on breastfeeding and dietary behaviors that may be potentially harmful during pregnancy and lactation.

5. CONCLUSION

The study revealed a large number of nursing women with food taboos. Health personnel should be aware of maternal food taboos and reasons for these taboos. A supportive approach and efficient communication might reduce the gap between scientific recommendations and daily feeding and nutritional practices of mothers willing to nurse their infants.

6. REFERENCES

Castro R. La lógica de una de las creencias tradicionales en salud, Eclipse y embarazo en Ocuituco, México. Salud Pública Méx 1995;37:329-338.

Fishman C, Evans R, Jenks E. Warm bodies, cool milk: Conflicts in post-partum food choice for Indochinese women in California. Soc Sci Med 1988;26:1125-1132.

Labbok M, Krasovec K. Toward consistency in breastfeeding definitions. Stud Fam Plann 1990;21:226-230.

Manderson L, Mathews M. Vietnamese attitudes towards maternal and infant health. Med J Aust 1981;1:69-72.

[WHO] World Health Organization. Infant and Young Children Feeding; WHO Resolution 39.28, adopted May 16,1986. Geneva: World Health Organization; 1986.

IMPACT OF CALCIUM SUPPLEMENTATION IN THE PRECEDING PREGNANCY ON THE HUMAN MILK CALCIUM CONCENTRATION OF GAMBIAN WOMEN

L.M.A. Jarjou, A. Prentice, and J. Bennett

1. INTRODUCTION

Following our detailed studies of human milk calcium concentration, we hypothesized that calcium intake in pregnancy may determine human milk calcium concentration and hence the calcium intake of breastfed infants (Prentice et al. 1994). To test this, we conducted a controlled calcium supplementation study in pregnant women accustomed to a low calcium intake.

2. METHODS

The study involved 124 women in a rural region of The Gambia, West Africa, where dietary calcium intake is 300 to 400 mg/day. The women were randomized, double-blind, to receive either 1500 mg Ca/day as the carbonate (S, n=62) or a matching placebo (Pl, n=62) from 20 weeks of pregnancy until delivery. At enrollment, the age and parity of the women were (mean±SD, range): 27.4±7.6 (15–46) years, parity 3.3±2.7 (0–10). The calcium-supplemented and placebo groups are characterized in Table 1. The women were a subset of a cohort participating in a study of the effect of calcium supplementation on blood pressure in pregnancy. All women in the human milk study had completed successfully the supplementation phase (tablet compliance=99±2%), were in good health and had delivered a singleton, healthy baby. Human milk samples were collected at 2, 13, and 52 weeks postpartum and analyzed for calcium and phosphorus using a standard method (Laskey et al. 1991).

MRC Keneba, PO Box 273, The Gambia and MRC Human Nutrition Research, Elsie Widdowson Laboratory, Fulbourn Road, Cambridge CB1 9NL, UK

3. RESULTS

No significant differences were observed in the human milk concentrations of calcium, phosphorus, or the calcium-to-phorphorus ratio at 2, 13, and 52 weeks of lactation, before or after adjustment for potential confounders. The calcium concentrations (mean±SEM, mg/L) in each group were: 2 weeks [S=248±7, Pl=250±6]; 13 weeks [S=231±4, Pl=234±3]; 52 weeks [S=187±4, Pl=183±3] (Fig. 1).

Table 1. Subject characteristics

	All n=124	Ca supplement n=61	Placebo n=63
At 20 weeks of pregnancy			
Parity	3.3 (2.7)	3.4 (2.7)	3.3 (2.8)
Age (y)	27.4 (7.6)	27.5 (7.4)	27.4 (7.8)
Weight (kg)	56.3 (6.7)	56.9 (6.6)	55.7 (6.8)
Height (m)	1.61 (0.05)	1.61 (0.05)	1.61 (0.05)
Dietary Ca intake (mg/d)	351 (186)	345 (206)	356 (166)
Intervention			
Days of tablet provision	136 (15)	137 (16)	135 (14)
Tablet compliance	99.3 (1.8)	99.1 (2.2)	99.5 (1.4)

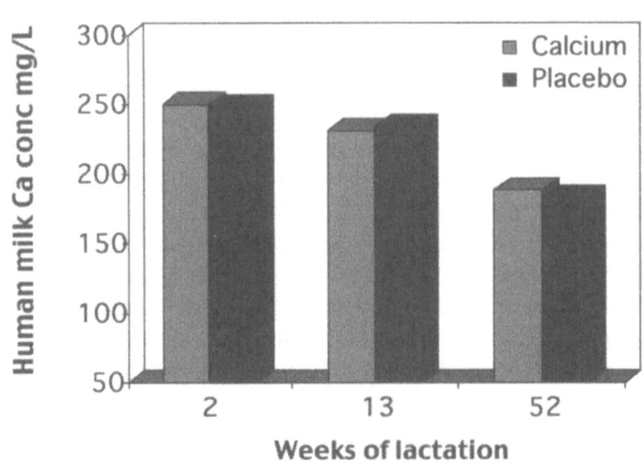

Figure 1. Human milk calcium concentrations in women who received (calcium) and did not receive (placebo) calcium supplementation in pregnancy.

4. CONCLUSION

This study shows that increasing the calcium intake of pregnant women accustomed to a low calcium intake does not significantly increase human milk calcium concentration during subsequent lactation.

5. ACKNOWLEDGMENT

The tablets were donated by Shire Pharmaceuticals and Nycomed Pharma.

6. REFERENCES

Laskey MA, Dibba B, Prentice A. A semi-automated micromethod for the determination of calcium and phosphorus in human milk. Ann Clin Biochem 1991;28:49-54.

Prentice A, Dibba B, Jarjou LMA, Laskey MA, Paul AA. Is breast milk calcium concentration influenced by calcium intake during pregnancy? Lancet 1994; 344: 411-412.

INFLUENCE OF RECENT DIETARY INTAKE ON PLASMA AND HUMAN MILK LEVELS OF CAROTENOIDS AND RETINOL IN BRAZILIAN NURSING WOMEN

Flavia Meneses, Alexandre G. Torres, and Nadia M.F. Trugo

1. INTRODUCTION

Retinol concentration in human milk is considered a better indicator of changes in maternal vitamin A status than serum levels (Rice et al. 2000). Carotenoid distribution pattern and concentrations in human milk vary widely worldwide and may be related to the characteristics of the local diet (Canfield et al. 2002). Although carotenoid concentrations in plasma may be used as biomarkers of dietary intake, correlations for individual carotenoids vary substantially (El-Sohemy et al. 2002). Supplementation of lactating women with single doses of vitamin A and β-carotene, in amounts several times higher than those obtained through daily dietary intake, increases plasma and milk levels of the respective nutrient (Stoltzfus et al. 1993; Canfield et al. 1997). However, the responses of retinol concentration in human milk and of carotenoid concentrations in both maternal plasma and milk to short-term changes in dietary intake have not been evaluated.

The aims of this study were to determine plasma and milk concentrations of retinol and of two classes of carotenoids (xanthophyl: lutein+zeaxanthin; carotene: β-carotene) in Brazilian nursing women; and to investigate the relationship of plasma and milk concentrations of retinol and carotenoids with their recent dietary intakes.

2. METHODS

2.1. Study Group and Sample Collection

Healthy nursing mothers (n=49; 26.6±0.9 years of age) of full-term infants, attending a public day care clinic, participated in the study after informed consent was obtained. Infants were exclusively or predominantly breastfeeding and were at 20 to 120 days

Laboratório de Bioquímica Nutricional e de Alimentos, Instituto de Química, Universidade Federal do Rio de Janeiro, Brazil

Protecting Infants through Human Milk, edited by Pickering *et al.*
Kluwer Academic/Plenum Publishers, 2004

postpartum. Fasting blood samples were obtained and plasma was separated by centrifugation. Milk samples were obtained with manual breast pumps. Total lipid content was determined immediately in milk (Lucas et al. 1978). Both plasma and milk aliquots were stored at –20°C until analyses.

2.2. Dietary Intake

Recent dietary intake was estimated through a 24-hour-recall questionnaire relative to the day before the sample collection. Habitual dietary intake also was assessed using a semiquantitative food frequency questionnaire. Retinol and carotenoid intakes were determined with the database from Mangels et al. (1993) updated with the USDA Nutrient Database for Standard Reference, Release 14.

2.3. Retinol and Carotenoid Analyses

Retinol and carotenoid concentrations in plasma and in milk were determined by reversed-phase HPLC, according to Hess et al. (1991) and Liu et al. (1998), respectively.

2.4. Statistical Analyses

The influence of the recent intake on plasma and milk levels of retinol and carotenoids was assessed by correlation analysis, controlling for habitual intakes, or by comparison (t-test) of groups with recent intakes above or below the mean (retinol) or the median (carotenoids) values. Data on carotenoid intake were log transformed before analyses.

3. RESULTS

Recent dietary intake of nutrients in the study group is shown in Table 1. Plasma and milk concentrations of retinol and carotenoids are shown in Table 2. The mean concentrations of carotenoids in plasma and milk of Brazilian lactating women were lower than the reported values for nursing women from developed countries, but plasma and milk retinol levels were similar (Canfield et al. 1997; Canfield et al. 2002). Plasma levels of lutein+zeaxanthin and β-carotene, evaluated by correlation analysis ($r = 0.39$ and 0.49, respectively) and by comparison of the groups with intakes above or below the median values (Fig. 1), were related to their recent intake.

4. DISCUSSION

Retinol concentration in plasma, as expected, and retinol and carotenoid milk levels, expressed either as μmol/L or nmol/g lipid, were not related to their respective recent dietary intake. Plasma levels of lutein+zeaxanthin and β-carotene may be used as appropriate markers for short-term (24 h) dietary intake in lactating women.

Table 1. Recent dietary intake of vitamin A and carotenoids in the study group[a]

	Dietary intake	Range
Vitamin A (µg RE[b])	1174±253[c]	66–4800
β-Carotene (µg)	2224[d]	0–18900
Lutein+zeaxanthin (µg)	1385[d]	0–9500

[a]n=49
[b]RE=retinol equivalents
[c]Mean±SEM
[d]Median

Table 2. Plasma and milk concentrations of retinol and carotenoids[a,b]

	Plasma, µmol/L	Milk, µmol/L (nmol/g lipid)
Retinol	1.70±0.1	1.4±0.1 (50.0±10.0)
β-Carotene	0.30±0.04	0.018±0.002 (0.6±0.1)
Lutein+zeaxanthin	0.06±0.01	0.006±0.001 (0.2±0.02)

[a]n=49
[b]Data expressed as mean±SEM

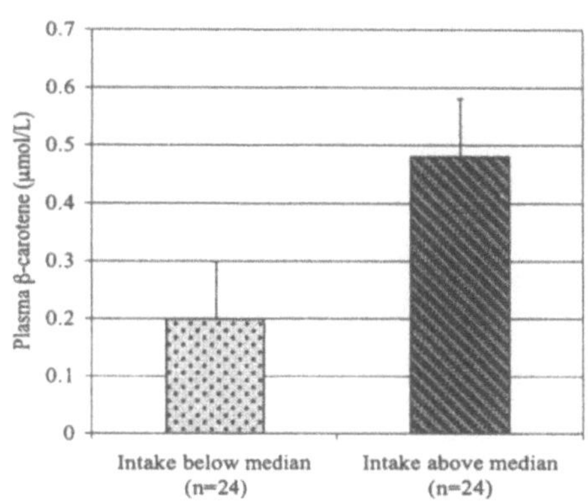

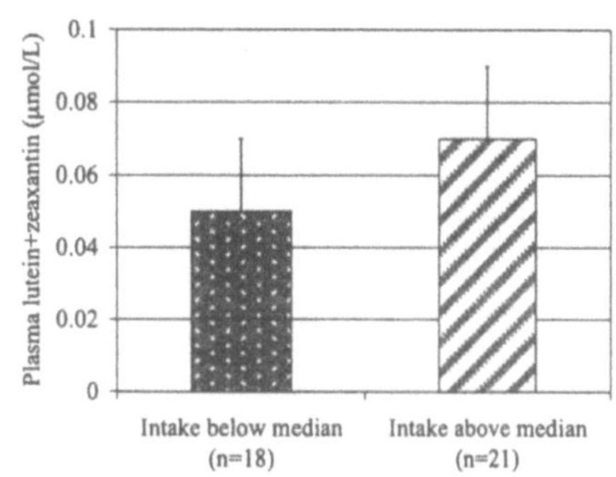

Figure 1. Influence of recent dietary intake on plasma levels of carotenoids (t-test; $P<0.05$)

5. ACKNOWLEDGMENTS

The authors thank CNPq, CAPES, FAPERJ and FUJB (Brazil) for financial support and CNPq for research fellowships.

6. REFERENCES

Canfield LM, Giuliano AR, Neilson EM, Yap HH, Graver EJ, Haiyan AC, Blashill BM. β-Carotene in breast milk and serum is increased after a single β-carotene dose. Am J Clin Nutr 1997;66:52-61.

Canfield LM, Liu M, Goldman WJ, Pramuk K. Major breast milk carotenoids of healthy mothers from nine countries. Adv Exp Med Biol 2002;503:235-236.

El-Sohemy A, Baylin A, Kabagambe E, Ascherio A, Spiegelman D, Campos H. Individual carotenoid concentrations in adipose tissue and plasma as biomarkers of dietary intake. Am J Clin Nutr 2002;76:172-179.

Hess D, Keller HE, Oberlin B, Bonfanti R, Schüep W. Simultaneous determination of retinol, tocopherols, carotenes and lycopene in plasma by means of High-Performance Liquid-Chromatography on reversed phase. Int J Vit Nutr Res 1991;61:232-238.

Liu Y, Xu MJ, Canfield LM. Enzymatic hydrolysis, extraction, and quantitation of retinol and major carotenoids in mature human milk. Nutr Biochem 1998;9:178-183.

Lucas A, Gibbs JAH, Lyster RLJ, Baum JD. Crematocrit: simple clinical technique for estimating fat concentration and energy value of human milk. Br Med J 1978;1:1018-1020.

Mangels SAR, Holden JM, Beecher GR, Forman MR, Lanza E. The carotenoid content of fruits and vegetables: an evaluation of analytical data. J Am Diet Assoc 1993;93:284-296.

Rice AL, Stoltzfus RJ, Francisco A, Kjolhede CL. Evaluation of serum retinol, the modified-relative-dose-response ratio, and breast milk vitamin A indicators of response to postpartum maternal vitamin A supplementation. Am J Clin Nutr 2000;71:799-806.

Stoltzfus RJ, Habicht JP, Rasmussen KM, Hakimi M. Evaluation of indicators for use in vitamin A intervention trials targeted women. Int J Epidemiol 1993;22:1111-1118.

FACTORS INFLUENCING CONCENTRATIONS OF IRON, ZINC, AND COPPER IN HUMAN MILK

Magnus Domellöf[1], Olle Hernell[1], Kathryn G. Dewey[2], Roberta J. Cohen[2], and Bo Lönnerdal[2]

1. INTRODUCTION

The World Health Assembly recommends exclusive breastfeeding of infants until 6 months of age and continued breastfeeding with appropriate complementary feeding until 2 years of age (WHA 2001). Iron deficiency as well as zinc deficiency are public health concerns during infancy, especially in developing countries (Domellöf & Hernell 2002). Copper deficiency, as well as copper toxicity, is a concern in infancy, although precise copper requirements have not been established for this age group (Lönnerdal 1998). Little is known about the mechanisms regulating the concentrations of iron, zinc, and copper in human milk (Lönnerdal 2000).

We previously have presented results from a randomized controlled trial of iron supplementation of >200 breastfed infants in Honduras and Sweden (Domellöf et al. 2001). The aim of the current study was to determine whether there were any associations between milk concentrations of iron, zinc, and copper at 9 months postpartum and maternal iron status or plasma zinc and copper concentrations in this unique group of lactating mothers with a wide range of nutritional status.

2. MATERIALS AND METHODS

This study was conducted at two sites: San Pedro Sula, Honduras and Umeå, Sweden. Inclusion criteria were: a) gestational age ≥37 weeks; b) birth weight >2500 g; c) no chronic illness in the infant; d) maternal age ≥16 years. Infants were exclusively breastfed until 6 months of age and at least partially breastfed until 9 months of age.

Human milk samples were collected at 9 months postpartum and iron, zinc, and copper concentrations were determined by atomic absorption spectrometry. Venous blood samples were obtained from the mothers at 9 months postpartum and were analyzed for hemoglobin (Hb). Plasma was analyzed for ferritin, zinc protoporphyrin (ZPP), soluble

[1]Department of Clinical Sciences, Pediatrics, Umeå University, Sweden
[2]Department of Nutrition, University of California, Davis, CA

Protecting Infants through Human Milk, edited by Pickering *et al.*
Kluwer Academic/Plenum Publishers, 2004

transferrin receptors (TfR), zinc, and copper. Nutrient intake from complementary food and infant weight were measured between 6 and 9 months.

Since distributions of plasma ferritin, ZPP, milk iron, milk zinc, milk copper, and complementary food energy intake were skewed, these variables were log-transformed in all calculations. For presentation, they were transformed back to the original scale and presented as geometric means.

3. RESULTS

Of the 263 mother-infant pairs recruited at 4 months postpartum, 214 remained in the study at 9 months of age. Sufficient human milk and blood samples were obtained from 191 mothers, and were included in the statistical analysis.

Infant complementary food energy intake was lower in Honduras than in Sweden (22 vs. 34 kcal/kg/day, $P<0.001$). There was a significantly higher proportion of Honduran than Swedish mothers with low Hb (12% vs. 0%), low ferritin (32% vs. 12%), and high ZPP (6% vs. 0%), whereas the proportions with high TfR were not significantly different between sites (6% vs. 4%). Honduran mothers had significantly lower mean (±SD) plasma zinc levels than Swedish mothers (0.61±0.09 vs. 0.94±0.11 mg/L, $P<0.001$), whereas mean maternal plasma copper value was similar at the two study sites (1.02±0.23 vs. 1.04±0.18 mg/L, $P=0.52$).

Honduran mothers had significantly lower milk iron concentrations than Swedish mothers (0.21 vs. 0.29 mg/L, $P<0.001$). Controlling for study site and complementary food energy intake, there were no significant correlations between milk iron concentration and any of the indices of maternal iron status: Hb ($r = -0.03$, $P=0.73$), ferritin ($r = -0.06$, $P=0.41$), ZPP ($r = 0.00$, $P=0.99$), and TfR ($r = -0.05$, $P=0.44$). However, there was a positive correlation between milk iron concentration and complementary food energy intake ($r = +0.24$, $P=0.001$), controlling for study site, suggesting that milk iron concentrations increase with weaning.

Honduran mothers had significantly higher human milk zinc concentrations than Swedish mothers (0.70 vs. 0.46 mg/L, $P<0.001$). Controlling for study site and complementary food energy intake, there was no significant correlation between milk zinc concentration and maternal plasma zinc ($r = -0.06$, $P=0.61$). Controlling for study site, milk zinc concentration was negatively correlated with complementary food energy intake ($r = -0.24$, $P=0.001$), suggesting that milk zinc concentrations decrease with weaning.

Honduran mothers had significantly higher milk copper concentrations than Swedish mothers (0.16 vs. 0.12 mg/L, $P=0.001$). In the multivariate analysis including maternal plasma copper, complementary food energy intake, and study site as explanatory variables, there was no significant correlation between milk copper concentration and maternal plasma copper ($r = +0.12$, $P=0.08$) or between milk copper concentration and complementary food energy intake ($r = +0.14$, $P=0.069$).

4. DISCUSSION

Most previous studies have shown no correlation between maternal iron status and milk iron concentration (Murray et al. 1978; Celada et al. 1982). Unlike previous studies, the current study included a larger number of lactating mothers, a wider range of maternal nutritional status and the analysis of TfR, a novel indicator of iron status. Similar to most previous studies, we found no correlation between milk iron and any of the iron status variables (Hb, ferritin, ZPP, and TfR). Our results suggest that the site difference in milk iron concentrations (lower in Honduras) was caused by differences in milk volume (higher in Honduras) rather than by differences in maternal iron status.

Our observation that milk zinc concentrations were more than 50% higher in Honduras than in Sweden was unexpected since Honduran mothers had significantly lower plasma zinc levels. However, the multivariate analysis showed that the site difference in milk zinc concentrations was attributable to differences in milk volume rather than by differences in maternal plasma zinc. It is interesting that prolonged breastfeeding and low complementary food intake in Honduras were associated with higher zinc concentrations in Honduran human milk in spite of lower maternal plasma zinc concentrations. This may be an important factor in the prevention of zinc deficiency among breastfed infants in developing countries. Most previous studies have found no correlation between maternal dietary zinc intake and milk zinc concentration (Lönnerdal 1986; Krebs et al. 1995). However, unlike our study, most of the women in those studies had adequate zinc status.

Previous studies have found no effect of dietary copper on the copper concentration of human milk (Lönnerdal 1986). In our study, we found no correlation between maternal plasma copper and milk copper. The observed site difference in milk copper (higher in Honduras) cannot be explained by the observed positive correlation between complementary food energy intake (lower in Honduras) and milk copper concentration in the Honduran subsample. We conclude that milk copper concentrations are determined by factors other than maternal plasma copper and milk volume.

If the passage of iron, zinc, and copper from plasma to milk in the mammary gland were the result of passive diffusion, positive correlations would be expected between plasma mineral status (concentration) and milk mineral concentration. Since we did not find such correlations, our results suggest a regulated transport of iron, zinc, and copper through the mammary gland epithelium. Recent animal studies are in agreement with such an interpretation (Kelleher & Lönnderal 2001).

We found that high complementary food energy intake (weaning) was associated with low milk zinc and high milk iron, suggesting that these two minerals are affected differently by weaning. This is supported by a previous study by our group in which human milk concentrations of zinc decreased and concentrations of iron increased in late lactation (Dewey et al. 1984). Decreased milk zinc and increased milk iron with increasing complementary food energy intake result in a decreased ratio between the concentrations of zinc and iron in human milk during the process of weaning (Fig. 1). The consequences of this change in ratio, if any, are unknown. Further studies of mammary gland physiology during weaning are needed to explain these observations.

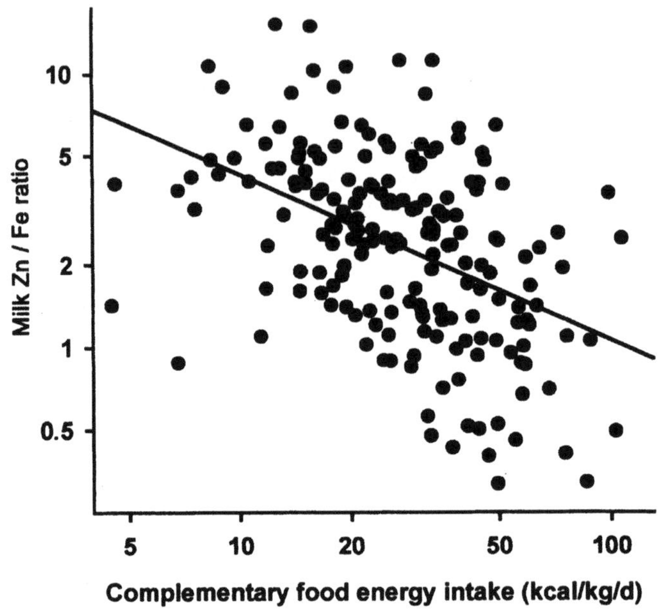

Figure 1. Significant correlation (r = –0.45, P<0.001) between infant complementary food energy intake (inverse proxy for human milk consumption) and the zinc-to-iron concentration ratio in human milk.

5. REFERENCES

Celada A, Busset R, Gutierrez J, Herreros V. No correlation between iron concentration in breast milk and maternal iron stores. Helv Paediatr Acta 1982;37:11-16.

Dewey KG, Finley DA, Lönnerdal B. Breast milk volume and composition during late lactation (7-20 months). J Pediatr Gastroenterol Nutr 1984;3:713-720.

Domellöf M, Hernell O. Iron-deficiency anaemia during the first two years of life. Scand J Nutr 2002;46:20-30.

Domellöf M, Cohen RJ, Dewey KG, Hernell O, Rivera LL, Lönnerdal B. Iron supplementation of breastfed Honduran and Swedish infants from 4 to 9 months of age. J Pediatr 2001;138:679-687.

Kelleher SL, Lönnerdal B. Long-term marginal intakes of zinc and retinol affect retinol homeostasis without compromising circulating levels during lactation in rats. J Nutr 2001;131:3237-3242.

Krebs NF, Reidinger CJ, Hartley S, Robertson AD, Hambidge KM. Zinc supplementation during lactation: effects on maternal status and milk zinc concentrations. Am J Clin Nutr 1995;61:1030-1036.

Lönnerdal B. Effects of maternal dietary intake on human milk composition. J Nutr 1986;116:499-513.

Lönnerdal B. Copper nutrition during infancy and childhood. Am J Clin Nutr 1998;67:1046S-1053S.

Lönnerdal B. Regulation of mineral and trace elements in human milk: exogenous and endogenous factors. Nutr Rev 2000;58:223-229.

Murray MJ, Murray AB, Murray NJ, Murray MB. The effect of iron status of Nigerien mothers on that of their infants at birth and 6 months, and on the concentration of Fe in breast milk. Br J Nutr 1978;39:627-630.

[WHA] World Health Assembly. Infant and young child nutrition. Resolution WHA 54.2; 2001.

POSITIVE EFFECT OF HUMAN MILK ON NEUROBEHAVIORAL AND COGNITIVE DEVELOPMENT OF PREMATURE INFANTS

Arthur I. Eidelman[1] and Ruth Feldman[2]

1. INTRODUCTION

Several large-scale studies have demonstrated that term infants who were breastfed scored higher on IQ tests in childhood, while other studies noted that once sociodemographic and parenting style factors are controlled, the effect of breastfeeding on intelligence is attenuated, suggesting that environmental conditions, not human milk per se, are the decisive factors (Jain et al. 2002). Evidence for the positive effects of human milk on the cognitive development of preterm infants is more conclusive (Horwood et al. 2001).

Mother-infant relationship following premature birth has been described as less optimal when compared with infants born at term. Mothers of preterm infants typically experience higher levels of anxiety and depression that may further impede development of the mother-infant relationship (Feldman et al. 1999). Thus, in addition to its nutritional benefit, milk provision possibly affects the psychobiology of maternal behavior. Prolactin and oxytocin, which are involved directly in the production and the reflex release of human milk, have been implicated in a range of maternal behavior. This oxytocin-mediated system is theorized to function as a feedback loop; mother-infant contact or breast stimulation stimulates oxytocin release, which in turn affects maternal mood and behavior. We thus hypothesized that given such a feedback loop, improvement in one component, i.e., the expression of human milk, would be related to improvements in other components (Matthiesen et al. 2001). Given the above postulated mechanisms it was expected that infants fed increased quantities of human milk would show a more mature neurobehavioral profile in the neonatal period and higher cognitive skills in infancy. In addition, mothers providing more human milk are hypothesized to be less depressed, demonstrate more affectionate touch, and their infants would be more alert during social interactions.

---

[1]Department of Neonatology, Shaare Zedek Medical Center, Hebrew University School of Medicine, Jerusalem, Israel
[2]Department of Psychology, Bar Ilan University, Ramat Gan, Israel

Protecting Infants through Human Milk, edited by Pickering *et al.*
Kluwer Academic/Plenum Publishers, 2004

2. METHODS

Eighty-six premature infants who were born before 33 weeks gestational age with a birth weight of below 1,750 g were studied; mean birth weight of 1,298 g (SD=336; range, 640–1720 g); mean gestational age of 30.5 weeks (SD=3.0; range, 26–33 weeks). Thirty-four infants received a substantial amount of human milk (>75% of nutrition); 21 received intermediate amounts of human milk supplemented by formula (between 25–75% of nutrition); and 31 infants received a minimal amount of human milk (<25% of nutrition). Infants were excluded from the study if they had IVH grades III or IV or suffered from perinatal asphyxia, metabolic, or genetic disease. Table 1 summarizes the clinical characteristics of the study population.

2.1. Procedure and Measures

The exact amount of human milk and formula an infant received was registered after each meal. The number of breastfeeding episodes was less than 5% of all feeding episodes for all infants, even for infants receiving a substantial amount of human milk. The number of breastfeeding episodes was used as a covariate in the analyses. Infant medical risk was measured according to the CRIB score. At 37 weeks of gestation, 10 minutes of mother-infant interaction were videotaped and coded. Coding was conducted using the Mother-Newborn Coding System (Feldman et al. 2002). Maternal depression was assessed with the Beck Depression Inventory (BDI). One to two days prior to discharge infants were tested with the Neonatal Behavioral Assessment Scale (NBAS). Infant cognitive development was assessed, by a psychologist blind to group assignment, with the Bayley Scale of Infant Development at corrected age 6 months.

3. RESULTS

Infants in the three groups spent the same number of days in the hospital and received a comparable number of feedings.

3.1. Mother-Infant Interactions

Infants in the substantial milk group were significantly more alert than infants in the other two groups, but no significant difference was found between the intermediate and minimal groups in infant alertness. No gender-related effects were found.

3.2. Neurobehavioral Maturation

A MANCOVA with the human milk group (substantial, intermediate, minimal) and infant gender as the between-subject factors and the number of breastfeeding episodes as the covariate was computed for the three NBAS clusters (habituation, motor maturity, range of states). Univariate tests (Table 2) revealed significant group differences in motor maturity and range of states but not in habituation. Post hoc comparisons showed a dose-response pattern for motor maturity; infants in the substantial human milk group scored the highest, infants in the intermediate group scored significantly less than infants in the substantial group, and infants in the minimal group showed lower motor maturity when compared with infants in the intermediate group. On the range of states cluster, differ-

Table 1. Family demographic and infant medical variables

	Substantial milk (n=34)		Intermediate milk (n=21)		Minimal milk (n=31)	
	M	SD	M	SD	M	SD
Birth weight (g)	1302.3	320.2	1298.5	309.5	1354.1	388.3
Gestational age (wks)	30.8	2.4	29.9	3.3	31.1	3.5
CRIB (score)	2.3	2.6	2.8	3.6	2.5	3.3
Mother's age (yrs)	28.6	5.4	29.1	6.1	29.9	5.8
Mother's education (yrs)	14.7	2.0	13.6	3.1	14.0	2.0
Father's age (yrs)	30.8	8.1	31.6	5.6	31.9	7.1
Father's education (yrs)	13.9	3.1	13.4	4.1	13.3	4.8
M/F ratio	19/17		12/9		15/17	
Primaparous/multiparous	15/21		9/12		13/19	
Apgar 1 min	7.9	1.9	7.3	2.7	7.9	1.7
Apgar 5 min	8.5	1.5	8.1	1.3	8.6	1.5

Table 2. Differences in mother-infant interaction, neurobehavior, and cognitive development

	Substantial milk (a)		Intermediate milk (b)		Minimal milk (c)		Univariate F
	M	SD	M	SD	M	SD	
Mother-infant interaction							
Maternal affect	16.1	10.6	14.1	11.6	12.6	9.4	1.0
Maternal talk	4.4	4.5	7.2	6.7	9.9	8.5	3.5* (a<b<c)
Maternal touch	21.5	11.8	17.8	9.0	13.1	9.5	3.7* (a>b>c)
Infant alert	9.5	8.0	4.1	3.8	4.2	5.0	4.4** (a>b,c)
Neurobehavioral maturation (NBAS)							
Habituation	6.4	1.0	6.3	1.3	6.4	0.8	0.7
Motor maturity	4.7	0.7	4.5	0.7	4.1	0.6	3.2* (a>b>c)
Range of state	4.0	0.5	3.5	0.7	3.6	0.6	3.4* (a>b,c)
Cognitive development							
MDI	94.2	8.8	91.7	7.2	90.5	8.5	3.3* (a>b,c)
PDI	85.8	11.5	78.6	12.6	78.0	11.4	5.2** (a>b,c)

*P<0.05; **P<0.01; MDI=Mental Development Index; PDI=Psychomotor Development Index

ences were found only between the substantial milk group and the other two groups, and no differences emerged between the intermediate and minimal groups.

3.3. Cognitive Development

A similar MANCOVA with human milk and infant gender as the between subject factors and the number of breastfeeding episodes as the covariate was computed for the two cognitive indices at 6 months of age (MDI, PDI). An overall main effect for the human milk group was found, *Wilks' F* (df=4, 156) = 3.14, P<0.05. Univariate analyses showed group differences on both the MDI and PDI scores (Table 2). Post hoc comparisons indicated that significant differences in mental and psychomotor development were found only between the substantial milk group and the other two groups, with no differences between the minimal and intermediate groups (Fig. 1). No differences were found as related to infant gender.

Maternal depression was related negatively to the amount of human milk (r = –0.31, P>0.01); significant negative correlations also were found between maternal depression and maternal affectionate touch (r = –0.24, P<0.05). Significant negative relations were found between maternal depression and infants' MDI scores at 6 months (r = –0.25, P<0.05), but not with their PDI scores (r = –0.11, P>0.10). Maternal depression was unrelated to neurobehavioral functioning. Maternal touch was related to higher motor maturity (r = 0.27, P<0.05), to increased infant alertness during the interaction (r = 0.36, P<0.01), and to better psychomotor skills at 6 months (r = 0.31, P<0.01). The range of states cluster was related to MDI at 6 months (r = 0.26, P<0.05).

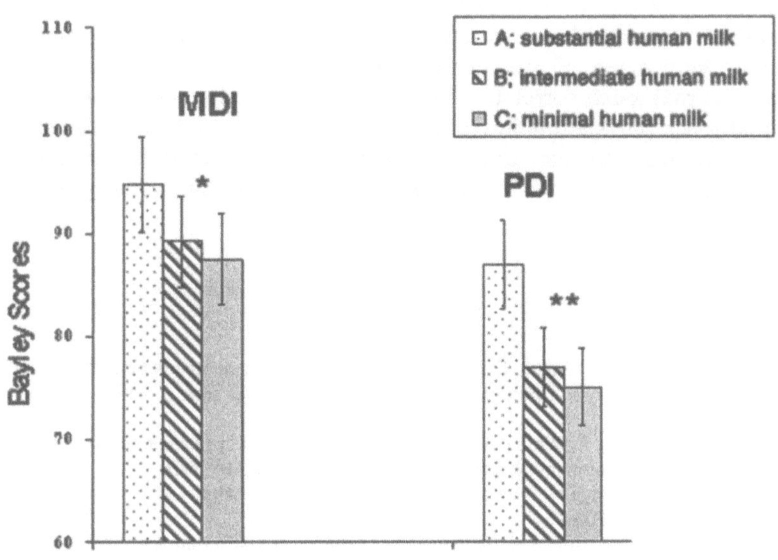

Figure 1. Congnitive indices (MDI and PDI) at 6 months of age show significant differences between group A and the other two groups in the MDI (*P<0.05) and PDI (**P<0.01).

4. DISCUSSION

Results of this study indicate that the amount of human milk ingested in the neonatal period is related to neurological and cognitive development in low-birth-weight premature infants. Infants who received a substantial amount of human milk (>75% of nutrition) showed a more mature neurodevelopmental profile at 37 weeks gestational age and higher mental and psychomotor skills at 6 months corrected age. In addition, human milk was associated with more optimal maternal-infant interactive patterns in terms of increased maternal affectionate touch and greater infant alertness during interactions, and with lower maternal depression. The results indicated that higher cognitive scores were found only for the group receiving a substantial amount of human milk, suggesting that there is a critical amount of human milk that must be supplied to make a lasting impact on the development of high-risk infants. Interestingly, on both the range of states and the MDI, only infants in the substantial milk group showed higher scores, which confirms the need for a critical amount of human milk for more optimal development in this neurodevelopmental process.

Motor maturity was related to the amount of human milk and to frequent maternal touch, pointing to links between motor development, touch, and feeding. Interestingly, both maternal touch and motor maturity showed a dose-response pattern, which may suggest that unlike the range of states and MDI, differential amounts of human milk differently affect the development of both maternal touch patterns and motor-neuro functions in a dose-response effect.

Human milk was related to better maternal mood and interactive behavior. Maternal depression was related to lower quantities of human milk and to longer latencies to the first breastfeeding, findings that may point to the existence of a time-window in the effects of human milk on maternal depression. Maternal depression also was related to reduced maternal touch and lower infant cognitive skills. Finally, the amount of human milk correlated with maternal affectionate touch during interactions. The results also indicate that maternal touch correlated with infants' visual alertness during interactions, suggesting that touch plays a role in the mother-infant earliest social relationship. Future research should delineate the amount, duration, and age of onset of human milk nutrition that is most beneficial for the physical, cognitive, and social-emotional growth of these vulnerable premature infants.

5. REFERENCES

Feldman R, Weller A, Leckman F, Kvint J, Eidelman AI. The nature of the mother's tie to her infant: Maternal bonding under conditions of proximity, separation, and potential loss. J Child Psychol Psychiatr 1999;40:929-940.

Feldman R, Eidelman AI, Sirota L, Weller A. Comparison of skin-to-skin (Kangaroo) and traditional care: Parenting outcomes and preterm infant development. Pediatrics 2002;110:16-26.

Horwood LJ, Darlow BA, Mogridge N. Breast milk feeding and cognitive ability at 7-8 years. Arch Dis Child Fetal Neonatal Ed 2001;84:F23-27.

Jain A, Concato J, Leventhal JM. How good is the evidence linking breastfeeding and intelligence? Pediatrics 2002;109:1044-1053.

Matthiesen AS, Ransjo-Arvidson AB, Nissen E, Uvnas-Moberg K. Postpartum maternal oxytocin release by newborns: effects of infant hand massage and sucking. Birth 2001;28:13-19.

BREASTFEEDING AND COGNITIVE DEVELOPMENT IN CHILDREN

W.H. Oddy[1,2], G.E. Kendall[1,2], E. Blair[1], N.H. de Klerk[1], S. Silburn[1,2], and S. Zubrick[1,2]

1. INTRODUCTION

The question of whether breastfeeding and formula feeding have differential effects on cognitive development has not been comprehensively answered in term infants (Drane & Logemann 2000). This has been due to lack of sample size resulting in inadequate statistical power and failure to obtain prospective data on a wide range of variables including infant feeding, the relevant covariates, and validated tests of cognitive outcomes later in childhood.

The aim of our study was to examine the association between the duration of full breastfeeding and cognitive outcome (verbal IQ and a Performance subtest) measured at 6 and at 8 years of age in a prospective population birth cohort of term infants, taking into account several perinatal, social, and family factors.

2. METHODS

A cohort study of 2,860 children enrolled prior to birth and followed prospectively (Newnham et al. 1993; Oddy et al. 1999) provided data from 2,393 term infants of English-speaking mothers. Of these, complete infant feeding data in the first year of life and verbal cognitive IQ [Peabody Picture Vocabulary Test—PPVT-R] (Dunn & Dunn 1981) were available for 1,450 children at 6 years of age, and a Performance subtest [Perceptual organization WISC- Block Design] (Wechsler 1991) for 1,375 children at 8 years of age. Full breastfeeding was categorized as none, >0 to <4 months, 4 to 6 months, and >6 months. Associations between breastfeeding duration and PPVT-R at 6 years and Block Design at 8 years were estimated before and after adjustment for gender, gestational age, maternal age, maternal education, parental smoking, and the presence of older siblings.

[1]Centre for Child Health Research, University of Western Australia, TVW Telethon Institute for Child Health Research, PO Box 855, West Perth, Western Australia, 6872 Australia
[2]Department of Nutrition, Dietetics and Food Science, Curtin University of Technology, Western Australia, 6845 Australia

2.1. Statistical Analysis

The numeric score for PPVT-R was factored into three levels (0=lowest 5%, 1=5th to 95th percentile, 2=highest 5%). There was a significant association between low PPVT-R and non-English maternal language ($P<0.0005$); therefore, children of non-English-speaking parents (n=100) were excluded from further analyses. Preterm infants also were excluded from statistical analysis due to their small number (<33 weeks, n=51 and 33–36 weeks, n=128). Therefore, our inferences are restricted to term infants with English-speaking parents.

Analyses were conducted using chi-square tests for association, Spearmans correlations, and multiple linear regression. The strength of the association between the cognitive measures and duration of full breastfeeding was indicated by a Linearity test. Adjustment was made in multiple linear regression for factors that were significantly correlated with each outcome independently and breastfeeding.

The ethics committees of King Edward and Princess Margaret Hospitals approved the study protocol. The parent or guardian of each child provided written consent for the child's participation.

3. RESULTS

Of this population, 90% of the children were breastfed at some time, and 28% were fully breastfed for more than six months; solid foods were introduced at or before six months in the great majority of infants (88%). There was propensity for the duration of breastfeeding to be longer in women who were older, better educated, nonsmokers, and who did not have other children ($P<0.0005$). Verbal IQ and the Performance subtest in children were correlated to full breastfeeding duration, gestational age, maternal age, maternal education, and parental smoking.

Table 1 gives the adjusted mean IQ scores for each level of breastfeeding, the F test for linearity from the fitted model, and the corresponding significance test. After adjustment for covariates, there remained a significant association between duration of receipt of human milk and verbal IQ ($F=8.59$, $P=0.003$) with a 3.56 point advantage for children fully breastfed for more than six months compared with children never breastfed. The association of full breastfeeding with the Performance subtest was weakened following adjustment ($F=1.49$, $P=0.223$).

4. DISCUSSION

We have shown a significant dose response relation between duration of full breastfeeding in infancy and verbal IQ as measured at six years. Children breastfed for longer than six months had adjusted mean verbal IQ scores that were 3.56 points higher than the scores for children never breastfed. After adjustment for the interaction terms of breastfeeding and maternal education, the effects of breastfeeding on verbal IQ remained. The associations were greater and more consistent for children whose mothers were in the highest education levels and who breastfed the longest.

There are a number of strengths of the Western Australian Pregnancy Cohort Study. It is a prospective birth cohort study that is representative of the general population. The follow-up of eligible children included 76% at six years and 72% at eight years. Children

Table 1. Mean (SD) standardized verbal and nonverbal IQ scores by duration of full breastfeeding after adjustment for covariates

		Duration of breastfeeding						
Measure	Total group	Never breastfed	Fully breastfed <4 mo	Fully breastfed 4–6 mo	Fully breastfed >6 mo	F test for linearity	P-value	Δ max-min
		(n=117)	(n=495)	(n=378)	(n=412)			
Verbal IQ[a]	106.9 (12.9)	105.2 (13.0)	105.6 (12.7)	107.2 (12.4)	108.7 (13.2)	8.59	0.003	3.56
		(n=79)	(n=348)	(n=272)	(n=299)			
Performance subtest[b]	12.4 (3.2)	12.1 (3.1)	12.3 (3.1)	12.5 (3.2)	12.5 (3.3)	1.49	0.223	0.39

[a]Verbal IQ measured by Peabody Picture Vocabulary Test – Revised at six years adjusted for gestational age, maternal age, maternal education, parental smoking, and older siblings.

[b]Aspect of Performance measured by Wechsler Block Design Test at eight years adjusted for gender, gestational age, maternal education, and parental smoking.

with non-English-speaking mothers were excluded from analysis as were preterm born children (<37 weeks gestation). Breastfeeding was measured prospectively as a continuous variable and the cognitive outcomes were defined operationally.

In prospective studies after adjustment for numerous confounding variables, children who were breastfed performed better on tests of cognition, verbal ability, and school performance. Similar results have been observed in term and preterm infants (Horwood & Fergusson 1998; Horwood et al. 2001; Lucas et al. 1992) and extend beyond adolescence (Lucas et al. 1994). The effects on verbal IQ are in the range of 2–5 points and may be as large as 10 points in low-birth-weight infants (Horwood et al. 2001; Lucas et al. 1992, 1994). The results of our study agree with this and other reports and add to a growing body of evidence for an association between breastfeeding and cognitive development.

Epidemiologic data do not allow certainty of knowledge that human milk exposure does or does not enhance neurodevelopmental outcome (Feldman & Feldman 1996). But Rogan and Gladen (1993) noted that even minor changes in the mean IQ can significantly alter the number of children falling below a cut-off level. The effect of full breastfeeding to at least six months on the verbal IQ score of a population can be conceptualized as shifting the score upward by 3.6 points for term infants as we have shown. If verbal IQ <75 is defined as being problematic, using 12.5 (conservative SD) for SD, predicts that 2.5% of the population would fall below a verbal IQ of 75 (with a mean of the standard 100). If the mean value of the population was increased from 100 to 105 by full breastfeeding for more than six months, only 1.1% would be below 75. Therefore, full breastfeeding for more than six months would be expected to reduce the number of children having a verbal IQ score of <75 by 56%.

The early introduction of milk other than human milk was associated with reduced verbal IQ after adjustment for social and perinatal confounders. Although these effects were interacting with maternal education, they may act through undefined mechanisms in human milk. Our prospective birth cohort study adds to the growing evidence from studies of term infants (Uauy & De Andraca 1995) that full breastfeeding for more than six months (WHO 2001) has beneficial effects on child cognitive development.

5. REFERENCES

Drane DL, Logemann JA. A critical evaluation of the evidence on the association between type of infant feeding and cognitive development. Paediatr Perinat Epidemiol 2000;14:349-356.

Dunn L, Dunn L. PPVT-R. Circle Pines, Minnesota, 55014-1796: American Guidance Service, 1981.

Feldman W, Feldman ME. The intelligence on infant feeding. Lancet 1996;347(9008):1057.

Horwood LJ, Darlow BA, Mogridge N. Breast milk feeding and cognitive ability at 7-8 years. Arch Dis Child 2001;84(Fetal Neonatal Edition):F23-F27.

Horwood LJ, Fergusson DM. Breastfeeding and later cognitive and academic outcomes. Pediatrics 1998;101:E91-E97.

Lucas A, Morley R, Cole TJ, Gore SM. A randomised multicentre study of human milk versus formula and later development in preterm infants. Arch Dis Child 1994;70:F141-F146.

Lucas A, Morley R, Cole TJ, Lister G, Leeson-Payne C. Breast milk and subsequent intelligence quotient in children born preterm. Lancet 1992;339:261-264.

Newnham JP, Evans SF, Michael CA, Stanley FJ, Landau LI. Effects of frequent ultrasound during pregnancy: a randomised controlled trial. Lancet 1993;342:887-891.

Oddy WH, Holt PG, Sly PD, Read AW, Landau LI, Stanley FJ, Kendall GE, Burton PR. Association between breastfeeding and asthma in 6 year old children: findings of a prospective birth cohort study. BMJ 1999;319:815-819.

Rogan WJ, Gladen BC. Breast-feeding and cognitive development. Early Hum Dev 1993;24:S21-S26.

Uauy R, De Andraca I. Human milk and breast feeding for optimal mental development. J Nutr 1995;125(8 Suppl):2278S-2280S.
Wechsler D. Wechsler Intelligence Scale for Children. 3rd Edition. San Antonio: Harcourt Brace; 1991.
[WHO] World Health Organization. The optimal duration of exclusive breastfeeding, Results of a WHO systematic review. Note for the Press 2001;7:(2 April).

BREASTFEEDING PROTECTS AGAINST THE ANORECTIC RESPONSE TO INFECTION IN INFANTS

Possible Role of DHA

M. López-Alarcón[1], P. García-Zuñiga[1], M. Del Prado[1], and C. Garza[2]

1. INTRODUCTION

Lower incidence and attenuated severity of infections are among the benefits of breastfeeding (Lopez-Alarcon et al. 1997). Breastfeeding also seems to protect against the anorexia that presents as a response to infections (Hoyle et al. 1980; Dickin et al. 1990; Lopez-Alarcon et al. 2002), but underlying mechanisms are not well understood. The polyunsaturated fatty acid α-linolenic and its derivatives docosahexaenoic acid (DHA) and eicosapenatenoic acid (EPA) may be involved in such protection because they participate in eicosanoid and cytokine synthesis that occurs during infection (Block et al. 1996; Calder 1997).

2. METHODS

Observational and experimental study designs were used to compare daily energy intakes, serum cytokine values (IL-1β and TNFα) and erythrocyte fatty acids of breast- and formula-fed infants. The observational study included 28 infants who were hospitalized with pneumonia and followed throughout hospitalization, until they were considered free of pneumonia and discharged. Most of them had been breastfed for certain periods of time before switching to formula (FF, n=17) and a small group continued to breastfeed at the time of hospitalization (BF, n=11).

The experimental study measured energy intake in infants immunized with the first dose of the tetravalent vaccine against diphtheria, pertussis, tetanus, and *Haemophilus influenzae* type b (DPTH). Participant infants were hospitalized 24 hours before immunization and followed for 24 hours post-immunization. Infants in the experimental study (age 3.3±0.4 mo) were stratified into three groups: infants who were breastfed from birth until the day of the study and who never received artificial formula (BF, n=6);

[1]Unity of Research in Medical Nutrition, Mexican Institute of Social Security, Av. Cuauhtemoc #330, Col Doctores, Mexico D.F. 06720
[2]Division of Nutritional Sciences, Cornell University, Ithaca, NY

infants who were fed formula since birth and who never received human milk (FF, n=5); and infants who never received human milk and who were fed a DHA-supplemented formula for at least one month before the study (SFF, n=9).

3. RESULTS

3.1. Observational Study

In this study both BF and FF infants decreased their energy intake at hospitalization compared with discharge. Although there was a trend for FF infants to decrease their energy intake more than BF infants, differences did not reach statistical significance (Table 1). At hospitalization compared with discharge, IL-1β increased similarly in both groups. In contrast, increases of TNFα were significantly lower in BF than in FF infants. The proportion of erythrocyte DHA was higher in BF than in FF infants (3.8±0.2 compared with 2.3±0.3, P=0.01).

The duration of lactation was associated positively with DHA concentration (r=0.71, P<0.001), and negatively associated with serum TNFα (r = –0.48, P=0.01) and increase of serum IL-β concentration (r = –0.44, P=0.04). The longer an infant received human milk, the higher the proportion of erythrocyte DHA and the lower the concentrations of IL-1β and TNFα in the acute phase of pneumonia.

Table 1. Main variables evaluated in infants with pneumonia, stratified by feeding mode[a]

Variables	BF, n=11	FF, n=17	P-value
Energy intake[b]	–17±23	–31±22	0.08
IL-1β[c]	112±37	122±6	0.22
TNFα[c]	90±15	120±21	<0.05
DHA[d]	3.9±0.2	2.3±0.3	<0.01

[a]Mean±SEM
[b]Difference between the day of hospitalization and the day of discharge, kcal/kg
[c]Percentage at hospitalization as compared with discharge
[d]Percentage of total content of fatty acids in erythrocytes

3.2. Experimental Study

The decreased energy intake by FF infants was significantly greater than that found in BF infants (–18±4.4% compared with –5±4.2%, P=0.04) following DPTH immunization. Decreases of energy intake in SFF infants (–11±5.2%) were intermediate to those found in BF and FF infants, but no statistical significance was found (Fig. 1).

Serum concentrations of IL-1β (200%, 308%, and 235%, for BF, FF, and SFF, respectively, P=0.47), and TNFα (176%, 131%, and 170%, respectively, P=0.32) increased in all the three groups (Fig. 2). BF and SFF infants tended to present similar

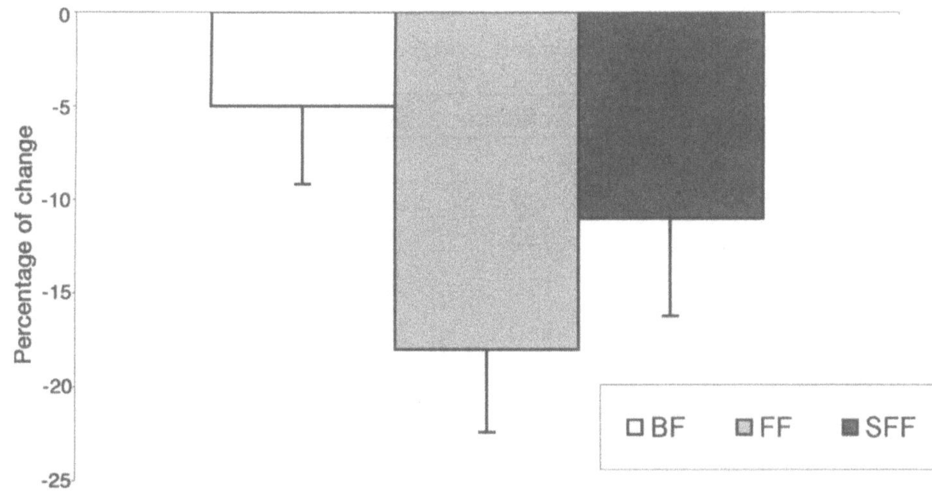

Figure 1. Relative changes of energy intake following DPTH immunization, stratified by feeding mode

changes of both cytokines, but the high variability among subjects did not permit enough power to detect possible differences with FF infants.

Fatty acid profile of SFF infants was similar to that of their BF counterparts. The total percentage of erythrocyte n-3 fatty acids and the proportion of DHA were significantly lower in FF infants than in BF and SFF groups. In a multiple regression model of the effect of cytokines on food intake, introducing feeding mode as a covariate, the decrease of energy intake after immunization was associated with an increase of serum TNFα. This association was present only in FF infants (Table 2).

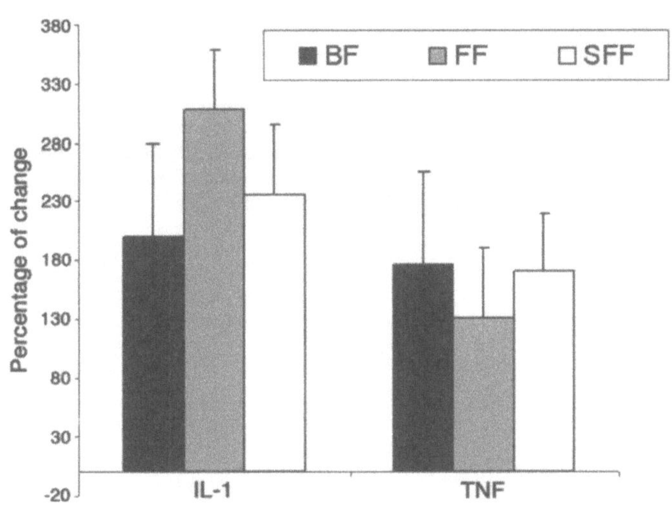

Figure 2. Relative changes of cytokines following DPTH immunization, stratified by feeding mode

Table 2. Variables associated with changes in energy intake following DPTH immunization

Variable	Coefficient	SD	P value	R^2
Changes in energy intake (%)			0.07	0.35
Intercept	7.7	27.2	0.78	
TNFα (pg/mL)	–128.6	65.4	0.06	
IL-1β (pg/mL)	13.7	55.6	0.81	
FF[a]	–86.2	33.6	0.02	
SFF[a]	–26.1	28.4	0.38	

[a]As compared with breastfed infants

4. CONCLUSION

In these models, breastfeeding protected infants against the anorectic response to infection. Such protection seems to be mediated by the amount of DHA infants receive from human milk. However, our results from the experimental model suggest that attenuation of anorexia during infections is explained only partially by differences in dietary DHA.

5. REFERENCES

Blok WL, Katan MB, van der Meer JWM. Modulation of inflammation and cytokine production by dietary (n-3) fatty acids. J Nutr 1996;126:1515-1533.

Calder PC. N-3 polyunsaturated fatty acids and cytokine production in health and disease. Ann Nutr Metab 1997;41:203-234.

Dickin KL, Brown K, Fagbule D, Adedoyani M, Gittelsohn J, Esrey A, Gbolahan AO. Effect of diarrhea on dietary intake by infants and young children in rural villages of Kwara State, Nigeria. Eur J Clin Nutr 1990;44:307-317.

Hoyle B, Yunus M, Chen L.C. Breast feeding and food intake among children with acute diarrhea disease. Am J Clin Nutr 1980;33:2365-2371.

López-Alarcón M, Villalpando S, Fajardo A. Breast-feeding lowers the frequency and duration of acute respiratory diarrhea in infants under six months of age. J Nutr 1997;127:436-443.

López-Alarcón MG, Garza C, Habicht JP, Martínez ML, Pegueros V, Villalpando S. Breastfeeding attenuates reductions in energy intake induced by a mild immunologic stimulus represented by DPTH immunization: possible roles of IL-1β, TNFα and leptin. J Nutr 2002;132:1293-1298.

EFFECT OF HUMAN HIND MILK ON PRETERM INFANT GROWTH

Mariela Bernabe-García[1], Ignacia Cisneros-Silva[2], Eduardo Rangel-Baltazar[1], María Luisa Cuevas-Urióstegui[3], and Samuel Flores-Huerta[4]

1. INTRODUCTION

Premature infants are a vulnerable population due to their high energy requirements and scarce nutritional reserves. Feeding of premature infants is a priority in neonatal nutrition; the goal is for their growth to approach intrauterine rates in order to maximize their development.

Mothers' hind milk has been proposed as a potentially important approach to feeding premature infants, because it contains a higher energy content than intact or "total" human milk (Valentine et al. 1994). Lipids of human milk are the main substrate of energy, but are also the most variable constituent of human milk. Further, hind milk has been defined in different ways, e.g., to extract the fore milk after 2 to 3minutes with an electric pump, or after 5 minutes when extraction is with a manual pump (Valentine et al. 1994; Kirsten & Bradford 1999). Based on our previous research, we systematized the extraction time in order to obtain a useful hind milk, defined by high energy content and high volume; milk obtained following a one-minute extraction had the highest proportion of energy density and volume, although there were no differences observed in hind milk samples in relation to lipids (g/dL) or energy content (kcal/dL) (Table 1).

In this study, we used hind milk to feed premature infants and compared the growth of infants who received either fortified hind milk or fortified total milk.

2. MATERIALS AND METHODS

A prospective, randomized, controlled trial was performed to evaluate weight, length, head circumference, and skin fold (triceps, biceps, suprailiac, subscapular, and suprapatellar) measurement increases in 20 clinically stabilized preterm infants whose

[1]Unidad de Investigación Médica en Nutrición, Hospital de Pediatría, C.M.N. Siglo XXI. Apartado postal C-029, C.S.P.I. "Coahuila". Coahuila N° 5, col. Roma. México, D.F. 06703
[2]Servicio de Prematuros, Hospital de Gineco-obstetricia " Luis Castelazo Ayala"
[3]Unidad de Investigación Médica en Epidemiología Clínica, Hospital de Pediatría, C. M. N. Siglo XXI
[4]División de Salud del Niño y del Adolescente, IMSS

birth weights were less than 1500 g. Infants received either fortified hind or fortified total own mothers' milk for three weeks using S26/SMA HMF (Wyeth Nutritionals, Inc.). Human milk was extracted with an electric pump (Medela, Inc.) at least seven times per day. The study started when the infants had an intake of at least 100 mL/kg/day and were followed until they reached 40 weeks of corrected gestational age.

The milk samples were analyzed for protein by micro-Kjeldahl, lipids by modified-Folch, lactose by the Trinder method, and energy was estimated by factorial estimation (Neville 1995).

The protocol and the informed consent process were approved by the Local and National Ethics and Research Committees of the Instituto Mexicano del Seguro Social, Mexico City. Data were compared using Student t-test or Mann-Whitney-U test, if applicable.

3. RESULTS

The composition of the fortified hind and total human milk samples were similar in energy (60 kcal/dL), lipids (2.6 g/dL), proteins (1.8 g/dL for hind milk and 1.9 g/dL for total milk), and lactose (5.8 g/dL for hind milk and 5.9 g/dL for total milk). There were no statistically significant differences in the characteristics of the preterm infants or their anthropometric measurements (Tables 2 and 3). However, Table 4 shows that the hind milk group had a lower intake of protein and human milk but a higher intake of dextrose solution than the total milk group.

Table 1. Composition of preterm human fore and hind milk

EXTRACTION TIME (minutes)	VOLUME (mL)			LIPIDS (g/dL)			PROTEINS (g/dL)			LACTOSE (g/dL)			ENERGY DENSITY (Kcal/dL)		
	Fore	Hind	Δ	Fore	Hind	Δ	Fore	Hind	Δ	Fore	Hind	Δ	Fore	Hind	Δ
1	10.3	31.0[a]	20.7	5.0	6.9[a]	1.9	1.4	1.5	0.1	5.5	5.1	-0.4	75.9	92.9[a]	17.0
	(5.7)	(21.5)		(1.4)	(2.4)		(1.5)	(0.4)		(0.9)	(1.0)		(12.9)	(22.1)	
2	19.3	17.4	-1.9	4.9	6.5[a]	1.6	1.3	1.4	0.1	6.1	6.0	-0.1	77.3	91.5[a]	14.2
	(12.3)	(13.9)		(1.1)	(1.5)		(0.3)	(0.4)		(1.2)	(0.9)		(12.9)	(13.2)	
3	24.8	19.3	-5.5	5.4	7.1[a]	1.7	1.4	1.3	-0.1	6.1	6.1	0	81.9	97.7[a]	15.8
	(16.0)	(20.2)		(1.8)	(2.1)		(0.7)	(0.3)		(1.0)	(0.9)		(18.4)	(20.0)	
4	33.8	20.1[a]	-13.7	5.6	7.1[a]	1.5	1.3	1.5	0.2	5.8	6.1	0.3	82.1	98.2[a]	16.1
	(16.8)	(19.0)		(2.3)	(2.2)		(0.3)	(0.4)		(0.8)	(1.1)		(23.9)	(22.4)	
5	40.7	18.7[a]	-22.0	5.6	7.7[a]	2.1	1.5	1.5	0	6.1	5.8	-0.3	84.7	102.8[a]	18.1
	(25.4)	(15.8)		(1.8)	(1.9)		(0.5)	(0.5)		(1.0)	(1.0)		(16.9)	(18.4)	

n=15; Mean (SD)

[a]Difference in concentration between hind and fore milk, $P<0.05$ (Paired Student t test or Wilcoxon signed-rank test)

Table 2. Characteristics of the preterm infants

Variable	Hind milk group[a]	Total milk group[a]
Weight[b] (g)	1358 (115.3)	1405 (163.2)
Length[b] (cm)	40.2 (0.87)	39.3 (2.06)
Head circumference[b] (cm)	30.3 (3.55)	29.0 (0.82)
Gestational age[b] (weeks)	31.5[c] (30-32)	31.0[c] (30–32)
Gender (male: female)	5 : 5	4 : 6
Minimal weight (g)	1255.7 (120.8)	1297.1 (194.3)
Age when the study began (days)	7.5 (1.4)	7.0 (1.3)
Weight at the study beginning (g)	1287.2 (123.4)	1324.4 (189.8)

n=10 in each group; [a]Mean (SD); [b]At birth; [c]Median (range)

Table 3. Anthropometric measurements of the preterm infants during intervention and following

Variable	Intervention		Following	
	Hind milk group[a]	Total milk group[a]	Hind milk group[a]	Total milk group[a]
Weight gain				
(g)	532.5[b] (340-582)	566.5[b] (373-801)	856.8 (345.9)	879.9 (248.1)
(g/kg/d)	17.07 (2.440)	18.31 (3.075)	13.34 (3.658)	13.09 (2.524)
Length gain				
(cm)	3.07 (0.490)	3.29 (1.010)	3.74 (1.180)	3.63 (0.916)
(cm/wk)	1.02 (0.163)	1.10 (0.337)	0.83 (0.202)	0.77 (0.121)
Head circumference				
(cm)	3.13 (0.397)	3.14 (0.556)	3.29 (1.188)	3.31 (0.783)
(cm/wk)	1.03 (0.110)	1.05 (0.185)	0.73 (0.153)	0.72 (0.118)
Skin fold sum gain				
(mm)	6.5 (1.414)	7.20 (3.630)	13.56 (9.194)	12.88 (6.175)
(mm/wk)	2.17 (0.471)	2.40 (1.210)	3.05 (1.588)	2.76 (1.249)

n=10 in each group; [a]Mean (SD); [b]Median (range)

Table 4. Intake of calories, protein, and fluids of preterm infants during intervention period

Variable	Hind milk group[a]	Total milk group[a]
Human milk (kcal/kg/d)	73.23 (8.536)	78.48 (8.234)
Dextrose infusion at 5% (kcal/kg/d)	8.57[b] (5.60-8.95)	7.22[b,c] (3.94-7.88)
Total calories: human milk+ dextrose infusion (kcal/kg/d)	81.33 (8.662)	85.47 (8.706)
Protein (g/kg/d)	2.26 (0.135)	2.56[d] (0.241)
Human milk (mL/kg/d)	123.02 (3.580)	129.53[c] (2.561)
Dextrose infusion at 5% (mL/kg/d)	50.39[b] (32.9-52.7)	42.46[b,c] (23.16-46.35)
Total fluids: human milk+ dextrose infusion (mL/kg/d)	172.76[b] (159.4-175.2)	172.64[b] (155.82-173.20)

n=10 in each group; [a]Mean (SD); [b]Median (range); [c]Hind milk group vs. total milk group, $P<0.005$; [d]Hind milk group vs. total milk group, $P<0.05$

4. DISCUSSION

The energy content of the fortified hind milk and fortified total milk obtained by factorial estimation was lower than the energy content of milk from other reports (Gross et al. 1980; Faerk et al. 2001; Reis et al. 2000). It may be that our study underestimated the lipid content, because the sample was taken from cold fortified human milk and the droplets of fat were not sufficiently emulsified. In addition, the yield of hind milk from the mothers was 537.2±71.4 mL/day, and we speculate that one minute of extraction was not sufficient to concentrate the lipids of human milk with high volumes, like the above, which resulted in similar composition of milk samples and cancelled the effect of higher energy density in hind milk.

The growth velocity of infants in both groups was greater than 15 g/kg/day, which has been suggested as the optimal nutritional goal for these infants (Nicholl & Gamsu 1999). Their growth velocity was similar to other reports [gain of: weight 17.6 g/kg/day, length 1.09 cm/week, and head circumference 1.04 cm/week] (Reis et al. 2000), which indicates that infants had an energy intake greater than that reported by the milk analysis.

Consistent with our prior study, during the intervention period premature infants were fed hind milk which was assumed to have had more energy (108 kcal/dL) than total milk (85 kcal/dL); therefore, to reach in theory a total energy intake of 130 kcal/kg/day infants of the hind milk group were fed 123 mL/kg/day while the total milk group had an intake of 130 mL/kg/day to reach 110 kcal/kg/day.

5. CONCLUSION

Because of possible problems with lipid separation, we may not have fed hind milk. The similarities in growth reflect the similar composition of the milk samples studied. A strict protocol is needed to ensure that hind milk is collected, stored, and fed to premature infants.

6. REFERENCES

Faerk J, Skafte L, Petersen S, Peitersen B, Michaelsen KF. Macronutrients in milk from mothers delivering preterm In: Newburg DS, editor. Bioactive Components of Human Milk. New York: Kluwer Academic/Plenum Publishers. Adv Exp Med Biol 2001;501:409-412.

Gross SJ, David RJ, Bauman L, Tomarelli RM. Nutritional composition of milk produced by mothers delivering preterm. J Pediatr 1980;96:641-644.

Kirsten D, Bradford L. Hindmilk feedings. Neonatal Netw 1999;18:68-70.

Neville M. Volume and caloric density of human milk In: Jensen RG, editor. Handbook of Milk Composition. San Diego: Academic Press, 1995; pp 99-113.

Nicholl RM, Gamsu HR. Changes in growth and metabolism in very low birthweight infants fed with fortified breast milk. Acta Paediatr 1999;88:1056-1061.Reis BB, Hall RT, Schanler RJ, Berseth CL, Chan G, Ernst JA, Lemons J, Adamkin D, Baggs G, O'Connor D. Enhanced growth of preterm infants fed a new powdered human milk fortifier: A randomized, controlled trial. Pediatrics 2000;106:581-588.

Valentine CJ, Hurst NM, Schanler RJ. Hindmilk improves weight gain in low-birth-weight infants fed human milk. J Pediatr Gastroenterol Nutr 1994;18:474-477.

IMPACT OF UNFORTIFIED HUMAN MILK FEEDING ON WEIGHT GAIN AND MINERAL STATUS OF VERY-LOW-BIRTH-WEIGHT INFANTS AFTER DISCHARGE FROM A KANGAROO MOTHER CARE UNIT

G. Kirsten, J. van Zyl, C. Kirsten, and E. Thompson

1. INTRODUCTION

Kangaroo mother care (KMC) and human milk feeding have significantly improved the neonatal survival of very- low-birth-weight infants in developing countries (Lincetto et al. 2000). These infants are discharged at low weights (1,800 g) and receiving only human milk, a multivitamin, and iron syrup. There is concern regarding the long-term effects of feeding these infants unfortified human milk. We hypothesized that the low caloric and low phosphorous content of human milk will result in hypophosphatemia and poor weight gain after discharge. The aim of our study was to determine the milk feeding pattern, weight gain, and calcium and phosphorous levels at 6 and 12 weeks corrected age of infants with birth weights <1,600 g who received intermittent KMC and whose mothers actively were encouraged to breastfeed during the hospitalization period.

2. METHODS

2.1. Study Design

This was a prospective, cohort analytical study.

2.2. Enrollment

Eighty healthy low-birth-weight infants (birth weight <1,600 g) from lower socioeconomic backgrounds were recruited upon admission to the KMC Unit at the Tygerberg Hospital. KMC was defined as skin-to-skin contact in a hospital setting between a mother and her low-birth-weight infant with exclusive human milk feeding (Kirsten et al. 2001). Milk intake was documented daily while postdischarge milk intake was obtained through weekly telephone interviews and during follow-up visits. The

Department of Paediatrics, Tygerberg Hospital and the University of Stellenbosch, Cape Town, South Africa

infants were weighed at discharge, and at 6 and 12 weeks corrected age. Blood was obtained for serum calcium, phosphorous, and alkaline phosphatase levels at discharge from hospital and at the 6- and 12-week corrected age follow-up visits. The infants were categorized after discharge as breast- or formula-fed.

3. RESULTS

Seven infants were excluded from the study. Sixty-six (90%) infants attended the follow-up at 12 weeks corrected age. Ninety percent of the infants were breastfed on discharge from the hospital, of which 75% were breastfed exclusively. There was a significant decrease in the percentage of exclusive breastfeeding after discharge from the hospital. Only 12 (18%) and 8 (12%), respectively, of the infants continued to be breastfed exclusively at 6 and 12 weeks corrected age.

3.1. Measurements

The mean phosphorous level (1.86 mmol/L) at 12 weeks corrected age and the mean daily weight gain between 6 and 12 weeks corrected age (20.9 g) of the breastfed infants were significantly lower compared with the formula-fed infants (phosphorous 2.06 mmol/L, P=0.02; weight gain 24.1 g, P=0.04). There were no significant differences in the mean calcium level (2.4 mmol/L, P=0.79) and the mean alkaline phosphatase levels (336 U/L, P=0.18) of the exclusively breast- and formula-fed infants (calcium 2.25 mmol/L; alkaline phosphatase 290 U/L) at 12 weeks corrected age.

4. CONCLUSION

Although some human milk feeding still occurred in 49% of the infants at 12 weeks corrected age, exclusive breastfeeding had decreased progressively from 75% to 12% after discharge from hospital. This could partly be due to the fact that none of the mothers in the study were actively encouraged to breastfeed after discharge.

Very-low-birth-weight infants have limited calcium and phosphorous stores (James et al. 1986). The lower phosphorous levels and inadequate weight gain of the breastfed infants at follow-up confirms the need for a human milk fortifier for very-low-birth-weight infants who receive KMC and are breastfed, especially where the mother continues to breastfeed after discharge from hospital. Lack of caloric and mineral supplementation could lead to hypophosphatemia and even rickets. Fortification should not be done in such a way that formula feeding is encouraged, as this is both undesirable and unaffordable for infants from lower socioeconomic backgrounds.

Of particular concern is the fact that very-low-birth-weight infants receiving KMC are discharged at progressively lower weights. Many of them are breastfed exclusively, and the mothers should be encouraged to continue breastfeeding. Their weight gain should, however, be monitored closely after discharge. Unfortunately, facilities for monitoring calcium and phosphorous levels are often lacking.

5. REFERENCES

James JR, Congdon PJ, Truscott J, Horsman A, Arthur R. Osteopenia of prematurity. Arch Dis Child 1986;61:871-876.

Kirsten GF, Bergman NJ, Hann FM. Kangaroo mother care in the nursery. Pediatr Clin North Am 2001;48:443-452.

Lincetto O, Nazir AI, Cattaneo A. Kangaroo mother care with limited resources. J Trop Pediatr 2000;46:293-295.

IS DURATION OF BREASTFEEDING INFLUENCING THE RISK OF OBESITY IN ADULT MALES?

L. Schack-Nielsen[1], K.F. Michaelsen[1], E.L. Mortensen[2], T.I.A. Sørensen[3], and J.M. Reinisch[4]

1. INTRODUCTION

Several large population studies have suggested that breastfeeding protects against obesity in childhood (Armstrong & Reilly 2002; Liese et al. 2001), but it is unknown if this effect persists into adulthood.

2. METHODS

The effect of breastfeeding on obesity was examined in The Copenhagen Perinatal Cohort (n=9125 individuals born in 1959-61). Information on breastfeeding was collected at the age of 1 year. For 2601 males, information was available on duration of breastfeeding, weight, and length at 12 months of age and as a young adult (mean 18.8 years, SD 1.3 years). Duration of breastfeeding was classified as ≤1 month (n=857), 2–3 months (n=833), 4–7 months (n=602), and >7 months (n=309). The effects of potential confounders, including parental social status and education, birth size, and maternal height and weight, were controlled for in statistical analyses.

3. RESULTS

Duration of breastfeeding had a highly significant dose-response effect on body mass index (BMI) at 12 months of age; infants breastfed for a longer period were leaner (BMI 15.0, 14.9, 14.6, and 14.4 in the four breastfeeding groups, respectively; P=0.009) (Fig. 1). There was no effect of breastfeeding on mean BMI or on the risk of overweight or obesity in childhood or young adulthood (Fig. 1 and Table 1).

[1]Department of Human Nutrition, The Royal Veterinary and Agricultural University, Copenhagen, Denmark
[2]Department of Health Psychology, Institute of Public Health, University of Copenhagen
[3]Danish Epidemiology Science Center, Institute of Preventive Medicine, Copenhagen University Hospital
[4]The Kinsey Institute for Research in Sex, Gender and Reproduction, Indiana University, USA

Table 1. Odds ratios (95% confidence interval) for the risk of being overweight or obese in the four breastfeeding groups

		BMI (kg/m^2)	n (%)	BF ≤1 mo	BF 2–3 mo	BF 4–7 mo	BF >7mo	P
7 Year	Overweight[a]	>17.9	30 (4)	1.0	1.3 (0.5-3.5)	0.7 (0.2-2.3)	2.4 (0.8-7.9)	0.26
13 Year	Overweight[a]	>21.9	50 (5)	1.0	0.8 (0.4-1.7)	0.4 (0.1-1.0)	1.3 (0.5-3.0)	0.12
Adulthood	Overweight	>25	263 (10.1)	1.0	1.2 (0.9-1.6)	0.8 (0.5-1.1)	1.2 (0.8-1.8)	0.10
Adulthood	Obesity	>30	39 (1.5)	1.0	1.2 (0.6-2.7)	1.0 (0.4-2.6)	0.8 (0.2-3.0)	0.92

[a]Cut-off values for overweight and obesity were defined according to Cole et al. (2000). In this study, at both the age of 7 and 13 years, only one boy (0.1%) was obese, thus odds ratios were not calculated for obesity at those ages.
BMI=body mass index; BF=breastfed

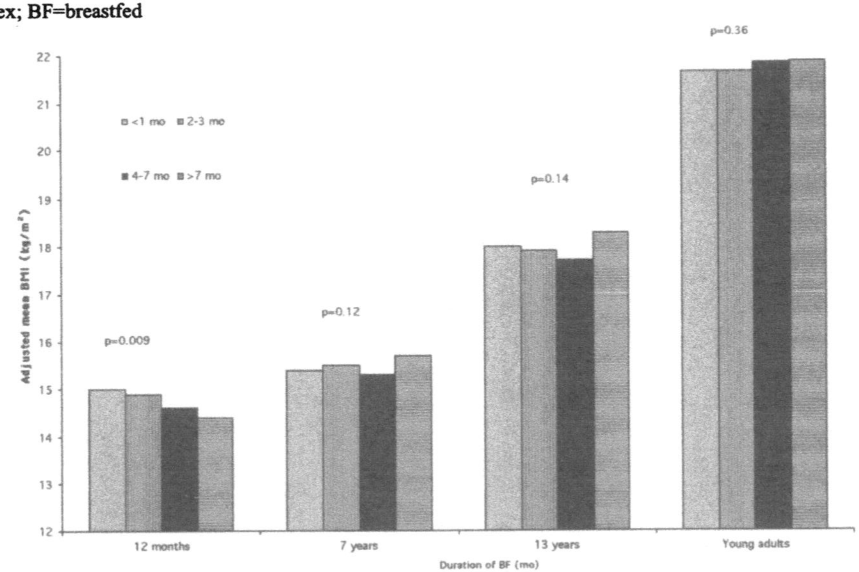

Figure 1. Mean body mass index in the four breastfed groups. Adjusted for potential confounders (see text)

4. CONCLUSION

Our data suggest that the protective effect of BF on being overweight and on obesity in early childhood does not persist into young adulthood in men.

5. REFERENCES

Armstrong J, Reilly JJ. Breastfeeding and lowering the risk of childhood obesity. Lancet 2002;359:2003-2004.

Cole TJ, Bellizzi MC, Flegal KM, Dietz WH. Establishing a standard definition for child overweight and obesity worldwide: international survey. BMJ 2000;320:1240-1243.

Liese AD, Hirsch T, von Mutius E, Keil U, Leupold W, Weiland SK. Inverse association of overweight and breast feeding in 9 to 10-y-old children in Germany. Int J Obes Relat Metab Disord 2001;25:1644-1650.

BREASTFEEDING, BODY MASS INDEX, AND ASTHMA AND ATOPY IN CHILDREN

W.H. Oddy[1,2], J.L. Sherriff[1], N.H. de Klerk[2], and G.E. Kendall[2]

1. INTRODUCTION

Asthma is the leading cause of hospitalization in Australian children and its prevalence is increasing worldwide (Peat & Li 1999). In developed nations the increase in prevalence of childhood asthma has been paralleled by an increase in childhood obesity (WHO 1998). There has been considerable debate as to whether formula-feeding is a risk factor for childhood obesity (von Kries et al. 2001). Furthermore, investigators have speculated that obesity may be a causal factor in the inception of childhood asthma and a number of studies have shown positive associations between body mass index (BMI=weight/(kg)/(m)^2) or obesity with asthma (von Mutius et al. 2001). Breastfeeding has been shown to protect against overweight and obesity (von Kries et al. 1999; Hediger et al. 2001) as well as asthma in childhood (Oddy et al. 1999), although the relationship between breastfeeding and childhood asthma remains speculative (Wright et al. 2001).

The aim of this study was to investigate whether the relationship of breastfeeding to asthma was influenced by BMI. The objectives were to determine the interrelationships between: a) breastfeeding and BMI; b) BMI with asthma and atopy; and c) breastfeeding with asthma and atopy after adjustment for BMI.

2. METHODS

The Western Australian Pregnancy Cohort Study cohort subjects were recruited serially from a public antenatal clinic or nearby private practice in Perth, Western Australia between 1989 and 1992 (Newnham et al. 1993). A total of 2,979 women were enrolled at 18 weeks gestation. Following loss to follow-up, 2,602 (91%) children remained available for study at six years.

At the time of enrollment, data were collected from parents about their general health and socioeconomic situation. Parents completed questionnaires following the first,

[1]Department of Nutrition, Dietetics and Food Science, Curtin University of Technology, Western Australia, 6845 Australia
[2]Centre for Child Health Research, University of Western Australia, TVW Telethon Institute for Child Health Research, PO Box 855, West Perth, Western Australia, 6872 Australia

Protecting Infants through Human Milk, edited by Pickering *et al.*
Kluwer Academic/Plenum Publishers, 2004

second, third, and sixth years of life. The sixth year assessment included a questionnaire and examination for clinical measures of asthma and atopy. An eight-year follow-up included measurement of maternal BMI, but not atopy.

Breastfeeding information was collected throughout the first year and on the first-, second-, and third-year questionnaires. Duration of any breastfeeding was defined as the age breastfeeding stopped and was expressed as a continuous variable (in months). Duration of exclusive breastfeeding was defined as the age that other milk was introduced and was expressed as a binary variable (exclusively breastfed for <4 months compared with exclusively breastfed ≥4 months).

The potential confounders for BMI were gender, gestational age, birth weight, smoking in pregnancy, breastfeeding, maternal education, maternal age at birth, and maternal BMI. The final model for BMI included gender, birth weight, smoking in pregnancy, breastfeeding per month, and maternal BMI. The confounders for current asthma were gender, gestational age, concurrent parental smoking, early infections, and maternal asthma status.

Current asthma was defined as asthma diagnosed by a physician ever *and* wheeze in the last year. Atopy was assessed by skin prick testing to four common environmental aeroallergens when the children attended the six-year clinical assessment. Analyses that included atopy were restricted to 1,595 children with skin tests. Height and weight measurements of all children were taken at 6 years of age and BMI [weight (kg) / height $(m)^2$] was calculated. Linear and logistic regression analyses were used with a series of categorical or continuous explanatory covariates.

2.1. Propensity Score

As a way of examining whether breastfeeding acts through BMI in an association with asthma and atopy or, conversely, whether BMI is associated with asthma or atopy only because of its common association with other factors, we created a propensity score. The propensity score was defined as the conditional exposure probability e(x) given a set of covariates (x) (Rosenbaum & Rubin 1983) for each individual and was based on the predicted value of the regression coefficients for these variables and BMI at 6 years of age (Drake & Fisher 1995). The score was used to adjust for the identified risk factors for BMI, thereby removing the adjusted effects of BMI from the final estimations. Informed consent was obtained for follow-up of the children from birth.

3. RESULTS

In a linear regression model, any breastfeeding (per additional month of feeding) was associated with decreased BMI in children (Coeff –0.013 95% CI –0.024, –0.001; P=0.030). The association was weakened following adjustment for gender, birth weight, maternal smoking during pregnancy, and concurrent maternal BMI (Coeff –0.012 95% CI –0.025, 0.002; P=0.083). The propensity score for BMI was generated from the adjusted data (Table 1).

The interaction between BMI and gender and its effect on asthma was not significant at either age; therefore, combined analyses were done. The odds ratio of current asthma, atopy, and BMI within unadjusted and adjusted analyses are shown in Table 2. All models were significant with the higher the BMI the greater the risk for current asthma (OR 1.12; 95% CI 1.06, 1.19; P<0.0001). The association of BMI with asthma was not

Table 1. Risk factors for BMI in six-year-old children

	Unstandardized coefficients for BMI at 6 years	Standard error	P-value	Confidence limits
Gender	.040	.095	.676	–.147, .227
Birth weight	.001	.000	<.0005	.000, .001
Smoking in pregnancy	.387	.103	<.0005	.186, .589
Breastfeeding per month	–.012	.007	.083	–.025, .002
Maternal BMI	.0075	.008	<.0005	.058, .091

Table 2. Odds ratios of current asthma and atopy, unadjusted and adjusted for known risk factors

	Current asthma, n=2,161		Atopy, n=1,595	
	Unadjusted β 95% CI P-value	Adjusted[a] β 95% CI P-value	Unadjusted β 95% CI P-value	Adjusted[a] β 95% CI P-value
Body mass index (per unit increase)	1.12 1.06, 1.19 <.0005	1.16 1.08, 1.25 <.0005	1.02 0.97, 1.08 .444	1.07 1.00, 1.15 .055
Exclusive breastfeeding <4 mo: ≥4 mo	1.29 1.02, 1.63 .032	1.40 1.03, 1.90 .033	1.22 0.99, 1.50 .061	1.43 1.11, 1.84 .005

[a]Adjusted for all other variables in the model (gender: male:female, gestational age: <37 weeks: ≥ 37 weeks, parental smoking: yes: no, childcare in the first 3 months of life: yes: no, maternal asthma yes: no) in addition to the propensity score for concurrent BMI (created from predicted values for BMI risk factors at six years—gender, birth weight, smoking in pregnancy, breastfeeding per month, maternal BMI)

altered by adjustment for other covariates or the propensity score (OR 1.16 95% CI 1.08, 1.25; P<0.0005). The association of BMI with atopy was bordering on significance following adjustment (P=0.055).

Following adjustment, the odds of current asthma at 6 years of age among children exclusively breastfed for less than four months compared with children exclusively breastfed for four months or more was significantly increased (OR 1.40; 95% CI 1.03, 1.90; P=0.033) as was atopy (OR 1.43; 95% CI 1.11, 1.84; P=0.005) (Table 2). Of the adjusted covariates for asthma, BMI, breastfeeding, gender, and maternal asthma were the only significant risk factors remaining. Of the adjusted covariates for atopy, BMI, breastfeeding, and gender were the significant remaining factors.

4. DISCUSSION

Our data provide robust evidence for an association between breastfeeding, BMI, and early childhood asthma. After taking account of BMI and its associated risk factors, a protective effect of exclusive breastfeeding against early asthma and atopy was evident. An increased BMI was a risk factor for childhood asthma and atopy. These findings suggest that public health interventions to optimize breastfeeding duration and reduce overweight and obesity in children may help to attenuate the community burden of wheezing illness early in life.

5. REFERENCES

Drake C, Fisher L. Prognostic models and the propensity score. Int J Epidemiol 1995;24:183-187.

Hediger ML, Overpeck MD, Kuczmarski RJ, Ruan WJ. Association between infant breastfeeding and overweight in young children. JAMA 2001;285:2453-2460.

Newnham JP, Evans SF, Michael CA, Stanley FJ, Landau LI. Effects of frequent ultrasound during pregnancy: a randomised controlled trial. Lancet 1993;342:887-891.

Oddy WH, Holt PG, Sly PD, Read AW, Landau LI, Stanley FJ, Kendall GE, Burton PR. Association between breastfeeding and asthma in 6 year old children: findings of a prospective birth cohort study. BMJ 1999;319:815-819.

Peat JK, Li J. Reversing the trend: reducing the prevalence of asthma. J Allergy Clin Immun 1999;103:1-10.

Rosenbaum PR, Rubin DB. The central role of the propensity score in observational studies for causal effects. Biometrika 1983;70:41-55.

von Kries R, Koletzko B, Sauerwald T, von Mutius E, Barnert D, Grunert V, von Vos H. Breastfeeding and obesity: cross sectional study. BMJ 1999;319:147-150.

von Kries R, Hermann M, Grunert VP, von Mutius E. Is obesity a risk factor for childhood asthma? Allergy 2001;56:318-322.

von Mutius E, Schwartz J, Neas LM, Dockery D, Weiss ST. Relation of body mass index to asthma and atopy in children: the National Health and Nutrition Examination Study III. Thorax 2001;56:835-838.

[WHO] World Health Organization. Obesity: preventing and managing the global epidemic. Geneva: World Health Organization; 1998.

Wright AL, Holberg CJ, Taussig LM, Martinez FD. Factors influencing the relation of infant feeding to asthma and recurrent wheeze in childhood. Thorax 2001;56:192-197.

ARTERIAL COMPLIANCE IN 10-YEAR-OLD CHILDREN IN RELATION TO BREASTFEEDING

L. Schack-Nielsen[1], C. Mølgaard[1], D. Larsen[1], C. Martyn[2], and K.F. Michaelsen[1]

1. INTRODUCTION

Reduced growth in early life increases the risk of cardiovascular disease (CVD) in later life, but studies of the consequences of early diet, especially breastfeeding and. formula feeding, on CVD or CVD risk factors have been conflicting (Owen et al. 2002, 2003; Leeson et al. 2001).

2. METHODS

A cohort, which included 93 children (44 boys), was followed during infancy and re-examined at 10 years of age. Duration of any breastfeeding was recorded at 9 months of age. Arterial compliance was measured as pulse wave velocity in the aorta-femoral and in the aorta-radial arterial segment by a noninvasive optical method. High pulse wave velocity indicates a stiffer arterial wall. Blood pressure was measured using automated methods. The effect of breastfeeding on pulse wave velocity was estimated in multiple regression analyses, all of which were adjusted for blood pressure, gender, height, and weight.

3. RESULTS

Basic characteristics of the 93 children studied are shown in Table 1. Duration of breastfeeding in months was associated positively with pulse wave velocity, but this association was significant only in the aorta-femoral arterial segment (regression coefficients (95% CI) 1.9 (0.2; 3.6) and 1.3 (–1.3; 3.9) cm/sec in the aorta-femoral and aorta-radial arterial segments, respectively). Further adjustments for lipid profile (triglyceride, low density lipoprotein- and high density lipoprotein-C), insulin resistance, current life style factors (physical activity, fat and energy intake), and birth weight did

[1]Department of Human Nutrition, The Royal Veterinary and Agricultural University, Copenhagen, Denmark
[2]MRC Environmental Epidemiology Unit, Southampton General Hospital, England

Protecting Infants through Human Milk, edited by Pickering *et al.*
Kluwer Academic/Plenum Publishers, 2004

Table 1. Basic characteristics of the study cohort at 10 years of age, shown as mean±SD, and breastfeeding duration as median (range)[a]

Height (cm)	Weight (kg)	BMI (kg/m^2)	PWV, AF (cm/sec)	PWV, AR (cm/sec)	SBP (mm Hg)	DBP (mm Hg)	PA (hours/day)	Diet (FE%)	BF (mo)
142.3±5.5	34.5±4.9	17.0±1.9	385±43	262±27	109±7	61±5	4.6±1.2	35.5±4.0	6 (0–9)

[a]BMI=body mass index, PWV=pulse wave velocity, AF=aorta-femoral, AR=aorta-radial, SBP=systolic blood pressure, DBP=diastolic blood pressure, PA=physical activity, FE%= fat energy percent, BF=breastfeeding (median duration)

Table 2. Coefficients from multiple regression models with pulse wave velocity (cm/sec) in the aorta-radial or aorta-femoral segment as dependent variable.

	AR-segment, β±SE (95% CI)	AF-segment, β±SE (95% CI)
Current systolic BP (mm Hg)	1.2±0.7 (0.1; 2.6)	0.7±0.5 (–0.2; 1.6)
Current diastolic BP (mm Hg)	2.3±1.2 (–0.2; 4.7)	1.0±0.8 (–0.7; 2.6)
Current fat intake (FE%)	2.7±1.1 (0.6; 4.9)	1.6±0.7 (0.2; 3.1)
Current physical activity (hours/day)	–7.9±2.2 (–12.3; –3.4)	–4.0±1.5 (–7.0; –1.0)
Duration of BF (mo)	1.6±1.2 (–0.9; 4.0)	2.0±0.8 (0.3; 3.7)

not change these estimates. In models including breastfeeding, current fat intake (fat energy percent) was positively (1.6 (0.2; 3.1) and 2.7 (0.6; 4.9) and physical activity (hours/day) negatively associated with pulse wave velocity (–4.0 (–7.0; –1.0) and –7.9 (–12.3; –3.4) cm/sec in the aorta-femoral and aorta-radial arterial segments, respectively) (Table 2).

4. CONCLUSION

Our results tend to support an earlier study of young adults showing that breastfeeding was associated with increased arterial stiffness (Leeson et al. 2001). This finding could be due to the higher cholesterol level during infancy observed in breastfed infants. However, the long-term consequences of breastfeeding on the risk of CVD and the predictive value of arterial compliance in relation to CVD is unknown, wherefore this finding should not be used to advocate against breastfeeding.

5. ACKNOWLEDGMENT

Financial support for this research was provided by the Danish Heart Foundation.

6. REFERENCES

Owen CG, Whincup PH, Odoki K, Gilg JA, Cook DG. Infant feeding and blood cholesterol: a study in adolescents and a systematic review. Pediatrics 2002;110:597-608.

Owen CG, Whincup PH, Gilg JA, Cook DG. Effect of breast feeding in infancy on blood pressure in later life: systematic review and meta-analysis. BMJ 2003;327:1189-1195.

Leeson CP, Kattenhorn M, Deanfield JE, Lucas A. Duration of breast feeding and arterial distensibility in early adult life: population based study. BMJ 2001;322:643-647.

DURATION OF EXCLUSIVE BREASTFEEDING AND RISK OF ANEMIA IN A COHORT OF MEXICAN INFANTS

Jareen K. Meinzen-Derr[1], M. Lourdes Guerrero[2], Mekibib Altaye[1], Guillermo M. Ruiz-Palacios[2], and Ardythe L. Morrow[1]

1. INTRODUCTION

Iron deficiency is the most common nutrient deficiency associated with anemia in childhood (CDC 1998), affecting more than half of infants in developing countries (WHO 2001). Bioavailability of iron in human milk is high, yielding about 50% absorption (Dallman 1988; Oski 1993; Saarinen et al. 1977; Krebs 2001). Iron available for absorption is at its highest in early transitional milk and steadily decreases over the course of lactation (Siimes et al. 1979). By six months, complementary foods are needed to provide the nutrients necessary for infant development (Picciano 2001; Dewey 2001). It is not known if a critical period of vulnerability towards iron deficiency exists in infants.

Varying degrees of anemia in young children have been associated with poor cognitive outcomes (Lozoff et al. 1991, 1996; Walter 1989; Walter et al. 1989; de Andraca et al. 1997). Anemia diagnosed at 9 months of age is associated with significantly lower achievement scores in second grade children compared with children who were not anemic at 9 months of age (Palti et al. 1985). Low concentrations of hemoglobin in 8-month-old children have been associated with impaired motor development at 18 months of age (Sherriff et al. 2001).

The World Health Organization has recommended exclusive breastfeeding to 6 months of age (2001) to prevent the major burden of morbidity and mortality due to infectious diseases in this age group. However, there is concern that longer duration of exclusive breastfeeding might increase the risk of infant anemia in populations in which iron deficiency is highly prevalent. Since 1998, we have conducted a cohort study of breastfeeding mother-infant pairs in Mexico City to examine bioactive factors in human milk that protect against diarrheal disease in infants. Following the protocol of our previous community-based efficacy trial of breastfeeding support (Morrow et al. 1999), we have provided peer counseling to all study mothers in this cohort with the goal of

[1]Cincinnati Children's Hospital Medical Center, 3333 Burnet Avenue, Cincinnati, OH 45229-3039
[2]Instituto Nacional de Ciencias Médicas y Nutrición, México City, México

Protecting Infants through Human Milk, edited by Pickering *et al.*
Kluwer Academic/Plenum Publishers, 2004

achieving WHO recommendations for exclusive breastfeeding. During the course of this project, the study physicians expressed concern about infant anemia. This study was undertaken to examine the association between the duration of exclusive breastfeeding and anemia in infants at 9 months of age in our cohort of Mexican children.

2. METHODS

From March 1998 to March 2003, 306 infants in San Pedro Martir, Mexico City, were monitored from birth to 2 years of age as part of an ongoing NIH-funded study on human milk. All were healthy, full-term infants whose mothers agreed to breastfeed. Mothers received home-based peer counseling to support exclusive breastfeeding and were visited in their homes weekly by a trained study worker. At all weekly visits, the diet of each infant for the previous 24 hours was recorded. Infant weight and length were recorded every three months.

Nurses collected a blood sample every three months from the infants, and hemoglobin values were determined at each occasion. Blood was drawn on the mothers at baseline, and hemoglobin values were measured. Hemoglobin concentration was measured using the HemoCue hemoglobin photometer. Due to the high altitude of Mexico City, anemia was defined as hemoglobin levels of <10 g/dL. All infants and mothers with low hemoglobin levels (<10 g/dL and <12.5g/dL, respectively) were referred for treatment. The duration of exclusive breastfeeding was defined as the number of days an infant was breastfed exclusively, receiving only human milk without any other fluid or supplementation. Exclusive breastfeeding was categorized as <4 months (<120 days), 4 to 6 months (120–179 days), and >6 months (179–218 days).

Statistical analyses were conducted using SAS® for Windows (version 8.2). Crude associations between anemia status and exclusive breastfeeding and confounding variables were tested using the two-sample t-test, Wilcoxon sum ranks test, and the Pearson's chi-square. Logistic regression was used to model the relation between anemia outcome and exclusive breastfeeding status while adjusting for possible confounders and other risk factors.

The study was approved by the institutional review boards of the Instituto Nacional de Ciencas Médicas y Nutrición and Cincinnati Children's Hospital Medical Center.

3. RESULTS

Data on hemoglobin levels at 9 months of age were available on 185 children, of whom 2 children did not initiate breastfeeding and were therefore removed from analysis. Among the 183 study infants at 9 months of age, the mean hemoglobin was 11.4 g/dL; 23 (11%) had a hemoglobin concentration <10 g/dL and were classified as anemic; none had a hemoglobin concentration <8 g/dL. No infant had a hemoglobin concentration <10 g/dL at birth.

There were no significant differences between the anemic and non-anemic infants with regard to birth weight, maternal age, maternal education, and duration of any breastfeeding. Compared with infants who were not anemic, infants who were anemic at 9 months tended to be male (68% anemic vs. 45% non-anemic), have a longer median duration of exclusive breastfeeding (18 weeks vs. 12 weeks), and to be previously anemic

Table 1. Multivariate logistic regression analysis of anemia at 9 months of age[a]

Risk factor	Odds ratio	95% Confidence interval
EBF ≥6 months[b]	12.2	2.4, 62.1
EBF 4–6 months	1.1	0.4, 3.3
EBF 0–4 months	1.0 (REF)[c]	
Previously anemic at 3 or 6 months	5.4	1.7, 17.6
Weight gain from birth to 9 months ≥4.9 kg (median)	2.9	0.997, 8.4

[a]Birth weight, gender, and maternal anemic status not significant in the model
[b]EBF=Exclusive breastfeeding
[c]REF=Reference

at either 3 or 6 months of age (18% vs. 4%). Eleven (9%) infants who were breastfed exclusively for <4 months were anemic; 7 (12%) infants exclusively breastfed for 4 to 6 months were anemic, and 5 (63%) infants who were breastfed exclusively for >6 months were anemic at 9 months of age. The trend towards increasing anemia with increasing duration of exclusive breastfeeding was significant (P=0.003).

In the multiple logistic regression analysis, infants who were breastfed exclusively for 6 to 7 months were more likely to be anemic than infants who were breastfed exclusively for <4 months (OR=12.2, 95% CI=2.4, 62.1). Other risk factors associated with anemia at 9 months of age were previous detection of anemia at 3 or 6 months of age (OR=5.4, 95% CI=1.7, 17.6) and gaining ≥4.9 kg (the median weight gain) between birth and 9 months of age (OR=2.9, 95% CI=0.997, 8.4). There was no association with risk of anemia and exclusive breastfeeding to 4 to 6 months of age (OR=1.1, 95% CI=0.4, 3.3) compared with infants who were breastfed exclusively for <4 months (Table 1). Birth weight, gender, the intake of iron supplementation by the infant, and maternal anemia status at delivery were not significant in the model.

4. CONCLUSION

The prevalence of anemia at 9 months of age is low in this population of full-term infants (12%), including infants who were breastfed exclusively. However, the risk of anemia at 9 months of age significantly increased among infants who exclusively breastfed for 6 to 7 months. This effect remained after controlling for the infant's previous hemoglobin status at 3 and 6 months of age, weight gain in kilograms from birth to 9 months of age, and potential intake of iron through formula or physician-prescribed iron supplements. Although the median birth weight differed by exclusive breastfeeding status, it did not differ by anemia status and was not a significant risk factor in the logistic regression model. Infant weight gain from 0 to 9 months was a significant risk factor, consistent with studies that have shown that a rapid rate of growth contributes to an increased depletion of iron stores (Leung & Chan 2001; Yip 1989; CDC 1998). Greater attention is needed to understand the relationship between duration of exclusive breastfeeding and risk of anemia, and the prevention of anemia in children.

5. ACKNOWLEDGMENT

This work was supported by a program project grant from the National Institute of Child Health and Human Development (HD13021).

6. REFERENCES

[CDC] Centers for Disease Control and Prevention. Recommendations to prevent and control iron deficiency in the United States. MMWR 1998;47(RR-3):1-36.

Dallman PR. Nutritional anemia of infancy: iron, folic acid, and vitamin B12. In: Tsang RC, Nichols BL, editors. Nutrition During Infancy. Philadelphia: Henley and Belfus, 1988; pp 216-235.

de Andraca I, Castillo M, Walter T. Psychomotor development and behavior in iron-deficient anemic infants. Nutr Rev 1997;55:125-132.

Dewey KG. Nutrition, growth, and complementary feeding of the breastfed infant. Pediatr Clin North Am 2001;48:87-104.

Krebs NF. Bioavailability of dietary supplements and impact of physiologic state: infants, children and adolescents. J Nutr 2001;131:1351S-1354S.

Leung AK, Chan KW. Iron deficiency anemia. Adv Pediatr 2001;48:385-408.

Lozoff B, Jimenez E, Wolf AW. Long-term developmental outcome of infants with iron deficiency. N Engl J Med 1991;325:687-694.

Lozoff B, Wolf AW, Jimenez E. Iron-deficiency anemia and infant development: effects of extended oral iron therapy. J Pediatr 1996;129:382-389.

Morrow AL, Guerrero ML, Shults J, Calva JJ, Lutter C, Bravo J, Ruiz-Palacios G, Morrow RC, Butterfoss FD. Efficacy of home-based peer counselling to promote exclusive breastfeeding: a randomised controlled trial. Lancet 1999;353:1226-1231.

Oski FA. Iron deficiency in infancy and childhood. N Engl J Med 1993;329:190-193.

Palti H, Meijer A, Adler B. Learning achievement and behavior at school of anemic and non-anemic infants. Early Hum Dev 1985;10:217-223.

Picciano MF. Nutrient composition of human milk. Pediatr Clin North Am 2001;48:53-67.

Saarinen UM, Siimes MA, Dallman PR. Iron absorption in infants: high bioavailability of breast milk iron as indicated by the extrinsic tag method of iron absorption and by the concentration of serum ferritin. J Pediatr 1977;91:36-39.

Sherriff A, Emond A, Bell JC, Golding J. Should infants be screened for anaemia? A prospective study investigating the relation between haemoglobin at 8, 12, and 18 months and development at 18 months. Arch Dis Child 2001;84:480-485.

Siimes MA, Vuori E, Kuitunen P. Breast milk iron—a declining concentration during the course of lactation. Acta Paediatr Scand 1979;68:29-31.

Walter T, De Andraca I, Chadud P, Perales CG. Iron deficiency anemia: adverse effects on infant psychomotor development. Pediatrics 1989;84:7-17.

Walter T. Infancy: mental and motor development. Am J Clin Nutr 1989;50:655-661; discussion 661-656.

[WHO] World Health Organization. The optimal duration of exclusive breastfeeding: Report of an expert consultation. Geneva: World Health Organization, 2001.

Yip R. The changing characteristics of childhood iron nutritional status in the United States. In Filer LJ Jr, editor. Dietary Iron: Birth to Two Years. New York: Raven Press, 1989; pp 37-61.

LONGITUDINAL STUDIES OF MOLYBDENUM BALANCES IN BREASTFED INFANTS

E. Sievers, U. Schleyerbach, and J. Schaub

1. INTRODUCTION

Recommendations for "adequate intake" of the essential trace element molybdenum (Mo) in infancy have been based on its supply by human milk [NAS 2001] and are set at 0.3 μg/kg/day. These recommendations were derived mainly from analysis of Mo concentrations in human milk. Longitudinal data reporting the range of Mo intake in breastfed infants are scarce. Therefore, longitudinal investigations of Mo intake and retention were performed in healthy breastfed infants.

2. METHODS

Nineteen Caucasian mothers with healthy term infants volunteered for participation in trace element balance studies at home. These studies were performed at the postnatal age of 3.6 (2.6–4.7), 8.4 (7.3–10.1), and 15.9 weeks (15.3–16.6). The infants were breastfed exclusively except for 6 of 43 collecting periods with a minor intake of tea, contributing <0.01 μg Mo per day to infant intake. Milk volume was assessed by test weighing the infant (electronic scales accurate to ±5 g). Fore- and hindmilk specimens were collected at each feed over a period of 72 hours, and an aliquot of the specimens of each feed was analyzed. Urinary collections were performed with pediatric-sized 24-hour collection bags (Hollister Inc., Ballina, Ireland). Feces were collected with diaper inserts (Blümia, Moltex Baby Hygiene GmbH, Mayen, Germany). Human milk, tea, urine and feces were analyzed by atomic absorption spectroscopy. The methods have been described in detail elsewhere (Sievers et al. 2000). Maternal nutrition was not within the scope of the investigation.

The results of intake and retention are presented as median and range of individual results obtained in 72 hours. Due to the individual variation of feeds per day, the data describing the molybdenum concentration in human milk were based on the median or mean results of all specimens of the individual mothers at the specific collecting period.

Department of Pediatrics, University of Kiel, Schwanenweg 20, D-24105 Kiel, Germany

The investigation was approved by the institutional ethics committee. Informed consent was obtained from the parents of all participants before their inclusion in the study.

3. RESULTS

A considerable intra- and interindividual range of Mo intake was observed in breastfed infants. The majority of the analyses rendered values <2.0 µg Mo/L, suggesting that representative assessments should consider all feeds. The highest Mo supply was provided by the same mother in all three investigation periods (1.6 µg/kg/day, 2.8 µg/kg/day, 0.8 µg/kg/day). There was more within-group variation of the Mo concentrations found in other mothers.

Table 1. Molybdenum intake and retention in breastfed infants (n=19)

Study participants	n=14[a]	n=15	n=14
Postnatal age, weeks	3.6 (2.6 to 4.7)	8.4 (7.3 to 10.1)	15.9 (15.3 to 16.6)
	Molybdenum, µg/kg/day (median, range)		
Intake	0.23 (0.01 to 1.58)	0.60 (0.0 to 2.8)	0.29 (0.12 to 0.83)
Retention	–0.02 (–0.99 to 1.27)	0.34 (–0.19 to 2.48)	0.23 (0.02 to 0.65)
	Molybdenum, µg/L, in human milk		
Median[b]	*<2.0 (<2.0 to 8.4)*	*<2.0 (<2.0 to 8.4)*	*<2.0 (<2.0 to 6.0)*
Mean[b]	*1.1±2.5*	*3.9±2.9*	*2.1±2.6*
Specimens analyzed	*n=254*	*n=258*	*n=287*

[a]Sievers et al. 2000
[b]Based on median results of each participant considered as one value (n=14, n=15, n=14)

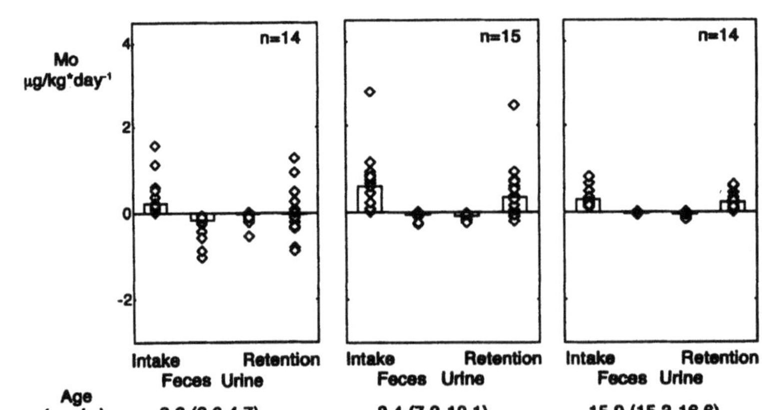

Figure 1. Molybdenum balance studies in breastfed infants data from the initial collecting period; Sievers et al. 2000)

The present results confirm that Mo intake from human milk is low. Despite the range of Mo intake (Table 1, Fig. 1), the median intake in the fourth and sixteenth weeks of life was close to the "adequate intake" of 0.3 µg/kg/day suggested by the National Academy of Sciences (NAS 2001).

The initial investigation period showed balanced Mo retention, and subsequently only three negative balances were recorded (Fig. 1, second investigation). This was predominantly a result of higher fecal Mo excretion observed at the age of 3.6 weeks, which exceeded the urinary Mo excretion.

4. DISCUSSION AND CONCLUSION

Nonsystematic intra-/interindividual variations may suggest that maternal Mo intake influences the Mo concentration in human milk. However, for the transfer of Mo from maternal food into human milk a transfer factor as high as 77.4 (Mo [g/kg] in food / Mo in human milk [g/L]) has been reported (Wappelhorst et al. 2002). *Regional differences of Mo in human milk* (NAS 2001) could reflect environmental concentrations, which may explain why the highest Mo intake was provided by the same mother in all three investigation periods.

All but three Mo balances at the ages 8.4 and 15.9 weeks were positive. The median intake assessed in the second investigation period was double the suggested adequate intake (NAS 2001). A considerable decrease of Mo plasma concentration in the infants studied here has been described previously (Sievers et al. 2000). Increased retention and high initial fecal Mo excretion support the existence of developmental changes in the Mo metabolism and requirements during infancy.

Although the median Mo intake analyzed was close to the suggested intake of 0.3 µg/kg/day (NAS 2001), the intake of many breastfed infants greatly exceeded the adequate intake proposed by the National Academy of Sciences. This finding should be considered in recommendations concerning the Mo intake of formula-fed infants.

5. ACKNOWLEDGMENT

The study was supported financially by the Deutsche Forschungsgemeinschaft (DFG Si 514).

6. REFERENCES

[NAS] National Academy of Sciences, Food and Nutrition Board. Dietary reference intakes for vitamin A, vitamin K, arsenic, boron, chromium, copper, iodine, iron, manganese, molybdenum, nickel, silicon, vanadium and zinc. Washington, DC: National Academies Press; 2001.

Sievers E, Arpe T, Schleyerbach U, Schaub J. Molybdenum supplementation in phenylketonuria diets: adequate in early infancy? J Pediatr Gastroenterol Nutr 2000;31:57-62.

Wappelhorst O, Kühn I, Heidenreich H, Markert B. Transfer of selected elements from food into human milk. Nutrition 2002;18:316-322.

ZINC CONCENTRATION IN HUMAN MILK

Longitudinal Studies in Consecutive Lactation Periods

E. Sievers and J. Schaub

1. INTRODUCTION

The concentration of zinc (Zn) in human milk declines during lactation with considerable interindividual range and diurnal variations being observed (Sievers et al. 1985). However, knowledge of Zn concentrations in comparable time intervals during consecutive lactation periods in the same individual is limited. Therefore, Zn concentrations were investigated in two exclusively breastfeeding mothers during two lactation periods.

2. METHODS

A 22-year-old primigravidous (M1) and a 24-year-old multiparous woman (M2) volunteered for collection of fore- and hindmilk specimens in the first lactation period (P1). The collecting periods comprised 72 hours at 5, 8, 12, and 16±1 weeks. In addition, after birth of their next child, both women participated in comparable collections in a second lactation period. However, it was not possible to include all feedings in the evaluation (sample numbers; Table 1). Specimens were collected using either breast pumps or manual expression. Mothers were instructed to carefully avoid sample contamination and used deionized water for cleaning procedures at home.

Milk specimens were stored at –20°C until analysis, when they were lyophilized, washed with nitric acid, and analyzed by atomic absorption spectroscopy. The methods have been described previously in detail (Sievers et al. 1992). Results are given as median (range). Statistical analysis was performed using nonparametric test procedures (U-test by Wilcoxon, Mann Whitney) and STATISTICA software (Stat. Soft. Corp., Tulsa, OK, USA). This investigation was approved by the institutional ethics committee, and informed consent obtained from the participants before their inclusion in the study.

Department of Pediatrics, University of Kiel, Schwanenweg 20, D-24105 Kiel, Germany

Protecting Infants through Human Milk, edited by Pickering *et al.*
Kluwer Academic/Plenum Publishers, 2004

3. RESULTS

Compared with Zn levels published previously [n=10; Fig. 1] (Sievers et al. 1985), the highest initial Zn concentration was observed in M2-P1; results for M2-P2 were lower (rank 5). Initial results of M1-P1 were the sixth highest and dropped only slightly at P2 to rank 8. At 16 weeks the position in both mothers remained constant in P1/P2. M2 had the highest Zn concentrations. Zn concentrations generally decreased during lactation.

Table 1. The longitudinal course of the zinc concentration in human milk of two mothers (M1, M2) in consecutive lactation periods (P1, P2). Values are the median (range).

Participant – lactation period investigated	Stage of lactation ± 1 week: week 5 (cp 1)[a]	week 8 (cp 2)	week 12 (cp 3)	week 16 (cp 4)
	Zn (mg/L) in human milk			
M1-P1	2.7 (1.0–4.4) n=54	2.9 (0.8–5.9)[b] n=47	1.8 (0.8–2.5) n=24	1.6 (0.6–4.0) n=29
M1-P2	2.5 (2.0–3.7) n=12	2.2 (1.4–3.1)[b] n=19	1.7 (0.3–2.1) n=13	1.7 (1.2–2.4) n=20
M2-P1	3.6 (2.9–4.2)[b] n=47	2.5 (1.2–3.3)[b] n=52	2.3 (1.4–3.3)[b] n=43	1.9 (1.0–3.4) n=54
M2-P2	2.9 (1.8–4.3)[b] n=14	2.9 (1.5–3.9)[b] n=44	1.5 (0.6–2.9)[b] n=43	2.0 (1.0–3.4) n=42

[a]cp=collecting period
[b]$P<0.05$; intraindividual comparison: P1 vs. P2

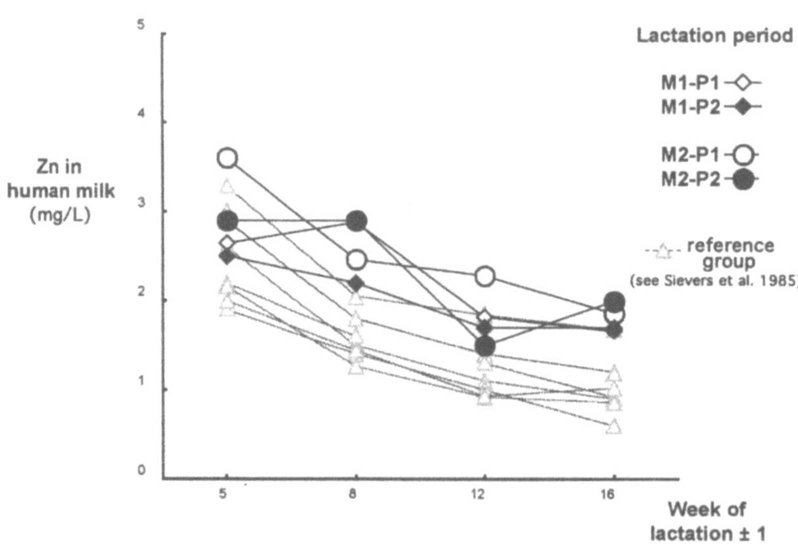

Figure 1. The longitudinal course of the zinc concentration in human milk of two mothers (M1, M2) in consecutive lactation periods (P1, P2). Values represent the median.

4. DISCUSSION AND CONCLUSION

Based on two case reports, the results suggest that a "specific" individual maternal Zn concentration may be reached by week 16. Diurnal variances of Zn concentration have been shown to follow a parallel course in human milk and serum (Sievers et al. 1985), but a greater decline of Zn concentrations is observed in human milk. These variances may be attributable to different mechanisms of Zn transport. We hypothesize that this also may be the reason for the initial difference of Zn in human milk and for its stability at four months. A potential intraindividual decrease of Zn concentration in consecutive lactation periods may be important for the future design of studies focusing on risk assessment for Zn deficiency (Krebs & Westcott 2002) in low-birth-weight infants of multiparous long-term breastfeeding mothers.

5. REFERENCES

Krebs NF, Westcott J. Zinc and breastfed infants: if and when is there a risk of deficiency? Adv Exp Med Biol 2002;503:69-75.

Sievers E, Oldigs H-D, Schulz-Lell G, Dörner K, Schaub J. Diurnal variations in the zinc concentrations of human milk. In: Schaub J, editor. Composition and Physiological Properties of Human Milk. Amsterdam: Elsevier Science Publishers, 1985; pp 65-75.

Sievers E, Oldigs H-D, Dörner K, Schaub J. Longitudinal zinc balances in breast-fed and formula-fed infants. Acta Paediatr 1992;81:1-6

CONCENTRATIONS OF EPIDERMAL GROWTH FACTOR AND TRANSFORMING GROWTH FACTOR-ALPHA IN PRETERM MILK

Bohuslav Dvorak[1,2], Camellia C. Fituch[3], Catherine S. Williams[1], Nancy M. Hurst[3], and Richard J. Schanler[3]

1. INTRODUCTION

Human milk is the major source of nutrients and growth promoting substances in the first weeks of life for the majority of neonates (Goldman 2000). As neonatal care has improved, survival of extremely prematurely born neonates has increased significantly. Yet these infants have the highest incidence of morbid events, such as necrotizing enterocolitis (NEC) (Lucas & Cole 1990). Questions have arisen about the most suitable and relevant nutritional support for these immature infants. Epidermal growth factor (EGF) and transforming growth factor-alpha (TGF-α) are trophic peptides present in human milk with significant healing effects on injured gastrointestinal tract mucosa. Human milk EGF levels are highest in the first days after parturition and then gradually decrease during the first two weeks of lactation (Read et al. 1984). Another structural homologue of EGF, TGF-α also is present in human colostrum and milk (Okada et al. 1991; Wagner et al. 1995), but at much lower concentrations than is EGF. However, neither peptide is found in commercial infant formulas. Decreasing gestational age of neonates is associated with higher risk to develop gastrointestinal tract disorders, and human milk provides better protection against these diseases compared with formula. The aim of this study was to determine whether the concentration of growth factors in human milk varies with gestation time. Concentrations of EGF and TGF-α in human milk collected during the first month of lactation from mothers with 1) extremely preterm born (EPT), 2) preterm born (PT), and 3) full-term born (FT) infants were measured. Because neonatal gastrointestinal tract diseases typically develop within the first postpartum weeks, milk EGF and TGF-α concentrations and protein content were evaluated longitudinally during the first month of lactation.

[1]Department of Pediatrics, University of Arizona, Tucson 85724
[2]Department of Cell Biology & Anatomy, University of Arizona, Tucson
[3]Department of Pediatrics, Baylor College of Medicine, Houston, 77030, TX

Protecting Infants through Human Milk, edited by Pickering *et al.*
Kluwer Academic/Plenum Publishers, 2004

2. METHODS

Human milk samples were obtained from mothers of infants born EPT (23–27 weeks gestational age; n=16), PT (32–36 weeks gestational age; n=16), and FT (38–42 weeks gestational age; n=15). Milk samples were collected in mid morning by a single expression from one breast at the end of the first (day 7), second (day 14), and fourth weeks (day 28) postpartum. Each mother supplied three samples, one for each time point. Milk concentrations of EGF and TGF-α were quantified with a homologous RIA.

3. RESULTS

Total protein concentration in all experimental groups was highest on day 7 of lactation and then gradually decreased during the first month of lactation. Concentrations of EGF in human milk from the EPT group (23–27 weeks) were significantly higher (135–165 μg/L) compared with values from the PT and FT groups (65–105 μg/L) throughout the first month of lactation. Longitudinally, there was no statistical difference in EGF concentration from the EPT group. However, the EGF concentration from the PT and FT groups did show statistically significant decrease over time. A similar pattern was observed with human milk TGF-α; however, the absolute values of milk TGF-α were 100 to 1,000 times less compared with the corresponding EGF data.

4. CONCLUSION

The present study describes EGF and TGF-α levels in human milk from mothers in EPT group (23–27 weeks gestation) and compares them with EGF and TGF-α levels in milk from mothers with PT (32–36 weeks) or FT (38–42 weeks) infants. Human milk EGF concentrations in the EPT group were significantly higher (60–80%) compared with the PT and FT groups. This trend was observed throughout the first month of lactation suggesting that increased secretion of EGF into EPT milk is a long-lasting phenomenon. A similar pattern was detected in milk TGF-α levels. Human milk or enteral formula are the neonate's sole nutritional sources in the early postnatal period. Because formula is devoid of peptide growth factors, a better understanding of the physiologic functions of milk-borne growth factors on the development of neonates is critical for future clinical use of these growth factors.

5. ACKNOWLEDGMENTS

This work was supported by the NIH Grants HD-39657 and HD-26013 (to B.D.).

6. REFERENCES

Goldman AS. Modulation of the gastrointestinal tract of infants by human milk. Interfaces and interactions. An evolutionary perspective. J Nutr 2000;130:426S-431S.

Lucas A, Cole TJ. Breast milk and neonatal necrotising enterocolitis. Lancet 1990;336:1519-1523.

Read LC, Upton FM, Francis GL, Wallace JC, Dahlenberg GW, Ballard FJ. Changes in the growth-promoting activity of human milk during lactation. Pediatr Res 1984;18:133-139.

Okada M, Ohmura E, Kamiya Y, Murakami H, Onoda N, Iwashita M, Wakai K, Tsushima T, Shizume K. Transforming growth factor (TGF)-alpha in human milk. Life Sci 1991;48:1151-1156.
Wagner CL, Forsythe DW, Pittard WB. Variation in the biochemical forms of transforming growth factor-alpha present in human milk and secreted by human milk macrophages. Biol Neonate 1995;68:325-333.

HIGHER MOLECULAR MASS FORMS OF TGFα IN HUMAN MILK

Carol L. Wagner and John E. Baatz

1. INTRODUCTION

Transforming growth factor-α (TGFα) has been identified in human milk by various methods, including Western blot analysis (Peptrides et al. 1984; Okada et al. 1991; Connolly & Rose 1988; Wagner et al. 1995). Human milk has been reported to contain higher molecular mass moieties of TGFα (Okada et al. 1991; Wagner et al. 1995), well above the 22-kD form that is predicted from primary translational production (Qian et al. 1993). Okada et al. (1991), in their study of TGFα fractions in human milk, reported that the majority of TGFα in aqueous samples eluted by Sephadex G-50 gel chromatography was of higher molecular mass than the ~6-kD mature form. There are numerous reports in other organ systems of higher molecular mass bands appearing that are immunoreactive with TGFα. In the past, these higher molecular mass bands have been attributed to nonspecific binding (Humphreys-Beher et al. 1994). To verify the existence of higher molecular mass TGFα moieties in human milk, a series of experiments were performed in our laboratory.

2. METHODS

Approval for this study was granted by the Human Subjects Committee at the Medical University of South Carolina. Lactating mothers were enrolled without regard to ethnicity or insurance status. Following patient consent, human milk samples (n=15) were obtained from 15 healthy mothers who had delivered infants at gestational ages greater than 35 weeks.

Following delivery, expressed milk was obtained as previously described (Wagner et al. 1995). To each 50-mL whole milk sample, 50 μL of antiprotease cocktail (Sigma, St. Louis, MO) was added. An aliquot of whole milk was set aside for later analysis, and the remaining volume was centrifuged at 3,000×g for 25 minutes at 4°C. Following centrifugation, milk was placed in a –20°C freezer for 2 to 5 minutes to achieve enhanced

Division of Neonatology, Department of Pediatrics, Medical University of South Carolina, Charleston, SC 29425

Protecting Infants through Human Milk, edited by Pickering *et al.*
Kluwer Academic/Plenum Publishers, 2004

separation of the fat fraction from the aqueous fraction. The fat layer was removed with a Teflon spatula, to which sodium taurocholate was added for emulsification. Fluid at the aqueous-fat interface was drawn off and the clear aqueous fraction below retrieved.

Following removal of the remaining aqueous fraction, the milk leukocyte pellet was washed twice in Hank's buffered saline. A portion of milk leukocytes was resuspended in DME-F12 media at a concentration of 1×10^6 cells/mL media and incubated at 37°C for 24 hours (Wagner et al. 1995). Conditioned media were collected to which 50 μL antiprotease cocktail was added/10 mL media. The conditioned media was centrifuged at 1,000×g for 6 minutes to remove cellular debris. The supernatant was frozen at –20°C until later analysis by Western blot.

After the milk leukocyte pellet was resuspended in phosphate buffered saline, antigen extraction buffer was added (20 μL/100 μL sample; Oncogene Science) to achieve cell membrane rupture, releasing both intracellular and membrane-bound pro-TGFα. The lysate then was centrifuged at 1,000×g for 10 minutes at 4°C, then frozen at –20°C until later Western blot analysis.

Total protein concentration (μg/sample) of whole milk and its fractions was determined by the BCA method using a commercially available kit (Sigma). A standard electrophoresis protocol for a SDS-polyacrylamide (SDS-PAGE) gel was followed (Wagner et al. 1995). To ascertain whether the binding of the primary (murine) or secondary (goat) antibodies was specific or nonspecific for TGFα, Western blot analysis was performed using different primary and secondary anti-TGFα antibody combinations. The first was substitution of a primary mouse antibody with different binding specificities (Oncogene Science). The second was substitution of the goat anti-mouse secondary antibody with donkey-anti-mouse (1:10,000; Jackson ImmunoResearch Laboratories, Inc., West Grove, PA) and rabbit-anti-mouse secondary antibodies (1:10,000; Jackson ImmunoResearch Laboratories).

In the second set of experiments, recombinant human TGFα, ranging from 100 ng/mL to 100 pg/mL, was added to samples of whole milk and the aqueous fraction. It was predicted that the ~6-kD band would become prominent with increasing concentration of recombinant TGFα added to the samples.

The last series of experiments were designed to determine if the higher molecular mass bands were aggregates of TGFα. To cleave the higher molecular mass forms of TGFα and release immunoreactive products of TGFα, human milk samples were incubated with trypsin insoluble beads (Sigma; 14-units/1-mL milk sample) for increasing incubation time points from 0-24 hours at 37°C. The milk samples were brought to pH 8 in order to activate trypsin. Following incubation, the bead-milk samples were spun at 1,000×g for 10 minutes at 4°C to remove the beads. The milk supernatants were frozen at –80°C until later analysis by Western blot.

3. RESULTS

Higher molecular mass forms of TGFα were detected in human milk and its fractions by Western blot analysis using two distinct antibody systems. Reproducible bands appeared consistently at 14, 21, 26–33, and 40–46 kD in whole milk and its aqueous fraction. When the secondary antibody was changed (goat, donkey, or rat anti-mouse antibodies), there were similar band patterns observed for whole milk and its aqueous fraction. Secondary Western blot analyses were negative for all antibodies tested. The negative control cytochrome C was not visualized with any TGFα detection antibody system used.

For higher resolution, whole milk and its fractions were run on a Bis-Tris gel, then blotted for TGFα using the same antibody system as described earlier. Similar lower molecular mass band patterns below 46 kD appeared as detected using the SDS-PAGE method. Higher bands above 46 kD could be visualized with the Bis-Tris gel for all samples (Fig. 1)

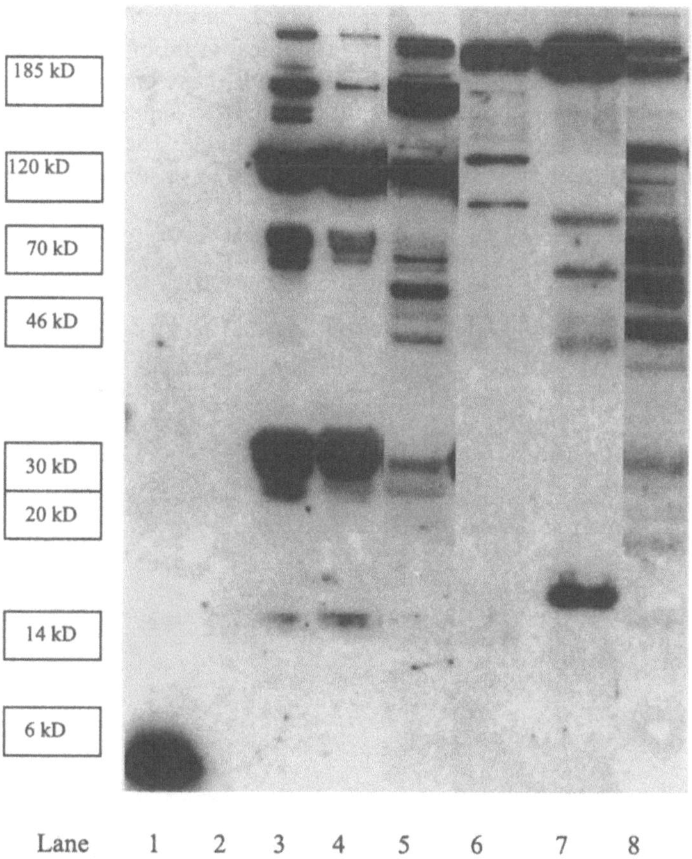

Figure 1. Western blot analysis for TGFα using a mouse-anti-human primary antibody (RDI) compared with a Distinct Mouse-Anti-Human Primary Antibody (Oncogene Science). Whole milk and its aqueous and fat fractions were electrophoresed then transferred to nitrocellulose for immunodetection of TGFα. Two distinct primary monoclonal antibodies were used to detect TGFα: both were mouse-anti-human antibodies (RDI and Oncogene Science) then probed with a secondary goat-anti-mouse polyclonal antibody (Pierce Diagnostics). Lane 1 represents recombinant TGFα (20 ng) from Research Diagnostics; Lane 2, blank; Lane 3, whole milk diluted 1:10 TBS; Lane 4, low-speed aqueous milk fraction (1:10); Lane 5, low speed fat fraction (1:10); Lane 6, milk leukocyte conditioned media; Lane 7, milk leukocyte conditioned media following concanavalin A exposure; Lane 8, lysed milk leukocyte supernatant.

Recombinant TGFα was then added to whole milk samples at increasing concentrations from 10 pg/mL to 100 ng/mL whole milk. With Western blot analysis, the ~6-kD band appeared at 1-ng TGFα/mL whole milk. Similarly, when r-TGFα was added to the aqueous fraction of human milk devoid of fat, the ~6-kD band appeared at 1 ng TGFα. With increasing concentration of r-TGFα added to either the whole milk or aqueous samples, the ~6-kD band became more prominent, with no change in the upper band pattern or densities for either whole milk or its aqueous fraction.

Following incubation of whole milk samples and fractions with insoluble trypsin beads for increasing lengths of time, Western blot analysis of the trypsin-insoluble bead treated milk samples for TGFα showed an increase in the density of the lower bands, including the ~6-kD-band (Fig. 2). Thus, with increasing exposure of the milk samples and their aqueous and fat fractions to insoluble trypsin beads, there was a shift from the higher to the lower molecular mass bands. This shift included the appearance of a ~6-kD band similar to that found in the control lane with r-TGFα alone. There was no further increase in the intensity of the lower bands beyond 12 hours of incubation with trypsin insoluble beads.

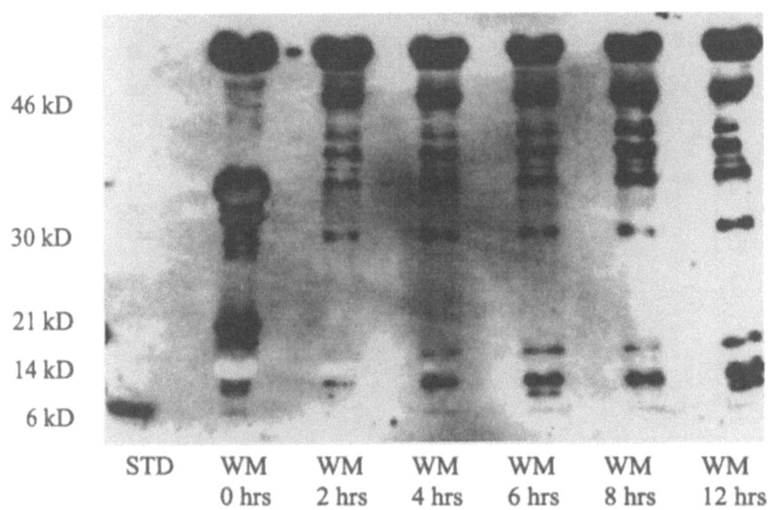

Figure 2. Western blot analysis of TGFα in whole milk samples following incubation with trypsin at increasing intervals (hours). Whole milk samples (WM) were incubated with insoluble trypsin beads for increasing periods from 0–24 hours (shown here 0–12 hours) at 37°C at pH 8. Bead-milk samples were centrifuged to remove beads and supernatant collected. Supernatants were analyzed for TGFα by Western blot analysis. Molecular mass markers are indicated on the left from 6–46 kD.

4. DISCUSSION

Our experiments confirmed the existence of higher molecular mass TGFα moieties in whole milk and its fractions above the predicted 22-kD band, and supported the premise that these moieties can be cleaved enzymatically to lower molecular mass forms. These findings by Western blot analysis suggest that ligomeric or preprocessed forms of TGFα predominate in whole milk and its fractions, including the cellular fraction.

Whether the higher molecular mass forms of TGFα represent noncovalent linkage with the EGF receptor remains to be studied.

5. ACKNOWLEDGMENT

This research was funded in part by NIH grant #3-MO1-RR01070-20S5.

6. REFERENCES

Connolly JM, Rose DP. Epidermal growth factor-like proteins in breast fluid and human milk. Life Sci 1988;42:1751-1756.

Humphreys-Beher MG, Macauley SP, Chegini N, van Setten G, Purushotham K, Stewart C, Wheeler TT, Schultz GS. Characterization of the synthesis and secretion of transforming growth factor-alpha from salivary glands and saliva. Endocrinology 1994;134:963-970.

Okada M, Ohmura E, Kamiya Y, Murakami H, Onoda N, Iwashita M, Wakai K, Tsushima T, Shizume K. Transforming growth factor (TGF)-alpha in human milk. Life Sci 1991;48:1151-1156.

Peptrides PE, Hosang M, Shooter EM, Bohlen P. Transforming growth factors in human milk: isolation and partial chemical and biological characterization. Proceedings of the 7th International Congress for Endocrinology, 1984; pp 1139.

Qian JF, Lazar-Wesley E, Breugnot C, May E. Human transforming growth factor alpha: sequence analysis of the 4.5-kb and 1.6-kb mRNA species. Gene 1993;132:291-296.

Wagner CL, Forsythe DW, Pittard WB. Variation in the biochemical forms of transforming growth factor-alpha present in human milk and secreted by human milk macrophages. Biol Neonate 1995;68:325-333.

TGFα WITHIN COMPARTMENTS OF HUMAN MILK

Carol L. Wagner and John E. Baatz

1. INTRODUCTION

Human milk plays a significant role in postnatal gut maturation and may serve as a vehicle for transmitting developmental signals from mother to neonate (Okada et al. 1991; Wagner et al. 1995). Various growth factors, cytokines, and gut peptides have been isolated from human milk, often in quantities that exceed maternal serum levels (Kudlow & Bjorge 1990; Coffey et al. 1992). There exists an interrelated system in which compartmentation of milk components leads to controlled release of nutrients and metabolites to the breastfed infant. Various proteins are sequestered differentially within the compartments of human milk. These proteins become sequentially processed within the gastrointestinal tract (Kudlow & Bjorge 1990). The majority of studies on human milk have focused on the aqueous (defatted) fraction of whole milk rather than the various compartments that include fat. Yet, the fat compartment composed of the milk fat globule with its associated plasma membrane appears to provide a unique delivery system of bioactive substances to the newborn gut (Okada et al. 1991; Wagner et al. 1995; Jensen et al. 1995).

A growth factor that is present in all compartments of human milk is transforming growth factor-α (TGFα), a member of the epidermal growth factor (EGF) family (Coffey et al. 1992). It has been proposed that the bioavailability of human growth factors, and thus their in vivo activity, can be affected by their compartmentation in milk (Jensen et al. 1995). Interleukin-10 (Garofalo et al. 1995) and TGFβ (McPherson & Wagner 2001), for example, are at higher concentrations in the fat, whereas vasoactive endothelial growth factor (VEGF) appears at higher concentration in the aqueous fraction (Siafakas et al. 1999). TGFα has been identified in the aqueous phase or whey portion of human milk and is secreted by milk macrophages (Okada et al. 1991; Wagner et al. 1995). Little is known about the biochemical characteristics of TGFα and its concentration gradient in whole milk and its cellular and noncellular compartments—including the milk fat globule (MFG) and the surrounding milk fat globule membrane (MFGM).

Division of Neonatology, Department of Pediatrics, Medical University of South Carolina, Charleston, SC 29425

Protecting Infants through Human Milk, edited by Pickering *et al.*
Kluwer Academic/Plenum Publishers, 2004

The objective of this study was to determine if there are differences in concentration and biochemical characteristics of TGFα within whole milk and its aqueous, liposome, MFG, MFGM, and milk leukocyte fractions. Based on the biophysical properties of TGFα (Kudlow & Bjorge 1990) and its transmembrane structure, it was hypothesized that when compared with whole milk and its aqueous fraction, the fat fraction would have a unique molecular mass profile and higher TGFα concentration. It was further hypothesized that disruption of the milk fat globule within the fat would result in enhanced release of TGFα from the intact membrane, leading to an increase in the concentration of immunoreactive TGFα.

2. METHODS

Approval for this study was granted by the Human Subjects Committee at the Medical University of South Carolina. Following delivery, expressed milk was obtained, the aqueous fraction removed, and the milk leukocyte pellet was prepared [Fig. 1] (Wagner et al. 1995). Conditioned media were collected, and a 50-μL antiprotease cocktail added per 10 mL media. The media were centrifuged at 1,500×g for 6 minutes at 4°C to remove cellular debris. The supernatant was frozen at –20°C until later analysis.

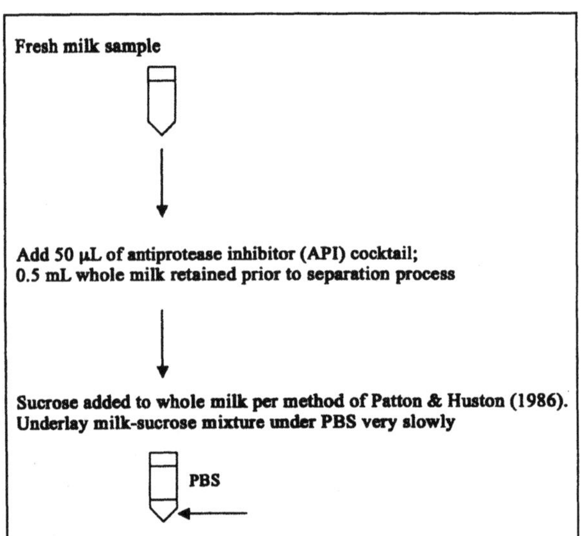

Figure 1. Schematic of milk fraction separation process

A second portion of milk leukocytes was resuspended in 500 μL PBS, washed to remove the residual fat layer; an antiprotease cocktail (50 μL/mL) was added to the cellular preparation. The supernatant was discarded and an additional 250 μL PBS with 12.5 μL antiprotease was added to the cellular preparation. Antigen Extraction Agent (Oncogene Science) at a concentration of 20 μL/100 μL was added to the cells to achieve lysis. Cells were incubated on ice for 30 minutes with occasional vortexing. The lysate was transferred to a polycarbonate tube for centrifugation at 80,000×g for 2 hours at 4°C. The lysate supernatant was aspirated from the residual pellet for later processing. The lysate pellet was washed with 1 mL PBS plus antiprotease (50 μL/1 mL PBS) then spun at 18,500×g for 1 hour at 4°C.

A chloroform-methanol extraction was performed on the cellular lysate as follows: 1 mL 2:1 chloroform:methanol+5% 0.1 N HCl was added to the lysate. Using a glass transfer pipette, the lysate solution was rinsed several times and vortexed between rinses.

In order to facilitate further separation of the fractions from whole milk and its cellular membrane component, whole milk samples were spun at 80,000×g for 1 hour at 4°C. The various fractions were removed as outlined for low-speed centrifugation. The liposomal pellet at the bottom of the test tube was washed with two 1-mL TBS aliquots to remove any residual aqueous fraction and then resuspended in 1 mL TBS. All samples were stored at –20°C until later analysis.

The MFGM was isolated from human milk samples according to the method of Patton and Huston (1986). Triton-X 100 (0.05% v/v; Sigma Chemicals, St. Louis, MO) or TBS (0.05% v/v) was added to paired whole milk samples (n=10) 2 hours prior to assay to disrupt the milk fat globule (Patton 1982). Subsequently, TGFα concentrations in the samples were measured by RIA.

The equivolume concentrations of TGFα in whole milk and its fractions were measured by RIA (Peninsula Laboratories, Belmont, CA; sensitivity 1 pg/100 μL sample; cross-reactivity with EGF 0%). Using methodology previously described (Wagner et al. 1995), a standard electrophoresis protocol for a SDS-polyacrylamide gel was followed (Laemmli 1970). Membranes were incubated with a primary monoclonal mouse-anti-human TGFα antibody (0.5 μg/mL; 0% EGF cross-reactivity; Research Diagnostics, Flanders, NJ) in Tween-TBS (TTBS) with 0.5% bovine serum albumin (BSA; Sigma) and secondary goat-anti-mouse HR-peroxidase conjugated polyclonal antibody (Pierce Chemical, Rockford, IL) 1:50,000 in 0.5% BSA buffer. Appropriate negative controls with secondary antibody alone were carried out to determine nonspecific binding. Subsequently, each membrane was treated with enhanced chemilluminescence specific for HR-peroxidase coupled to biotin/avidin (Amersham).

3. RESULTS

Forty-five whole milk samples were collected from 38 lactating mothers on postpartum days 3–30. The gestational age of infants at delivery ranged from 26 to 42 weeks. The mean (±SD) concentration of TGFα in whole milk samples was 310±214 pg/mL. The TGFα concentration of the fractions by low-speed centrifugation was higher in all fat samples compared with their paired aqueous fractions. Specifically, while the mean TGFα concentration in the aqueous samples was 188±168 pg/mL (range, 25–680 pg/mL), the mean concentration in the fat samples was 599±361 pg/mL (range, 170–1280 pg/mL). TGFα concentration in the milk leukocyte media was 18±9 pg/mL.

While a similar pattern in TGFα concentration was noted between low- and high-speed centrifugation samples, there were important differences (refer to Higher molecular mass forms of TGFα in human milk, Wagner & Baatz 2004, Fig. 1; this volume). The mean TGFα concentration per volume for the aqueous high-speed fraction was 386±109 pg/mL, 854±92 pg/mL for the fat fraction, and 89±31 pg/mL for the liposomal pellet. As with the low-speed samples, the mean TGFα concentration was greatest in the high-speed fat fraction. The mean TGFα concentration in the aqueous fraction of milk was 37% (range, 5– 79%) of the TGFα concentration in the fat fraction per volume.

In a subsequent experiment to further define the characteristics of TGFα within human milk, ten paired whole milk samples were mixed with 0.05% (v/v) Triton-X 100 to achieve disruption of the MFG. When Triton-X 100 was added to whole milk samples to disrupt the MFG, there was an increase in the TGFα concentration of all 10 samples when compared with untreated whole milk samples. Specifically, TGFα concentration in the 10 samples increased from a mean concentration of 270±84 pg/mL in the untreated whole milk samples to 347±86 in the Triton-X 100 treated samples. Triton-X 100 resulted in a mean increase in TGFα of 32.6±4.2% (range, 7.5–80.2%).

Western blot analysis for TGFα in whole milk samples and fractions was performed. A representative Western blot is presented in (refer to Higher molecular mass forms of TGFα in human milk, Wagner & Baatz 2004, Fig. 1; this volume). The TGFα banding patterns in whole milk and its aqueous and liposomal pellet samples were similar (11, 17, 25, 52, 70, 120, and 185).

4. CONCLUSIONS

Our findings support the premise of compartmentation of a bioactive substance, namely TGFα, within human milk and its biochemical variation within those compartments. The significance of these differences in TGFα's concentration, biochemistry, and associated bioavailability within those compartments, and their role as a site-specific delivery system to various regions in the newborn gut must be explored.

5. ACKNOWLEDGMENT

This research was funded in part by NIH grant #3-MO1-RR01070-20S5.

6. REFERENCES

Coffey RJ, Romano M, Polk WH, Dempsey PJ. Roles for transforming growth factor-alpha in gastric physiology and pathophysiology. Yale J Biol Med 1992;65:693-704; discussion 621-693.

Garofalo R, Chheda S, Mei F, Palkowetz KH, Rudloff HE, Schmalstieg FC, Rassin DK, Goldman AS. Interleukin-10 in human milk. Pediatr Res 1995;37:444-449.

Jensen RG, Blanc B, Patton S. Particulate constituents in human and bovine milks. In: Jensen RG, editor. Handbook of Milk Composition. San Diego: Academic Press, 1995; pp 50-61.

Kudlow JE, Bjorge JD. TGF alpha in normal physiology. Semin Cancer Biol 1990;1:293-302.

Laemmli UK. Cleavage of structural proteins during the assembly of the head of bacteriophage T4. Nature 1970;227:680-685.

McPherson RJ, Wagner CL. The effect of pasteurization on TGFα and TGFβ concentrations in human milk. Adv Exp Med Biol 2001;501:559-566.

Okada M, Ohmura E, Kamiya Y, Murakami H, Onoda N, Iwashita M, Wakai K, Tsushima T, Shizume K. Transforming growth factor (TGF)-alpha in human milk. Life Sci 1991;48:1151-1156.

Patton S. Release of remnant plasma membrane from milk fat globules by Triton X-100. Biochim Biophys Acta 1982;688:727-734.

Patton S, Huston GE. A method for isolation of milk fat globules. Lipids 1986;21:170-174.

Siafakas CG, Anatolitou F, Fusunyan RD, Walker WA, Sanderson IR. Vascular endothelial growth factor (VEGF) is present in human breast milk and its receptor is present on intestinal epithelial cells. Pediatr Res 1999;45:652-657.

Wagner CL, Forsythe DW, Pittard WB. Variation in the biochemical forms of transforming growth factor-alpha present in human milk and secreted by human milk macrophages. Biol Neonate 1995;68:325-333.

Wagner CL, Baatz JA. Higher molecular mass forms of TGFα in human milk. In: Pickering LK, Morrow AL, Ruiz-Palacios GM, Schanler RJ. Protecting Infants through Human Milk: Advancing the Scientific Evidence. Advances in Experimental Medicine and Biology Series. New York: Kluwer Academic/Plenum Publishers, 2004; this volume.

VARIATIONS IN CONCENTRATIONS OF LACTOFERRIN IN HUMAN MILK: A NINE COUNTRY SURVEY

E. Lien[1], J. Jackson[1], C. Kuhlman[1], K. Pramuk[1], B. Lönnerdal[2], and D. Janszen[3]

1. INTRODUCTION

Lactoferrin (Lf), an 80-kD glycoprotein, is a major whey protein in human milk (HM). The structure of Lf is similar to that of transferrin and ovotransferrin. Lactoferrin binds iron tightly and releases it at a pH less than 3.0 (Lönnerdal & Iyer 1995), has anti-inflammatory and antibacterial properties (Goldman et al. 1990), and has antioxidant properties (Huang et al. 1999).

Although concentrations of Lf in HM have been evaluated previously, many studies reported results from analysis of only a limited number of samples or from pooled HM. In addition, most of the analytical techniques were immunologic methods (Lönnerdal et al. 1976; Zavaleta et al. 1995; Montagne et al. 2000; Ronayne de Ferrer et al. 2000). The present study analyzed HM samples from nine countries located on five continents using high performance liquid chromatography (HPLC).

2. METHODS

A complete breast expression containing a minimum of 50 mL of mature HM was collected from women who had delivered full-term healthy infants. Additional maternal criteria included parity less than five; 18 to 40 years of age; more than five breast-feeds per day; and no ingestion of antimicrobial agents, steroids, stool softeners, or anti-inflammatory medications. Samples were collected in Australia, China, Chile, Canada, Mexico, Japan, Philippines, the United Kingdom, and the United States.

The HM samples were analyzed by a HPLC instrument (Agilent Technologies, Wilmington, DE) equipped with a Jupiter C4 column using gradient elution with water-acetonitrile-trifluroacetic acid and diode array detection at 280 nm. All data were

[1]Wyeth Nutrition, Philadelphia, PA
[2]Department of Nutrition, University of California, Davis, CA
[3]Wyeth Pharmaceuticals, Philadelphia, PA

Protecting Infants through Human Milk, edited by Pickering *et al.*
Kluwer Academic/Plenum Publishers, 2004

analyzed using analysis of covariance with means of each country expressed as least square means and also by analysis of variance. Total nitrogen was determined by complete combustion of the sample using a LECO FP-528L Determinator instrument (LECO Corp., St. Joseph, MI) with thermoelectric determination of combusted nitrogen.

3. RESULTS

The overall mean milk Lf concentration was 1.83±0.67 g/L (±SEM). Mean concentrations of Lf ranged from 1.37 g/L in Mexico to 2.12 g/L in China (Fig. 1). Milk Lf levels in Mexico and Australia were significantly lower than in all other countries.

Milk Lf concentration declined over the duration of lactation. Three patterns were apparent and representative relationships are shown in Figure 2. Concentrations of Lf in milk samples from women in Australia remained fairly consistent over the duration of lactation, but samples from women in the United Kingdom showed a sharp decline. The patterns for the remaining countries were similar to that of Canada.

Milk Lf was correlated positively to total nitrogen in all countries, but this was significant only for Japan, the Philippines, and the United States ($P<0.05$). There was also a significant correlation between Lf and α-lactalbumin for milk from Canada, China, Japan, the Philippines, and the United States. These correlations are illustrated in Table 1.

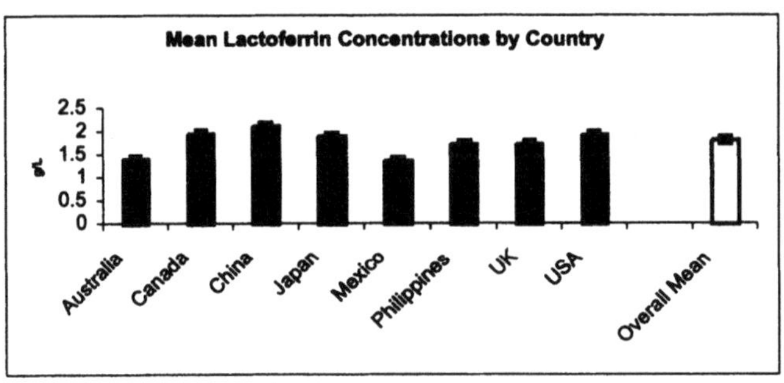

Figure 1. Mean lactoferrin concentrations by country

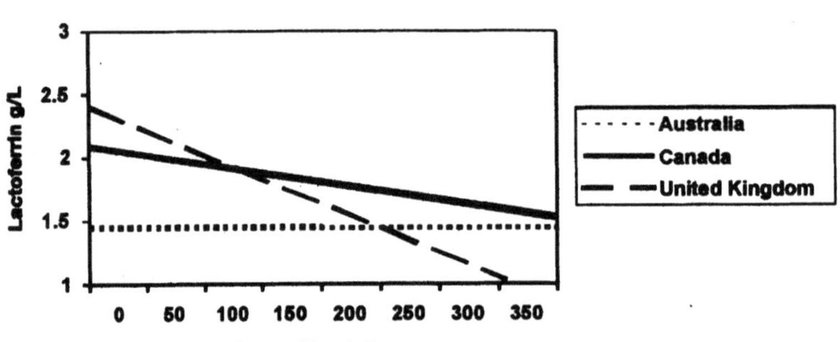

Figure 2. Duration of lactation vs. lactoferrin concentration

Table 1. Correlations (r) between lactoferrin, nitrogen and α-lactalbumin

Country	Nitrogen	α-Lactalbumin
Australia	0.267	0.175
Canada	0.203	0.366[a]
China	0.085	0.300[a]
Japan	0.422[a]	0.296[a]
Mexico	0.178	0.238
Philippines	0.540[a]	0.452[a]
United Kingdom	0.214	−0.077
United States	0.560[a]	0.706[a]

[a]$P<0.05$

4. DISCUSSION AND CONCLUSIONS

Lf, one of the most abundant proteins in human milk, has been shown to have many beneficial activities, which include bacteriostatic and bactericidal properties, regulation of immune response and possibly participating in iron absorption (Conneely 2001). The present study was designed to evaluate Lf levels in HM collected from women living in a variety of locations. All subjects were from a middle socioeconomic background except the Philippines and China, but the data did not suggest a relationship between socio-economic status and Lf concentrations. Variations existed among countries, with milk from Mexico and Australia being significantly lower in Lf than milk from the other countries. Our data compared favorably with other publications, although most published methods of analysis for Lf were immunologic (Lönnerdal et al. 1976; Zavaleta et al. 1995; Montagne et al. 2000; Ronayne de Ferrer et al. 2000). Our HPLC method was less cumbersome and sample preparation was minimal.

Total nitrogen concentration decreased over the duration of lactation, and so did the concentration of Lf. This correlation was positive for every country, although the correlation was significant only for the United States, Japan, and the Philippines. The correlation between the concentration of Lf, a major milk protein, and that of milk nitrogen was expected, and has been reported previously (Nagasawa et al. 1972; Lönnerdal et al. 1976). The concentration of Lf also was positively correlated to that of α-lactalbumin for all the countries except the United Kingdom. Several whey proteins show a declining pattern during lactation (Sanchez-Pozo et al. 1986) and they likely are under similar hormonal control.

In conclusion, the present study evaluated human milk levels of Lf from women living in eight countries distributed on five continents. The concentrations showed only modest variability and were correlated to both total nitrogen and to α-lactalbumin levels. While the role of Lf in infancy remains to be delineated, these data will prove useful for evaluation of functional hypotheses and for design of improved infant formulas.

5. REFERENCES

Conneely OM. Antiinflammatory activities of lactoferrin. J Am Coll Nutr 2001;20:389S-395S; discussion 396S-397S.

Goldman AS, Goldblum RM, Hanson LA. Anti-inflammatory systems in human milk. Adv Exp Med Biol 1990;262:69-76.

Huang SW, Satue-Gracia MT, Frankel EN, German JB. Effect of lactoferrin on oxidative stability of corn oil emulsions and liposomes. J Agric Food Chem 1999;47:1356-1361.

Lonnerdal B, Forsum E, Hambraeus L. A longitudinal study of the protein, nitrogen, and lactose contents of human milk from Swedish well-nourished mothers. Am J Clin Nutr 1976;29:1127-1133.

Lonnerdal B, Iyer S. Lactoferrin: molecular structure and biological function. Annu Rev Nutr 1995;15:93-110.

Montagne P, Cuillière M, Molé C, Béné M, Faure G. Dynamics of the Main Immunologically and Nutritionally Available Proteins of Human Milk during Lactation. J Food Comp Anal 2000;13:127-137.

Nagasawa T, Kiyosawa I, Kuwahara K. Amounts of lactoferrin in human colostrum and milk. J Dairy Sci 1972;55:1651-1659.

Ronayne de Ferrer PA, Baroni A, Sambucetti ME, Lopez NE, Ceriani Cernadas JM. Lactoferrin levels in term and preterm milk. J Am Coll Nutr 2000;19:370-373.

Sanchez-Pozo A, Lopez J, Pita ML, Izquierdo A, Guerrero E, Sanchez-Medina F, Martinez Valverde A, Gil A. Changes in the protein fractions of human milk during lactation. Ann Nutr Metab 1986;30:15-20.

Zavaleta N, Nombera J, Rojas R, Hambraeus L, Gislason J, Lönnerdal B. Iron and lactoferrin in milk of anemic mothers given iron supplements Nutr Res. 1995;15:681-690.

FUCOSYLATED OLIGOSACCHARIDES IN HUMAN MILK IN RELATION TO GESTATIONAL AGE AND STAGE OF LACTATION

Barbara Davidson[1], Jareen K. Meinzen-Derr[1], Carol L. Wagner[2], David S. Newburg[3], and Ardythe L. Morrow[1]

1. INTRODUCTION

Breastfeeding is known to offer significant protection against infectious diarrhea. Oligosaccharides, the third largest solid component of human milk, constitute a major mechanism of innate defense of breastfed infants against infectious diarrhea (Morrow et al. 2004; Jiang et al. 2004; Newburg et al. 2004; Ruiz-Palacios et al. 2003). The fucosylated oligosaccharides of human milk comprise the majority of milk oligosaccharides and have been shown to inhibit host cell binding to specific enteric pathogens (Crane et al. 1994; Newburg et al. 1990; Ruiz-Palacios et al. 2003). Mothers vary in the quantity and type of oligosaccharides found in their milk, which may influence the degree to which their milk offers protection of their infants against specific pathogens. Human milk fucosylated oligosaccharide synthesis is controlled by the same fucosyltransferase genes (FUT2 and FUT3) that control secretor and Lewis blood group types (Newburg et al. 2004; Viverge et al. 1990). Oligosaccharide expression in human milk also may be affected by gestational age and stage of lactation.

Total oligosaccharide concentration has been shown to decline over the course of lactation (Coppa et al. 1993; Brand et al. 1994; Nakhla et al. 1999). The relative amount of α1,2-linked fucosylated oligosaccharide also appears to decline over the course of lactation. In the milk of 11 Mexican mothers studied longitudinally, the ratio of α1,2-linked to non-α1,2-linked fucosylated oligosaccharides was 5:1 in the first few weeks postpartum, which decreased to 1:1 by the end of one year of lactation (Chaturvedi et al. 2001).

The relationship between gestational age and the oligosaccharide composition of human milk is not clear. Investigators have reported differences in lactose concentration between preterm and term milk (Gross et al. 1980; Dawodu et al. 1990), suggesting that the oligosaccharide concentration of preterm and term milk also might vary. However,

[1]Cincinnati Children's Hospital Medical Center, 3000 Burnet Avenue, Cincinnati, OH 45229-3039
[2]Division of Neonatology, Department of Pediatrics, Medical University of South Carolina, Charleston, SC
[3]Program in Glycobiology, Shriver Center, University of Massachusetts Medical School, Waltham, MA

only two limited studies have been published previously on this topic. In contrast, based on analyses of milk from mothers of 13 preterm infants and 2 term infants, Nakhla et al. (1999) reported that the neutral oligosaccharide content did not differ between preterm and term milk. Miller et al. (1994) analyzed serial milk samples from mothers of two preterm infants and eight term infants to determine the concentration of lactose, fucose, sialic acid, and *N*-acetylglucosamine. They noted that preterm milk appeared to have higher concentrations of these components, but given the small sample size this observation was not statistically testable (Miller et al. 1994).

The purpose of the current study was to examine (1) gestational age and (2) stage of lactation in relation to the concentration (a) of total fucosylated oligosaccharide in human milk and (b) the percentage of total fucosylated oligosaccharide that contains an α1,2-linked fucose.

2. METHODS

Study participants were 18 lactating mothers whose infants were admitted to a neonatal intensive care unit in South Carolina. Approval for the analysis of the milk samples was granted by the university's IRB under exempt status because the samples had no patient identifiers except for maternal blood type, gestational age of infant at delivery, and days postpartum. Women had consented previously to have their samples analyzed for another IRB approved protocol. For each study mother, a single milk sample with >2 mL volume collected one to five weeks postpartum was selected and sent to Boston for analysis. Milk samples were analyzed by HPLC. The concentration of total fucosylated oligosaccharides (μmol/mL) and the percentage of α1,2-linked fucosyloligosaccharides were compared by infant gestational age (<31 weeks, n=7; 31–36 weeks, n=6; >36 weeks, n=5) and stage of lactation (week 1 vs. weeks 2–5 postpartum).

3. RESULTS

The concentration of total fucosylated oligosaccharide in the 18 milk samples was 6.96±1.69 (mean±SEM) μmol/mL, with individual samples ranging from 0.57 to 24.50 μmol/mL. Two of the 18 (11%) subjects had no α1,2-linked fucosyloligosaccharides in their milk. In the remaining 16 subjects whose milk contained α1,2-linked fucosyloligosaccharide, the percentage of total fucosylated oligosaccharide that contained an α1,2-linked fucose was 41±7.5% (mean±SEM) with individual samples ranging from 4.2% to 79.8%.

As shown in Figure 1, total fucosylated oligosaccharides in maternal milk was observed to increase with gestational age, although this trend was not statistically significant ($P=0.25$). The percentage of total oligosaccharide that was α1,2-linked did not differ by gestational age. Total fucosylated oligosaccharide content did not differ by stage of lactation. However, the percentage of total oligosaccharide that contained an α1,2-linked fucose, as shown in Figure 2, differed significantly ($P<0.001$) between the milk collected from four mothers in the first week postpartum (days 1–7) compared with the milk collected from 14 mothers during weeks 2 to 5 (7.4±3.1 vs. 44.9±8.2; mean±SEM).

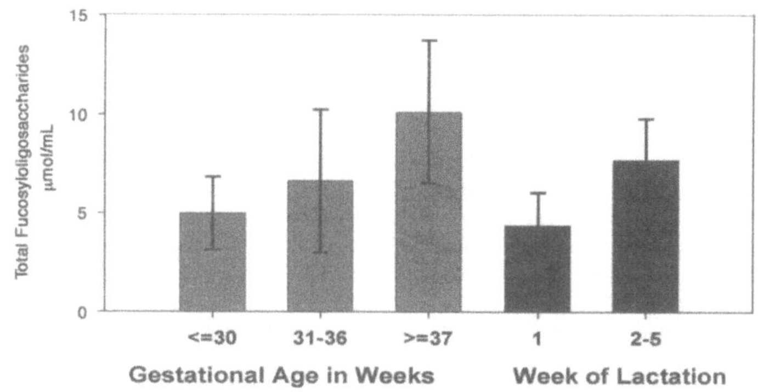

Figure 1. Total fucosyloligosaccharides in milk

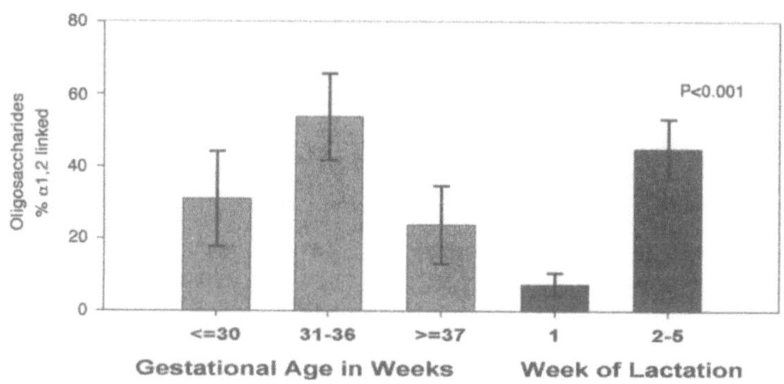

Figure 2. Mean percentage of α1,2 fucosylated oligosaccharides

4. CONCLUSIONS

Our data indicate that the percentage of total fucosylated oligosaccharide that has an α1,2-linked fucose is significantly lower in colostrum (days 1–7) than milk from weeks 2 to 5 postpartum, but does not differ by gestational age. Our data also suggest that total fucosylated oligosaccharide in human milk may increase with gestational age, but there was no evidence of association with stage of lactation. However, a larger study of this question may be warranted.

5. ACKNOWLEDGMENT

This work was supported by a program project grant from the National Institute of Child Health and Human Development (HD13021).

6. REFERENCES

Chaturvedi P, Warren CD, Altaye M, Morrow AL, Ruiz-Palacios G, Pickering LK, Newburg DS. Fucosylated human milk oligosaccharides vary between individuals and over the course of lactation. Glycobiology 2001;11:365-372.

Coppa GV, Gabrielli O, Pierani P, Catassi C, Carlucci A, Giorgi PL. Changes in carbohydrate composition in human milk over 4 months of lactation. Pediatrics 1993;91:637-641.

Crane JK, Azar SS, Stam A, Newburg DS. Oligosaccharides from human milk block binding and activity of the Escherichia coli heat-stable enterotoxin (Sta) in T84 intestinal cells. J Nutr 1994;124:2358-2364.

Dawodu AH, Osibanjo O, Damole IO. Nutrient composition of milk produced by mothers of preterm infants in Nigeria. East Afr Med J 1990;67:873-877.

Gross SJ, David RJ, Bauman L, Tomarelli RM. Nutritional composition of milk produced by mothers delivering preterm. J Pediatr 1980;96:641-644.

Miller JB, Bull S, Miller J, McVeagh P. The oligosaccharide composition of human milk: Temporal and individual variation. J Pediatr Gastroenterol Nutr 1994;19:371-376.

Nakhla T, Fu D, Zopf D, Brodsky NL, Hurt H. Neutral oligosaccharide content of preterm human milk. Br J Nutr 1999;82:361-367.

Newburg DS, Pickering LK, McCluer RH, Cleary TG. Fucosylated oligosaccharides of human milk protect suckling mice from heat-stable enterotoxin of Escherichia coli. J Infect Dis 1990;162:1075-1080.

Ruiz-Palacios GM, Cervantes LE, Ramos P, Chavez-Munguia, Newburg DS. Campylobacter jejuni binds intestinal H(O) antigen (Fucα1,2Galβ1,4GlcNAc), and fucosyloligosaccharides of human milk inhibit its binding and infection. J Biol Chem 2003;278:14112-14120.

Viverge D, Grimmonprez L, Cassanas G, Bardet L, Solere M. Variations in oligosaccharides and lactose in human milk during the first week of lactation. J Pediatr Gastroenterol Nutr 1990;11:361-364.

VARIATION IN PROLACTIN CONSUMPTION BY FULLY BREASTFED INFANTS

M.D. Cregan, L.R. Mitoulas, and P.E. Hartmann

1. INTRODUCTION

Animal studies have shown that biologically active prolactin from milk is transferred to the circulation of the neonate following suckling, and that prolactin assists in the development of the pituitary and adrenal glands, reproductive organs, gastrointestinal and respiratory tracts, and modulates the acquired immune system (Ellis et al. 1996). The aim of this study was to determine the amount of prolactin consumed by a breastfed human infant.

2. METHODS

Exclusively breastfeeding women (n=15; 1–6 months postpartum) measured their milk production over a 24-hour period (Arthur et al. 1989), collecting fore- and hind-milk samples at each feed. The prolactin concentration of each sample was determined by IRMA, and a mean fore- and hind-milk value was calculated to determine the amount of prolactin consumed by the infant at each feed. Data analysis was performed using SuperAnova and SPSS software. All data are expressed as mean±SEM.

3. RESULTS

3.1. Variation over a 24-hour Period

Over the course of a 24-hour period the highest volume of milk was removed from a breast by the infant between 2 AM and 10 AM. Concurrently, the mean concentration of prolactin in milk was higher at these times, resulting in the infant receiving the greatest amount of prolactin between 2 AM and 10 AM (Table 1).

Biochemistry and Molecular Biology, School of Biomedical and Chemical Sciences, Faculty of Life and Physical Sciences, The University of Western Australia, 35 Stirling Highway, Crawley, Western Australia, 6009. (Mark Cregan is the corresponding author.)

Protecting Infants through Human Milk, edited by Pickering *et al.*
Kluwer Academic/Plenum Publishers, 2004

Table 1. Variation in the infant feed volume, prolactin concentration in milk, and the amount of prolactin received by the infant over a 24-hour period (24-hour clock)

	22.01 to 02.00	02.01 to 06.00	06.01 to 10.00	10.01 to 14.00	14.01 to 18.00	18.01 to 22.00
Number of Observations	10	12	15	15	14	14
Feed Volume (mL)	72 ± 7^{a}	91 ± 6^{b}	98 ± 6^{b}	66 ± 6^{a}	72 ± 6^{a}	64 ± 6^{a}
Prolactin Concentration (μg/L)	17.5 ± 1.3^{a}	24.3 ± 1.2^{b}	21.8 ± 1.0^{b}	14.2 ± 1.0^{ac}	14.0 ± 1.1^{c}	15.6 ± 1.1^{ac}
Prolactin Received by Infant (μg)	1.35 ± 0.18^{a}	2.16 ± 0.16^{b}	2.07 ± 0.14^{b}	0.96 ± 0.14^{a}	1.01 ± 0.15^{a}	1.09 ± 0.15^{a}

Identical superscripts indicate time periods where there were no significant (p>0.05) differences between groups

Table 2. Variation in the 24-hour milk production, the mean prolactin concentration of milk over a 24-hour period, and the amount of prolactin received by the infant over a 24-hour period over the first six months of lactation

	Months Post-Partum 1 to 2	3 to 4	5 to 6
Number of Observations	4	8	3
24h Milk Production (mL)	749 ± 89^{a}	841 ± 64^{a}	801 ± 104^{a}
Mean 24h Prolactin Concentration (μg/L)	31.3 ± 4.3^{a}	13.7 ± 3.1^{b}	10.0 ± 4.9^{b}
Prolactin Received by Infant Over 24h (μg)	23.3 ± 4.1^{a}	10.2 ± 2.9^{b}	7.7 ± 4.7^{b}

Identical superscripts indicate time periods where there were no significant differences (p>0.05) between groups

3.2. Variation during the First Six Months of Lactation

Despite there being no significant ($P>0.05$) difference in 24-hour milk production during the first six months of lactation, the amount of prolactin received by the infant over a 24-hour period was greater in the first two months of lactation than between three and six months, due to a progressive decline in the concentration of prolactin in milk (Table 2).

4. CONCLUSIONS

We conclude that an infant receives the greatest amount of prolactin in the early morning period and during early lactation. Therefore, developmental benefits of milk prolactin to the pituitary and adrenal glands, reproductive organs, gastrointestinal and respiratory tracts, and the acquired immune system of the infant will be conferred at these times.

5. ACKNOWLEDGMENTS

The authors would like to thank the mothers who participated in this study and the Australian Breastfeeding Association for assisting us in their recruitment. This study was approved by the Human Research Ethics Committee of the University of Western Australia and was supported by Medela AG and the Women and Infants Research Foundation at King Edward Memorial Hospital for Children.

6. REFERENCES

Arthur PG, Jones TR, Spruce J, Hartmann PE. Measuring short-term rates of milk synthesis in breastfeeding mothers. Q J Exp Physiol 1989;74:419-428.

Ellis LA, Mastro MA, Picciano MF. Milk-borne prolactin and neonatal development. J Mammary Gland Biol Neoplasia 1996;1:259-269.

TRANSFER OF METFORMIN INTO HUMAN MILK

T. Hale, J. Kristensen, L. Hackett, R. Kohan, and K. Ilett

1. INTRODUCTION

In the past decade Type II diabetes has increased by 30%, particularly in younger people, including pregnant women (Rosenbloom et al. 1998, 1999). In addition, the use of metformin for treating polycystic ovarian syndrome (PCOS) has increased (Knockenhauer et al. 1998). PCOS affects approximately 5% of reproductive age patients. Metformin has been found to improve ovulatory function in insulin-resistant women with PCOS, to reduce first trimester miscarriage (Glueck et al. 2001), and to decrease the progression from impaired glucose tolerance to Type II diabetes mellitus (Inzucchi 2002). Therefore using metformin while breastfeeding is important, although to date no data are available on transfer of metformin into human milk or to the breastfed infant. The aim of this study was to characterize milk/plasma ratio (M/P) and infant dose for metformin in breastfeeding women and determine plasma concentrations and any effects in their infants. The hypothesis is that maternal metformin use is safe for the breastfed infant.

2. METHODS

Seven women taking metformin (median dose 1500 mg orally daily) and their infants were studied. Metformin concentrations in plasma and milk were measured by high-performance liquid chromatography. Infant exposure was estimated as the product of estimated milk production rate and average drug concentration in milk, and also expressed as a percentage of the weight-normalized maternal dose.

3. RESULTS

The mean M/P for metformin was 0.35 (95% CI 0.2–0.5). The mean of its average concentrations in milk over the dose interval was 0.27 mg/L (0.15–0.39 mg/L). The absolute infant dose averaged 0.04 mg kg^{-1} day^{-1} (0.02–0.06 mg kg^{-1} day^{-1}), and the mean

---

Texas Tech University Health Sciences Center, King Edward Memorial & Princess Margaret Hospital, The Western Australian Centre for Pathology, University of Western Australia

Protecting Infants through Human Milk, edited by Pickering *et al.*
Kluwer Academic/Plenum Publishers, 2004

relative infant dose was 0.28% (0.16%–0.4%). Metformin was present in low or undetectable concentrations in the plasma of four of the infants who were sampled. No health problems were found in the six infants who were evaluated.

4. CONCLUSIONS

The concentrations of metformin in human milk were generally low and the mean infant exposure to the drug was only 0.28% of the weight-normalized maternal dose. Since this is well below the 10% level of concern for breastfeeding, and the infants were healthy, we conclude that metformin use by breastfeeding mothers is safe. Nevertheless, each decision to breastfeed should be made after conducting a risk:benefit analysis for the individual mother and her infant.

5. REFERENCES

Glueck CJ, Phillips H, Cameron D, Sieve-Smith L, Wang P. Continuing metformin throughout pregnancy in women with polycystic ovary syndrome appears to safely reduce first-trimester spontaneous abortion: a pilot study. Fertil Steril 200;175:46-52.

Inzucchi SE. Oral antihyperglycemic therapy for type 2 diabetes: scientific review. JAMA 2002;287:360-372.

Knochenhauer ES, Key TJ, Kahsar-Miller M, Waggoner W, Boots LR, Azziz R. Prevalence of the polycystic ovary syndrome in unselected black and white women of the southeastern United States: a prospective study. J Clin Endocrinol Metab 1998;83:3078-3082.

Rosenbloom AL, House DV, Winter WE. Non-insulin dependent diabetes mellitus (NIDDM) in minority youth: research priorities and needs. Clin Pediatr (Phila) 1998;37:143-152.

Rosenbloom AL, Joe JR, Young RS, Winter WE. Emerging epidemic of type 2 diabetes in youth. Diabetes Care 1999;22:345–354.

PSEUDOEPHEDRINE EFFECTS ON MILK PRODUCTION IN WOMEN AND ESTIMATION OF INFANT EXPOSURE VIA HUMAN MILK

T. Hale, K. Ilett, P. Hartmann, K. Aljazaf, L. Mitoulas, J. Kristensen, and L. Hackett

1. INTRODUCTION

There have been numerous anecdotal reports that pseudoephedrine use results in decreased milk production (Anderson 2000). This study was carried out to determine milk production, plasma prolactin levels, blood flow to the breast, and milk levels of pseudoephedrine following a maternal dose of 60 mg. Pseudoephedrine is a sympathomimetic amine (alpha-adrenoceptor agonist) that enjoys wide use as a nasal mucous membrane and sinus decongestant. The drug has been detected in the milk of three nursing mothers (at 3, 3, and 18 months of lactation) after ingestion of a single dose of a combined pseudoephedrine HCl 60 mg /triprolidine HCl 2.5 mg tablet (Findlay et al. 1984). The average concentration in milk over 24 hours was 264 μg/L. Although milk production was not measured, it was calculated that this would correspond to a relative infant dose of around 5% of the weight-adjusted maternal dose.

2. METHODS

Eight breastfeeding mothers received either a 60 mg pseudoephedrine hydrochloride tablet or an identical placebo tablet orally. Plasma prolactin levels were drawn at zero time and at 60 minutes following the dose of pseudoephedrine or placebo. Twenty-four hour milk production studies were done during the treatment and placebo phases. On both study days, fore- and hind-milk samples (1–5 mL) were collected from both breasts using an electric pump immediately before dose administration and again at 1, 2, 3, 4, 5, 8, 12, and 24 hours after dose. Aliquots of each sample were reserved for analysis of fat content and pseudoephedrine analysis. Blood flow in both breasts was measured on both study

Texas Tech University Health Sciences Center, University of Western Australia, Curtin University of Technology, King Edward Memorial & Princess Margaret Hospital, The Western Australian Centre for Pathology and Medical Research

days before drug/placebo administration and again after 1, 2, 3, and 4 hours after dose using an ultrasound machine.

3. RESULTS

At the time of peak drug concentration in milk, breast blood flow was not different from control. Plasma prolactin levels were similar for placebo and active drug periods. However, average milk volume was reduced by a mean of 21% from 784±288 mL/day in the placebo period to 623±300 mL/day in the active drug period (t=2.6, P=0.005). The estimated infant dose of pseudoephedrine at the usual maximum of 60 mg four times daily to steady-state was 4.3±1.3% of the weight-adjusted maternal dose.

4. CONCLUSION

A single dose of pseudoephedrine significantly reduced milk production; this effect was not attributable to changes in blood flow or prolactin secretion. At maximum pseudoephedrine doses given to steady-state, the calculated infant dose via milk was <10% of the maternal dose, and breastfeeding is unlikely to adversely affect the infant. Nevertheless, decreased milk production may be unwanted and the drug, therefore, should be used cautiously. However, in select instances the drug may be useful to suppress lactation.

5. REFERENCES

Anderson PO. Decongestants and milk production. J Hum Lact 2000;16:294.

Findlay JW, Butz RF, Sailstad JM, Warren JT, Welch RM. Pseudoephedrine and triprolidine in plasma and breast milk of nursing mothers. Br J Clin Pharmacol 1984;18:901-906.

THE ANTI-INFECTIVE ACTIVITY OF HUMAN MILK IS POTENTIALLY GREATER THAN THE SUM OF ITS MICROBICIDAL COMPONENTS

C.E. Isaacs and J.H. Jia

1. INTRODUCTION

The immune system present in human milk must inactivate a wide spectrum of microorganisms. In order to accomplish this function milk contains multiple protective factors, many of which interact in an additive or synergistic manner. Antimicrobial factors in human milk provide layers of protection using multiple, often redundant, mechanisms that attack pathogens by various mechanisms. As a result of milk containing combinations of protective factors with complementary properties, the total antimicrobial activity provided to the infant's gastrointestinal tract is likely to be significantly greater than is suggested by measuring microbicidal components individually. The present study was undertaken to determine the effect of using antiviral lipids and peptides alone and in combination on the minimum concentrations of each factor required to inactivate herpes simplex virus (HSV).

2. METHODS

Approximately 10^5 50% tissue culture infective doses of HSV-1 or HSV-2 were mixed with lipid, peptide, or a lipid plus peptide mixture in RPMI-1640 tissue culture medium at the indicated concentration. Incubations were for 1 hour at 37°C. Virus mixed only with medium was used as a control. Following incubation, the infectivity of each mixture was titered by the serial dilution end point method. Dilutions (10-fold) in medium were inoculated into monolayers of Vero (HSV-1) or CV-1 (HSV-2) cells. Virus titers were determined by measuring the cytopathic effect at each dilution. The difference between the titer ($\log_{10}$) of the control virus and the titers of treated virus was used as a measure of antiviral activity.

Institute for Basic Research in Developmental Disabilities, Department of Developmental Biochemistry, 1050 Forest Hill Road, Staten Island, NY 10314

Protecting Infants through Human Milk, edited by Pickering *et al.*
Kluwer Academic/Plenum Publishers, 2004

3. RESULTS

Of five peptides tested against HSV-1, D2A21 (Demegen, Pittsburgh, PA) was the most effective in inactivation of HSV-1 (Table 1). Both magainins and the lentivirus lytic peptide (LLP) did not display significant antiviral activity. The human defensin (HNP-1) inactivated HSV-1 but less strongly than D2A21. The results with D2A21 and HNP-1 showed that in the presence of serum, relatively high concentrations of peptide were required to reduce HSV-1 titers by 3 $\log_{10}$ (1,000-fold) or greater.

When the monoglyceride ether octyl glycerol was utilized by itself, a concentration of 10 to 15 mM was required to inactivate ≥3 $\log_{10}$ of HSV-1. This effective antiviral range of lipid is the same as has been found in previous studies with *Chlamydia trachomatis* (Lampe et al. 1998), as well as *Neisseria gonorrhoeae* and *Trichomonas vaginalis*. Experiments were then done combining D2A21 and octyl glycerol to determine whether their antiviral activities were additive.

Octyl glycerol (3 mM) reduced the titer of HSV-1 by 1 to 1.5 $\log_{10}$ (10- to 30-fold) over a 1-hour incubation period. When D2A21 (20 µg/mL) was added to the mixture an additional drop in virus titer of 3 $\log_{10}$ (1,000-fold) was found at 1 hour when compared with the lipid only effect. Raising the peptide concentration to 50 µg/mL in combination with octyl glycerol reduced the HSV-1 titer by 4 $\log_{10}$ (10,000-fold) after 1 hour and by at least 6 $\log_{10}$ (1,000,000-fold) by 2 hours.

Mixtures of octyl glycerol and D2A21 also inactivated HSV-2. A D2A21 concentration of 10 µg/mL combined with lipid reduced the titer of HSV-2 by 2 $\log_{10}$ (100-fold) between 1 and 3 hours of incubation. Doubling the D2A21 concentration to 20 µg/mL reduced the concentration of HSV-2 by 3 to 4 $\log_{10}$ (1,000–10,000 fold) after 1 hour incubation and by more than 10,000-fold by 2 hours.

Table 1. Inactivation of HSV-1 and HSV-2 by antimicrobial peptides and lipid[a]

Lipid[b]	Peptide	Peptide concentration (µg/mL)	Viral titer reduced by ≥1,000-fold	Virus
–	D2A21	200	Yes	HSV-1
–	HNP-1	400	Yes	HSV-1
–	Magainin I	1,000	No	HSV-1
–	Magainin II	1,000	No	HSV-1
–	LLP	200	No	HSV-1
+	–	–	No	HSV-1
+	D2A21	20	Yes	HSV-1
+	D2A21	20	Yes	HSV-2

[a]Incubations were done in the presence of 10% fetal bovine serum for 1 hour at 37°C.
[b]1-O-octyl-sn-glycerol (3 mM)

4. CONCLUSIONS

When the lipid ether 1-O-octyl-sn-glycerol was used in combination with the antimicrobial peptide D2A21, the peptide concentration could be reduced by at least 90 percent and still decrease the titers of HSV-1 and HSV-2 by >1,000-fold in 1 hour. These results suggest that antimicrobial compounds in human milk (lipids) can potentiate the activity of other protective compounds found both in milk and in the infant's gastro-intestinal tract (antimicrobial peptides).

Antimicrobial substances present in human milk at suboptimal levels may still contribute to the protective function of milk. The true antimicrobial potential of human milk may only be determined by assaying protective factors in combination microbicidal mixtures.

5. ACKNOWLEDGMENTS

This work was supported in part by grant AI39061-08 from the NIH and the New York State Office of Mental Retardation and Developmental Disabilities.

6. REFERENCE

Lampe MF, Ballweber LM, Isaacs CE, Patton DL, Stamm WE. Killing of *Chlamydia trachomatis* by novel antimicrobial lipids adapted from compounds in human breast milk. Antimicrobial Agents Chemother 1998;42:1239-1244.

HUMAN MILK OLIGOSACCHARIDE BLOOD GROUP EPITOPES AND INNATE IMMUNE PROTECTION AGAINST CAMPYLOBACTER AND CALICIVIRUS DIARRHEA IN BREASTFED INFANTS

A.L. Morrow[1], G.M. Ruiz-Palacios[2], M. Altaye[1], X. Jiang[1], M.L. Guerrero[2], J.K. Meinzen-Derr[1], T. Farkas[1], P. Chaturvedi[3], L.K. Pickering[4], and D.S. Newburg[3]

1. INTRODUCTION

Human milk contains a variety of bioactive agents, including oligosaccharides, which are part of the innate defense system (Hanson et al. 1991; Zopf & Roth 1996; Newburg et al. 1998; Erney et al. 2000; Hamosh 2001; Chaturvedi et al. 2001). Oligosaccharides are the third largest solid constituent of human milk after lactose and lipids (Stahl et al. 1994; Zopf & Roth 1996; Erney et al. 2000; Chaturvedi et al. 2001; Hamosh 2001). α1,2-Linked fucosylated oligosaccharides in human milk have been shown to inhibit host ligand binding to campylobacter, caliciviruses, and other enteric pathogens (Newburg et al. 1990; Crane et al. 1994; Marionneau et al. 2002; Ruiz-Palacios et al. 2003; Huang et al. 2003). Significant variation exists between mothers in the quantity of α1,2-linked fucosylated oligosaccharides in their milk. We conducted this study in breastfed infants to determine the clinical relevance of the observed variation in human milk fucosylated oligosaccharides in relation to protection offered infants against diarrhea due to *Campylobacter jejuni* and caliciviruses.

2. METHODS

We analyzed samples and data from 93 breastfeeding mother-infant pairs included in a cohort study conducted in San Pedro Martir, Mexico City. These study pairs were followed from birth to two years postpartum. Infant illness and feeding history were

[1]Center for Epidemiology & Biostatistics (ALM, MA, JKM-D) and Division of Infectious Diseases (XJ, TF), Cincinnati Children's Hospital Medical Center, 3333 Burnet Avenue, Cincinnati, OH 45229-3039
[2]Departamento de Infectología, Instituto Nacional de Ciencias Médicas y Nutrición, México City, México
[3]Program in Glycobiology, Shriver Center, University of Massachusetts Medical School, Waltham, MA
[4]National Immunization Program, Centers for Disease Control and Prevention, Atlanta, GA

collected by trained field workers who made weekly home visits. Milk samples were collected from mothers weekly in the first month, and monthly thereafter. Diarrhea was attributed to campylobacter or calicivirus if the pathogen was detected in a stool sample collected during or within seven days of an episode of diarrhea. Diarrhea episodes associated with two or more pathogens were excluded from pathogen-specific analyses. Concentrations of fucosylated oligosaccharides were determined by HPLC from milk samples collected one to five weeks postpartum. Data were analyzed by Poisson regression.

3. RESULTS

The 93 mother-infant pairs in this study were monitored for 857 breastfeeding infant-months and 765 post-breastfeeding infant-months between birth and 2 years of age. None practiced exclusive breastfeeding. Milk oligosaccharide concentrations ranged from 1.0 to 36.1 nmol/L. Total 2-linked fucosylated oligosaccharide concentrations ranged from 0.8 to 20.8 nmol/L (50 to 92 percent of milk oligosaccharide). Milk from all study mothers contained α1,2-linked fucosyloligosaccharides, including: lacto-*N*-fucopentaose I (LNF-I), 2′-fucosyllactose (2′-FL), lacto-*N*-difucohexaose I (LDFH-I), and lactodifucotetraose (LDFT) [Table 1]. A total of 234 diarrhea episodes were identified during breastfeeding (median, 2 diarrhea episodes per child; range, 0–12 episodes per child). The incidence of all diarrhea was 28.8 cases per 100 child-months of breastfeeding. A total of 77 (33%) diarrhea episodes were moderate-to-severe; the incidence of moderate-to-severe diarrhea during breastfeeding was 9.5 cases per 100 child-months. During breastfeeding, protection against diarrhea due to *C. jejuni* (n=31 cases) was significantly (P=0.004) associated with 2′-FL; protection against calicivirus diarrhea (n=16 cases); was significantly (P=0.012) associated with LDFH-I; and protection against moderate-to-severe diarrhea was associated with LNF-I (P<0.001), 2′-FL (P<0.001), and LDFH-I (P=0.002) as percentages of total milk oligosaccharides [Table 2]. Post-breastfeeding, no

Table 1. Characterization of the concentration (mean±SD) and percent of specific and total α1,2-linked fucosylated oligosaccharides in maternal milk

Milk oligosaccharide	Concentration (nmol/L)	Percent of milk oligosaccharides[a]
	Mean±SD	
Lacto-*N*-fucopentaose I (LNF-I)	3.21±1.75	25.1±9.9
2'-Fucosyllactose (2'-FL)	3.85±1.04	33.7±10.4
Lacto-*N*-difucohexaose I (LDFH-I)	1.26±1.00	9.5±5.7
Lactodifucotetraose (LDFT)	0.70±0.72	5.1±3.4
Total 2-linked fucosyloligosaccharide	9.02±3.23	73.3±8.8
Total milk oligosaccharide[b]	12.44±4.8	100

[a]Percent of milk oligosaccharide is the quantity of each specific oligosaccharide divided by the total quantity of the milk oligosaccharides measured in this study.

[b]Total milk oligosaccharide includes eight oligosaccharides: the four 2-linked fucosylated oligosaccharides, two non-2-linked fucosylated oligosaccharides (3-FL and LNF-II) and their two precursors.

association was observed between maternal milk oligosaccharides and infant risk. These relationships were not confounded by maternal, infant, or other factors.

Table 2. Univariate analyses of specific α1,2-linked fucosylated oligosaccharides as a percent of milk oligosaccharide and protection against *C. jejuni*-associated diarrhea and calicivirus-associated diarrhea in study children, by Poisson regression[a]

Pathogen	No. Cases[b]	Milk oligosaccharide	β (SE)[a]	P
Campylobacter	31	2′-FL	–5.6 (1.9)	0.004
Calicivirus	16	LDFH-I	–13.3 (5.3)	0.012

[a]The model included only one independent variable, a specific 2-linked fucosylated oligosaccharide, as a percent of milk oligosaccharide, and pathogen-specific diarrhea as the dependent variable. Negative beta coefficients indicate protection.

[b]22 subjects had 31 cases of campylobacter diarrhea, 13 subjects had 16 cases of calicivirus diarrhea.

4. CONCLUSIONS

This is the first study to provide evidence that variation in specific human milk oligosaccharides is associated with protection of infants against specific pathogens and all causes of diarrhea. Our findings underscore the importance of breastfeeding, define specific protective factors, and suggest the potential to develop novel oral agents that prevent diarrhea caused by different pathogens.

5. ACKNOWLEDGMENT

This work was supported by a program project grant from the National Institute of Child Health and Human Development (HD13021).

6. REFERENCES

Chaturvedi P, Warren CD, Altaye M, Morrow AL, Ruiz-Palacios G, Pickering LK, Newburg DS. Fucosylated human milk oligosaccharides vary between individuals and over the course of lactation. Glycobiology 2001;11:365-372.

Crane JK, Azar SS, Stam A, Newburg DS. Oligosaccharides from human milk block binding and activity of the *Escherichia coli* heat-stable enterotoxin (STa) in T84 intestinal cells. J Nutr 1994;124:2358-2364.

Erney RM, Malone WT, Skelding MB, Marcon AA, Kleman-Leyer KM, O'Ryan ML, Ruiz-Palacios G, Hilty MD, Pickering LK, Prieto PA. Variability of human milk neutral oligosaccharides in a diverse population. J Pediatr Gastroenterol Nutr 2000;30:181-192.

Hamosh M. Bioactive factors in human milk. Pediatr Clin North Am 2001;48:69-86.

Hanson LA, Jalil F, Ashraf R, Bernini S, Carlsson B, Cruz JR, Gonzalez T, Hahn-Zoric M, Mellander L, Minoli Y, Moro G, Nave F, Zaman S, Mata L, Karlberg J, Lindblad BS. Characteristics of human milk antibodies and their effect in relation to the epidemiology of breastfeeding and infections in a developing country. Adv Exp Med Biol 1991;310:1-15.

Huang P, Farkas T, Marionneau S, Zhong W, Ruvoen-Clouet DVM, Morrow AL, Altaye M, Pickering LK, Newburg DS, LePendu J, Jiang X. Noroviruses bind to human ABO, Lewis and secretor histo-blood group antigens: identification of 4 distinct strain-specific patterns. J Infect Dis 2003;188:19-31.

Marionneau S, Ruvoen N, Le Moullac-Vaidye B, Clement M, Cailleau-Thomas A, Ruiz-Palacois G, Huang P, Jiang X, Le Pendu J. Norwalk virus binds to histo-blood group antigens present on gastroduodenal epithelial cells of secretor individuals. Gastroenterology 2002;122:1967-1977.

Newburg DS, Pickering LK, McCluer RH, Cleary TG. Fucosylated oligosaccharides of human milk protect suckling mice from heat-stabile enterotoxin of *Escherichia coli.* J Infect Dis 1990;162:1075-1080.

Newburg D, Peterson J, Ruiz-Palacios G, Matson D, Morrow A, Shults J, Guerrero M, Chaturvedi P, Newburg S, Scallan C, Taylor M, Ceriani R, Pickering L. Role of human-milk lactadherin in protection against symptomatic rotavirus infection. Lancet 1998;351:1160-1164.

Ruiz-Palacios GM, Cervantes LE, Ramos P, Chavez-Munguia B, Newburg DS. Campylobacter jejuni binds intestinal H(O) antigen (Fucα1,2Galβ1,4GlcNAc), and fucosyloligosaccharides of human milk inhibit its binding and infection. J Biol Chem 2003;278:14112-14120.

Stahl B, Thurl S, Zeng J, Karas M, Hillenkamp F, Steup M, Sawatzki G. Oligosaccharides from human milk as revealed by matrix-assisted laser desorption/ionization mass spectrometry. Anal Biochem 1994;223:218-226.

Zopf D, Roth S. Oligosaccharide anti-infective agents. Lancet 1996;347:1017-1021.

HUMAN MILK CONTAINS ELEMENTS THAT BLOCK BINDING OF NOROVIRUSES TO HISTO-BLOOD GROUP ANTIGENS IN SALIVA

Xi Jiang[1], Pengwei Huang[1], Weiming Zhong[1], Ardythe L. Morrow[1], Guillermo M. Ruiz-Palacios[2], and Larry K. Pickering[3]

1. INTRODUCTION

Noroviruses (NORs), previously known as Norwalk-like viruses, belong to one of four genera of caliciviruses. NORs mainly cause epidemics of acute gastroenteritis in humans. We found that NORs recognize human histo-blood group antigens as receptors. Recombinant virus-like particles (VLPs) of the prototype Norwalk virus (NV) specifically bind to human intestinal sections and saliva of secretors but not of nonsecretors (Marionneau et al. 2002). Human volunteer studies showed that nonsecretors who do not express the receptor antigens were naturally resistant to NV challenge (Lindesmith et al. 2002). Extended studies with additional NOR strains showed that different NOR strains recognize different receptors defined by the ABO, Lewis, and secretor types (Huang et al. 2003). Four binding patterns of NORs have been described based on studies of saliva samples. Three patterns bind to saliva of secretors with ABO, AO, and AB types, and one pattern binds to saliva containing Lewis epitopes. The sugar moiety of these antigens are believed to be involved in NOR binding.

Human milk is rich in oligosaccharides that are either in free forms or conjugates of glycoproteins or glycolipids. It also is known that human milk expresses histo-blood group antigens similar to those in other body fluids such as saliva and on mucosal epithelial cells. In this study we characterized human milk for expression of histo-blood group antigens and for their interaction with NOR.

2. METHODS

A total of 60 milk samples from 60 women, 30 from Mexico and 30 from the United States, involved in a rotavirus vaccine study, were evaluated. The baculovirus-expressed

[1]Division of Infectious Diseases (XJ, PH, WZ), and Center for Epidemiology & Biostatistics (ALM), Cincinnati Children's Hospital Medical Center, 3333 Burnet Avenue, Cincinnati, OH 45229-3039
[2]Departamento de Infectologia, Instituto Nacional de Ciencias Médicas y Nutrición, México City, México
[3]National Immunization Program, Centers for Disease Control and Prevention, Atlanta, GA

Protecting Infants through Human Milk, edited by Pickering *et al.*
Kluwer Academic/Plenum Publishers, 2004

recombinant VLPs representing the four binding patterns (NV, VA387, MOH, and VA207 that bind to AO, ABH, AB, and Lewis antigens, respectively) to human saliva samples were studied (Huang et al. 2003). Monoclonal antibodies (MAbs) specific for human histo-blood group antigens were used to determine the blood types of milk donors by enzyme immunoassays (EIAs) (Huang et al. 2003). To determine NOR binding to milk samples, the EIAs to measure NOR VLP binding to histo-blood group antigens in saliva were followed (Huang et al. 2003). The same EIAs also were used to test milk samples blocking NOR binding to human histo-blood group antigens. Milk samples used in these assays were boiled to inactivate antibodies that may interfere with the assays.

3. RESULTS

Six (11%) mothers had high levels (OD>0.2) of Le^a and low or undetectable Le^b in their milk samples, and these six mothers were assigned as nonsecretors (Le^{a+b-}). Forty-nine (82%) mothers had high levels (OD>0.4) of Le^b and low or undetectable Le^a in their milk, and these 49 mothers were assigned as secretors (Le^{a-b+}). The remaining five (8%) mothers had low levels of both Le^a and Le^b (Le^{a-b-}) but detectable H-type 1 antigen in their milk, and these five mothers were assigned as Lewis negative secretors. The number of subjects with a nonsecretor phenotype was slightly lower in these two populations (13% in Norfolk, Virginia, and 7% in Mexico City) compared with that of the European and North American populations (20%).

When the milk samples were tested for type A and type B antigens, none of the 60 milk samples revealed a positive reaction, suggesting the A and B antigens were not expressed in milk. This result was confirmed by later findings that none of the 60 milk samples reacted with the A and B antigen-binding strain (MOH, see results below). However, when serum samples from the 60 mothers were tested for ABO types using the immune hemagglutination assay, a normal distribution of ABO types among the 60 mothers was found. Sixteen mothers were type A, four type B, one type AB, and the remaining 39 were type O.

Milk samples from all 54 secretors, but none of the six nonsecretors, blocked the bindings of VA387 and NV to a secretor saliva sample (Fig. 1). Milk samples from all six nonsecretors blocked VA207 binding to a nonsecretor saliva sample. Milk samples from the 54 secretors revealed variable lower blocking activity against VA207, consistent with the previous observation that VA207 also binds to saliva of secretors (Huang et al. 2003). None of the 60 milk samples blocked MOH binding to a type A saliva (data not shown), consistent with the above observation of lack of expression of type A and type B antigens in human milk. Cow milk did not show any blocking activity (data not shown).

Milk samples with high blocking activity also had high binding activity with VA387 and NV. None of the six nonsecretors bound to these two strains (Fig. 1). Milk samples from five of the six nonsecretors reacted with VA207. None of the 60 milk samples bound to MOH (data not shown). These results are consistent with the above milk typing and blocking results. However, due to some unknown factors in the milk that might interfere with the direct binding EIAs, the binding results were not as clear as those of the blocking experiments. Significant numbers of milk samples from secretors did not react with VA387 and NV. Milk samples from four secretors apparently had higher binding activity with VA387 and NV than the remaining secretors. The same four mothers also were high-binders to VA207. Different treatments of milk samples (freezing/thawing,

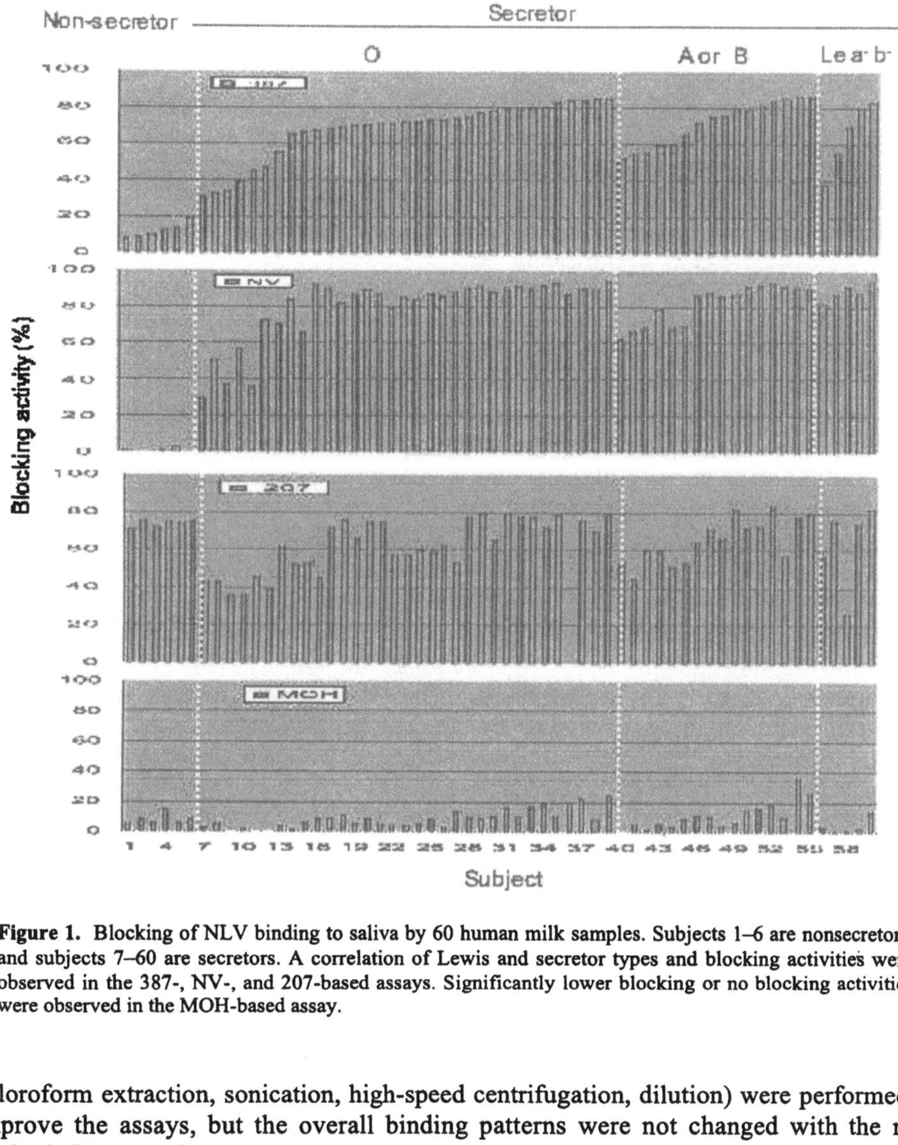

Figure 1. Blocking of NLV binding to saliva by 60 human milk samples. Subjects 1–6 are nonsecretors, and subjects 7–60 are secretors. A correlation of Lewis and secretor types and blocking activities were observed in the 387-, NV-, and 207-based assays. Significantly lower blocking or no blocking activities were observed in the MOH-based assay.

chloroform extraction, sonication, high-speed centrifugation, dilution) were performed to improve the assays, but the overall binding patterns were not changed with the new methods (data not shown).

Milk secretory IgAs against the four strains of rNORs (NV, VA387, MOH and VA207) were tested to determine the exposure history of the mothers to NORs. Significant numbers of secretors, but none of the six nonsecretors, had antibodies (titers >1:160) against NV and VA387 (19 [35%] and 23 [43%] of the 54 secretor women, respectively). One [17%] nonsecretor woman and 18 [33%] secretor women had antibodies (titer >1:160) against VA207. Milk antibodies against MOH were detected in 14 [26%] secretors but in none of the 6 nonsecretors. Three [17%] of 18 type A and/or type B secretors and 11 [31%] of the 36 type O secretors had antibodies against MOH. All of the 14 mothers who had antibodies against MOH also had antibodies against VA387, suggesting shared antigenic epitopes may exist between MOH and VA387.

4. DISCUSSION

In summary, human milk contains the Lewis and secretor antigens, and these antigens potentially are responsible for blocking NOR VLP binding to histo-blood group antigens. In a separate study we observed that breastfed infants were less likely to have NOR diarrhea when the concentrations of secretor antigens (Lewis b antigens) of their mothers' milk were high (Morrow et al. 2004; this volume). Thus, we hypothesize that the soluble human blood group antigens (HBGA) in human milk may provide protective effects to breastfed infants against NOR infection by acting as decoy receptors to block NOR attachment to the HBGA receptors on the intestinal epithelial cells.

The biological significance of lack of expression of the A and B antigens in human milk is unclear. The A and B antigens are strong immunogens that can cause antibody-related hemolysis in blood transfusion. This could be a selective pressure to avoid early induction of the antibody response in breastfed infants. It also sacrifices the infants from lack of protection against the infection with the MOH-like strains by their mothers' milk. A report of failure of human milk protecting a child from diarrhea caused by a genogroup II NOR supports this hypothesis. MOH also is a genogroup II virus.

This is the first report of histo-blood group antigen in human milk that is related to binding with NORs. There are still many questions that need to be addressed. The hypothesis of milk histo-blood group antigens protecting infants from NOR infection remains to be confirmed. The methods for treatment of milk samples for characterization of histo-blood group antigens also need to be improved. Further studies to address these issues are necessary for better understanding of the NOR/receptor interaction, which may result in development of strategies to control and prevent NOR infection.

5. ACKNOWLEDGMENT

This work was supported by a program project grant from the National Institute of Child Health and Human Development (HD13021).

6. REFERENCES

Huang P, Farkas T, Marionneau S, Zhong W, Ruvoën-Clouet DVM, Morrow AL, Altaye M, Pickering LK, Newburg DS, LePendu J, Jiang X. Noroviruses bind to human ABO, Lewis and secretor histo-blood group antigens: identification of 4 distinct strain-specific patterns. J Infect Dis 2003;188:19-31.

Lindesmith L, Moe C, LePendu J, Jiang X, Baric R. Determinants of susceptibility and protective immunity to Norwalk virus infection. International Congress of Virology, Annual Meeting, Paris, France, July 27-August 2, 2002.

Marionneau S, Ruvoen N, Le Moullac-Vaidye B, Clement M, Cailleau-Thomas A, Ruiz-Palacios G, Huang PW, Jiang X, Le Pendu J. Norwalk virus binds to H typeS 1/3 histo-blood group antigens present on gastro-duodenal epithelial cells of "secretor" individuals. Gastroenterology 2002;122:1967-1977.

Morrow AL, Ruiz-Palacios GM, Altaye M, Jiang X, Guerrero ML, Meinzen-Derr JK, Farkas T, Chaturvedi P, Pickering LK, Newburg DS. Human milk oligosaccharide blood group epitopes and innate immune protection against campylobacter and calicivirus in breastfed infants. In: Pickering LK, Morrow AL, Ruiz-Palacios GM, Schanler RJ. Protecting Infants through Human Milk: Advancing the Scientific Evidence. Advances in Experimental Medicine and Biology Series. New York: Kluwer Academic/Plenum Publishers, 2004; this volume.

BREASTFEEDING AND NATURAL COLONIZATION WITH *LACTOBACILLUS* SPP AS PROTECTION AGAINST ROTAVIRUS-ASSOCIATED DIARRHEA

M.L. Guerrero, S. Moreno-Espinosa, F. Tuz-Dzib, J. Solís-Albino, H. Ortega-Gallegos, and G.M. Ruiz-Palacios

1. INTRODUCTION

Group A human rotavirus (HRV) is the leading cause of severe diarrhea among infants and young children throughout the world (Parashar et al. 2003). Each year, HRV causes approximately 111 million episodes of gastroenteritis, 2 million hospitalizations, and an estimated 352,000 to 592,000 deaths in children under 5 years of age. The lower incidence of disease in breastfed infants may be due to a variety of reasons, but the most important determinant may be the composition of bioactive protective factors in human milk. These protective factors can be grouped into those that: (a) inhibit attachment and invasion of pathogens, such as secretory antibodies, multifunctional agents, including fatty acids and lactoferrin, and homologs of host cell-surface glycoconjugates; and (b) factors that promote development of the infant's enteric flora (Newburg 2000).

Intestinal colonization starts immediately after delivery and is a dynamic process modified by diverse factors. The type of diet influences the composition of the intestinal microflora. The intestinal flora of breastfed infants is dominated by *Bifidobacterium* and *Lactobacillus* species, in contrast to formula-fed infants, whose pattern of intestinal colonization is closer to that of an adult, including anaerobes, enterococcus, and Gram-negative bacilli (Walker 2000; Salminen & Deighton 1992). The effect of human milk on the intestinal flora is caused in large part by oligosaccharides, which are a major component of human milk. Intestinal flora play an important role in protection against enteric infections, competing with pathogens for attachment sites and nutrients, producing antimicrobial substances, and stimulating immune response (Salminen & Deighton 1992).

Several studies have found that, although HRV infection occurs in breastfed infants, the severity of disease is substantially less than that in formula-fed children (Newburg et al. 1998). Clinical and experimental studies have shown that intake of viable *Lactobacillus* spp induces intestinal colonization and protects against HRV diarrhea (Kaila et al. 1992; Yasui et al. 1995). The disease burden of HRV is so great that the search for

Departamento de Infectologia, Instituto Nacional de Ciencias Médicas y Nutrición – Salvador Zubirán, Vasco de Quiroga No. 15, Delegacion Tlalpan, México D.F. V 14000, México

Protecting Infants through Human Milk, edited by Pickering *et al.*
Kluwer Academic/Plenum Publishers, 2004

low-cost and effective methods to prevent this disease is a global priority for public health. The aim of the present study was to determine whether breastfeeding and the natural intestinal colonization with *Lactobacillus* spp protect children against HRV-associated diarrhea.

2. METHODS

2.1. Design

We conducted a case-control study nested within a prospectively designed cohort study. Children were followed longitudinally during a winter season. Trained field workers visited each household once a week to interview each child's mother, collecting information about changes in feeding patterns and daily occurrence of diarrhea, including stool frequency, number, and consistency since the previous visit. Cases of diarrhea were monitored by a pediatrician during the first 24 hours of disease until 7 days after the end of the episode. Whenever diarrhea occurred, a stool sample was tested for HRV. A stool sample was collected every other week and tested qualitatively and quantitatively for *Lactobacillus* spp. Children with HRV-associated diarrhea were age-matched with children without HRV infection in a three controls per each case ratio.

2.2. Setting

This study was conducted in San Pedro Martir, a low-income periurban area on the southwestern outskirts of Mexico City, where physicians, nurses, and field workers from the Instituto Nacional de Ciencias Médicas y Nutrición have been providing health care for families enrolled in community-based studies since 1983.

2.3. Participants

Children from 0 to 18 months of age were eligible for enrollment if they were full-term and had no underlying disease, no history of neonatal hospitalization, a normal immune system, no other factor that would modified intestinal colonization, and belonged to a family that planned to remain in the community during the study period.

2.4. Main Outcome Measure

We compared the *Lactobacillus* spp counts in stool specimens from children with HRV-associated diarrhea and *Lactobacillus* spp counts in children not infected with HRV, adjusted by age.

3. RESULTS

One hundred fifty-seven infants were included (51% female) and 132 (84%) children completed the study. All children were monitored from October 1998 to May 1999, for a total of 1,029 child-months (mean 6.5 months, SD 2.22). A total of 169 episodes of diarrhea were identified. The overall incidence of diarrhea, irrespective of etiology was 17.8 episodes/100 child-months. HRV was identified in 16 episodes of diarrhea. The overall incidence of HRV-associated diarrhea was 1.56 episodes/100 child-months.

Fifteen children (54% female) with HRV-associated diarrhea were age-matched with 45 children (60% female) not infected with HRV. *Lactobacillus* spp counts were done in samples obtained 15 days prior to HRV-associated diarrhea episodes.

Total *Lactobacillus* spp counts were lower in children with HRV-associated diarrhea (geometric mean 4.19) than in HRV-free infants (geometric mean 5.7, P=0.01). Breastfed children had higher *Lactobacillus* spp counts than nonbreastfed children (Log likelihood ratio X^2=4.73, P=0.02). Due to the high correlation among different types of feeding and age (r = 0.70, P<0.001) in the bivariate model of logistic regression, one of the variables should have been excluded in order to make possible the estimation of the model. Furthermore, we observed an important instability in the iterative estimation of the model that could be explained by the existing colinearity and the reduced sample size. Due to these factors, and in order to use detailed information of these variables, avoiding the existing colinearity, and taking advantage of all the collected information about the number of times that the child consumed the different types of foods in 24 hours, Principal Component Analysis was conducted instead of analyzing data as dichotomous variables (Johnson 2000; SPSS 2002). The suspected colinearity in the multivariate correlation analysis was confirmed in the correlation matrix realized as the first step of the Principal Component Analysis. We observed a negative correlation between breastfeeding and consumption of formula (r = –0.78, P<0.001), breastfeeding and consumption of solid foods (r = –0.61, P<0.001), and a positive correlation between age and consumption of solid food (r = –0.70, P<0.001).

We obtained five principal components that explained 100% of variance. We considered the two first components because together they explained more than 75% of the total variance explained. The first component showed that 47% of the total variance was explained by variables associated with more or less risk of developing HRV-associated diarrhea, including human milk, formula, solid foods, and age in months. The second component was related to the grade of intestinal colonization by *Lactobacillus* spp

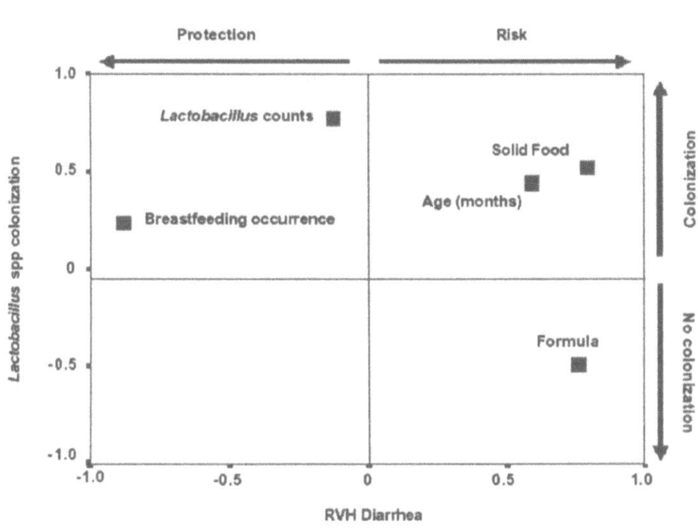

Figure 1. Graphic of components in rotated space

and showed 28% of the total variance explained. The graphic representation of the component analysis shows that higher occurrence of breastfeeding is associated with lower risk of HRV-associated diarrhea, and with a higher level of *Lactobacillus* spp colonization: higher level of *Lactobacillus* spp colonization diminishes the risk of having HRV-associated diarrhea; higher occurrence of bottle-feeding increases the risk of HRV-associated diarrhea and diminishes the probability of being colonized by *Lactobacillus* spp; higher frequency of feeding with solid foods, and older age, increase the risk of HRV-associated diarrhea and increase mildly the probability of being colonized by *Lactobacillus* spp (Fig. 1).

4. DISCUSSION

In this nested case-control study of 157 children from 0 to 18 months of age monitored during a winter season, we found an incidence of HRV-associated diarrhea of 1.56 episodes/100 child-months, which is low if compared with the incidence reported in the same community in a previous study (3.2 episodes/100 child-months), where children were followed during two years, including the winter season (Velazquez et al. 1993). This low incidence was similar to the one observed for another medical group in Mexico City (data unpublished), during the same winter season. Breastfeeding was a common practice in the studied community. Studies that showed differences of intestinal colonization pattern between breastfed and formula-fed children emphasize *Bifidobacterium* colonization and, to a lesser extent, colonization by *Lactobacillus* spp (Walker 2000). The reason we chose to quantify *Lactobacillus* instead of *Bifidobacterium* was because the reported experimental studies that show protection against HRV-associated diarrhea were done using *Lactobacillus* (Kaila et al. 1992). Several protector mechanisms had been proposed for *Lactobacillus* against gastroenteritis. We do not know precisely which mechanism is involved in protection against HRV, but the most likely mechanism is its role as an immunomodulator, as shown in previous studies in which *Lactobacillus* was administered to patients with HRV-associated diarrhea.

Principal Component Analysis allowed us to analyze each of the different variables independently, nullifying the effect of colinearity and giving specific value to each variable. We determined that breastfeeding protects against HRV-associated diarrhea proportionally to the number of feedings, with more feedings giving more protection. This protection against HRV-associated diarrhea conferred by breastfeeding occurred independently of the grade of intestinal colonization by *Lactobacillus* spp. Even colonization with *Lactobacillus* spp is proportional to the magnitude of exposure. *Lactobacillus* spp confer notably less protection than breastfeeding. While one of the protective mechanisms of breastfeeding is promotion of adequate and protective intestinal colonization, human milk also has other protective mechanisms including secretion of polymeric IgA and IgM, lactoferrin, lysozyme, cytokines, growth factors, and oligosaccharides (Newburg 1998; 2000). This existence of other protective elements can explain the independence of both variables. Although the mechanism of these effects are complex and not fully understood, dietary intervention to establish an intestinal microflora dominated by *Bifidobacterium* and *Lactobacillus* and breastfeeding promotion is recommended.

5. ACKNOWLEDGMENTS

We are indebted to the people of San Pedro Martir who participated in this study. This study was funded by a Program Project Grant mechanism through NICHD (HD13021).

6. REFERENCES

Johnson D. Análisis de componentes principales. In: Editores T, editor. Métodos multivariados aplicados al análisis de datos. México: Thomson Editores, 2000; pp 93-145.

Kaila M, Isolauri E, Soppi E, Virtanen E, Laine S, Arvilommi H. Enhancement of the circulating antibody secreting cell response in human diarrhea by a human Lactobacillus strain. Pediatr Res 1992;32:141-144.

Newburg DS. Are all human milks created equal? Variation in human milk oligosaccharides. J Pediatr Gastroenterol Nutr 2000;30:131-133.

Newburg D, Peterson J, Ruiz-Palacios G, Matson D, Morrow A, Shults J, Guerrero M, Chaturvedi P, Newburg S, Scallan C, Taylor M, Ceriani R, Pickering L. Role of human-milk lactadherin in protection against symptomatic rotavirus infection. Lancet 1998;351:1160-1164.

Parashar UD, Hummelman EG, Bresee JS, Miller MA, Glass RI. Global illness and deaths caused by rotavirus disease in children. Emerg Infect Dis 2003;9:565-572.

Salminen S, Deighton M. Lactic acid bacteria in the gut in normal and disordered states. Dig Dis 1992;10:227-238.

SPSS 11.5 Syntax Reference Guide, Base System, Advanced Models, Regression Models [program]. 11.5 version. Chicago: SPSS, Inc., 2002.

Velazquez FR, Calva JJ, Lourdes Guerrero M, Mass D, Glass RI, Pickering LK, Ruiz-Palacios GM. Cohort study of rotavirus serotype patterns in symptomatic and asymptomatic infections in Mexican children. Pediatr Infect Dis J 1993;12:54-61.

Walker WA. Role of nutrients and bacterial colonization in the development of intestinal host defense. J Pediatr Gastroenterol Nutr 2000;30(Suppl 2):S2-S7.

Yasui H, Kiyoshima J, Ushijima H. Passive protection against rotavirus-induced diarrhea of mouse pups born to and nursed by dams fed Bifidobacterium breve YIT4064. J Infect Dis 1995;172:403-409.

HUMAN MILK α1,2-LINKED FUCOSYLATED OLIGOSACCHARIDES DECREASE RISK OF DIARRHEA DUE TO STABLE TOXIN OF *E. COLI* IN BREASTFED INFANTS

David S. Newburg[1], Guillermo M. Ruiz-Palacios[2], Mekibib Altaye[3], Prasoon Chaturvedi[1], M. Lourdes Guerrero[2], Jareen K. Meinzen-Derr[3], and Ardythe L. Morrow[3]

1. INTRODUCTION

Breastfed infants have a lower risk of diarrhea than infants fed artificial formula. Human milk components, including oligosaccharides, inhibit pathogens in vitro and are postulated to protect infants from disease. Most human milk oligosaccharides are fucosylated. The fucose terminus may be connected by an α1,2 linkage catalyzed by a fucosyltransferase produced by the secretor gene (*FUT2*), or by an α1,3 or α1,4 linkage catalyzed by fucosyltransferases produced by the Lewis gene (*FUT3*) or other α1,3 transferase genes (*FUT4,5,6,7,9*) of this family. The secretor and Lewis genes also control expression of the Lewis blood group type (Erney et al. 2000, Henry et al. 1995). Some women are nonsecretors, i.e., they do not secrete 2-linked fucosyloligosaccharides into their milk and other bodily fluids. Even among secretors, however, the expression of milk fucosyloligosaccharides varies significantly (Chaturvedi et al. 2001, Erney et al. 2000, Thurl et al. 1997, Viverge et al. 1990). Enterotoxigenic *Escherichia coli* that produce stable toxin (ST-*E. coli*) is a common cause of diarrhea; the ability of stable toxin to cause diarrhea is inhibited by human milk α1,2-linked fucosyloligosaccharides in vitro and in vivo.

We investigated variation of α1,2 fucosyloligosaccharide expression in human milk with respect to maternal determinants and any effect this variation in milk might have on the risk of diarrhea among breastfed infants. These questions were addressed by measuring: 1) The relationship between expression of the major fucosyloligosaccharides in milk and maternal Lewis blood group type, and 2) the relationship between individual expres-

[1]Shriver Center of the University of Massachusetts Medical School, 200 Trapelo Road, Waltham, MA 02452
[2]Instituto Nacional de Ciencias Medicas y Nutricion, Mexico City, Mexico
[3]Cincinnati Children's Hospital Medical Center, Cincinnati, Ohio

Protecting Infants through Human Milk, edited by Pickering *et al.*
Kluwer Academic/Plenum Publishers, 2004

sion of 2-linked fucosyloligosaccharides in milk and the degree of protection of the breastfed infant against diarrhea, particularly ST-*E. coli*-associated diarrhea.

2. METHODS

A cohort of Mexican breastfeeding mother-infant pairs was followed for up to two years postpartum, with feeding and illness data collected weekly.

2.1. Oligosaccharide Levels

Oligosaccharide levels were measured in milk samples collected 1 to 5 weeks postpartum; oligosaccharides were isolated, perbenzoylated, resolved by reversed-phase HPLC, and detected at 229 nm (Chaturvedi et al. 1997). The Lewis synthetic pathway contains divergent pathways between the 2-linked fucosyloligosaccharides and fucosyloligosaccharides that contain only 3- and 4- linkages, which are thought to compete for common substrates. This complex reciprocal relationship can be summarized in a single measure as the ratio of the 2-linked oligosaccharides (LNF-I+2'-FL+LNDFH-I+LDFT [H-1+H-2+Le^b+Le^y]), whose synthetic pathway is initiated by the secretor gene product, to those containing only 3- and 4- linkages (LNF-II + 3-FL [Le^a+Le^x]), whose synthesis is initiated by (and limited to) the Lewis gene product. This ratio of 2-linked to non-2-linked fucosyloligosaccharides was used as a measure of the relative quantities of these distinct oligosaccharides in the milk of each mother.

2.2. Lewis Blood Group Types

Maternal Lewis blood group types were determined by hemagglutination assays using specific monoclonal antibodies.

2.3. Statistical Analysis

Incidence rates of diarrhea were calculated as the total number of cases per 100 child-months at risk (i.e., birth to the end of breastfeeding or termination from study). The effect of milk oligosaccharide ratio on risk of moderate-to-severe diarrhea of any cause was examined by using a generalized linear model with a Poisson link function. All diarrhea episodes were treated as independent events. For comparisons involving data that were not distributed normally, a median two-sample test was used.

3. RESULTS

Lewis blood group types were distributed in our cohort of lactating mothers as follows: 67 were Le^{a-b+}, 24 were Le^{a-b-}, and 2 were indeterminate. The ratios of 2-linked fucosyloligosaccharides to fucosyloligosaccharides containing only 3- and 4- linkages were determined in the milks of each of these mothers. The ratios were sorted from the highest to the lowest and grouped by quartile. The distribution of mothers' Lewis blood group types by quartiles of their milk ratios (Table 1) was asymmetric: All 23 mothers whose milk was in the lowest quartile belonged to Lewis blood group type Le^{a-b+}, which represents approximately one-third of the mothers of the Le^{a-b+} blood group phenotype.

Table 1. Distribution of Lewis blood group types[a]

Oligosaccharide ratios: Quartile (range)	Blood group type Le^{a-b+}	Le^{a-b-}
Lowest (1.16–3.92)	23	0
Middle Two (3.93–10.09)	37	8
Highest (10.10–42.36)	7	16

[a]Fisher's exact test, P<0.01

Conversely, 74% of the mothers whose milk oligosaccharide ratios were in the highest quartile belonged to Lewis blood group type Le^{a-b-}. These data suggest that the relative amounts of 2-linked fucose in milk relate to specific Lewis and secretor genotypes of the mother.

3.1. Relationship of Milk Fucosyloligosaccharide Ratios to *E. coli* ST Diarrhea in Nursing Infants

A specific oligosaccharide of human milk that contains a 2-linked fucose is able to inhibit *E. coli* ST in vitro and in vivo. If the enzymes (i.e., secretor and Lewis gene products) that control the synthesis of the 2-linked fucosyloligosaccharides early in lactation likewise control the synthesis of the particular 2-linked fucosyloligosaccharide structure that protects against ST, then a positive relationship might be expected between the ratios of 2- to 3/4-linked oligosaccharides and protection against ST-associated diarrhea in breastfeeding infants.

Figure 1 shows ratios of fucosyloligosaccharides in milk being consumed by four infants who exhibited symptoms of diarrhea concurrent with infection by ST-*E. coli* (symptomatic infected) compared with ratios of milk consumed by the 43 infants who did not exhibit symptoms of diarrhea while infected by ST-*E. coli* (asymptomatic infected). For comparison, the ratios of milk consumed by 46 uninfected healthy control infants are shown.

The oligosaccharide ratios were significantly lower (median 4.9, n=4) in milk consumed by infants infected with ST-producing *E. coli* and suffering moderate-to-severe diarrhea than the ratios in milk consumed by asymptomatic infected infants (7.1, n=43; P=0.04 by the median two-sample test) or uninfected controls (6.4, n=46; P =0.04). Thus, even among this population of mothers who are secretors and all produce 2-linked fucosyloligosaccharides, lower relative amounts of these 2-linked oligosaccharides were associated with increased risk of ST-associated diarrhea.

Other pathogens, such as campylobacter and noroviruses, also are inhibited *in vitro* and *in vivo* by other fucosyloligosaccharides, and especially by fucosyloligosaccharides containing the α1,2 linkage. To test whether this same ratio of fucosyloligosaccharides in milk might be associated with protection of breastfeeding infants from other pathogens, we investigated the relationship between values of this ratio in milk and the incidence of moderate-to-severe cases of diarrhea by any cause. By Poisson regression, this ratio in milk samples was significantly related to protection against moderate-to-severe diarrhea in the breastfeeding infants: relative risk was 0.90 (95% CI 0.83, 0.96); P=0.002. This suggests that the ratio is indicative of the presence of other specific 2-linked fucosyloligosaccharides in milk that protect against some of the more common enteropathogens in this population.

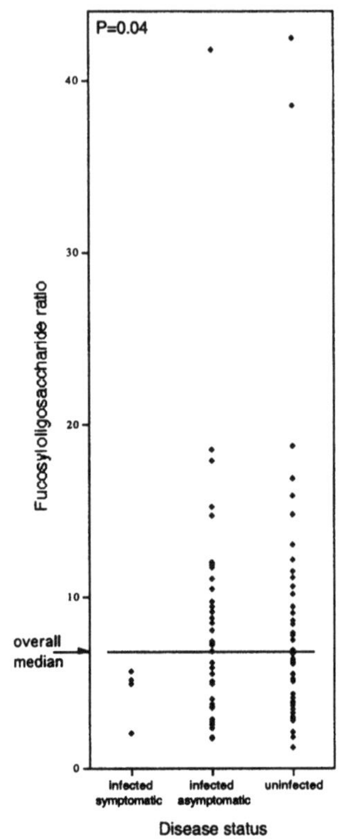

Figure 1. Fucosyloligosaccharide ratios

4. CONCLUSION

The major human milk fucosyloligosaccharides are Lewis and H epitopes and their expression varies by maternal Lewis blood group type. The complex variation in individual expression of these oligosaccharides can be distilled into a single measure for each milk sample, the ratio of the four major 2-linked oligosaccharides to the two major fucosyloligosaccharides that do not contain any 2-linkages. Variation in this oligosaccharide ratio, reflecting individual differences in milk oligosaccharide expression, relates to a different risk for heat-stable enterotoxigenic *E. coli*-associated diarrhea in breastfed infants.

The observation that a high ratio of 2-linked oligosaccharides in maternal milk is associated with decreased risk of diarrhea in breastfed infants is consistent with previous reports that human milk 2-linked fucosylated oligosaccharides can inhibit binding of specific pathogens to their host cell receptors, notably stable toxin of *E. coli* in vitro and in vivo (Newburg et al. 1995). Inhibition of stable toxin would be expected to decrease the symptoms of diarrhea among children infected by ST-*E. coli*. Because diarrhea associated with ST-*E. coli* accounts for less than 2% of total diarrhea cases in our population, our finding an association between these ratios and diarrhea of any etiology suggest the presence of a family of 2-linked fucose-containing oligosaccharides and/or glycoconjugates in milk that protect against a variety of enteric pathogens. For example, some strains of noroviruses also use 2-linked fucosylated glycoconjugates as receptors (Huang et al. 2003). Similarly, 2-linked fucosylated oligosaccharides and glycoconjugates inhibit binding and colonization by *Campylobacter jejuni* (Ruiz-Palacios et al. 2003).

Differential innate expression of oligosaccharides and their related glycoconjugates in human milk suggests that breastfeeding provides differential protection to infants against specific pathogens. In general, the findings of this study provide evidence for a significant role of milk oligosaccharides to protect breastfed infants against enteric pathogens. Our findings imply that milk from mothers with specific secretor and Lewis genotypes may be most protective against specific pathogens. This phenomenon may explain why in central Mexico, where enterotoxigenic *E. coli* is endemic, over 99% of the indigenous population are secretors.

5. ACKNOWLEDGMENT

This work was supported by a program project grant from the National Institute of Child Health and Human Development (HD13021).

6. REFERENCES

Chaturvedi P, Warren CD, Ruiz-Palacios GM, Pickering LK, Newburg DS. Milk oligosaccharide profiles by reversed-phase HPLC of their perbenzoylated derivatives. Anal Biochem 1997;251:89-97.

Chaturvedi P, Warren CD, Altaye M, Morrow AL, Ruiz-Palacios G, Pickering LK, Newburg DS. Fucosylated human milk oligosaccharides vary between individuals and over the course of lactation. Glycobiology 2001;11:365-372.

Erney RM, Malone WT, Skelding MB, Marcon AA, Kleman-Leyer KM, O'Ryan ML, Ruiz-Palacios G, Hilty MD, Pickering LK, Prieto PA. Variability of human milk neutral oligosaccharides in a diverse population. J Pediatr Gastroenterol Nutr 2000;30:181-192.

Henry S, Oriol R, Samuelsson B. Lewis histo-blood group system and associated secretory phenotypes. Vox Sang 1995;69:166-182.

Huang P, Farkas T, Marionneau S, Zhong W, Ruvoen-Clouet DVM, Morrow AL, Altaye M, Pickering LK, Newburg DS, LePendu J, Jiang X. Noroviruses bind to human ABO, Lewis and secretor histo-blood group antigens: identification of 4 distinct strain-specific patterns. J Infect Dis 2003;188:19-31.

Newburg DS, Chaturvedi P, Crane JK, Cleary TG, Pickering LK. Fucosylated oligosaccharide(s) of human milk inhibits stable toxin of *Escherichia coli*. In: Agrawal VP, Sharma CB, Sah A, Zingde MD, editors. Complex Carbohydrates and Advances in Biosciences. Muzaffarnagar, India: Society of Biosciences; 1995; pp 199-226.

Ruiz-Palacios GM, Cervantes LE, Ramos P, Chavez-Munguia B, Newburg DS. Campylobacter jejuni binds intestinal H(O) antigen (Fucal,2Gal b1,4GlcNAc), and fucosyloligosaccharides of human milk inhibit its binding and infection. J Biol Chem 2003;278:14112-14120.

Thurl S, Henker J, Siegel M, Tovar K, Sawatzki G. Detection of four human milk groups with respect to Lewis blood group dependent oligosaccharides. Glycoconj J 1997;14:795-799.

Viverge D, Grimmonprez L, Cassanas G, Bardet L, Solere M. Discriminant carbohydrate components of human milk according to donor secretor types. J Pediatr Gastroenterol Nutr 1990;11:365-370.

LACTOFERRIN BLOCKS THE INITIAL HOST CELL ATTACHMENT MECHANISM OF ENTEROPATHOGENIC *E. COLI* (EPEC)

Theresa J. Ochoa, Marita Noguera-Obenza, and Thomas G. Cleary

1. INTRODUCTION

Enteropathogenic *Escherichia coli* (EPEC) is a major cause of infantile diarrhea. The initial event in pathogenesis of EPEC and many other bacterial enteropathogens (*Shigella, Salmonella, Yersinia,* and Shiga toxin-producing *E. coli*) involves production and translocation of bacterial proteins through a needle complex. In EPEC, multimers of *E. coli* secreted protein A (EspA) assemble into a transiently expressed tube between the bacteria and the host cell. Secreted proteins (EspB, EspD, and others) are introduced into host cells via this conduit, triggering cytoskeletal events that lead to the intimate attachment of bacteria to the epithelial surface, effacement of host microvilli and pedestal formation ["attaching and effacing" lesion] (Vallance & Finlay 2000; Sekiya et al. 2001).

Immunologic and nonimmunologic factors present in human milk protect infants from intestinal infections. Lactoferrin, a glycoprotein present in most human mucosal secretions including milk, protects against Gram-negative bacteria in multiple ways. Milk immunoglobulins, free secretory component, and lactoferrin inhibit EPEC adherence to HeLa cells (de Araujo & Giugliano 2001).

The purpose of this study was to investigate the effect of lactoferrin on the initial attachment step of EPEC. To focus on the first host cell interactions we evaluated EPEC-induced hemolysis and production of secreted *E. coli* proteins.

2. METHODS

For the hemolysis assay (Shaw et al. 2001), an overnight growth of EPEC O127:H6 strain E2348/69 was incubated with human erythrocytes (20%) and recombinant human lactoferrin (Agennix, Houston, TX) in conditions known to induce the formation of the needle complex (Kenny et al. 1997) [DMEM/HEPES, pH 7.4, at 37°C in a 5% CO_2

University of Texas Medical School at Houston, Department of Pediatrics, Division of Infectious Diseases, 6431 Fannin, Houston, TX 77030

Protecting Infants through Human Milk, edited by Pickering *et al.*
Kluwer Academic/Plenum Publishers, 2004

incubator]. After a 6-hour incubation, hemoglobin release was measured spectrophotometrically (OD_{543}).

For measurement of the secreted proteins, EPEC was incubated in DMEM/HEPES without erythrocytes in the presence or absence of lactoferrin (10 mg/mL). The amount of protein secreted into the supernatants was measured by EIA using affinity purified anti-EspA from human milk and monoclonal antibodies to EspB and EspD.

3. RESULTS

Lactoferrin did not impair growth of EPEC in DMEM/HEPES. Lactoferrin (1.25, 2.5, 5, and 10 mg/mL) incubated with 20% erythrocytes and bacteria in DMEM/HEPES for 6 hours, blocked EPEC-induced hemolysis in a dose-dependent manner ($P<0.01$).

Secretion of EspABD by EPEC occurred at 3 to 4 hours of incubation with a peak at 6 to 7 hours. There was no detection of EspB when EPEC were grown in the presence of lactoferrin ($P<0.0001$). Lactoferrin also decreased the amount of EspA, but less dramatically, and delayed the release of EspD. Saturation with iron (2:1 molar ratio of iron to lactoferrin) did not affect these results (Fig. 1).

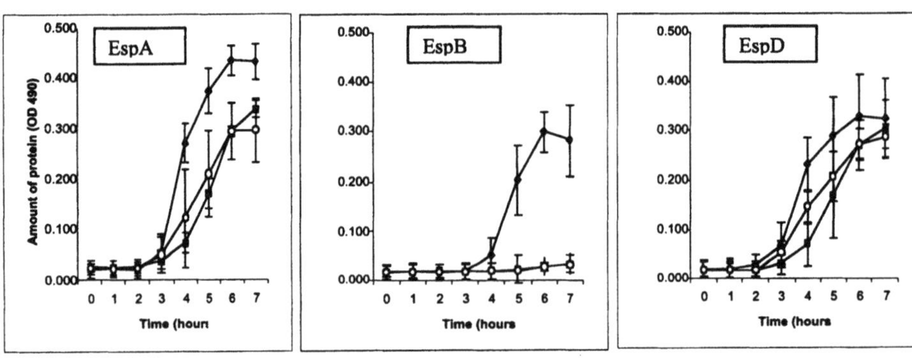

Figure 1. Effect of lactoferrin on the amount of EspABD in supernatant of EPEC. Bacteria grown in DMEM/HEPES [O] and in lactoferrin [▲] (3 experiments, mean±SD).

To evaluate the immediate effect of lactoferrin, bacteria were grown in DMEM/HEPES for 5 hours before lactoferrin (10 mg/mL) was added to the media; 15 minutes later the amount of EspABD in the supernatant was measure by EIA. EspB rapidly disappeared ($P<0.03$); the decrease in EspA and EspD was less dramatic (Fig. 2).

These data suggest that lactoferrin might be degrading the secreted proteins. We therefore determine whether lactoferrin had a proteolytic effect using purified protein in the absence of bacteria. Lactoferrin (1 mg/mL) was incubated with pure EspB (2 µg/mL) for 4 hours at 37°C in a 5% CO_2 incubator. A Western blot was done using monoclonal antibody to EspB. Lactoferrin degraded EspB into three faint bands in comparison with the single band of EspB in the control with DMEM/HEPES (data not shown).

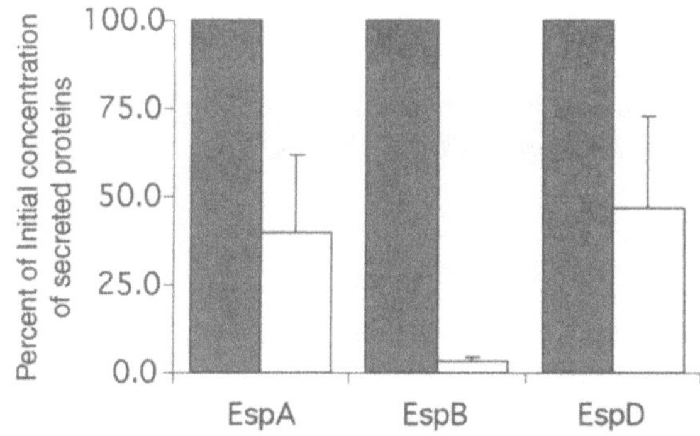

Figure 2. Effect of lactoferrin on extracellular EspABD. Amount of protein prior to adding lactoferrin [■] and 15 minutes after adding lactoferrin [□] (3 experiments, mean±SEM).

4. DISCUSSION

Lactoferrin blocks the initial step in EPEC mammalian cell attachment as indicated by its prevention of hemolysis and by decreasing the amount of proteins necessary for bacterial contact and pore formation. The secreted proteins disappear in the presence of lactoferrin because of a proteolytic effect. The type III secretory system is necessary to cause hemolysis in vitro (Shaw et al. 2001). The ability of lactoferrin to block EPEC-induced hemolysis implies an effect of lactoferrin on the components of the type III secretory system, especially the secreted proteins EspABD that are known to be key elements of EPEC hemolytic activity.

Lactoferrin is an iron-binding protein with antimicrobial, anti-inflammatory, and immunomodulatory functions (Brock 2002). Antimicrobial activity of lactoferrin is not due solely to its iron-binding capacity. Lactoferrin binds to the lipid A portion of lipopolysaccharide (LPS) to disrupt the bacterial cell membrane (Applemelk 1994). We speculate that the binding of lactoferrin to LPS interferes with the type III secretory machinery allowing the secreted proteins to be released and digested. We have observed a similar event regarding the effect of lactoferrin on *Shigella flexneri*. Lactoferrin induces loss and degradation of the two key virulent proteins, IpaB and IpaC, necessary for invasion of mammalian cells by *Shigella* (Gomez et al. 2003).

A proteolytic activity of lactoferrin in *Haemophilus influenzae* also has been described. Lactoferrin degrades IgA1 and Hap, two autotransporters proteins that are important colonization factors of *H. influenzae*. Degradation is inhibited by serine protease inhibitors (Qiu et al. 1998). Thus, lactoferrin triggers similar events in *Haemophilus,* a bacteria that lacks a type III secretory system. Therefore, the type III secretory dysfunction induced by lactoferrin that we describe is related to interaction with LPS rather than with one of the protein components of the secretory machinery.

This disruption of the needle complex/type III secretory system in two models (EPEC and *Shigella*) implies that lactoferrin could provide broad cross-protection against many enteropathogens that share this mechanism.

5. ACKNOWLEDGMENT

This work was supported by a program project grant from the National Institute of Child Health and Human Development (HD13021).

6. REFERENCES

Appelmelk BJ, An YQ, Geerts M, Thijs BG, de Boer HA, MacLaren DM, de Graaff J, Nuijens JH. Lactoferrin is a lipid A-binding protein. Infect Immun 1994;62:2628-2632.

Brock JH. The physiology of lactoferrin. Biochem Cell Biol 2002;80:1-6.

de Araujo AN, Giugliano LG. Lactoferrin and free secretory component of human milk inhibit the adhesion of enteropathogenic Escherichia coli to HeLa cells. BMC Microbiol 2001;1:25.

Gomez H, Ochoa T, Carlin L, Cleary T. Human lactoferrin impairs virulence of *Shigella flexneri*. J Infect Dis 2003;187:87-95.

Kenny B, Abe A, Stein M, Finlay BB. Enteropathogenic Escherichia coli protein secretion is induced in response to conditions similar to those in the gastrointestinal tract. Infect Immun 1997;65:2606-2612.

Qiu J, Hendrixson DR, Baker EN, Murphy TF, St Geme JW 3rd, Plaut AG. Human milk lactoferrin inactivates two putative colonization factors expressed by Haemophilus influenzae. Proc Natl Acad Sci USA 1998;95:12641-12646.

Sekiya K, Ohishi M, Ogino T, Tamano K, Sasakawa C, Abe A. Supermolecular structure of the enteropathogenic Escherichia coli type III secretion system and its direct interaction with the EspA-sheath-like structure. Proc Natl Acad Sci USA 2001;98:11638-11643.

Shaw RK, Daniell S, Ebel F, Frankel G, Knutton S. EspA filament-mediated protein translocation into red blood cells. Cell Microbiol 2001;3:213-222.

Vallance BA, Finlay BB. Exploitation of host cells by enteropathogenic Escherichia coli. Proc Natl Acad Sci USA 2000;97:8799-8806.

CELLS FROM MATURE HUMAN MILK ARE CAPABLE OF CYTOKINE PRODUCTION FOLLOWING IN VITRO STIMULATION

Joanna Hawkes, Dani-Louise Bryan, and Robert Gibson

1. INTRODUCTION

Leukocytes in milk may contribute to development of mucosal defense mechanisms in the recipient infant (Hanson 1999). The principal types of leukocytes found in human milk are granulocytes, monocytes/macrophages, and lymphocytes. Each of these cell types could be responsible for production of a variety of cytokines, and a number of investigators have examined this possibility using cells isolated from colostrum (Rudloff et al. 1992; Subiza et al. 1988; Skansen-Saphir et al. 1993). In contrast, little information is available regarding cytokine production by cells obtained from mature milk or the relationship between milk cell and peripheral blood cell cytokine production. The aim of this study was to determine the capacity of a mixed population of human milk cells (HMC) to produce the potentially pro-inflammatory cytokines IL-1β, IL-6, and TNF-α and compare the cytokine profile with that obtained from peripheral blood mononuclear cells (PBMC) collected from the same mothers.

2. METHODS

2.1. Subjects

Consent was obtained from 120 healthy women who had delivered full-term, singleton infants. At 5 weeks postpartum, a milk sample of 50 mL (n=80) expressed into a sterile polypropylene container and a peripheral blood sample (20 mL, n=82) were collected on the day of the appointment.

2.2. Cell Culture and Cytokine Assays

Human milk cells were isolated by centrifugation and cultured at 5×10^6 cells/mL with or without lipopolysaccharide (LPS; 500 ng/mL). After 24 hours, cell culture

Child Nutrition Research Centre at Child Health Research Institute, Flinders Medical Centre and Flinders University, Adelaide, Australia

Protecting Infants through Human Milk, edited by Pickering *et al.*
Kluwer Academic/Plenum Publishers, 2004

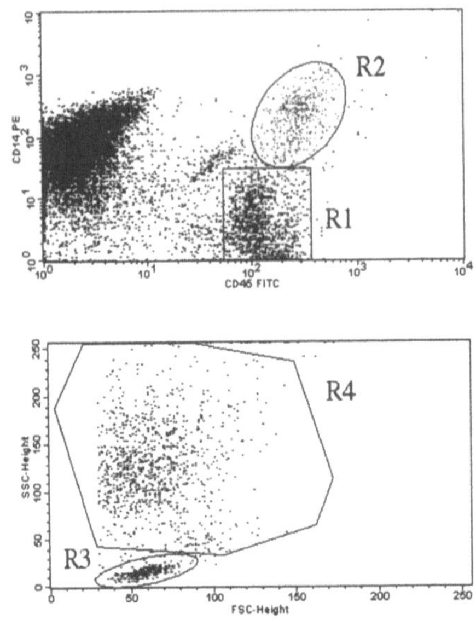

Figure 1. Analysis of a representative sample of human milk cells by flow cytometry. Top: Distribution by CD45/CD14 fluorescence; R1=lymphocytes+granulocytes ($CD14^-/CD45^+$), R2=monocytes/macrophages ($CD14^+/CD45^+$). Bottom: Distribution of cells in R1 based on forward scatter/side scatter parameters; R3=lymphocytes, R4=granulocytes.

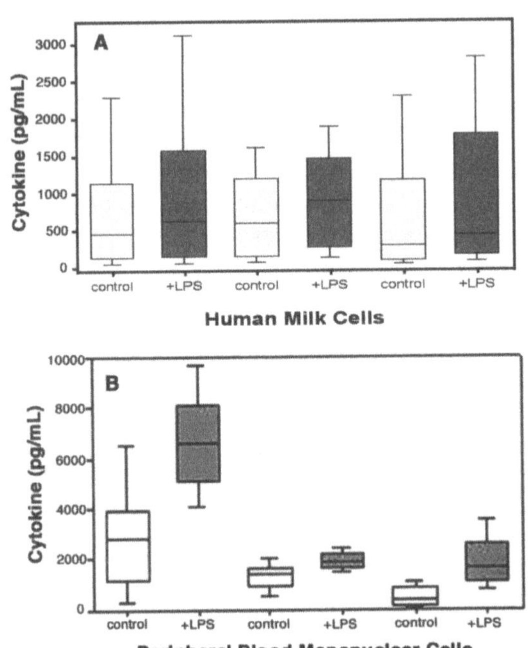

Figure 2. Cytokine production by expressed HMC and paired PBMC. Box plots show medians and upper and lower quartiles, with the 10th and 90th percentiles extending either side. (*P<0.001, Wilcoxon signed ranks test.)

supernatants were harvested for analysis of secreted cytokines. The cells were resuspended in fresh media, lysed by one freeze-thaw cycle and the lysates harvested for analysis of intracellular cytokines. PBMC (1×10^6 cells/mL) were cultured with or without LPS (200 ng/mL) and supernatants and lysates collected as described for the HMC. Cell culture supernatants (intracellular and secreted cytokine) were analyzed for IL-1β, IL-6, and TNF-α using double antibody sandwich enzyme immunosorbent assay (Hawkes et al. 1999).

2.3. Analysis of HMC by Flow Cytometry

Human milk cells (1×10^6 cells) were stained with fluorochrome-labeled monoclonal antibodies against CD45 (leukocyte common antigen) and CD14 (monocytes/macrophages) and analyzed by two-color direct immunofluorescence. The percentages of monocytes, lymphocytes, and granulocytes were determined on the basis of CD45/CD14 fluorescence and forward/side scatter parameters and results are given as a percentage of total leukocytes.

3. RESULTS

There was considerable variation in the total yield and proportion of individual cell types between donors (Fig. 1). The major cell types represented were monocytes/macrophages 3–80% (35±17, mean%±SD), granulocytes 1–92% (40±22) and lymphocytes 1–94% (25±18).

HMC spontaneously produced significantly less IL-1β, IL-6, and TNF-α than PBMC in the absence of stimulation (Fig. 2). In vitro stimulation of HMC with LPS increased cytokine production by approximately 40–50%, whereas PBMC responded to LPS with increased cytokine production of up to 350%.

Regardless of stimulation conditions, the majority of IL-6 and TNF-α was secreted into the culture supernatant by both HMC and PBMC (Table 1). In contrast, although almost 60% of IL-1β was secreted by PBMC, <20% of HMC IL-1β was secreted into the extracellular compartment following stimulation with LPS.

Table 1. Distribution of intracellular and secreted cytokines in cultured HMC and PBMC[a]

		IL-1β		IL-6		TNF-α	
		control	+LPS	control	+LPS	control	+LPS
HMC[b]	intracellular	85	82	2	4	3	3
	secreted	15	18	98	96	97	97
PBMC[c]	intracellular	68	43	8	22	3	3
	secreted	32	57	92	78	97	97

[a]Results are expressed as % of total cytokine detected.
[b]HMC=human milk cells
[c]PBMC=peripheral blood mononuclear cells

4. CONCLUSIONS

This study has shown that cells isolated from mature milk samples obtained from healthy women have the capacity to spontaneously produce IL-1β, IL-6, and TNF-α in cell culture, whereas earlier studies using cells isolated from colostrum usually have described minimal production of these cytokines in the absence of in vitro stimulation (Niklova et al. 1990; Sone et al. 1997). LPS stimulation significantly increased production of each of these potentially pro-inflammatory cytokines. These observations suggest that mature milk cells (obtained at 5 weeks postpartum) maintain their capacity to participate in the production of cytokines well after the colostral phase of lactation is over. This report demonstrates differences in the amount of intracellular and secreted cytokines produced in vitro by HMC. Although the vast majority of both TNF-α and IL-6 was secreted by HMC with <5% remaining in the intracellular compartment, IL-1β may be induced in HMC mainly in a nonsecreting form.

In conclusion, these observations suggest that cells in mature human milk are capable of active involvement in production of cytokines in the mammary gland and have the capacity to respond to further stimulation after leaving the breast.

5. ACKNOWLEDGMENT

These data have been published in full in The Journal of Clinical Immunology 2002;22: 338-344.

6. REFERENCES

Hanson LA. Human milk and host defence: immediate and long-term effects. Acta Paediatr 1999;88:42-46.

Hawkes JS, Bryan D-L, James MJ, Gibson RA. Cytokines (IL-1β, IL-6, TNF-α, TGF-β1 and TGF-β2) and prostaglandin E2 in human milk during the first three months postpartum. Pediatr Res 1999;46:194-199.

Nikolova E, Staykova M, Raicheva D, Karadjova M, Neronov A, Ivanov I, Goranov I. Interleukin production by human colostral cells after in vitro mitogen stimulation. Am J Reprod Immunol 1990;23:104-106.

Rudloff HE, Schmalstieg FC Jr, Mushtaha AA, Palkowetz KH, Liu SK, Goldman AS. Tumor necrosis factor-alpha in human milk. Pediatr Res 1992;31:29-33.

Skansen-Saphir U, Lindfors A, Andersson U. Cytokine production in mononuclear cells of human milk studied at the single-cell level. Pediatr Res 1993;34:213-216.

Sone S, Tsutsumi H, Takeuchi R, Matsuda K, Imai S, Ogra PL, Chiba S. Enhanced cytokine production by milk macrophages following infection with respiratory syncytial virus. J Leukoc Biol 1997;61:630-636.

Subiza JL, Rodriguez C, Figueredo A, Mateos P, Alvarez R, de la Concha EG. Impaired production and lack of secretion of interleukin 1 by human breast milk macrophages. Clin Exp Immunol 1988;71:493-496.

RAT MILK DECREASES NECROTIZING ENTEROCOLITIS IN A RAT MODEL

Bohuslav Dvorak[1,2], Melissa D. Halpern[1], Hana Holubec[3], Katerina Dvorakova[3], Jessica A. Dominguez[1], Catherine S. Williams[1], and Yolanda G. Meza[1]

1. INTRODUCTION

Neonatal necrotizing enterocolitis (NEC) is the most common and devastating gastrointestinal tract (GI) disease of prematurely born infants. The pathogenesis of NEC is unknown, but intestinal immaturity, enteral feeding, intestinal hypoxia/ischemia, and bacterial colonization are considered the major risk factors for development of NEC (Caplan & Jilling 2001). Clinical studies indicate that human milk, which provides hormones, cytokines, growth factors, and nucleotides that facilitate maturation of the intestinal mucosal barrier and other essential intestinal functions, plays a protective role against this disease (Schanler 2001; Lucas & Cole 1990). However, factor(s) responsible for the protective effect remain to be identified. We have shown that supplementation of formula with epidermal growth factor (EGF), a peptide normally present in human milk but absent in infant formula, is highly protective against NEC in a rat experimental model (Dvorak et al. 2002; Crissinger 1995). In this model, NEC is induced in neonatal rats via enteral feeding of cow milk-based formula coupled with asphyxia and cold stress. Using this method, approximately 80% of neonatal rats develop NEC within 4 days (Dvorak et al. 2002; Halpern et al. 2002). The aim of this study was to examine the effect of artificial feeding of rat milk versus cow milk-based formula on development of NEC in a neonatal rat model.

2. METHODS

Newborn rats were fed artificially with either collected rat milk (RM) or cow milk-based formula (RMS). To induce development of clinical and pathological signs of NEC, neonatal rats were stressed twice daily with asphyxia [breathing 100% nitrogen gas for 60 seconds] followed by cold stress [4°C for 10 minutes] (Dvorak et al. 2002; Halpern et al.

[1]Department of Pediatrics, University of Arizona, Tucson, AZ 85724
[2]Department of Cell Biology & Anatomy, University of Arizona
[3]Department of Microbiology & Immunology, University of Arizona

Protecting Infants through Human Milk, edited by Pickering *et al.*
Kluwer Academic/Plenum Publishers, 2004

2002). Rats in the RMS and RM groups were hand-fed every 3 to 4 hours during the first 48 hours. The hand-feeding method was then replaced with mechanized artificial feeding for an additional 48 hours. Body weight gain was recorded daily. After 96 hours, all surviving animals were terminated via decapitation. A 2-cm section of distal ileum proximal to the ileocecal valve from each animal was fixed overnight in 70% ethanol, paraffin-embedded, sectioned at 4 to 6 μm, and stained with hematoxylin and eosin for histological evaluation of NEC. The rest of the ileum was snap frozen in liquid nitrogen for further biochemical and gene expression analysis. Histological changes in ileal architecture were evaluated using our previously published scoring system (Dvorak et al. 2002; Halpern et al. 2002) and scanning electron microscopy (EM). Intestinal cytokine mRNA expression was determined by the Real-time PCR assay. Cytokine histological localization was performed by confocal microscopy.

3. RESULTS

Similar to human NEC, artificial feeding of rat milk reduces the incidence and severity of NEC. The overall incidence of NEC revealed that 81% of RMS pups developed significant intestinal abnormalities described as moderate, severe, or full necrosis. In contrast, artificial feeding of RM significantly reduced the incidence of NEC to 26% ($P<0.001$). Freezing and thawing of collected rat milk did not eliminate the protective effect of maternal milk. Scanning EM of the ileum from the RMS group confirmed pathological changes: damaged villi architecture, loss of epithelial integrity, and enterocyte ruptures. Ileal anti-inflammatory interleukin-10 (IL-10) expression was increased significantly in the RM group compared with RMS. Increased IL-10 peptide production was detected in the RM group with signal localized predominantly in the cytoplasm of villus epithelial cells.

4. CONCLUSION

Artificial feeding of rat milk collected during the early postnatal period significantly reduced the incidence and severity of NEC-like injury in the neonatal rat model. Similar to human NEC, enteral feeding of rat milk decreased, but did not completely eliminate development of disease. The mechanism by which this protection occurs is associated with increased endogenous production of anti-inflammatory IL-10 cytokine in the site of injury. Better understanding of the mechanisms underlying these protective effects could be beneficial either in the prevention of NEC or in the development of future therapeutic strategies to cure NEC.

5. ACKNOWLEDGMENTS

This work was supported by the NIH grants HD39657 and HD26013 (to B.D.).

6. REFERENCES

Caplan MS, Jilling T. New concepts in necrotizing enterocolitis. Curr Opin Pediatr 2001;13:111-115.

Crissinger KD. Animal models of necrotizing enterocolitis. J Pediatr Gastroenterol Nutr 1995;20:17-22.

Dvorak B, Halpern MD, Holubec H, Williams CS, McWilliam DL, Dominguez JA, Stepankova R, Payne CM, McCuskey RS. Epidermal growth factor reduces the development of necrotizing enterocolitis in a neonatal rat model. Am J Physiol Gastrointest Liver Physiol 2002;282:G156-164.

Halpern MD, Holubec H, Dominguez JA, Williams CS, Meza YG, McWilliam DL, Payne CM, McCuskey RS, Besselsen DG, Dvorak B. Upregulation of IL-18 and IL-12 in the ileum of neonatal rats with necrotizing enterocolitis. Pediatr Res 2002;51:733-739.

Lucas A, Cole TJ. Breast milk and neonatal necrotising enterocolitis. Lancet 1990;336:1519-1523.

Schanler RJ. The use of human milk for premature infants. Pediatr Clin North Am 2001;48:207-219.

EFFORTS TO PREVENT MOTHER-TO-CHILD TRANSMISSION OF HUMAN IMMUNODEFICIENCY VIRUS TYPE 1 THROUGH HUMAN MILK

Past, Present, and Future

S. Urdaneta[1], C.M. Berlin[2,3], and M.K. Howett[1,4]

1. INTRODUCTION

About a third of mothers who are positive for human immunodeficiency virus (HIV) infect their newborn infants (UNAIDS/WHO 2002). Most vertical transmission occurs during gestation and delivery (Edgeworth & Ugen 2000). Breastfeeding by an HIV-positive woman adds an additional 14% to the risk of in utero and intrapartum transmission (Dunn et al. 1992). Alternatives to breastfeeding or modulation of breastfeeding techniques that are accessible, acceptable, and safe to use in low- and middle-income countries are in demand. Thus, research on making breastfeeding safer is a high priority. The purpose of this chapter is to review treatment approaches to decrease or eliminate HIV in human milk.

2. METHODS

We searched for English publications using the keywords *HIV, prevention, vertical, mother-to-child, transmission, breast milk* and *breastfeeding*. The search engine was PubMed (www.ncbi.nih.gov/entrez/query.fcgi?db=PubMed), a service of the United States National Library of Medicine, which allows access to MEDLINE citations (starting in the mid 1960s) and additional life science journals. Additional information was obtained from the Internet. Identified methods currently under study or published for prevention of mother-to-child transmission of HIV-1 through human milk were classified into groups according to the treatment method.

[1]Departments of Microbiology and Immunology, Pennsylvania State University, College of Medicine, M.S. Hershey Medical Center, Hershey, PA 17033
[2]Department of Pediatrics, Pennsylvania State University, College of Medicine, Hershey, PA
[3]Department of Pharmacology, Pennsylvania State University, College of Medicine, Hershey, PA
[4]Department of Obstetrics & Gynecology, Pennsylvania State University, College of Medicine, Hershey, PA

3. RESULTS

A total of six treatment approaches to decrease or eliminate infectious HIV in human milk were identified and will be discussed. These include: 1) modified feeding practices, 2) heat treatment of milk, 3) lipolysis, 4) treatment of the breastfeeding mother with antimicrobial agents, 5) AIDS vaccine, and 6) treatment of infected human milk with microbicides.

3.1. Modified Feeding Practices

According to the World Health Organization (WHO), "when replacement feeding is accessible, feasible, affordable, sustainable and safe, avoidance of breastfeeding by HIV-infected mothers is recommended" and nursing mothers should follow proposed alternatives [Table 1] (UNFPA/UNICEF/WHO/UNAIDS 2000; WHO/UNAIDS/UNICEF 1998). The most widely used and 100%-effective method to prevent mother-to-child transmission of HIV through breastfeeding is complete substitution of formula for human milk. In resource-constrained countries, the epicenter of the HIV/AIDS pandemic, the use of formula is neither feasible nor safe. Of the proposed alternatives, exclusive breastfeeding with early weaning after six months and heat treatment of expressed milk might be more applicable. Exclusive breastfeeding for the first six months of life represents no greater risk of HIV transmission than formula feeding (Coovadia & Coutsoudis 2001). Women represent about 50% of the HIV-infected population worldwide (UNAIDS/WHO 2002), plus the social stigma surrounding the diagnosis of HIV infection in African countries makes it difficult to identify an HIV-negative wet nurse within the family or to use a milk bank, other alternatives to breastfeeding. The WHO guidelines do not specify heat treatment conditions to be used, but several approaches have/are being tested.

Table 1. Modified breastfeeding options recommended by the WHO for HIV-infected mothers

1. Formula feeding
2. Exclusive breastfeeding with abrupt early weaning after 3–6 months
3. HIV-negative wet nurse within the family
4. Human milk bank
5. Expression and heat treatment of milk

3.2. Heat Treatment of Human Milk

In light of susceptibility of HIV to heat (Pennypacker et al. 1995), heat treatment of infected human milk seems to be a simple, inexpensive strategy, applicable in impoverished areas [Table 2]. Holder Pasteurization (62°C for 30 minutes) is used in milk banks (Lawrence & Lawrence 1999) to clear potentially contaminated donor milk from pathogens, including HIV. Orloff and colleagues reported decreased cell-free and cell-associated HIV in spiked human milk samples, 5 logs and 6 logs, respectively (Orloff et al. 1993). With this treatment, however, there is significant loss of immunoglobulin M (IgM), lactoferrin, and the saturated iron binding capacity. Holder pasteurization also reduces IgA levels by 20% (Ford et al. 1977). If milk is treated, instead, at 56°C for 30 minutes (Orloff et al. 1993), IgA, IgM, and iron binding capacity are conserved (Ford et al. 1977), but cell-associated HIV still is detectable.

Table 2. Heat treatment options of HIV-infected human milk

1. Holder pasteurization
2. Heating of milk in a water bath
a. Boiling of human milk
b. Pretoria pasteurization
3. Solar-powered pasteurization device

Chantry et al. (2000) boiled human milk from four HIV-positive mothers in a small water bath. Upon reaching the boiling point, the human milk was removed from the heat source. None of the cellular fractions of boiled milk samples were positive for HIV-1 proviral DNA as tested by qualitative PCR analysis. This report did not specify volumes of milk or water used or temperature controls. Boiling human milk destroys 100% of its immunologic activity (Lawrence & Lawrence 1999).

Pretoria pasteurization (Jeffery & Mercer 2000; Jeffery et al. 2001), similar to Holder pasteurization, heats human milk to 56°C–62°C for up to 15 minutes. Of 51 samples tested (human milk of HIV-positive women and spiked milk samples), none had evidence of persistence of infectious HIV using p24 or by PCR analyses of human milk cells exposed to treatment. However, the lack of consistency among the positive controls makes it hard to clearly determine the efficacy of this method. Only 9 of 51 control samples were positive for infectious virus. Pretoria pasteurization, however, offers the advantage of using simple utensils accessible to most households (i.e., a peanut butter jar and an aluminum pot).

A solar-powered pasteurizer device was proposed by Boisen and Jorgensen (2000); this device may be used to heat expressed human milk to 60°C for 30 minutes. Besides bacteria, the authors claim that the device also can destroy HIV in human milk as determined by culture of the cell-free fraction and cells in human milk. The lack of need for electricity makes this device attractive to use in rural areas. Caveats are its cost of $100 per child and that it is not discreet (Madsen 2000). This would require a community-based approach as well as education of the community to overcome the social stigma.

Heat treatment methods in practice are cumbersome in areas without a readily available heat source (Papathakis & Rollins 2002). The potentially negative impact of heating human milk should be studied further.

3.3. Lipolysis

Human milk lipase normally releases free fatty acids that have intrinsic antiviral activity against some enveloped viruses (Thormar et al. 1987). These lipases are active in milk stored at room temperature. Thus, Chantry et al. (2000) also tested the effect of this natural event on HIV. This simple, practical method unfortunately did not destroy HIV-1 proviral DNA. Therefore, this has been discarded as a method to prevent mother-to-child transmission of HIV through human milk.

3.4. Treatment of the Breastfeeding Mother with Antimicrobial Agents

Perinatal transmission of HIV can be prevented with short-course antiretroviral (ARV) treatment of the mother and the newborn. However, the efficacy of these regimens to reduce mother-to-child transmission through human milk remains a high research priority (UNFPA/UNICEF/WHO/UNAIDS 2000). The protection offered by Zidovudine (ZDV) and Nevirapine regimens continues despite exposure to HIV during breastfeeding for up to 12 to 24 months (UNFPA/UNICEF/WHO/UNAIDS 2000; Leroy et al. 2002). The long-term efficacy of a combined ZDV with Lamivudine (3TC) is in progress (UNFPA/UNICEF/WHO/UNAIDS 2000). The long-term safety for children exposed to ARV remains undetermined (Bultreys et al. 2002). The antimalarial chloroquine (CQ) inhibits post-translational modification of newly produced viral gp120 of HIV-1 and HIV-2 (Savarino et al. 2001). After treating women during the last 10 days of pregnancy and first 10 days postpartum (100 mg/day), CQ accumulated in unspecified human milk cells (Boelaert et al. 2001). CQ is absorbed from human milk by the neonate, with a maximum safe dose of 4.4±2.6 mg (Ogunbona et al. 1987). The effects of CQ on the emergence of HIV resistance and its possible toxicity need to be addressed further.

3.5. AIDS Vaccine

The search for an HIV/AIDS vaccine started in 1987 (UNAIDS 2001) and remains under study. Over 100 trials for preventive or therapeutic vaccination against HIV/AIDS have taken place or are currently in progress (ACTIS 2002). However, less than 10% of the trials are directed to prevent mother-to-child transmission through breastfeeding. Strategies proposed to develop a vaccine that would protect a child from mother-to-child transmission include the use of the third variable region (V3) of gp120 to induce neutralizing antibodies to HIV-1 (Mofenson & Burns 1991) or the use of the controversial anti-idiotypic antibody network (Denisova et al. 2000). The conserved V3 region among different HIV strains has been associated with decreased risk of mother-to-child transmission (Mofenson & Burns 1991). Denisova et al. (2000) showed in vitro that an anti-idiotypic antibody that identifies the antigen/antibody complex of the V3 loop with its corresponding anti-V3 antibody, renders the anti-V3 antibody cross-reactive and allows it to neutralize an otherwise resistant strain of HIV. The first clinical trial in neonates was conducted in 1993 by Borkowsky and colleagues with two different recombinant gp120 vaccines (Bass 2001). A Phase I clinical trial in nursing newborns with a canarypox-based vaccine (ALVAC vCP1452) has been proposed by Laura Guay and Francis Mimro (Bass 2001). A Phase I/II study of the effects of giving two anti-HIV vaccines to infants of HIV-positive mothers is recruiting subjects (ACTIS 2002). However, nursing infants are not eligible to enroll. A vaccine is not likely to be available any time soon. Until then, other alternatives to prevent HIV transmission are in high demand.

3.6. Treatment of Infected Human Milk with Microbicides

Alkyl sulfates are chaotropic agents and anionic surfactants widely used in cosmetics and personal care products (e.g., soaps, lotions, toothpaste, baby wipes). The prototype of this chemical family is sodium dodecyl sulfate (SDS). We previously have reported that SDS is microbicidal against sexually transmitted agents, such as HIV-1, herpes simplex virus type 2 (HSV-2), human papillomavirus and chlamydia (Howett et al. 1999). This broad-spectrum activity is observed with concentrations as low as 0.025%. SDS is of low toxicity with a maximum safe dose for children of up to 1 g/kg (Dreisbach & Robertson 1987). SDS (≥0.1–1%) inactivates HSV-2 and HIV-1-spiked human milk, and can be removed from milk without recovery of infectious HSV-2 (Urdaneta et al., unpublished data). Very importantly, SDS treatment/removal did not affect significantly nutritional and protective functions (proteins, lipids, immunoglobulins) of human milk. Monocaprin, a related and potentially edible compound, also was effective in inactivating HSV-2 added to human milk. Further study of inactivation of human milk naturally or artificially infected with HIV is in progress. SDS has the advantage of rapid inactivation of viruses and bacteria (i.e., within minutes upon contact with the agents); SDS does not require a heat source and is inexpensive. A decontamination device could be designed so that infected human milk may be hand-expressed or pumped into a recipient (i.e., nursing bottle or sac) containing SDS. A nipple manifold would have incorporated a filter that would remove the microbicide as the child sucks the milk from the bottle. As a result, the child would receive nutritionally and immunologically sound human milk, free from HIV-1 and other contaminants, and virtually free of microbicides. Microbicidal inactivation of HIV-1 is an attractive alternative to prevent mother-to-child transmission through human milk. However, its application would require education of stigmatized and extremely resource-poor areas of the world.

4. CONCLUSIONS

Research to prevent mother-to-child transmission through human milk has been particularly active during the past decade with no definite results. Hopes for an HIV/AIDS vaccine are high, but this is a long-term goal. In the mean time, palliative measures are in urgent need to prevent continued transmission of HIV. In the context of mother-to-child transmission, great progress has been achieved in preventing/reducing antenatal and intrapartum transmission. Human milk-borne transmission remains a difficult issue to tackle in resource-poor areas of the world, such as the African continent. Here, the health benefits of breastfeeding outweigh the risk of HIV transmission. Strong social and cultural boundaries do not make the task any easier. An ideal option to prevent mother-to-child transmission through human milk would effectively reduce/inactivate HIV infectivity, maintain milk's nutritional and protective value, be inexpensive and socially/culturally acceptable.

5. REFERENCES

[ACTIS] AIDS Clinical Trials Information Service. Available at www.actis.org. Accessed 12/2/02.

Bass E. AIDS vaccines and HIV transmission via breastfeeding. Is there a role for vaccines in protecting infants against HIV in breast milk? *AIDScience* Vol. 1, No. 14, November 8, 2001. Available at http://aidscience.org.

Boelaert JR, Yaro S, Augustijns P, Meda N, Schneider YJ, Schols D, Mols R, De Laere EA, Van de Perre P. Chloroquine accumulates in breast-milk cells: potential impact in the prophylaxis of postnatal mother-to-child transmission of HIV-1. AIDS 2001;15:2205-2207.

Boisen F, Jorgensen AF. Pasteurization of HIV contaminated breast milk. Abstract No. LbPp122. XIII International AIDS Conference. Durban, South Africa; 2000.

Bultreys M, Nolan ML, Jamieson DJ, Dominguez K, Fowler MG. Advances in the prevention of mother-to-child HIV-1 transmission: Current issues, future challenges. *AIDScience* Vol. 2, No. 4, February 28, 2002. Available at http://aidscience.org.

Chantry CJ, Morrison P, Panchula J, Rivera C, Hillyer G, Zorilla C, Diaz C. Effects of lipolysis or heat treatment on HIV-1 provirus in breast milk. J Acquir Immune Defic Syndr 2000;24:325-329.

Denisova GF, Zerwanitzer M, Denisov DA, Spectorman E, Mondor I, Sattentau Q, Gershoni JM. Expansion of epitope cross-reactivity by anti-idiotype modulation of the primary humoral response. Mol Immunol 2000;37:53-58.

Dreisbach RH, Robertson WO. Handbook of Poisoning: Prevention, Diagnosis and Treatment. 12th Edition. Norwalk, CT: Appleton & Lange, 1987.

Dunn DT, Newell ML, Ades AE, Peckham CS. Risk of human immunodeficiency virus type 1 transmission through breastfeeding. Lancet 1992;340:585-588.

Edgeworth RL, Ugen KE. Immunopathological factors for vertical transmission of HIV-1. Pathobiology 2000;68:53-67.

Ford JE, Law BA, Marshall VM, Reiter B. Influence of the heat treatment of human milk on some of its protective constituents. J Pediatr 1977;90:29-35.

Howett MK, Neely EB, Christensen ND, Wigdahl B, Krebs FC, Malamud D, Patrick SD, Pickel MD, Welsh PA, Reed CA, Ward MG, Budgeon LR, Kreider JW. A broad-spectrum microbicide with virucidal activity against sexually transmitted viruses. Antimicrob Agents Chemother 1999;43:314-321.

Jeffery BS, Mercer KG. Pretoria pasteurisation: a potential method for the reduction of postnatal mother to child transmission of the human immunodeficiency virus. J Trop Pediatr 2000;46:219-223.

Jeffery BS, Webber L, Mokhondo KR, Erasmus D. Determination of the effectiveness of inactivation of human immunodeficiency virus by Pretoria pasteurization. J Trop Pediatr 2001;47:345-349.

Leroy V, Karon JM, Alioum A, Ekpini ER, Meda N, Greenberg AE, Msellati P, Hudgens M, Dabis F, Wiktor SZ. Twenty-four month efficacy of a maternal short-course zidovudine regimen to prevent mother-to-child transmission of HIV-1 in West Africa. AIDS 2002;16:631-641.

Madsen BF. Solar-powered device inactivates HIV in breast milk. AIDS Education Global Information System (AEGIS). Available at www.aegis.com/news/ads/2000/AD001616.html; 2000.

Mofenson LM, Burns DN. Passive immunization to prevent mother-infant transmission of human immunodeficiency virus: current issues and future directions. Pediatr Infect Dis J 1991;10:456-462.

Ogunbona FA, Onyeji CO, Bolaji OO, Torimiro SE. Excretion of chloroquine and desethylchloroquine in human milk. Br J Clin Pharmacol 1987;23:473-476.

Orloff SL, Wallingford JC, McDougal JS. Inactivation of human immunodeficiency virus type I in human milk: effects of intrinsic factors in human milk and of pasteurization. J Hum Lact 1993;9:13-17.

Papathakis PC, Rollins NC. Adequacy of feeding recommendations for infants of HIV-infected mothers: assessment of nutrient content, cost and preparation time of breastmilk replacements in the South African context. Oral Presentation (MoOrF1030). XIV International AIDS Conference. Barcelona, Spain; 2002.

Pennypacker C, Perelson AS, Nys N, Nelson G, Sessler DI. Localized or systemic in vivo heat inactivation of human immunodeficiency virus (HIV): a mathematical analysis. J Acquir Immune Defic Syndr Hum Retrovirol 1995;8:321-329.

Savarino A, Gennero L, Chen HC, Serrano D, Malavasi F, Boelaert JR, Sperber K. Anti-HIV effects of chloroquine: mechanisms of inhibition and spectrum of activity. AIDS 2001;15:2221-2229.

Thormar H, Isaacs CE, Brown HR, Barshatzky MR, Pessolano T. Inactivation of enveloped viruses and killing of cells by fatty acids and monoglycerides. Antimicrob Agents Chemother 1987;31:27-31.

UNAIDS. Fact Sheet. The Search for an HIV Vaccine. United Nations Special Session on HIV/AIDS. New York, June 2001.

UNAIDS/WHO. AIDS Epidemic Update: December 2000. Geneva: World Health Organization; 2000.

UNAIDS/WHO. AIDS Epidemic Update: December 2002. Geneva: World Health Organization; 2002.

UNFPA/UNICEF/WHO/UNAIDS. New data on the prevention of mother-to-child transmission of HIV and their policy implications—Conclusions and recommendations. Report No. WHO/RHR/01.28; Geneva: World Health Organization; October 2000.

WHO/UNAIDS/UNICEF. Technical consultation on HIV and infant feeding implementation guidelines. Report of a meeting. Geneva, 20-22 April 1998. Geneva: World Health Organization; 1998.

INHIBITION OF HIV-1 INFECTION IN VITRO BY HUMAN MILK SULFATED GLYCOLIPIDS AND GLYCOSAMINOGLYCANS

M. Viveros-Rogel[1], L. Soto-Ramirez[1], P. Chaturvedi[2], D.S. Newburg[2], and G.M. Ruiz-Palacios[1]

1. INTRODUCTION

Sulfated glycolipids (SG) and glycosaminoglycans (GAG) present on the surface of colonic, vaginal epithelial, and neuroglial cells bind to HIV gp120, suggesting that these glycoconjugates may have a role in HIV infection. The major goal of our study was to test the ability of SG and GAG from human milk to inhibit HIV-1 infection in vitro. SG and GAG were purified from pooled human milk and characterized by high pressure liquid chromatography (HPLC) and mass spectrometry. Eight different preparations of SG and one of GAG were tested for inhibition of infection. Two laboratory isolates, HIV-1_{ADA} (macrophage-tropic virus) and HIV-1_{SF2} (lymphotropic virus), were used for inhibition assays using peripheral blood mononuclear cells (PBMC) and monocyte-derived macrophages (MDM). Inhibition assays were performed by preincubation of serial dilutions of glycoconjugates with each virus before infecting the monolayer of cultured MDM and PBMC. After 4 days, HIV p24 antigen was quantified by enzyme immunoassay (EIA) in culture supernatants. Significant inhibition of viral infectivity was defined as >80% reduction in p24 concentration. GAG showed a low inhibitory effect (8–44%) in HIV-1 infection of PBMC. Table 1 shows the minimal amounts of the most active SG fractions, expressed as volumes of human milk from which they were extracted, that inhibit >80% HIV-1 infection.

Table 1. HIV infection of dendritic cells is inhibited by human milk sulfatides (mL)

Target cells	HIV-1_{ADA}	HIV-1_{SF2}
MDM	0.5	0.5
PBMC	0.25	0.25

HIV=human immunodeficiency virus; MDM=monocyte-derived macrophages; PBMC=peripheral blood mononuclear cells

[1]Department of Infectious Diseases, Instituto Nacional de Ciencias Médicas y Nutrición Salvador Zubirán, Mexico City, Mexico
[2]Shriver Center, University of Massachusetts Medical School, Waltham, MA, USA

Protecting Infants through Human Milk, edited by Pickering *et al.*
Kluwer Academic/Plenum Publishers, 2004

These results show that sulfated glycolipids from human milk inhibit infection of PBMC and MDM by HIV-1 laboratory isolates in vitro.

2. BACKGROUND

The global epidemic of AIDS has become one of the most pressing public health emergencies of the last 20 years. The Joint United Nations Programme on HIV/AIDS (UNAIDS) and the World Health Organization (WHO) at the end of December 2002 recorded 42 million people living with HIV/AIDS worldwide (UNAIDS 2002).

Transmission of HIV can occur through contact with infected body fluids. Vertical transmission of HIV from an infected mother to her child is a special problem. Almost all HIV-infected children acquire the virus from their mothers either before or during birth or from ingestion of milk from their mothers (Schwartz et al. 1999). WHO has estimated that up to one-third of all cases of transmission of HIV-1 from an infected mother to her child may occur via human milk (Nicoll et al. 2000; Richardson et al. 2003).

Although maternal milk can serve as a source of virus transmission to the newborn, this fluid also contains many substances that can block virus infection. Human milk contains large numbers and amounts of complex carbohydrates including glycoconjugates and oligosaccharides that protect infants against a variety of infectious pathogens (Zopf et al. 1996; Newburg et al. 1996, 1999).

Glycoconjugates, including glycoproteins, glycolipids, mucins, and glycosaminoglycans, contain complex oligosaccharide structures attached to proteins, lipids, and other molecular backbones. Complex carbohydrate moieties of glycoconjugates and oligosaccharides are synthesized by the many glycosyltransferases in the mammary gland; those with homology to cell surface glycoconjugate pathogen receptors may inhibit pathogen binding, thereby protecting the nursing infant (Yarema et al. 1998; Bertozzi et al. 2001). Sulfated glycolipids have been reported to be receptors for a variety of microbes, included HIV-1 virus (Kamisago et al. 1996; Suzuki et al. 1996; Yahi et al. 1992; Bath et al. 1993; Schneider-Schaulies et al. 2000).

Glycolipids are ubiquitous in cell surface membranes, and importantly, the glycolipid-enriched membrane domain also includes proteins related to signal transduction. Several investigations suggest that sulfated glycolipids perform important functions in the areas of cellular recognition, cell-cell adhesion, migration, and receptor-mediated signal transduction (Vos et al. 1994; Hirabayashi et al. 1999). The negative charge of the sulfated glycolipids allows them to bind to positively charged amino acid side-chains of proteins. By imparting a negative charge to the glycoconjugates, the sulfated groups may promote concentration of negative charges at the cell surface in proximity to the lipid bilayer, thereby helping processes such as cell adhesion, cell invasion, cell fusion, and endocytosis.

Evidence suggests that glycosaminoglycans (a class of compounds characterized by large sulfated polysaccharides) of human milk also inhibit HIV infection in vitro by binding to the CD4 host cell receptor (Newburg et al. 1995).

Sulfated glycolipids and glycosaminoglycans present on the surface of colonic and vaginal epithelium and neuroglial cells bind to gp120, the outer membrane protein of HIV, suggesting that these glycoconjugates may have a role in HIV infection (Furuta et al. 1994; Harouse et al. 1991). Human milk contains both GAGs and sulfatides that inhibit the binding of gp120 to CD4 in an EIA. Therefore, the GAGs and sulfatides of human milk could influence the rate of vertical transmission of this virus through breast-feeding if they are present in human milk in biologically relevant concentrations.

The purpose of this study was to test the ability of several sulfated glycolipid species and glycosaminoglycans from human milk to inhibit the infection of human MDM and PBMC cells by laboratory strains of HIV-1. Human MDM and PBMC cells are good models to study HIV infection in vitro because they are primary target cells of HIV.

3. OBJECTIVES

We tested the ability of the human milk GAGs and SG to inhibit the infection of primary human MDM and PBMC cells by HIV-1 in vitro.

4. MATERIALS AND METHODS

4.1. Isolation and Purification of Sulfated Glycolipids from Human Milk

Purified individual sulfated glycolipid species from pooled human milk were obtained as follows: human milk was obtained from the New England Milk Bank and was kept frozen at –80°C until use. Lipids were extracted from milk using chloroform/methanol/water, and the lipids of the organic lower phase were partitioned between 90% aqueous methanol and hexane. The hexane phase containing the bulk of triglycerides was discarded and the lipid extract was subjected to alkaline hydrolysis with 0.6 N methanolic sodium hydroxide to eliminate phospholipids. After neutralization with hydrochloric acid, the sample was desalted on a C-18 column followed by ion-exchange chromatography on a DEAE-Sephadex column (acetate form) equilibrated with chloroform. The sample was loaded in chloroform and the column was washed with 8 column volumes of chloroform to remove neutral glycolipids. The sulfated glycolipids were eluted with a 0.5 M potassium acetate solution in chloroform/methanol (4:1) containing 10 mL of ammonium hydroxide per 500 mL of solution, followed by desalting on a C-18 column. This sulfatide sample, designated 1, was dried under nitrogen and stored at –20°C until testing.

The individual sulfated glycolipid species were purified using a combination of normal and reversed-phase HPLC. The normal-phase HPLC was carried out on a silica column using a gradient elution with methylene chloride/methanol/0.1 M ammonium acetate (pH 4.0). Absorption at 200 nm was used to detect glycolipids, and peak fractions were collected on the basis of their correspondence to authentic sulfated glycolipids available, or by the number of sugar moieties or type of fatty acid chain in the ceramide part of the molecule as determined by mass spectrometry. The fractions were further purified based on the fatty acid length on a reversed-phase column with methanol/methylene chloride as the mobile phase. Individual peaks corresponding to pure molecular species were collected, dried, and stored. In order to confirm the presence of sulfated glycolipids, the sample was analyzed by direct-injection negative-ion electrospray mass spectrometry.

The sulfatides of sample 1 were further purified on a silicic acid column. Sample 1, dissolved in chloroform, was loaded onto a silicic acid column that had been equilibrated with chloroform. After rinsing the column with an aliquot of chloroform, the sulfatides were eluted from the column with acetone, and this purified sulfatide fraction, designated

2, was dried under nitrogen and stored at –20°C until testing. Sample 1 was subfractionated on an aminopropyl silica column (100 mg Bond-Elut cartridge, Varian, Harbor City, CA) that had been conditioned with hexane. Sample 1 was dissolved in chloroform and loaded onto the column. Fractions were eluted sequentially from the column with: ethyl acetate/hexane (15:85), yielding sample 3; chloroform/methanol (23:1), sample 4; di-isopropylether/acetic acid (98:5), sample 5; acetone/methanol (9:1.35), sample 6; chloroform/methanol (2:1), sample 7; and chloroform/methanol/3.6 M ammonium acetate (30:60:8), sample 8. All samples were dried under nitrogen and stored at –20°C until testing. The glycosaminoglycan fraction was prepared from pooled human milk as described previously (Newburg et al. 1995).

4.2. Cell-Based Assay for Inhibition of HIV-1 Infection

Human milk SG and GAG were tested for their ability to inhibit infection by HIV. The above eight different preparations of SG and the GAG preparation were tested by first dissolving (with vortexing) the glycoconjugates in a volume of sterile PBS (phosphate buffer saline) equal to 0.05 times the volume of human milk from which it was isolated (20×) to obtain a stock solution.

Two laboratory isolates, HIV-1_{ADA} (macrophage-tropic virus) and HIV-1_{SF2} (lymphotropic virus), were used for inhibition assays; concentration of HIV-1 p24 antigen was determined by a HIV-1 p24 EIA. Virus stock concentration was adjusted to 1 ng/mL for the inhibition assay. PBMCs from an HIV-1 seronegative individual were purified by the Ficoll/Hypaque method, stimulated with 5 μg/mL of phytohemagglutinin A (PHA) and activated with 10 U/mL of recombinant human interleukin 2 (IL-2) for 48 h at 37°C and 5% CO_2. PBMCs were cultured with RPMI 1640 medium containing 20% fetal bovine serum and 1% of antibiotics (100 U/mL of penicillin and 100 μg/mL of streptomycin). MDM cells were isolated by their adherence to plastic using 4×10^6 PBMCs per well in a 48-well cell culture plate. MDM were maintained in RPMI 1640 plus 5% human serum and 20% fetal bovine serum at 37°C and 5% CO_2. After 5 days, cells were washed twice with PBS and maintained in RPMI 1640 with 20% fetal bovine serum and 1% antibiotics at 37°C and 5% CO_2 until a monolayer of MDM was formed (10–12 days).

Serial dilutions of glycoconjugates were preincubated with each viral stock (1 ng/mL of HIV-1 p24 antigen) for 3 h at 37°C prior to their addition to monolayers of cultured MDC or PBMC (5×10^5 cells/well). This mixture of cells, virus, and glycoconjugates was incubated overnight (16 h) at 37°C and 5% CO_2. After overnight incubation, cells were washed twice with PBS and maintained with RPMI 1640 medium with 20% fetal bovine serum and 1% antibiotics (500 μL/well) for 4 days. At day 4 postinfection, culture supernatant was collected to quantify HIV p24 antigen by EIA. Significant inhibition of viral infectivity was defined as >80% reduction in p24 concentration. The percent of inhibition was calculated as follows:

a) p24 concentration from the sample (virus+cells+glycolipid) / p24 concentration from the positive control (virus+cells) * 100 = x% infection

b) 100% infection – x% = % inhibition.

5. RESULTS

We found low inhibition (8–44%) with the human milk GAG preparation in HIV-1 infection of PBMC. Glycosaminoglycans were tested in a range of concentration of 0.03× to 3.3×, 1× being the equivalent concentration in PBS as it is found in pooled human milk. In six of the eight preparations of SG tested, we found a high inhibitory effect (>80%) on HIV-1 infection of PBMC and MDM cells; fractions 6 and 7 did not inhibit HIV-1_{ADA} infection of PBMCs. Table 2 shows the minimal amounts of SG expressed in equivalent amounts per volume of human milk that inhibit >80% infection of HIV-1_{ADA} and HIV-1_{SF2} laboratory isolates.

Table 2. Inhibition of HIV infection by human milk sulfatide fractions

		HIV-1_{ADA}		HIV-1_{SF2}	
Target cells	Preparation of sulfated glycolipids	Amount of sulfated glycolipids expressed as equivalent volumes of human milk	Percent inhibition	Amount of sulfated glycolipids expressed as equivalent volumes of human milk	Percent inhibition
MDM	1	13	99	13	86
	2	3.6	100	3.6	95
	3	1	97	0.5	100
	4	0.5	100	0.5	100
	5	1	100	0.5	100
	6	7.4	100	0.5	100
	7	1	96	0.5	100
	8	1	85	4	100
PBMC	1	24	100	4	100
	2	0.25	100	0.25	84
	3	2	92	2	88
	4	2	89	4	99
	5	2	83	2	93
	6	----	0	2	95
	7	----	0	2	90
	8	4	100	2	93

Sulfated glycolipid fractions from human milk inhibited HIV-1 infection of PBMC and MDM in vitro, even at low concentrations, indicating high biologic potency. The inhibition of virus infectivity was independent of virus strain (HIV-1_{ADA} and HIV-1_{SF2}) or cell type used as infection target.

6. DISCUSSION

All of the human milk fractions were tested at concentrations that would be relevant to breastfed infants. The human milk glycosaminoglycan fractions, even in high concentrations, show only low inhibition of HIV-1 infection in PBMC cells. The range of concentrations that the GAG fraction contributes to the inhibition of HIV-1 infection of target cells should be further evaluated. It is possible that individual GAGs might more strongly inhibit HIV-1 infection in vitro.

The sulfated glycolipid fraction of human milk contains sulfated glycolipids that vary in fatty acid chain length, sugar residues and sulfate groups, as identified by normal and reversed-phase HPLC and mass spectrometric analysis. The heterogeneity and structural complexity of the human milk sulfated glycolipids, in conjunction with our finding that different purified fractions have highest activity with MDM and PBNCs, suggest the possibility that some individual glycolipid species may be highly potent, as the absolute amounts of individual active species present in the glycolipid fraction could be extremely minute.

Despite the presence of human milk glycoconjugates with antiviral activity, including active sulfated glycolipid species, the continuous exposure to HIV in children nursing HIV-positive mothers can lead to HIV transmission through breastfeeding being a significant cause of HIV infection in some children. However, exclusive breastfeeding is considered the best form of feeding for the child during the early months of life, and in the case of HIV transmission for populations where the infant mortality rate is high, the risk of death associated with the lack of breastfeeding may be greater than the risk of HIV infection acquired through human milk.

In summary, sulfated glycolipids in human milk have biologic functions, and may play a role in protection against viral pathogens. Furthermore, the sulfated glycolipid fraction of human milk can be a useful source from which to characterize the biological role of sulfated glycolipids.

The identification of human milk components that protect against HIV infection would contribute significantly to the information regarding breastfeeding and vertical transmission of HIV. The strong inhibitory activity against HIV-1 infection in vitro by human milk sulfated glycolipids support the possibility that these glycoconjugates may act as soluble receptor homologues, preventing HIV-1 interaction with target cells. Knowing the precise structure/function relationship could lead to future generations of highly selective and potent therapeutic and pharmaceutical reagents.

7. ACKNOWLEDGMENT

This work was supported by a program project grant from the National Institute of Child Health and Human Development (HD13021).

8. REFERENCES

Bertozzi CR, Kiessling LL. Chemical glycobiology. Science 2001;291:2357-2364.

Bhat S, Mettus RV, Reddy EP, Ugen KE, Srikanthan V, Williams WV, Weiner DB. The galactosyl ceramide/sulfatide receptor binding region of HIV-1 gp120 maps to amino acids 206-275. AIDS Res Hum Retroviruses 1993;9:175-181.

Furuta Y, Eriksson K, Svennerholm B, Fredman P, Horal P, Jeansson S, Vahlne A, Holmgren J, Czerkinsky C. Infection of vaginal and colonic epithelial cells by the human immunodeficiency virus type 1 is neutralized by antibodies raised against conserved epitopes in the envelope glycoprotein gp120. Proc Natl Acad Sci USA 1994;91:12559-12563.

Harouse JM, Bhat S, Spitalnik SL, Laughlin M, Stefano K, Silberberg DH, Gonzalez-Scarano F. Inhibition of entry of HIV-1 in neural cell lines by antibodies against galactosyl ceramide. Science 1991;253:320-323.

Hirabayashi Y, Ichikawa S. In: Fukuda M, Hindsgaul O, editors. Roles of Glycolipids and Sphingolipids in Biological Membrane. The Frontiers in Molecular Biology Series. Oxford: IRL Press at Oxford University Press, 1999; pp 220-248.

Kamisago S, Iwamori M, Tai T, Mitamura K, Yazaki Y, Sugano K. Role of sulfatides in adhesion of Helicobacter pylori to gastric cancer cells. Infect Immun 1996;64:624-628.

Newburg DS. Human milk glycoconjugates that inhibit pathogens. Curr Med Chem 1999;6:117-127.

Newburg DS. Oligosaccharides and glycoconjugates in human milk: their role in host defense. J Mammary Gland Biol Neoplasia 1996;1:271-283.

Newburg DS, Linhardt RJ, Ampofo SA, Yolken RH. Human milk glycosaminoglycans inhibit HIV glycoprotein gp120 binding to its host cell CD4 receptor. J Nutr 1995;125:419-424.

Nicoll A, Newell ML, Peckham C, Luo C, Savage F. Infant feeding and HIV-1 infection. AIDS 2000;14 Suppl 3:S57-74.

Richardson BA, John-Stewart GC, Hughes JP, Nduati R, Mbori-Ngacha D, Overbaugh J, Kreiss JK. Breast-milk infectivity in human immunodeficiency virus type 1-infected mothers. J Infect Dis 2003;187:736-740.

Schneider-Schaulies J. Cellular receptors for viruses: links to tropism and pathogenesis. J Gen Virol 2000;81:1413-1429.

Schwartz SA, Nair MP. Current concepts in human immunodeficiency virus infection and AIDS. Clin Diagn Lab Immunol 1999;6:295-305.

Suzuki T, Sometani A, Yamazaki Y, Horiike G, Mizutani Y, Masuda H, Yamada M, Tahara H, Xu G, Miyamoto D, Oku N, Okada S, Kiso M, Hasegawa A, Ito T, Kawaoka Y, Suzuki Y. Sulphatide binds to human and animal influenza A viruses, and inhibits the viral infection. Biochem J 1996;318(Part 2):389-393.

UNAIDS. AIDS Epidemic Update, December 2002.

Vos JP, Lopes-Cardozo M, Gadella BM. Metabolic and functional aspects of sulfogalactolipids. Biochim Biophys Acta 1994;1211:125-149.

Yahi N, Baghdiguian S, Moreau H, Fantini J. Galactosyl ceramide (or a closely related molecule) is the receptor for human immunodeficiency virus type 1 on human colon epithelial HT29 cells. J Virol 1992;66:4848-4854.

Yarema KJ, Bertozzi CR. Chemical approaches to glycobiology and emerging carbohydrate-based therapeutic agents. Curr Opin Chem Biol 1998;2:49-61.

Zopf D, Roth S. Oligosaccharide anti-infective agents. Lancet 1996;347:1017-1021.

TRANSMISSION OF CYTOMEGALOVIRUS (CMV) THROUGH HUMAN MILK

Are New Breastfeeding Policies Required for Preterm Infants?

Andrea Willeitner

1. INTRODUCTION

Nine out of ten mothers with positive cytomegalovirus (CMV) serology shed CMV in their milk at some time during lactation. CMV is transmitted readily through human milk. Although the majority of acquired CMV infections cause little or no symptoms, there is an association between CMV infection and severe disease in small premature infants. Pasteurization damages some of the anti-infective properties of untreated human milk but is the only reliable and feasible method to destroy CMV infectivity. The current practice of feeding untreated human milk may require reevaluation for seropositive mothers of very immature infants.

2. BACKGROUND

Postnatally acquired CMV infection has rarely, if ever, been associated with significant disease in healthy term infants. However, case reports of serious disease and death from CMV infections acquired in the early postnatal period have been reported in immunocompromised infants, and human milk has been suggested as a possible route of transmission (Richter et al. 1997; Jonkhoff-Slok et al. 1997). Preterm infants are physiologically immunodeficient due to their immaturity, and the potential clinical relevance of CMV transmission through human milk has raised questions about the appropriateness of feeding strategies currently applied in this population.

Neonatal/Perinatal Medicine, University of Wisconsin–Madison, Meriter Hospital, 6 Center, 202 S. Park Street, Madison, WI 53715

Protecting Infants through Human Milk, edited by Pickering *et al.*
Kluwer Academic/Plenum Publishers, 2004

3. METHODS

A review of the literature published between 1966 and January 31, 2003 was performed using the Medline database with the PubMed interface. The main search keyword was *cytomegalovirus,* additional search parameters were *serologic tests, vertical disease transmission, premature, milk, lactation, human milk,* and *breast milk.* The search was limited to "human studies" and "infants (birth to 23 months of age)."

Of the 426 original references identified, 205 contained information on postnatally acquired CMV infection, 86 of these dealt with premature infants, and 39 addressed CMV in human milk.

4. RESULTS

4.1. Epidemiology of CMV

In pregnant women, the seroprevalence of CMV IgG antibodies is between 48 percent [France] and 100 percent [Thailand] (Gambarotto et al. 1997; Tantivanich et al. 1999). In our experience, between 49 percent [Munich, Germany] and 71 percent [Madison, WI, USA] of pregnant women are seropositive for CMV IgG (unpublished data). Reactivation and intermittent CMV shedding seems to occur in 20 percent of pregnancies and in the postnatal period (Shen et al. 1993; Kumar et al. 1985; Doerr 1987). CMV is found in saliva, tears, urine, cervical secretions, and human milk of women before and after delivery, but the frequency and duration of postpartum virus reactivation is largely unknown (Stagno 1995).

4.2. CMV in Human Milk

CMV shedding in human milk was described in 16 to 70 percent of seropositive mothers at some time during lactation (Pana et al. 1981; Dworsky et al. 1983; Ahlfors & Ivarsson 1985). The wide variation may be explained by varying frequency of milk sampling and different sensitivities of assay methods used. Clinical studies using PCR as the gold standard for viral detection found CMV DNA in the milk of more than 90 percent of seropositive mothers, with over 75 percent shedding infectious virus (Hamprecht et al. 2001).

4.3. CMV Transmission

In cross-sectional studies, the major predictors of CMV infection of children at age one year were maternal serostatus and whether or not the infant was breastfed (Peckham 1989; Minamishima et al. 1994). Infection rates between 37 and 79 percent have been reported for infants receiving CMV-positive milk (Hamprecht et al. 2001; Vochem et al. 1998; Wu et al. 1989). The role of cervical secretions seems to be less important, because in two of these studies (Hamprecht et al. 2001; Vochem et al. 1998) in which infection rates were 37 and 59 percent, the rate of cesarean section was more than 80 percent, and intrapartum contact with CMV was ruled out by negative CMV cultures obtained from the infant immediately after birth. Low infection rates in infants of seropositive mothers who do not shed CMV in their milk, or chose not to breastfeed, suggest that vertical transmission through saliva or horizontal transmission is of minor significance in the first months postpartum (Wu et al. 1989).

4.4. Clinical Impact

Hamprecht and coworkers monitored infants under 1500 g birth weight or 32 weeks gestational age for acquired CMV infection after intrauterine infection and intranatal exposure had been ruled out (Hamprecht et al. 2001; Maschmann et al. 2001). Of 90 infants born to mothers with a positive CMV serology, 33 (37%) became infected (evidenced by positive urine culture), and 16 (18%) had symptoms of CMV disease. Neutropenia (88%) was the most frequent symptom, followed by elevated liver function tests (31%) and thrombocytopenia (25%). No infant died, but four infants (25%) had sepsis-like disease, requiring reintubation in two cases. The sepsis-like disease occurred in the absence of systemic bacterial infection, but was coincidental with detection of CMV DNA in blood or urine. A cross-sectional study found clinical symptoms in 88 percent of small premature infants (mean gestational age 28.5 weeks) with postnatally acquired CMV infection (Ballard et al. 1979). Another report found symptomatic infection in 34 percent of preterm infants exposed to CMV in their mothers' milk, but of the five infected infants under 26 weeks gestational age, four (80%) developed severe sepsis-like disease (Vochem et al 1998). A study on older premature infants (mean gestational age 30.4 weeks) found a transmission rate of 25 percent in exposed infants, and none of them had clinical symptoms (Mosca et al. 2001). Little is known about the long-term impact of early acquired CMV infection; however, one case-control study found a higher risk of severe neurologic sequelae and mental handicap in infants under 2000 g birth weight (Paryani et al. 1985).

5. DISCUSSION

The high incidence of CMV transmission through human milk has been well established in term infants, with rates of infection observed between 35 and 80 percent. In healthy term infants, infection is almost always asymptomatic or subclinical, and no long-term sequelae have been seen on follow-up examinations (Wu et al. 1989; Dworsky et al. 1983; Peckham et al. 1987; Gentile et al. 1989). Transmission of CMV through human milk seems to be similarly frequent in preterm infants, and in the majority of cases infection appears to cause little if any clinical disease. The youngest and smallest premature infants, however, may have a significant risk of developing serious clinical symptoms, including sepsis-like systemic illness. The largest study published monitored 176 preterm infants under 32 weeks of gestation for acquired CMV infection. Acquisition of CMV from sources other than human milk was virtually excluded (Hamprecht et al. 2001). Of the 90 breastfed infants of CMV-seropositive mothers, 33 acquired CMV, 16 had clinical symptoms, and 4 developed severe systemic disease. While the mean birth weight for the entire sample was 1100 g, infants who developed symptomatic CMV infection had a mean birth weight of 935 g, and the sickest infants, i.e., those who had sepsis-like disease, had a mean birth weight of 795 g. In another prospective study by the same group of investigators, 80 percent of infants under 26 weeks of gestation who acquired CMV from human milk developed sepsis-like disease (Vochem et al. 1998). An earlier report found clinical disease (respiratory deterioration, hepatosplenomegaly, pallor) in 88 percent of sick preterm infants who acquired CMV infection, but blood transfusions were not ruled out as a source of infection (Ballard et al. 1979). In a study including more mature preterm infants, rates of transmission and disease were significantly lower (Mosca et al. 2001).

While the numbers are still small, there is enough clinical evidence to suggest that for a subset of very immature preterm infants, CMV infection acquired through human milk is not only a frequent event, but also associated with severe disease in a considerable number of cases. Studies that include infants under 1000 g birth weight are needed to define more clearly the population of infants at the highest risk for a severe clinical course of acquired CMV infection.

Prevention of CMV transmission through human milk can be achieved most reliably by heat treatment (pasteurization at 62.5°C, 30 minutes), which has been shown to completely destroy infectious CMV (Welsh et al. 1979; Bjorksten et al. 1980; Dworsky et al. 1982). However, pasteurization also damages many of the anti-infective properties of human milk, and pasteurized milk loses all of its antibacterial antibody activity against pathogenic *Escherichia coli* or group B streptococci in vitro (Liebhaber et al. 1977; Hernandez et al. 1979; May 1988). Moreover, a study in preterm infants found higher rates of bacterial infection when pasteurized human milk or formula was given than when untreated human milk was fed (Narayanan et al. 1984). Alternative heating methods may be gentler, but require more study (Goldblum et al. 1984).

Freezing human milk for 12 hours destroyed infectivity in nine out of ten samples (Dworsky et al. 1982), and freezing for three days or longer has been shown to reduce titers of viable CMV by 99 percent, but the virus could still be grown in cell cultures (Friis & Andersen 1982; Bryant et al. 2002). Whether the reduction of CMV achieved by freezing can reduce the clinical risk of infection remains to be established. A clinical trial found only one case of CMV infection in 18 infants fed frozen milk from their seropositive mothers (Sharland et al. 2002). However, the case number was small, and the follow-up period of 67 days may have been too short to detect all cases of infection. A prospective randomized clinical trial is warranted to compare CMV infection rates in infants fed untreated, pasteurized, and frozen milk from their CMV positive mothers to establish the clinical value of freezing for prevention of CMV infection. Formula feeding has multiple disadvantages and generally should not be encouraged.

The association of human milk-acquired CMV infection with significant disease in a substantial percentage of very small premature infants, and the availability of primary prevention through pasteurized human milk or formula raises the issue of whether mothers of infants at risk who intend to breastfeed should be tested for CMV IgG status. At present, it is unknown whether the disadvantages of pasteurization outweigh the risks of contracting CMV for these infants. However, the question of whether or not mothers with a positive CMV serology should be provided with this information should be addressed.

Finally, although the prospective studies on CMV transmission have been methodologically sound and comprehensive, they lack a clinical control group. The symptoms of acquired CMV infection are nonspecific. Neutropenia, thrombocytopenia, abnormal liver function tests, and sepsis-like disease can be caused by a multitude of factors in sick premature infants. The exclusion of systemic bacterial infection in cases of sepsis-like disease, and the observed temporal relationship between the onset of symptoms and the demonstration of CMV infection is indicative but not evidentiary for a causative relation. It could be argued that infants who are sick or unstable for reasons other than CMV are more prone to contract the virus, and that CMV is an innocent bystander rather than a pathogenic factor for their disease. A prospective study of premature infants of mothers seropositive and seronegative for CMV is required in order to compare the frequency of symptoms compatible with CMV infection between exposed and unexposed, but otherwise comparable infants. The seropositivity rate of 50 to 70 percent in many industrialized countries provides the ideal setting for such an investigation.

6. ACKNOWLEDGMENTS

The author wishes to express her gratitude to Dr. Frank Greer and Dr. David Carlton for the critical review of the manuscript.

7. REFERENCES

Ahlfors K, Ivarsson SA. Cytomegalovirus in breast milk of Swedish milk donors. Scand J Infect Dis 1985;17:11-13.

Ballard RA, Drew WL, Hufnagle KG, Riedel PA. Acquired cytomegalovirus infection in preterm infants. Am J Dis Child 1979;133:482-485.

Bjorksten B, Burman LG, De Chateau P, Fredrikzon B, Gothefors L, Hernell O. Collecting and banking human milk: to heat or not to heat? Br Med J 1980;281:765-769.

Bryant P, Morley C, Garland S, Curtis N. Cytomegalovirus transmission from breast milk in premature babies: does it matter? Arch Dis Child Fetal Neonatal Ed 2002;87:F75-77.

Doerr HW. Cytomegalovirus infection in pregnancy. J Virol Methods 1987;17:127-132.

Dworsky M, Stagno S, Pass RF, Cassady G, Alford C. Persistence of cytomegalovirus in human milk after storage. J Pediatr 1982;101:440-443.

Dworsky M, Yow M, Stagno S, Pass RF, Alford C. Cytomegalovirus infection of breast milk and transmission in infancy. Pediatrics 1983;72:295-299.

Friis H, Andersen HK. Rate of inactivation of cytomegalovirus in raw banked milk during storage at -20 degrees C and pasteurisation. Br Med J (Clin Res Ed) 1982;285:1604-1605.

Gambarotto K, Ranger-Rogez S, Aubard Y, Piver P, Duffetelle B, Delpeyroux C, Roussanne MC, Nicot T, Denis F. [Primary cytomegalovirus infection and pregnant women: epidemiological study on 1100 women at Limoges]. Pathol Biol (Paris) 1997;45:453-461.

Gentile MA, Boll TJ, Stagno S, Pass RF. Intellectual ability of children after perinatal cytomegalovirus infection. Dev Med Child Neurol 1989;31:782-786.

Goldblum RM, Dill CW, Albrecht TB, Alford ES, Garza C, Goldman AS. Rapid high-temperature treatment of human milk. J Pediatr 1984;104:380-385.

Hamprecht K, Maschmann J, Vochem M, Dietz K, Speer CP, Jahn G. Epidemiology of transmission of cytomegalovirus from mother to preterm infant by breastfeeding. Lancet 2001;357:513-518.

Hernandez J, Lemons P, Lemons J, Todd J. Effect of storage processes on the bacterial growth-inhibiting activity of human breast milk. Pediatrics 1979;63:597-601.

Jonkhoff-Slok TW, Veenhoven RH, de Graeff-Meeder ER, Buller HA. An immunocompetent infant with cow's milk allergy and cytomegalovirus colitis. Eur J Pediatr 1997;156:528-529.

Kumar ML, Jenson HB, Dahms BB. Fatal staphylococcal epidermidis infections in very low-birth-weight infants with cytomegalovirus infection. Pediatrics 1985;76:110-112.

Liebhaber M, Lewiston NJ, Asquith MT, Olds-Arroyo L, Sunshine P. Alterations of lymphocytes and of antibody content of human milk after processing. J Pediatr 1977;91:897-900.

Maschmann J, Hamprecht K, Dietz K, Jahn G, Speer CP. Cytomegalovirus infection of extremely low-birth weight infants via breast milk. Clin Infect Dis 2001;33:1998-2003.

May JT. Microbial contaminants and antimicrobial properties of human milk. Microbiol Sci 1988;5:42-46.

Minamishima I, Ueda K, Minematsu T, Minamishima Y, Umemoto M, Take H, Kuraya K. Role of breast milk in acquisition of cytomegalovirus infection. Microbiol Immunol 1994;38:549-552.

Mosca F, Pugni L, Barbi M, Binda S. Transmission of cytomegalovirus. Lancet 2001;357:1800.

Narayanan I, Prakash K, Murthy NS, Gujral VV. Randomised controlled trial of effect of raw and holder pasteurised human milk and of formula supplements on incidence of neonatal infection. Lancet 1984;2:1111-1113.

Pana A, Santi AL, Grassi M, Divizia M, Assumma M, Carratu A. On the presence of cytomegalovirus in the milk of normal women; correlation between breast feeding and virus excretion in infants. Boll Ist Sieroter Milan 1981;60:85-88.

Paryani SG, Yeager AS, Hosford-Dunn H, Johnson SJ, Malachowski N, Ariagno RL, Stevenson DK. Sequelae of acquired cytomegalovirus infection in premature and sick term infants. J Pediatr 1985;107:451-456.

Peckham CS. Cytomegalovirus in the neonate. J Antimicrob Chemother 1989;23 Suppl E:17-21.

Peckham CS, Johnson C, Ades A, Pearl K, Chin KS. Early acquisition of cytomegalovirus infection. Arch Dis Child 1987;62:780-785.

Richter D, Hampl W, Pohlandt F. Vertical transmission of cytomegalovirus, most probably by breast milk, to an infant with Wiskott-Aldrich syndrome with fatal outcome. Eur J Pediatr 1997;156:854-855.

Sharland M, Khare M, Bedford-Russell A. Prevention of postnatal cytomegalovirus infection in preterm infants. Arch Dis Child Fetal Neonatal Ed 2002;86:F140.

Shen CY, Chang SF, Chao MF, Yang SL, Lin GM, Chang WW, Wu CW, Yen MS, Ng HT, Thomas JC, et al. Cytomegalovirus recurrence in seropositive pregnant women attending obstetric clinics. J Med Virol 1993;41:24-29.

Stagno S. Cytomegalovirus. In: Remington JS, Klein JO, editors. Infectious Diseases of the Fetus and Newborn Infant. Philadelphia: WB Saunders, 1995.

Tantivanich S, Suphadtanaphongs V, Siripanth C, Desakorn V, Suphanit I, Phromin S, Panakitsuwan S, Amarapand P. Prevalence of cytomegalovirus antibodies among various age groups of Thai population. Southeast Asian J Trop Med Public Health 1999;30:265-268.

Vochem M, Hamprecht K, Jahn G, Speer CP. Transmission of cytomegalovirus to preterm infants through breast milk. Pediatr Infect Dis J 1998;17:53-58.

Welsh JK, Arsenakis M, Coelen RJ, May JT. Effect of antiviral lipids, heat, and freezing on the activity of viruses in human milk. J Infect Dis 1979;140:322-328.

Wu J, Tang ZY, Wu YX, Li WR. Acquired cytomegalovirus infection of breast milk in infancy. Chin Med J (Engl) 1989;102:124-128.

MULTIPLE NEW ISOFORMS OF THE HUMAN PROLACTIN RECEPTOR GENE

Josephine F. Trott[1], Russell C. Hovey[1], Sailaja Koduri[2], and Barbara K. Vonderhaar[2]

1. INTRODUCTION

Prolactin (PRL) is a polypeptide hormone with a clear role in promoting mammary gland growth, differentiation, and lactogenesis. In addition, endocrine and/or autocrine/ paracrine PRL (Clevenger et al. 1995; Ginsburg & Vonderhaar 1995) promotes mammary carcinogenesis in rodents (Wennbo et al. 1997) and also may contribute to the initiation and progression of human breast cancer (Hankinson et al. 1999).

PRL acts through the prolectin receptor (PRLR), a member of the large class-1 cytokine receptor superfamily (Bole-Feysot et al. 1998). The PRLR is composed of an extracellular ligand binding domain, a transmembrane region, and an intracellular domain (Kelly et al. 1989). To date the human gene has been known to contain ten exons, including five alternative exon 1 sequences, where only exons 3 through 10 are coding exons (Hu et al. 1999, 2002). Different isoforms of the PRLR have been named for the length of their intracellular domain generated by alternative 3′ splicing of a single PRLR gene (Ormandy et al. 1998; Hu et al. 1999). Until recently, two such isoforms had been cloned from humans; a long form [hPRLR-LF; exons 1 to 10] (Boutin et al. 1989) and an intermediate form [same as hPRLR-LF but lacking part of exon 10] (Kline et al. 1999). Short isoforms of the PRLR have been cloned from the rat (Boutin et al. 1988), mouse (Davis & Linzer 1989), sheep, cow, and goat (Bignon et al. 1997), although their roles largely are unknown. We tested the hypothesis that short isoforms of the PRL receptor (PRLR) exist in human tissue and regulate the actions of PRL (Trott et al. 2002).

[1]Current address: Lactation and Mammary Gland Biology Group, Department of Animal Science, University of Vermont, Burlington, VT 05405-1710

[2] Molecular and Cellular Endocrinology Section, Mammary Biology and Tumorigenesis Laboratory, National Cancer Institute, Room 5B47, 10 Center Drive, Bethesda, MD 20892-1402 (Dr. Vonderhaar is corresponding author.)

Protecting Infants through Human Milk, edited by Pickering *et al.*
Kluwer Academic/Plenum Publishers, 2004

2. METHODS

A new exon 11 of hPRLR was identified using 3′ RACE performed on human ovary cDNA. Five full-length novel isoforms of the PRLR containing this exon were found by RT-PCR; two short forms named SF1a and SF1b (cloned from placenta mRNA), a soluble form (lacking the transmembrane domain) named Δ7/11 (cloned from breast tumor mRNA) and two splice variants, Δ4-SF1b and Δ4-Δ7/11 (cloned from breast tumor mRNA) that are exon 4 deletion variants of SF1b and Δ7/11, respectively (Fig. 1). The cDNA for SF1a, SF1b, LF and Δ7/11 isoforms was tagged with a C-terminal FLAG epitope by RT-PCR and inserted behind the elongation factor-α1 promoter (pEF; Invitrogen), then expressed in Chinese hamster ovary (CHO-K1) cells, and both RNA and protein products analyzed. The expression level of SF1a, SF1b, LF and Δ7/11 isoform mRNAs in human tissues was analyzed by semiquantitative RT-PCR.

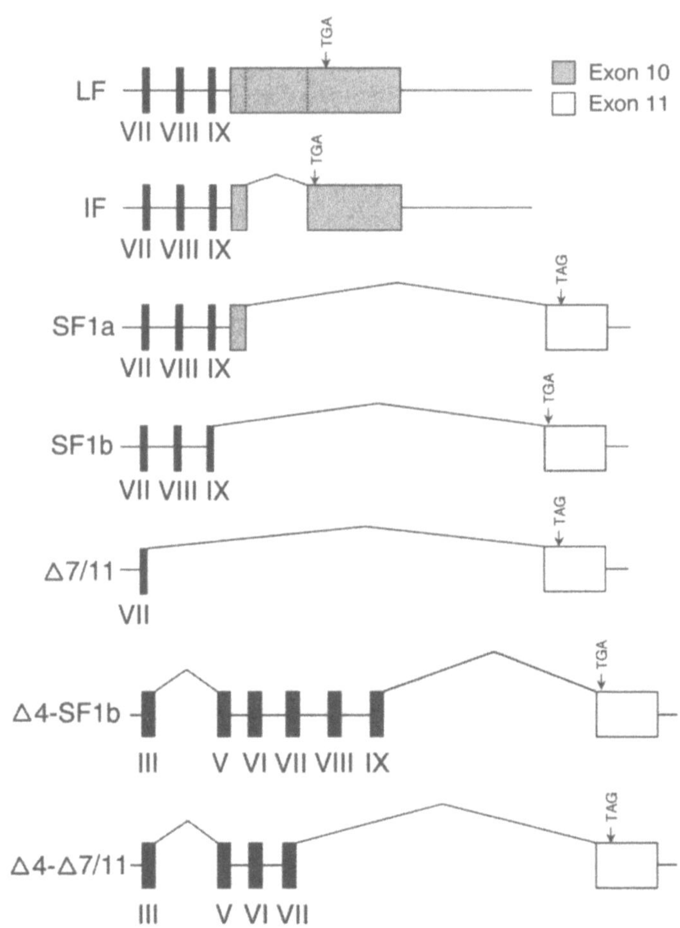

Figure 1. Exon structure of the seven hPRLR isoforms. Four isoforms share coding exons 3 to 9 (long {LF}, intermediate {IF}, short form 1a {SF1a} and short form 1b {SF1b}). Roman numerals delineate exon numbers. The position of each stop codon is indicated with an arrow. Reproduced from Trott et al. 2003 by permission of the Society for Endocrinology.

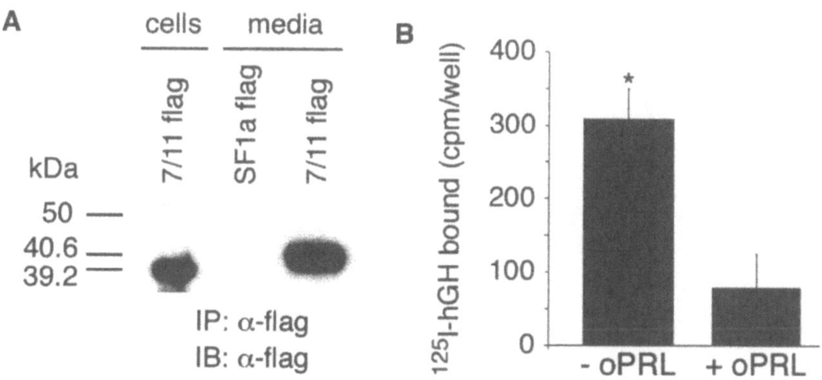

Figure 2. Δ7/11 is a secreted PRL binding protein. (A) CHO-K1 cells were transfected with SF1a-FLAG or Δ7/11-FLAG. Both media and cell lysates were immunoprecipitated with α-FLAG mAb and immunoblotted with α-FLAG-HRP mAb. Each lane has the equivalent of either 250 μL media or 200 μg total protein. (B) Δ7/11-FLAG and LF-FLAG transfected CHO-K1 cells were incubated for 24 hours at 37°C, 5% CO_2 with ^{125}I-hGH, then the medium immunoprecipitated with α-FLAG mAb and the precipitates counted in a γ-counter (Perkin-Elmer). No specific binding was obtained with media from cells transfected with LF-FLAG (data not shown). The specific ^{125}I-hGH-binding by the media of Δ7/11-FLAG transfected cells was corrected for the non-specific binding of media from LF-FLAG transfected cells. *$P<0.005$. Data are expressed as mean±SEM (n=4). Reproduced from Trott et al. 2003 by permission of the Society for Endocrinology.

3. RESULTS

Western analysis of intracellular FLAG-tagged proteins expressed by transfected CHO cells indicated that SF1a-FLAG, SF1b-FLAG and LF-FLAG encoded translation products of approximately 57, 38, and 93 kDa, respectively. The Δ7/11-FLAG protein was found in both media and cells (Fig. 2A), consistent with the lack of a transmembrane domain. The 7/11FLAG protein in media was slightly larger than the cellular protein (40.6 kDa compared with 39.2 kDa). Using fluorescent immunocytochemistry against the FLAG epitope, LF-FLAG protein was localized as cytoplasmic with perinuclear concentration, while the intracellular distribution of Δ7/11 was vesiculated, consistent with the fact that it is secreted.

Cells transfected with the same amount of DNA for the membrane proteins SF1a-FLAG, SF1b-FLAG and LF-FLAG all bound human growth hormone (hGH) with similar affinity but expressed different numbers of binding sites; SF1b had the greatest number, SF1a the lowest number and LF an intermediate number of sites (Trott et al. 2002). The secreted Δ7/11-FLAG also specifically bound hGH, indicating that it is a secreted PRL binding protein (Fig. 2B). Neither SF1a nor SF1b was capable of transducing a differentiative signal to the β-casein gene promoter (Fig. 3A). However, SF1b functions as a strong dominant negative to the differentiative function of the LF, irrespective of binding site number (Fig. 3B), while SF1a is a weaker dominant negative (Fig. 3C).

Expression of SF1a, SF1b, and LF mRNAs was detected in samples of human breast, placenta, kidney, liver, and pancreas. No expression of Δ7/11 was evident in these tissues; however, it was expressed in breast tumors. We also found differential expression of the short isoforms (SF1a and SF1b) in samples of normal and cancerous breast tissue (Trott et al. 2003).

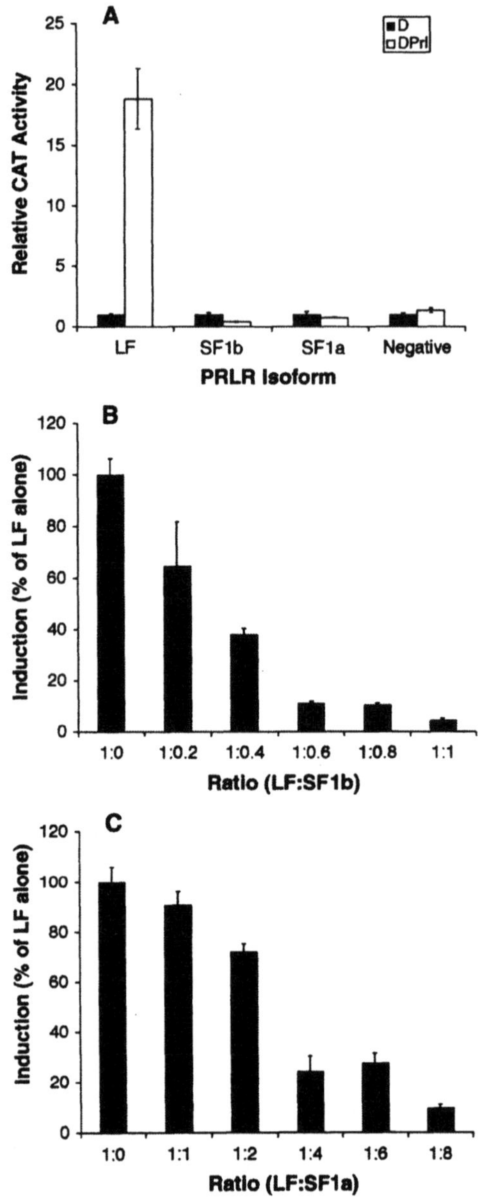

Figure 3. hPRLR-SF1a and -SF1b do not transduce a differentiative signal but both are dominant negatives to the hPRLR-LF. CHO-K1 cells were co-transfected transiently with β-casCAT (β-casein promoter with chloramphenicol acetyl transferase cDNA), pEFLacZ and combinations of short form 1a (SF1a), short form 1b (SF1b), long form (LF) or pEF6C (Negative). The levels of CAT activity (mean±SEM) were normalized for LacZ activity. (A) β-casein promoter activity in transfected CHO-K1 cells after 48-hour treatment with either dexamethasone (D) alone or D plus prolactin (DPrl). (B) and (C) A constant mass of LF DNA was transfected with different amounts of SF DNA, and the total mass of transfected DNA held constant by adding pEF6C DNA. (B) SF1b is a strong dominant negative against LF-transduced PRL-stimulation of the β-casein promoter. (C) SF1a is a weak dominant negative against the LF-transduced PRL-stimulation of the ß-casein promoter. Reproduced from Trott et al. 2003 by permission of the Society for Endocrinology.

4. DISCUSSION

Autocrine PRL has a function in breast tumorigenesis (Vonderhaar 1999), and serum PRL levels have been linked to increased breast cancer risk (Hankinson et al. 1999). The actions of the dominant negative isoform SF1b on hPRLR-LF may be important in PRL-regulated differentiation of breast epithelium. Likewise, it is possible that the prolactin binding protein Δ7/11 may be important in regulating the function of PRL in breast tumorigenesis. Further studies to elucidate the effects of SF1a and SF1b on PRL-induced mitosis will help to define whether these isoforms play a role in endocrine or autocrine PRL-stimulated normal and/or breast cancer growth.

5. REFERENCES

Bignon C, Binart N, Ormandy C, Schuler LA, Kelly PA, Djiane J. Long and short forms of the ovine prolactin receptor: cDNA cloning and genomic analysis reveal that the two forms arise by different alternative splicing mechanisms in ruminants and in rodents. J Mol Endocrinol 1997;19:109-120.

Bole-Feysot C, Goffin V, Edery M, Binart N, Kelly PA. Prolactin (PRL) and its receptor: actions, signal transduction pathways and phenotypes observed in PRL receptor knockout mice. Endocr Rev 1998;19:225-268.

Boutin JM, Jolicoeur C, Okamura H, Gagnon J, Edery M, Shirota M, Banville D, Dusanter-Fourt I, Djiane J, Kelly PA. Cloning and expression of the rat prolactin receptor, a member of the growth hormone/prolactin receptor gene family. Cell 1988;53:69-77.

Boutin JM, Edery M, Shirota M, Jolicoeur C, Lesueur L, Ali S, Gould D, Djiane J, Kelly PA. Identification of a cDNA encoding a long form of prolactin receptor in human hepatoma and breast cancer cells. Mol Endocrinol 1989;3:1455-1461.

Clevenger CV, Chang WP, Ngo W, Pasha TL, Montone KT, Tomaszewski JE. Expression of prolactin and prolactin receptor in human breast carcinoma. Evidence for an autocrine/paracrine loop. Am J Pathol 1995;146:695-705.

Davis JA, Linzer DI. Expression of multiple forms of the prolactin receptor in mouse liver. Mol Endocrinol 1989;3:674-680.

Ginsburg E, Vonderhaar BK. Prolactin synthesis and secretion by human breast cancer cells. Cancer Res 1995;55:2591-2595.

Hankinson SE, Willett WC, Michaud DS, Manson JE, Colditz GA, Longcope C, Rosner B, Speizer FE. Plasma prolactin levels and subsequent risk of breast cancer in postmenopausal women. J Natl Cancer Inst 1999;91:629-634.

Hu ZZ, Zhuang L, Meng J, Leondires M, Dufau ML. The human prolactin receptor gene structure and alternative promoter utilization: the generic promoter hPIII and a novel human promoter hP(N). J Clin Endocrinol Metab 1999;84:1153-1156.

Hu ZZ, Zhuang L, Meng J, Tsai-Morris CH, Dufau ML. Complex 5' genomic structure of the human prolactin receptor: multiple alternative exons 1 and promoter utilization. Endocrinology 2002;143:2139-2142.

Kelly PA, Boutin JM, Jolicoeur C, Okamura H, Shirota M, Edery M, Dusanter-Fourt I, Djiane J. Purification, cloning, and expression of the prolactin receptor. Biol Reprod 1989;40:27-32.

Kline JB, Roehrs H, Clevenger CV. Functional characterization of the intermediate isoform of the human prolactin receptor. J Biol Chem 1999;274:35461-35468.

Ormandy CJ, Binart N, Helloco C, Kelly PA. Mouse prolactin receptor gene: genomic organization reveals alternative promoter usage and generation of isoforms via alternative 3'-exon splicing. DNA Cell Biol 1998;17:761-770.

Trott JF, Hovey RC, Koduri S, Vonderhaar BK. Alternative splicing to exon 11 of human prolactin receptor gene results in multiple isoforms including a secreted prolactin-binding protein. J Mol Endocrinol 2003;30:31-47.

Vonderhaar BK. Prolactin involvement in breast cancer. Endocr Relat Cancer 1999;6:389-404.

Wennbo H, Gebre-Medhin M, Gritli-Linde A, Ohlsson C, Isaksson OG, Tornell J. Activation of the prolactin receptor but not the growth hormone receptor is important for induction of mammary tumors in transgenic mice. J Clin Invest 1997;100:2744-2751.

BIOIMPEDANCE VECTOR ANALYSIS IN BREASTFED AND FORMULA-FED INFANTS IN THE FIRST SIX MONTHS OF LIFE

F. Savino, S. Maccario, F. Cresi, G. Grasso, R. Oggero, L. Silvestro, and G.C. Mussa

1. INTRODUCTION

During the first months of life, modification of body composition occurs rapidly. Studies have reported that breastfed (BF) infants show a different growth pattern than formula-fed (FF) infants, particularly in the first years of life. Methods have been developed for estimating body composition. Even though the majority of these methods, such as isotope dilution techniques, total body nitrogen, and densitometry, provide precise analyses and estimations of the body mass, the use of invasive methods, which lead to an increasing risk of radiation exposure, cause difficulties, especially in pediatrics. Bioelectrical Impedance Analysis (BIA) estimates body composition in children and adults by measuring electrical impedance of body tissue. BIA has been accepted as a body composition measurement by the U.S. National Institutes of Health (NIH 1996). This test consists of applying an alternative current of 800 μA and 50 kHz, which is not perceivable and not dangerous. This technique is based on equations that translate the electrical signals in terms of body composition. The related theoretical assumptions and reference models are applicable and accurate only on selected groups of healthy adults and children.

Bioimpedance vector analysis is derived from plotting direct measurements of reactance (Xc) and phase angle (Pa) from the analyzer. These analyses are independent from anthropometric parameters of subjects. For this reason the R-Xc graph method should be a new clinical approach for evaluating the nutritional status and fluid shifts for the pediatric population (De Palo et al. 2000; Piccoli et al. 2002; Savino et al. 2003).

2. AIM

The present study was performed to evaluate the differences of bioimpedance vector between BF and FF infants.

Department of Pediatrics, University of Turin, Italy

Protecting Infants through Human Milk, edited by Pickering *et al.*
Kluwer Academic/Plenum Publishers, 2004

Table 1. Anthropometric parameters of the study population[a]

	Breastfed, n=22	Formula-fed, n=22
Age (days)	69.0±41	87.7±30
Birth weight (g)	3240±345.3	3323±345.3
Weight (g)	5119±1080	5431±846.6
Length (cm)	58±4.6	60.7±3.6
Cranial circumference (cm)	38.8±1.7	39.8±1.8

[a]Student t-test: no differences between the two group of infants

Table 2. Impedance measurements[a]

	Breastfed	Formula-fed
Pa	2.4±1.4	2.2±1.0
Xc	22.4±14.5	23.1±12.3
BMI	15.1±2	14.6±1.2
TBW	4.06±0.69	4.31±0.51
R/H (m)	16.7±3.1	15.6±2.3
Xc/H (m)	7.9±5.4	7.5±3.5

[a]Student t-test: no differences between the two group of infants

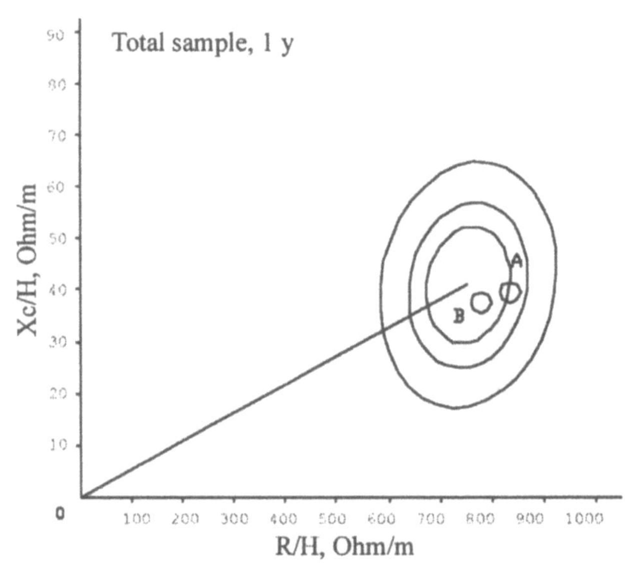

Figure 1. R-Xc graph in the study population: A=breastfeeding, B=formula-feeding

3. METHODS

Sixty-four healthy infants, 33 exclusively BF (average age of 70±41 days) and 31 FF (average age of 77±29 days), were enrolled in the study. The evaluation of anthropometric parameters, including weight, length, and cranial circumference were taken by the same operator following standard procedures. Impedance measurements were conducted in all subjects with the same single frequency phase-sensitive impedance analyzer (STA BIA, Akern System Srl; Florence, Italy/Clinton Township, MI, USA). Before each testing session the instrument was checked by a calibration circuit of known impedance value (R=380 Ω, Xc=47 Ω). The current applied on the patient normally is transmitted by four electrodes, which are placed according to the common tetrapolar analysis. Two outer distal electrodes were placed on the dorsal surface of the right hand and foot, next to the metacarpal-phalangeal and metatarsal-phalangeal joints; two inner electrodes were placed proximally on the right forearm and leg, leaving 5.5 cm of free skin around the outer electrodes. The placement of the sensor electrode, particularly in very young infants, has been reported as the major cause of technical bias. In fact, a minimal inter-electrode distance of 5.5 cm must be taken between pairs of electrodes in order to avoid alteration in the electrical transmission (Gartner et al. 1992, 1993, 1994; Barillas-Mury et al. 1987). Two hours postfeeding, the patient must be placed on a nonconductive surface without direct contact to conductive material or to the parents. The patient must be naked except for dry diapers.

Impedance values normally are divided into two main categories: *direct* parameters such as resistance (R), reactance (Xc), phase angle (Pa); *indirect* parameters such as total body water (TBW) calculated by an equation (i.e., Field equation), and body mass index (BMI). Bioimpedance vector analysis followed the R-Xc graph method, which uses the plot of direct measurements of Xc and R standardized by the infant's length (Piccoli et al. 1994; Vienna & Hauser 1999). The statistical analysis was performed by the Student t-test.

4. RESULTS

The anthropometric parameters (weight, length, and cranial circumference) were similar for both the samples of infants [P>0.05] (Table 1). The direct impedenziometric values showed not significant differences between the two groups of subjects (Table 2). However, the R-Xc graph was different between the samples as depicted in Figure 1. BF infants (A) can be considered leaner than the reference population, whose average impedance vector is marked in the center of the graph (distribution in the first years of life), and with a normal nutritional status. On the other hand, FF infants (B) marked an area that is lower than that for BF infants.

5. CONCLUSION

Body growth in the first six months of life involves not only quantitative changes but also qualitative changes in composition, which could explain our results (Butte et al. 2000). Anthropometric data between the two groups of infants were similar, as were the evaluated impedance parameters. R-Xc graph showed a different position for the two studied populations: according to this method BF infants appear qualitatively different and may be considered leaner than the FF infants. Further studies are needed to confirm these data and to provide a correct interpretation of nutritional differences.

6. REFERENCES

Barillas-Mury C, Vettorazzi C, Molina S, et al. Experience with bioelectrical impedance analysis in young children: sources of variability. In: Ellis KJ, Yasumura S, Morgan WD, editors. In Vivo Body Composition Study. London: IPSM 3, 1987; p 87.

Butte NF, Hopkinson JM, Wong WW, Smith EO, Ellis KJ. Body composition during the first 2 years of life: an updated reference. Pediatr Res 2000;47:578-585.

De Palo T, Messina G, Edefonti A, Perfumo F, Pisanello L, Peruzzi L, Di Iorio B, Mignozzi M, Vienna A, Conti G, Penza R, Piccoli A. Normal values of the bioelectrical impedance vector in childhood and puberty. Nutrition 2000;16:417-424.

Gartner A, Maire B, Delpeuch F, Sarda P, Dupuy RP, Rieu D. Importance of electrode position in bioelectrical impedance analysis. Am J Clin Nutr 1992;56:1067-1068.

Gartner A, Maire B, Delpeuch F, Sarda P, Dupuy RP, Rieu D. The use of bioelectrical impedance analysis in newborns. The need for standardization. Basic Life Sci 1993;60:165-168.

Gartner A, Sarda P, Dupuy RP, Maire B, Delpeuch F, Rieu D. Bioelectrical impedance analysis in small- and appropriate-for-gestational-age newborn infants. Eur J Clin Nutr 1994;48:425-432.

[NIH] National Institutes of Health. Bioelectrical impedance analysis in body composition measurement: National Institutes of Health Technology Assessment Conference Statement. December 12-14, 1994. Am J Clin Nutr 1996;64 (Suppl):524S-532S.

Piccoli A, Rossi B, Pillon L, Bucciante G. A new method for monitoring body fluid variation by bioimpedance analysis: the RXc graph. Kidney Int 1994;46:534-539.

Piccoli A, Fanos V, Peruzzi L, Schena S, Pizzini C, Borgione S, Bertino E, Chiaffoni G, Coppo R, Tato L. Reference values of the bioelectrical impedance vector in neonates in the first week after birth. Nutrition 2002;18:383-387.

Savino F, Grasso G, Cresi F, Oggero R, Silvestro L. Bioelectrical impedance vector distribution in the first year of life. Nutrition 2003;19:492-496.

Vienna A, Hauser G. A qualitative approach to assessing body compartments using bioelectrical variables. Coll Antropol 1999;23:461-472.

WEIGHING DIAPERS FOR INTAKE ASSESSMENT AFTER EARLY DISCHARGE

E. Sievers[1], S. Haase[2], and J. Schaub[1]

1. INTRODUCTION

Human milk is regarded as the ideal nutrition for newborns and young infants, and exclusive breastfeeding is recommended (WHO 2003). Lactation consultation may benefit from a simple approach to evaluate the intake in exclusively breastfed infants.

Twenty-four-hour test-weighing is difficult under home conditions and is not very suitable as a routine method. Weighing diapers is a simple pediatric approach for assessment of quantitative excretion in infancy. Both methods have been applied previously in scientific investigations of infants at home (Sievers et al. 1992). This study was performed to determine whether weighing diapers is useful for determining the intake of neonates in the first days of life.

2. METHODS

Ten healthy infants born by caesarean section (birth weight 2500–4000 g) were included in the investigation during the first six days of life. The intake was assessed by weighing breastfed infants before and after breastfeeding and weighing bottles before and after each feed for infants who were not exclusively breastfed. Diapers were weighed before and after use. The scales had an accuracy of ±5 g for infant weight or ±1 g for bottle and diaper weights. The body weights of the infants were assessed daily at 6:00–7:00 AM, evaluations were based on complete 24-hour periods except for day 1.

Data are presented as median (range); statistical analysis was performed using nonparametric test procedures (Spearman's rank correlation). STATISTICA (Stat. Soft. Corp., Tulsa, OK, USA) was applied for computer analysis. Informed consent was obtained from the parents of all participants before their inclusion in the study. The investigation had been approved by the institutional ethics committee.

[1]Department of Pediatrics, University of Kiel, Schwanenweg 20, D-24105 Kiel, Germany
[2]Municipal Hospital, Kiel, Germany

Table 1. Intake and corresponding (fecal/urinary) excretion in the first six days of life

Day of life	1	2	3	4	5	6
Infants investigated, n=10			Median (range)			
Infant weight (kg)	2.90 (2.58-3.95)	2.88 (2.53-3.91)	2.78 (2.44-3.74)	2.81 (2.54-3.67)	2.82 (2.55-3.70)	2.79 (2.58-3.77)
Day-to-day weight gain (%)	−2.65 (−5.14 to +0.54)	−2.89 (−5.05 to 1.5)	0.36 (−1.74 to 4.11)	−0.19 (−1.91 to 3.31)	0.76 (−1.41 to 3.06)	0.91 (−0.9 to 3.6)
Intake (g)	22 (12-68)	127 (76-157)	155 (79-188)	230 (122-305)	298 (205-528)	317 (223-600)
Excretion (g)	18 (1-117)	86.5 (55-152)	83.0 (46-159)	111 (66-257)	221 (181-282)	155 (116-246)
Intake (g/kg/d)	7.0 (4.0-24.9)	41.5 (22.0-59.8)	53.6 (21.2-77.2)	81.3 (50.4-106.9)	100.1 (62.2-188.2)	109.6 (63.6-159.2)
Excretion (g/kg/d)	10.4 (0.4-30.1)	27.4 (19.1-41.1)	28.8 (15.3-58.6)	31.7 (25.0-77.5)	67.3 (50.3-76.2)	63.6 (41.4-122.0)
Percent excretion % of intake	125 (7-264)	74 (52-121)	58 (31-105)	48 (30-84)	81 (53-89)	59 (41-77)

3. RESULTS

The *absolute* daily intake volume did not correlate with infant body weight, nor with the absolute weight gain within the total study period (P>0.05). However, it did correlate with weight gain from day to day (Table 1).

A daily intake of 80±5 g/kg body weight resulted in an excretion between 24 and 57 g/kg/day. At an excretion of >60 g/kg/day the intake exceeded 90 g/kg/day. A significant correlation of intake and excretion was observed if days 1 to 6 of all infants studied were considered (Fig. 1, P<0.01, r=0.85, n=45); the evaluation of single days rendered a significant correlation only on day 6.

A significant correlation (P<0.05) between *percent excretion* and intake was observed on days 2/3, but not between percent excretion and absolute body weight nor between percent excretion and weight gain of the infants. Daily assessment and intake per kilogram body weight and weight development did not show a correlation until day 6.

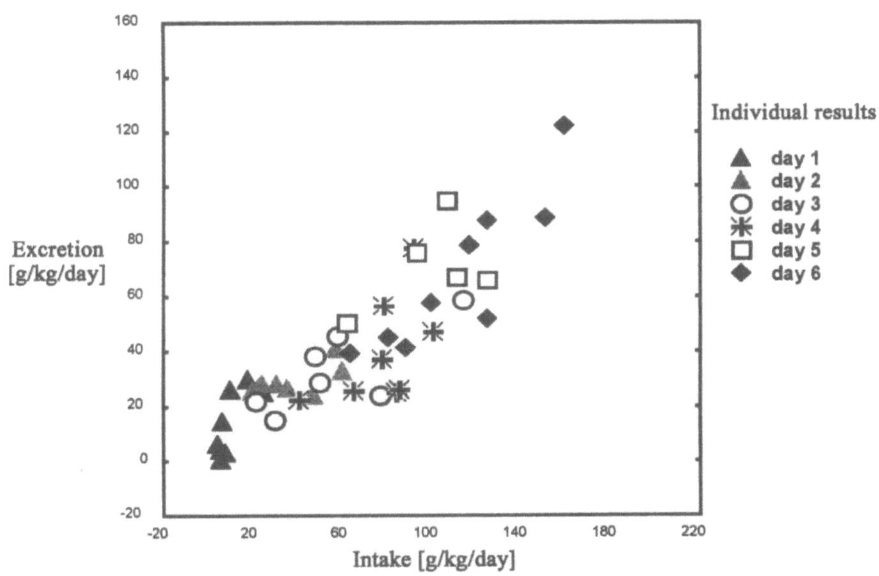

Figure 1. Intake and corresponding (fecal/urinary) excretion in the first six days of life

4. CONCLUSION

The assessment of fecal and urinary excretion by weighing diapers may confirm sufficient *excretion*. It is, however, of limited value for the deduction of *intake* in clinical practice. This applies primarily to low intake volumes (<90 g/kg/day), which are relevant at the initial postnatal period after early discharge. In the first five days of life, the approach studied does not render results with sufficient precision for the individual mother-infant pair. The results suggest, however, a limited applicability thereafter and at higher intake volumes. Therefore, longitudinal data of healthy exclusively breastfed infants are required.

5. REFERENCES

Sievers E, Oldigs H-D, Dörner K, Schaub J. Longitudinal zinc balances in breast-fed and formula-fed infants. Acta Paediatr 1992;81:1-6

[WHO] World Health Organization. Global strategy for infant and young child feeding. Geneva: World Health Organization, 2003.

DONOR MILK FOR PRETERM AND SICK CHILDREN

Human Milk Banking in Germany

S. Springer

1. HUMAN MILK BANKS IN GERMANY

Human milk banking is common in many European countries. In Germany, a survey conducted in 2001 showed the high acceptance of donor milk among parents of patients in need of human milk. In addition, when a mother who delivers a preterm infant is able to provide a surplus of human milk beyond the needs of her own infant, this milk is preferred by NICU staff for early feedings of other preterm infants because of the special needs of premature infants.

In 2001, the 15 German milk banks were able to supply about 6500 liters of donor milk from more than 300 nursing mothers. The collection capacity varies widely, from 20 to 2500 liters per year. The purpose of this manuscript is to provide information about human milk banks in Germany.

2. INDICATIONS FOR DONOR MILK

One of the most important German milk banks is at the Children's Hospital at Leipzig University. In 2001, more than 1800 liters of human milk were provided for preterm infants in the neonatal units of the region, for older infants in intensive care units, and for children in pediatric surgical clinics. The donor milk was provided for in- and out-patients (Table 1).

The Leipzig Milk Bank collects human milk on a daily basis. This makes it possible, in very special cases, to provide fresh milk with its clear advantages, especially its immunological and anti-infective properties. Necrotizing enterocolitis is extremely rare in the neonatal unit of our hospital in part because we use fresh human milk. Collection and storage procedures are vital to providing safe, high quality donor milk to infants who need it.

University of Leipzig, Children's Hospital, Oststraße 21-25, D - 04317 Leipzig, Germany

Protecting Infants through Human Milk, edited by Pickering *et al.*
Kluwer Academic/Plenum Publishers, 2004

Table 1. Indications for banked donor milk at Leipzig University, Germany

Location	Indications
In-patients	Preterm infants
	Lactation delay on the postpartum unit
	Kidney disease
	Infants after intestinal surgery
	Infants with serious infections
	Short bowel syndrome
	Cow milk intolerance
Out-patients	Formerly preterm infants
	Multiple births
	Dystrophy
	During chemotherapy
	Intractable diarrhea
	Short bowel syndrome
	Cow milk intolerance

3. OUTLOOK

Some milk banks provide training facilities to help ensure safe collection, storage, and appropriate use of donor milk. There are guidelines for German milk banks such as those that exist in the United States and the United Kingdom. These recommendations include criteria for selection of donors (Springer et al. 1998), the basics of collecting milk and storing it, and pasteurization of donor milk. Conferences are held to share information, optimize the workload, and increase cooperation among the individual human milk banks. The interest in feeding human milk to very-low-birth-weight newborns has increased steadily in other countries. Along with this interest is the need to learn management of human milk banks in the modern world. Collaboration among staff and standardization of guidelines for human milk banks in Europe and worldwide will help to ensure the ability of all milk banks to provide safe, high quality donor milk to all preterm or sick children in need.

4. REFERENCE

Springer S, Bannert N, Boettcher M, Dittmer C, Handrick W, Heine W, Henker J, Pustowoit B, Spencker FB, Vogtmann C. Guidelines for the Establishment and Operation of Human Milk Banks. Leipziger Universitätsverlag, 1998.

PLASMA NON-ESTERIFIED FATTY ACID COMPOSITION IS DIFFERENT IN LACTATING AND IN NONPREGNANT NONLACTATING WOMEN

Alexandre G. Torres, Jacqueline G. Ney, Mirna Ribeiro, and Nadia M.F. Trugo

1. INTRODUCTION

The endocrine changes that occur in human lactation lead to increased mobilization of fatty acids from adipose tissue and may result in altered plasma levels of non-esterified fatty acids (NEFA) (Neville et al. 1994). Fasting total NEFA concentration in plasma is elevated in lactating compared with nonlactating women three to six months postpartum (Butte et al. 1999), but the composition of individual NEFA in plasma from lactating women has not been determined. Fatty acid mobilization from adipose tissue is a selective process, influenced by the fatty acid structure (Raclot et al. 1997). During lactation, mobilization of individual fatty acids might be selectively affected and result in altered plasma NEFA composition. Since adipose tissue seems to be the most important source of polyunsaturated fatty acids (PUFA) in human milk (Demmelmair et al. 1998), these alterations could affect PUFA transfer to milk.

The aims of this study were to determine individual NEFA concentrations in plasma of lactating women and to compare these NEFA concentrations with those of nonpregnant nonlactating (NPNL) women.

2. METHODS

Twenty-two healthy nursing women, between 20 and 120 days postpartum, and a matched (age, body mass index, and dietary habits) control group of 11 NPNL women participated in the study after informed consent. All nursing women had term gestation, were exclusively or predominantly breastfeeding, and attended a public daycare clinic in Rio de Janeiro.

Data collection involved: weight and height measurements, a questionnaire of general data, and two 24-hour recall questionnaires. Dietary intake of lipid-related nutri-

Laboratório de Bioquímica Nutricional e de Alimentos, Departamento de Bioquímica, Instituto de Quimica, Universidade Federal do rio de Janeiro, Brazil

Protecting Infants through Human Milk, edited by Pickering *et al.*
Kluwer Academic/Plenum Publishers, 2004

ents was quantified from the 24-hour recall questionnaires using the software Nutrisurvey™ (Dr. J. Erhardt, Germany). Blood samples were taken by venipuncture after an overnight fast. Plasma was separated by centrifugation, and after addition of the internal standard (C17:0), NEFA were isolated from the other classes of lipids by treatment with fumed silicon dioxide (Polette et al. 1992). After lyophilization, fatty acids were esterified to methanol (Lepage & Roy 1986). Fatty acid methyl esters were analyzed by capillary gas-chromatography in a polar column (Omegawax-320, Supelco) and their absolute (μg/mL) and relative concentrations (wt%) were determined.

3. RESULTS

Lactating and NPNL women were 26.1±6.1 and 24.6±2.6 years of age, respectively, with body mass index of 23.7±0.5 and 21.3±2.2 kg/m^2 (mean±SEM), respectively. Daily intake of energy, lipids (en%), and total and individual saturated, monounsaturated, and polyunsaturated fatty acids were similar between lactating and NPNL women.

Table 1. Relative contents (wt%) of plasma NEFA of lactating and nonpregnant nonlactating (NPNL) women

Fatty acid	Relative concentration (Mean±SD; wt%)		P[a]
	Lactating women (n=22)	NPNL women (n=11)	
14:0	1.43 ± 0.20	2.03 ± 0.41	0.00001
15:0	0.43 ± 0.08	0.66 ± 0.38	0.01
16:0	34.4 ± 2.19	30.5 ± 1.17	0.0001
18:0	13.2 ± 1.67	12.0 ± 2.43	n.s.[b]
16:1n-7	2.96 ± 0.77	2.92 ± 0.75	n.s.
18:1n-9	21.4 ± 3.62	24.2 ± 5.35	0.08
18:1n-7	2.62 ± 0.33	1.64 ± 1.08	0.001
20:1n-9	0.29 ± 0.21	0.98 ± 1.06	0.01
22:1n-9	1.38 ± 0.39	0.48 ± 0.23	0.0001
24:1n-9	0.44 ± 0.11	0.51 ± 0.29	n.s.
18:2n-6	17.9 ± 1.91	22.1 ± 3.61	0.0001
20:3n-6	0.52 ± 0.25	0.71 ± 0.41	n.s.
20:4n-6	2.38 ± 0.57	1.97 ± 0.69	0.09
18:3n-3	0.64 ± 0.08	1.18 ± 0.84	0.01
20:5n-3	0.38 ± 0.19	ND[c]	—
Total n-6	20.8 ± 2.12	24.3 ± 3.70	0.01
Total n-3	1.00 ± 0.22	1.18 ± 0.84	n.s.
n-6/n-3	21.6 ± 9.18	27.4 ± 12.2	0.07
PUFA	21.8 ± 2.14	25.5 ± 4.04	0.001
Total	100	100	—

[a]Significantly different when P<0.05 (unpaired t-test)
[b]n.s.=not significant
[c]ND=not detected

Fifteen fatty acids were identified in plasma of lactating women and 14 in plasma of the NPNL women, with 20:5n-3 being detected only in the former. Absolute concentrations (μg/mL) of most of the individual fatty acids were significantly higher in the lactating women, resulting in higher ($P<0.005$; t-test) total NEFA concentration (424±159 μg/mL; mean±SD) than in the control group (210±34.9 μg/mL).

In order to evaluate whether fat mobilization would discriminate between the different fatty acids, as a result of a selective process, the relative concentrations of fatty acids were calculated (Table 1). Lactating women had higher levels of palmitic acid and tended to have lower levels of monounsaturated 1n-9 fatty acids than the NPNL controls. For the n-6 and n-3 PUFA an interesting result was obtained. The relative amounts of both 18C essential fatty acids were higher in NPNL than in lactating women, whereas their longer chain metabolites, 20:4n-6 and 20:5n-3, tended to be lower or were undetectable in the control group, respectively.

The differences between the two study groups in plasma NEFA composition also could be identified after Pearson correlation analyses between fatty acids in each group. Twenty-one significant correlations were found between the plasma NEFA of lactating women and twenty-four for that of NPNL women. Most of the correlations could be explained by metabolic interactions between fatty acids such as: precursor-product relationships and competition for metabolic pathways. Nevertheless, most of correlations were not common between both study groups or had opposite signals. Furthermore, there were neither significant correlations involving 18:2n-6 nor any of the n-3 fatty acids (18:3n-3 and 20:5n-3) in lactating women, which might be attributed to a lower dependence of n-6 and n-3 metabolism on the metabolism of the other fatty acids. Selected correlations are shown in Table 2.

Table 2. Selected significant correlations[a] were found between plasma NEFA concentrations (wt%) from lactating and nonpregnant nonlactating (NPNL) women

Plasma NEFA		Lactating women (n=22)		NPNL women (n=11)	
		r	P	r	P
18:1n-9	18:1n-7	0.7	0.01	–0.7	0.01
16:1n-7	20:4n-6	–0.6	0.01	—	—
18:1n-9	20:4n-6	–0.5	0.02	—	—
20:3n-6	20:4n-6	0.5	0.01	—	—
18:1n-9	18:2n-6	—	—	–0.8	0.01
18:1n-9	18:3n-3	—	—	–0.7	0.01
18:2n-6	20:3n-6	—	—	0.8	0.02
18:3n-3	20:1n-9	—	—	0.9	0.01

[a]Pearson analysis, $P<0.05$

4. DISCUSSION

The higher individual fatty acids in lactating women may be attributed to the increased fatty acid mobilization during lactation. Interestingly, plasma NEFA levels of lactating women were two times higher than those of NPNL controls, even with the very efficient uptake of fatty acids from blood by the mammary gland. Since relative contents of most fatty acids were different between both groups, it seems that the selectivity of one or more of the metabolic processes involved in fatty acid mobilization from adipose tissue, as well as fatty acid metabolism in liver or muscle, are affected during lactation. The finding of higher 18C essential fatty acids and lower long-chain metabolites in NPNL women indicates that an adaptation process is taking place in one or more metabolic pathways during human lactation that ultimately results in higher long-chain PUFA (LC-PUFA) availability for transfer to human milk.

5. CONCLUSIONS

The endocrine and metabolic changes of lactation caused alterations in the total and the relative concentrations of plasma NEFA, and in correlations between individual NEFA. These changes ensure a higher availability of fatty acids, especially of LC-PUFA, for human milk production.

6. ACKNOWLEDGMENTS

The authors thank CNPq, CAPES, FAPERJ and FUJB (Brazil) for financial support and CNPq for research fellowships.

7. REFERENCES

Butte NF, Hopkinson JM, Mehta N, Moon JK, Smith EOB. Adjustments in energy expenditure and substrate utilization during late pregnancy and lactation. Am J Clin Nutr 1999;69:299-307.

Demmelmair H, Baumheuer M, Koletzko B, Dokoupil K, Kratl G. Metabolism of $U^{13}C$-labeled linoleic acid in lactating women. J Lipid Res 1998;39:1389-1396.

Lepage G, Roy CC. Direct transesterification of all classes of lipids in a one-step reaction. J Lipid Res 1986;27:114-120.

Neville MC, Casey C, Hay WW Jr. Endocrine regulation of nutrient flux in the lactating woman. Do the mechanisms differ from pregnancy? Adv Exp Med Biol 1994;352:85-98.

Polette A, Durand P, Floccard B, Blache D. A method for specific analysis of free fatty acids in biological samples by capillary gas-chromatography. Anal Biochem 1992;206:241-245.

Raclot T, Langin D, Lafontan M, Groscolas R. Selective release of human adipocyte fatty acids according to molecular structure. Biochem J 1997;324:911-915.

GLOSSARY

2′-FL	2′-fucosyllactose
ADPH	adipophilin
ALT	alanine aminotransferase
ANOVA	analysis of variance
ARA	arachidonic acid, 20:4n-6
BCG	Bacillus Calmette-Guérin
BDI	Beck Depression Inventory
BF	breastfeeding; breastfed
BFHI	Baby Friendly Hospital Initiative
BHITS	Breastfeeding and HIV International Transmission Study
BIA	bioelectrical impedance analysis
BMD	bone mineral density
BMI	body mass index
Btn	butyrophilin
BW	body weight
CDI	MacArthur Communicative Developmental Inventories
CI	confidence interval
CLD	cytosolic lipid droplet
CMV	cytomegalovirus
C-section	caesarian section
CT	cholera toxin
CVD	cardiovascular disease
DHA	docosahexaenoic acid, 22:6n-3
DHS	demographic and health surveys
DI	dietary intake
DPA	dual photon absorptiometry
DPTH	diphtheria, pertussis, tetanus, and *Haemophilus influenzae* type b tetravalent vaccine
DXA	dual energy x-ray absorptiometry
EBF	exclusive breastfeeding; exclusively breastfed
EGF	epidermal growth factor
EIA	enzyme immunoassay
EIEC	enteroinvasive *Escherichia coli*
EM	electron microscopy
EPA	eicosapentaenoic acid, 20:5n-3

EPEC	enteropathogenic *Escherichia coli*
EPT	extremely preterm
ER	endoplasmic reticulum
EspA, EspB, EspD	secreted proteins
ETEC	enterotoxigenic *Escherichia coli*
FF	formula-fed
FFM	fat free mass
FT	full-term
FTE	full-time equivalent
FUT2	secretor gene
FUT2,3,4,5,6,7	fucosyltransferase genes
FUT3	Lewis gene
FUT4,5,6,7	α1,3 transferase genes
GAG	glycosaminoglycan
GEE	generalized estimating equation
GEMM	genetically engineered mouse models
GH	growth hormone
GI	gastrointestinal tract
GLUT1	a plasma membrane glucose transporter
Hb	hemoglobin
HBGA	human blood group antigens
HCV	hepatitis C virus
HGF	hepatocyte growth factor
HM	human milk
HMC	human milk cells
HNP-1	human defensin
HPLC	high performance liquid chromatography
HRV	human rotavirus
HSV-1	Herpes simplex virus 1
HSV-2	Herpes simplex virus 2
HTLV-1	human T-cell lymphotropic virus type 1
IBFAN	International Baby Food Action Network
IGF	insulin-like growth factor
ILO	International Labor Organization
IMCI	Integrated Management of Childhood Illness program
IRS	Insulin receptor substrates
KMC	kangaroo mother care
LC-PUFA	long-chain polyunsaturated fatty acids
LDFH-I	lacto-*N*-difucohexaose I
LDFT	lactodifucotetraose
Lf	lactoferrin
LLP	lentivirus lytic peptide
LNF-I	lacto-*N*-fucopentaose I
LPS	lipopolysaccharide
LS-II	lactogenesis stage II
MBF	mixed breastfeeding; foods in addition to human milk
MDI	Mental Development Index
MDM	monocyte-derived macrophages
MEC	mammary epithelial cells

MFG	milk fat globule
MFGM	milk fat globule membranes
MFP	mammary fat pad
MMTV	mouse mammary tumor virus long terminal repeat
MTCT	mother-to-child transmission
NBAS	Neonatal Behavioral Assessment Scale
NEC	necrotizing enterocolitis
NEFA	non-esterified fatty acids
NORs	noroviruses
NPNL	nonpregnant nonlactating
NV	Norwalk virus
Pa	phase angle
PAL	physical activity level
PBI	preceding birth interval
PBMC	peripheral blood mononuclear cells
PCOS	polycystic ovary syndrome
PDI	Psychomotor Development Index
PE	red blood cell phosphatidylethanolamine
PHA	phytohemagglutinin A
PPARγ	peroxisome proliferator activated-receptor gamma
PPVT-R	Peabody Picture Vocabulary Test
PR	progesterone receptor
PRL	prolactin
PRLR	prolactin receptor
PSS:NICU	Parental Stressor Scale: Neonatal Intensive Care Unit
PT	preterm
PUFA	polyunsaturated fatty acids
QCT	quantitative computed tomography
QTL	quantitative trait loci
R	resistance
RCT	randomized controlled trial
RDA	Recommended Dietary Allowances
REA	rapid ethnographic assessment
RHDV	rabbit haemorrhagic diarrhea virus
RR	relative risk
SG	sulfated glycolipid
SPA	single photon absorptiometry
ST-*E. coli*	stable toxin-producing enterotoxigenic *Escherichia coli*
STEC	Shiga toxin-producing *Escherichia coli*
TBW	total body water
TDLU	terminal duct lobular unit
TEB	terminal end bud
TfR	transferrin receptors
TGF-α	transforming growth factor-alpha
Th1, Th2	T-helper cells
TIP-47	mannose-6 phosphate receptor targeting protein
USAID	United States Agency for International Development
USF	upstream stimulatory factor

VEGF	vascular endothelial growth factor
VLBW	very-low-birth-weight; ≤1,500 g
VLPs	virus-like particles
VSV	vesicular stomatitus virus
WAP	whey acidic protein
WFS	World Fertility Surveys
WHA	World Health Assembly
WHO	World Health Organization
WMD	weighted mean difference
Xc	reactance
XOR	xanthine oxidoreductase
Zn	zinc
ZPP	zinc protoporphyrin

AUTHOR INDEX

SUBJECT INDEX

MIX
Papier aus verantwortungsvollen Quellen
Paper from responsible sources
FSC® C105338

If you have any concerns about our products,
you can contact us on
ProductSafety@springernature.com

In case Publisher is established outside the EU,
the EU authorized representative is:
Springer Nature Customer Service Center GmbH
Europaplatz 3, 69115 Heidelberg, Germany

Printed by Libri Plureos GmbH
in Hamburg, Germany